The Nursing Profession
TURNING POINTS

DATE DUE

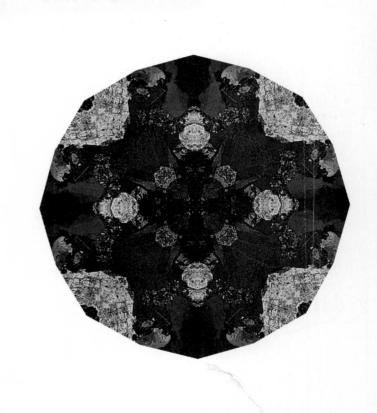

The Nursing Profession

TURNING POINTS

Edited by

Norma L. Chaska, Ph.D., R.N., F.A.A.N.

Professor, Department of Nursing Administration
School of Nursing
Indiana University
Indianapolis, Indiana

Illustrated

The C.V. Mosby Company

St. Louis • Baltimore • Philadelphia • Toronto   1990

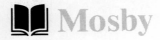

Editor: Darlene Como
Developmental Editor: Laurie Sparks
Project Manager: Carol Sullivan Wiseman
Designer: Susan E. Lane
Editing and Production: Editing, Design, & Production Inc.

The C. V. Mosby Company
11830 Westline Industrial Drive, St. Louis, Missouri 63146

Library of Congress Cataloging-in-Publication Data

The Nursing profession : turning points / edited by Norma L. Chaska. p.   cm.
    Companion v. to: The Nursing profession : views through the mist and the Nursing
profession : a time to speak.
    Includes bibliographical references.
    ISBN 0-8016-6067-X
    1. Nursing.   2. Nursing—United States.   I. Chaska, Norma L.
[DNLM: 1. Nursing.   WY 16 N97418]
   RT82.N869   1990
   610.73—dc20
   DNLM/DLC
   for Library of Congress   89-13140
                                              CIP

C/D/D   9 8 7 6 5 4 3 2 1

Contributors

Judith W. Alexander, Ph.D., R.N.
Associate Professor
College of Nursing
University of South Carolina
Columbia, SC

Kathleen G. Andreoli, D.S.N., R.N., F.A.A.N.
Vice President, Nursing Affairs and Dean of
   the College of Nursing of Rush University
Rush-Presbyterian-St. Lukes Medical Center
Chicago, IL

Myrtle K. Aydelotte, Ph.D., R.N., F.A.A.N.
Professor and Dean Emerita
University of Iowa
Iowa City, IA
Former Executive Director
American Nurses' Association

Constance M. Baker, Ed.D., R.N.
Professor and Dean
School of Nursing
Indiana University
Indianapolis, IN

Sr. Rose Therese Bahr, A.S.C., Ph.D., R.N.,
   F.A.A.N.
Professor of Nursing and Associate Director
Life Cycle Institute and Director
Gerontology Center
The Catholic University of America
Washington, DC

Violet H. Barkauskas, Ph.D., R.N., F.A.A.N.
Associate Professor, Community Health Nursing
Associate Dean for Administration
School of Nursing
The University of Michigan
Ann Arbor, MI

Elaine E. Beletz, Ed.D., R.N., F.A.A.N.
Associate Professor of Nursing
College of Nursing
Villanova University
Villanova, PA

Em Olivia Bevis, M.A., R.N., F.A.A.N.
Consultant in Nursing Education
Adjunct Professor, Research
Georgia Southern College
Statesboro, GA

Marjorie Beyers, Ph.D., R.N., F.A.A.N.
Associate Vice-President
Nursing and Allied Health Services
Mercy Health Services
Farmington Hills, MI

Barbara J. Brown, Ed.D., R.N., F.A.A.N.
Associate Executive Director
King Faisal Specialist Hospital and Research Centre
Riyadh 11211, Saudi Arabia

Johnna Sue Brown, M.S., R.N.
Instructor, Nursing and Health Technologies
Long Beach City College
Long Beach, CA

Bonnie Bullough, Ph.D., R.N., F.A.A.N.
Professor and Dean Emerita
School of Nursing
State University of New York
Buffalo, NY

Norma L. Chaska, Ph.D., R.N., F.A.A.N.
Professor, Department of Nursing Administration
School of Nursing
Indiana University
Indianapolis, IN

Olga Maranjian Church, Ph.D., R.N., F.A.A.N.
Professor and Chair, Graduate Program
School of Nursing
The University of Connecticut
Storrs, CT

Diana Clark, M.H.A., R.N.
Vice President, Academic Affairs
Methodist Hospital of Indiana, Inc.
Indianapolis, IN

Joyce C. Clifford, M.S.N., R.N., F.A.A.N.
Vice President for Nursing and Nurse-in-Chief
Beth Israel Hospital
Boston, MA

Jacqueline F. Clinton, Ph.D., R.N., F.A.A.N.
Professor and Director
Center for Nursing Research and Evaluation
University of Wisconsin — Milwaukee
Milwaukee, WI

Colleen Conway-Welch, Ph.D., R.N., C.N.M., F.A.A.N.
Professor and Dean, School of Nursing
Vanderbilt University
Nashville, TN

Anne J. Davis, Ph.D., R.N., F.A.A.N.
Professor, Mental Health and Community Nursing
University of California SF
San Francisco, CA

Carol A. Deets, Ed.D., R.N.
Professor, Department of Nursing Administration
Interim Associate Dean for Graduate Programs
School of Nursing
Indiana University
Indianapolis, IN

Elizabeth C. Devine, Ph.D., R.N.
Assistant Professor, School of Nursing
University of Wisconsin — Milwaukee
Milwaukee, WI

Sr. Rosemary Donley, Ph.D., R.N., F.A.A.N.
Executive Vice-President
The Catholic University of America
Washington, DC

Eleanor Donnelly, Ph.D., R.N.
Associate Professor, Department of Psychiatric-Mental Health Nursing
School of Nursing
Indiana University
Indianapolis, IN

Kathleen Dracup, D.N.Sc., R.N., F.A.A.N.
Associate Professor, School of Nursing
University of California
Los Angeles, CA

Kathleen M. Driscoll, J.D., M.S., R.N.
Associate Professor, Department Head
Community Health Nursing
College of Nursing and Health
University of Cincinnati
Cincinnati, OH

Linda A. Dudjak, M.S.N., R.N., O.C.N.S.
Clinical Director Inpatient Services
Pittsburgh Cancer Institute
Pittsburgh, PA

Mary E. Duffy, Ph.D., R.N.
Associate Professor
School of Nursing
The University of Texas Health Science Center at Houston
Houston, TX

Claire M. Fagin, Ph.D., R.N., F.A.A.N.
Professor and Dean
School of Nursing
University of Pennsylvania
Philadelphia, PA

Joan Farrell, Ph.D., R.N.
Professor and Dean
College of Health
University of North Florida
Jacksonville, FL

Jacqueline Fawcett, Ph.D., R.N., F.A.A.N.
Professor
School of Nursing
University of Pennsylvania
Philadelphia, PA

Geraldene Felton, Ed.D., R.N., F.A.A.N.
Professor and Dean
College of Nursing
The University of Iowa
Iowa City, IA

Joyce J. Fitzpatrick, Ph.D., R.N., F.A.A.N.
Professor and Dean of Nursing
Frances Payne Bolton School of Nursing
Case Western Reserve University
Administrative Associate in Nursing
University Hospitals of Cleveland
Cleveland, OH

Sr. Mary Jean Flaherty, Ph.D., R.N.,
    F.A.A.N.
Associate Professor and Chair,
    Division of Maternal–
    Child Health Nursing
School of Nursing
The Catholic University of America
Washington, DC

Patricia A.R. Flynn, M.S., R.N.
University of California SF
San Francisco, CA

Marsha Fowler, Ph.D., R.N.
Professor
School of Nursing and
    Graduate School of Theology
Azusa Pacific University
Azusa, CA

Sara T. Fry, Ph.D., R.N.
Associate Professor
Doctoral Program
School of Nursing
University of Maryland
Baltimore, MD

Nancy Graham, Dr. P.H., R.N.
Vice President of Nursing
Lenox Hill Hospital
New York, NY

Karen Haller, Ph.D., R.N.
Director of Nursing for Research and Education
The John Hopkins Hospital
Baltimore, MD

Edward J. Halloran, Ph.D., R.N., C.N.A.A.,
    F.A.A.N.
Associate Professor
School of Nursing
University of North Carolina
    at Chapel Hill
Chapel Hill, NC

Evelyn Hartigan, Ed.D., R.N.
Associate Administrator, Patient Care Services
University of Utah Hospital and Associate Dean
College of Nursing
University of Utah
Salt Lake City, UT

Sue T. Hegyvary, Ph.D., R.N., F.A.A.N.
Professor and Dean
School of Nursing
University of Washington
Seattle, WA

Nancy K. Hester, Ph.D., R.N.
Assistant Professor, Senior Faculty Associate
Center of Nursing Research, School of Nursing
University of Colorado Health Sciences Center
Denver, CO

William L. Holzemer, Ph.D., R.N., F.A.A.N.
Professor and Director, Office of Research,
    Evaluation and Computer Resources
School of Nursing
University of California
San Francisco, CA

Donna B. Jensen, Ph.D., R.N.
Associate Professor
Community Health Care Systems
School of Nursing
Oregon Health Sciences University
Portland, OR

Virginia A. Kemp, Ph.D., R.N.
Associate Professor, Director of Research
School of Nursing
Medical College of Georgia
Augusta, GA

Maeona K. Kramer, Ph.D., R.N.
Professor
College of Nursing
University of Utah
Salt Lake City, UT

Rosemary A. Langston, Ph.D., R.N.
Dean
College of Nursing and Health Sciences
Winona State University
Winona, MN

Elizabeth R. Lenz, Ph.D., R.N., F.A.A.N.
Professor and Associate Dean for Graduate Studies
School of Nursing
University of Maryland
Baltimore, MD

Carol A. Lindeman, Ph.D., R.N., F.A.A.N.
Professor and Dean
School of Nursing
Oregon Health Sciences University
Portland, OR

Brenda Lyon, D.N.S., R.N.
Associate Professor and Chair
Department of Nursing of Adults with Biodissonance
School of Nursing
Indiana University
Indianapolis, IN

Violet M. Malinski, Ph.D., R.N.
Assistant Professor
Hunter-Bellevue School of Nursing
Hunter College-CUNY
New York, NY

Celine Marsden, M.N., R.N.
Cardiac Patient and Family Project
School of Nursing
University of California
Los Angeles, CA

Edna M. Menke, Ph.D., R.N.
Associate Professor and Associate Dean
College of Nursing
The Ohio State University
Columbus, OH

Doris M. Modly, Ph.D., R.N.
Assistant Professor
Frances Payne Bolton School of Nursing
Case Western Reserve University
Cleveland, OH

Mary H. Mundt, Ph.D., R.N.
Associate Professor, School of Nursing
University of Wisconsin—Milwaukee
Milwaukee, WI

Ellen K. Murphy, J.D., M.S., R.N., F.A.A.N.
Associate Professor, School of Nursing
University of Wisconsin—Milwaukee
Milwaukee, WI

Margaret A. Newman, Ph.D., R.N., F.A.A.N.
Professor
School of Nursing
University of Minnesota
Minneapolis, MN

Carol A. Soares O'Hearn, Ph.D., R.N.
Associate Professor
Department of Nursing
Stonehill College
North Easton, MA

Marian Martin Pettengill, Ph.D., R.N.
Executive Director for MAIN (Midwest Alliance in
    Nursing) and Adjunct Assistant Professor
Department of Nursing Administration, School of Nursing
Indiana University
Indianapolis, IN
Adjunct Assistant Professor
Department of Administrative Studies
College of Nursing
University of Illinois at Chicago
Chicago, IL

Anne Lynn Porter, Ph.D., R.N.
Director, Nursing and Allied Health Services
Mercy Health Services
Farmington Hills, MI

Tim Porter-O'Grady, Ed.D., R.N., C.N.A.A.
Senior Partner, Affiliated Dynamics, Inc.
Atlanta, GA

Mary Fry Rapson, Ph.D., R.N.
Associate Dean, Undergraduate Studies
School of Nursing
University of Maryland
Baltimore, MD

Marilyn A. Ray, Ph.D., R.N.
Eminent Scholar, Christine E. Lynn—Endowed Chair in
   Nursing
Florida Atlantic University
Division of Nursing
Boca Raton, FL

Suzanne M. Rogers, M.S.N., R.N.
Senior Vice President of Nursing
Butterworth Hospital
Grand Rapids, MI

Estelle H. Rosenblum, Ph.D., R.N.
Professor and Dean, College of Nursing
University of New Mexico
Albuquerque, NM
Director, Continuing Nursing Education
Professional Seminar Consultants, Inc.
Albuquerque, NM

Barbara J. Sarter, Ph.D., R.N.
Assistant Professor of Nursing
School of Nursing
University of Southern California
Los Angeles, CA

Christine Sheppard, R.N.
Director of Nursing, Labor Relations
Recruitment and Retention
Lenox Hill Hospital
New York, NY

Marian B. Sides, Ph.D., R.N.
Assistant Professor
School of Nursing
University of Wisconsin—Milwaukee
Milwaukee, WI

Mariah Snyder, Ph.D., R.N., F.A.A.N.
Professor, School of Nursing
University of Minnesota
Minneapolis, MN

Patricia L. Starck, D.S.N., R.N.
Professor and Dean
School of Nursing
The University of Texas Health Science Center at
   Houston
Houston, TX

Marilyn Stember, Ph.D., R.N.
Professor and Executive Associate Dean
School of Nursing
University of Colorado Health Sciences Center
Denver, CO

Joanne S. Stevenson, Ph.D., R.N., F.A.A.N.
Professor, Department of Life Span Process
College of Nursing
The Ohio State University
Columbus, OH

Jane E. Tarnow, D.N.Sc., R.N.
Assistant to the V.P./Dean
College of Nursing of Rush University
Rush-Presbyterian-St. Lukes Medical Center
Chicago, IL

Mary K. Wakefield, Ph.D., R.N.
Chief-of-Staff
Senator Quentin N. Burdick, North Dakota
Washington, DC

Jean Watson, Ph.D., R.N., F.A.A.N.
Professor and Dean, School of Nursing
Associate Director, Nursing Service
Director, Center for Human Caring
University of Colorado Health Sciences Center
Denver, CO

Diana Weaver, D.N.S., R.N.
Associate Hospital Director
Director of Nursing, University Hospital
University of Kentucky
Lexington, KY

Fay W. Whitney, Ph.D., R.N., C.R.N.P., F.A.A.N.
Assistant Professor, Director Primary Health Care Graduate Program
School of Nursing
University of Pennsylvania
Philadelphia, PA

Gail A. Wolf, D.N.S., R.N.
Vice President, Nursing Administration
Shadyside Hospital
Pittsburgh, PA

Joyce M. Yasko, Ph.D., R.N., F.A.A.N
Professor and Program Director, Medical–Surgical Nursing
School of Nursing, University of Pittsburgh
Associate Director Nursing, Pittsburgh Cancer Institute
Pittsburgh, PA

Rosalee Yeaworth, Ph.D., R.N., F.A.A.N.
Professor and Dean
College of Nursing
University of Nebraska Medical Center
Omaha, NE

Foreword

A couple of decades ago most Americans might have been assured when they were informed that the American health system was still superior to any other and that the system was fundamentally sound except for a few problems that require minor adjustments or palliatives. Over the years, however, the American people have grown more skeptical, disenchanted and perhaps even envious as they learn how their Canadian neighbors provide easier access to care at lower cost and with greater consumer satisfaction. Despite the presence of a highly trained work force, a growingly impressive technology and a tremendous outlay of funds, the public has become convinced that there are better ways of deploying our resources to provide more effective and humane health care.

The magnitude of the health care problem is highlighted in the growing discontent of the two major health professions, medicine and nursing. The continued if not worsening plight of the nursing profession is perhaps a symptom as well as a contributor to our general predicament. Any improvement in the health care picture would have to come to terms with some of the salient concerns of nursing.

Like the previous two volumes edited by Norma Chaska, this volume is very ambitious, broad in scope, and provides a wide spectrum of articles by some of the outstanding leaders in the nursing profession. Many issues are addressed, such as the theoretical and knowledge bases of nursing practice, the unique contribution of nursing to health care, the minimal educational requirements for all nurses, the pathways and opportunities for various nursing specialties, the development of appropriate professional norms and behavior, and the ways of structuring the role of nursing in the delivery system to make it more effective for patients and gratifying for nurses.

Some dominant concerns of the nursing profession that are discussed in this book mirror those of other health care professions, particularly medicine. These include problems of providing holistic care, the provision of care to critically ill patients, and legal and moral issues in the prolongation of life. The authors consider social, economic, and administrative influences on the nursing profession as well as defensive strategies that are available to the profession. The contributors make use of a wide range of methodological strategies including historical, phenomenological and quantitative approaches.

This book will be of interest to nursing students, educators, clinicians, and administrators. Indeed, all health professionals and administrators, as well those who are deliberating on the future directions of the health delivery system, will find in this huge volume much that is informative and stimulating.

Sol Levine, PhD
Vice President
The Henry J. Kaiser Family Foundation
Menlo Park, California
University Professor
    and Professor of Sociology and Community Medicine,
Boston University, Boston, Massachussets
June 1, 1989

Preface

"After a time of decay comes a turning point. The powerful light that has been banished returns. There is movement, but it is not brought about by force . . . The movement is natural, arising spontaneously. For this reason the transformation of the old becomes easy. The old is discarded and the new is introduced. Both measures accord with the time; therefore no harm results."

I Ching

This quote reported to be from *The I Ching* illustrates the predominant theme through this volume. Although few persons would suggest that nursing is in a state of decay, many would propose that nursing has remained stagnant in its endeavor toward professionalization. In examining nursing as a profession, it is clear now that nursing is in the midst of advancing major change. Many of the contributing authors portray transformations and turning points that are occurring simultaneously in the profession, as in nursing education and practice. Others take the view that nursing is at one critical turning point in progressing toward full professional status. Regardless of how nursing becomes firmly established as a full profession, the alterations and development must be made uniformly. As *The I Ching* advises, a turning point is met easily and smoothly if it is to be achieved successfully. No harm should result.

As in a kaleidoscope, change becomes a thing of beauty gradually unveiled. The kaleidoscope serves as an appropriate vehicle to illustrate nursing in all of its ramifications present and future. The kaleidoscope functions on the principle of multiple reflection, as invented and patented by Sir David Brewster in 1817.* Inside, two glass plates work as mirrors. The plates are placed down the entire length of a small tube and slant toward each other. Both ends of the tube are enclosed. One end of the tube has a small peephole. At the far end of the kaleidoscope are two more plates. One is made of clear glass, which is closer to the eyehole, and the other is ground glass. Pieces of colored beads, glass, shells, or other objects are placed between the plates. These objects are reflected in the mirrors. The ground glass throws the reflections in many forms. Many patterns are then formed. When the viewer turns the kaleidoscope wheel, the objects inside shift and the patterns change. Designers have used the kaleidoscope to discover new patterns for fabrics, wallpaper, and artifacts. The contributing authors in this volume have used the kaleidoscope to suggest and refashion new patterns for nursing.

Thus, the purpose of this book is to provide an in-depth global scope and study of nursing as a profession. Specifically it is to display numerous reflections and patterns of thought and considerations about the state of nursing now and for the future. Many prisms are needed to assess accurately and plan for advancement of the profession. The reader

---

(Reprinted in *The Turning Point Science, Society and The Rising Culture* by Fritjof Capra; New York: Simon & Schuster, 1982)

The world book encyclopedia, (1989). World Book, Inc.: Chicago, IL

will find viewpoints that are agreeable, troubling, disconcerting, stimulating, and refreshing. It is intended that the content cause one to ruminate, dialogue, and further discuss the "pieces" in this volume as a kaleidoscope of nursing. Only then can nursing come clearly into focus to be followed by action and acceleration within the kaleidoscope for nursing as a profession.

This book is a companion to *The Nursing Profession: Views Through The Mist*, published by McGraw-Hill in 1978 and *The Nursing Profession: A Time To Speak*, published by McGraw-Hill in 1983. The first text is out of print. The second will remain available as long as there is a demand. This volume is similar in format to the last, with one difference. Each of the contributor's chapters is introduced in the descriptions to each part of the book, rather than at the beginning of each chapter. Thus, linkages are further established throughout the book. The section on Nursing Administration was divided into two distinct parts: Service and Academic. This separation allowed for both sub-specialty areas in Nursing Administration to be represented sufficiently. For the first time in this series of books with the main title *The Nursing Profession*, international nursing is addressed with substantive content. This addition represents an effort to meet expanding needs in the professional development of nursing internationally. Further content, such as ethics and legal concerns, were significantly increased in this book as a result of a survey conducted by McGraw-Hill in 1987.

For each book persistent effort was made to provide original writing by nurse authors who represent diverse disciplines in their doctoral preparation. Thus, this volume contains *original* chapters by 79 contributors. All of the *primary* contributors (first authors) are doctorally prepared with the exception of one. Seventy-eight contributors hold doctoral degrees representing the disciplines of nursing, sociology, psychology, anthropology, philosophy, education, and law. Thirteen contributors were contributing authors in either the *Views Through the Mist* or *A Time To Speak*. Sixty-six of the contributors are new to this book. The contributors represent all of the geographic regions of the United States and include one person who is currently professionally employed in Saudi Arabia. The contributors are recognized leaders in the profession of nursing. Thirty-four of the contributors are elected fellows in the American Academy of Nursing.

The book is divided into nine parts. The first eight parts contain chapters dealing with critical aspects of nursing as a profession: professionalization, nursing education, nursing research, nursing theory, nursing practice, nursing administration: service, nursing administration: academic, and the future of nursing. To facilitate the process of reflection and dialogue, questions for discussion are raised by the editor at the end of each chapter. In part nine, the current state of the profession is summarized—in general—highlighting particular points of the contributing authors. The focus is placed predominantly on nursing education. In addition, the summary chapter offers some specific reflections, suggestions, and conclusions to stimulate further questions and potential resolution to the challenges. Finally, the analogy of the kaleidoscope is suggested as a means for projecting nursing in its completeness into the future.

The questions that are posed throughout the volume may be helpful in a number of ways. Agencies or institutions employing nurses may use them in planning and establishing long-range goals. The questions may help identify and solve problems in organizations. They should provide a means for analyzing and formulating nursing and health policy. It is hoped that they will greatly assist nursing educators for all programs to conduct discussion seminars for nursing students and further, to serve as the basis for specific course content. The questions may assist nurses in international nursing education to plan effective programs that will facilitate high quality nursing practice. The questions should be of value to those interested in continuing education, whether they are instructors, practicing nurses, or nonpracticing nurses returning to practice. By reading the volume, reflecting on the questions, and positing possible answers, the reader should be able to gain a comprehensive perspective of the profession. The volume should help the reader to develop his or her own global view of the profession, to build a foundation for assessing possible future changes, enhance unity, and plan for the full actualization of the profession.

Additional comments are in order. First, the term "man" is used as a universal theoretical concept in discussions of nursing theory. Second, this volume does not necessarily reflect the views or opinions of the School of Nursing, Indiana University-Purdue University at Indianapolis (IUPUI) or Indiana University.

Finally, in reading this volume it seems appropriate to heed a particular excerpt from Scripture. That passage is: ". . . make yourselves a new heart and a new spirit! [Turn] and live."—Ezekiel, 18:31-32*

ACKNOWLEDGMENTS

This volume owes its existence to significant shared interest and concern for nursing on the part of the contributors, who had the difficult task of addressing complex subjects in nursing within the confines of minimal pages. Their patience and good will in responding to stringent deadlines are gratefully appreciated.

I am indebted to Margaret A. Newman, PhD, RN, FAAN, Professor, School of Nursing, University of Minnesota, Minneapolis who suggested the subtitle for the book. I am grateful to Leah L. Curtin, MS, MA, RN, FAAN, Editor, *Nursing Management* for sharing beauty from her kaleidoscope collection and a discussion about kaleidoscopes. I am much indebted to Cozy Baker, whose volume *Through The Kaleidoscope . . . And Beyond†* suggested the predominant theme, imagery, and artistic representation for the summary chapter and the book.

I am thankful for the library assistance of Elizabeth Heckathorn, MS, RN in choosing a subtitle and theme. I am most grateful to Carol L. Miller, EdD, RN, Professor, Department of Primary Health Care Nursing, School of Nursing, Indiana University who

volunteered for a major responsibility in the primary review of the galleys and page proofs. She faithfully, thoroughly, expertly, and conscientiously completed the task.

I gratefully acknowledge the assistance of a pool of colleagues who reviewed some of the chapters in this volume and made helpful suggestions. Specifically, Joyce S. Martin, MSN, RN, EdD Candidate, Associate Professor, Department of Parent-Child Nursing, School of Nursing, Indiana University reviewed the chapters by Langston (Chapter 8), Beletz (Chapter 9), Rapson (Chapter 10), Mundt (Chapter 11), Duffy (Chapter 12), Fitzpatrick and Modly (Chapter 13), Watson and Bevis (Chapter 14), Snyder (Chapter 15), and Conway-Welch (Chapter 65).

Brenda Lyon, DNS, RN, Associate Professor and Chair, Department of Nursing of Adults with Biodissonance, School of Nursing, Indiana University reviewed and suggested some "Editor's Questions for Discussion" for the chapter by Soares O'Hearn (35). Carol A. Deets, EdD, RN, Professor, Department of Nursing Administration and Interim Associate Dean for Graduate Programs, School of Nursing, Indiana University, critiqued the chapter by Chaska and Alexander (57).

Jan Beckstrand, PhD, MS, MS, RN, Associate Professor, Assistant Dean for Clinical Research, School of Nursing, Indiana University and Director of Clinical Research for Nursing Services, Indiana University Hospitals offered significant comments pertaining to nursing theory in the summary chapter. Eleanor Donnelly, PhD, RN, Associate Professor, Department of Psychiatric-Mental Health Nursing, School of Nursing, Indiana University reviewed all of the chapters in this volume that pertain to nursing theory and suggested some of the "Editor's Questions for Discussion" for those chapters. Moreover, she held many hours of shared discussion, critique, and debate regarding knowledge development and nursing science.

Linda A. Ellis, EdD, RN, Associate Professor and Associate Dean Graduate Program, School of Nursing, Medical College of Georgia offered beneficial comments in her review of the Chaska chapter (63) pertaining to search and screen committees. In

---

*The Jerusalem Bible. (1968). Reader's Edition. NY: Doubleday, p. 1191.
†Baker, C. (1987). *Through the Kaleidoscope . . . And Beyond*. Annapolis, MD: Beechcliff Books.

addition, she provided other suggestions related to the book.

Appreciation is extended to my friends and colleagues in the School of Nursing, Indiana University who advocated the completion of this third book. Rebecca T. Markel, EdD, RN, Associate Professor and Assistant Dean for Development, Beverly Richards, DNS, RN, Associate Professor and Interim Chair, Department of Psychiatric-Mental Health Nursing, and Jeanne M. Pontious, MSN, RN Associate Professor, Department of Community Health Nursing, provided helpful-suggestions from using the previous books in teaching. Constance M. Baker, EdD, RN, Professor and Dean, School of Nursing, Doris J. Froebe, PhD, RN, FAAN, Interim Executive Associate Dean for Academic Affairs and Chair, Department of Nursing Administration, and my department colleagues offered consistent interest and encouragement.

Acknowledgement is due a support network who helped ease the development of this manuscript. Particular thanks are due Roberta Fisher, MSN, RNC; Betty Sorg, MSN, RN, CPNP: Jean Parks, MS; and Mr. and Mrs. Edward Elliott.

I am most indebted to Shirley Chaska Baird, EdD, RD, LD for her invaluable comments and supportive suggestions related to the total manuscript. Finally, I am significantly indebted to my family— Marge, Shirley, Jim, Willy, Paul, and Vivian—for their sustained support, concern, encouragement, and interest; without them this volume would not have been possible.

I extend special appreciation to Sally J. Barhydt, Senior Editor, College Division, McGraw-Hill Book Company and McGraw-Hill for initially encouraging me to edit these volumes titled *The Nursing Profession*. The association with them throughout the production of the volumes has been highly valued.

Appreciation is extended to the publisher for this third volume and to Darlene Como, Nursing Editor at C.V. Mosby Company. Her sustained support throughout the transfer of nursing textbooks and nursing authors' contracts from McGraw-Hill to C.V. Mosby was encouraging. Her interest and counsel in the production of this volume were most helpful. I look forward to continued fruitful association with Darlene Como and C.V. Mosby in the future.

Norma L. Chaska

Introduction

Norma Chaska presents a wide ranging compendium of facts, perceptions, and interpretations of the contemporary nursing scene. Contributors introduce diverse points of view that include numerous approaches as well as contradictions to challenge readers to think carefully about what nursing is or might be in the not-too-distant future.

The book is aptly titled *Turning Points*. As planet Earth and its peoples move into the 21st century there is no turning back. Concomitantly an unknown future is sweeping nurses and nursing across new thresholds and into new domains. Meanwhile, nurses continue to debate definitions of nursing, entry levels, purposes of nursing, where nursing is learned, where it is practiced, and by whom.

Of continued concern are such questions as: does nursing have a body of knowledge specific to nursing or is nursing content borrowed from other fields? Is nursing practice based on a science of knowing or a science of doing? Are criteria for excellence in practice rooted in skills and experience or is it determined by knowledgeable utilization of a body of theoretical knowledge deriving from a science of nursing?

How long will the old cliché of "a nurse is a nurse is a nurse" continue? Nurses have yet to achieve professional status. How do nurses define "professional?" Is "professional" a status term or should it signify a "learned profession," peer of other learned professions? More than one contributor questions whether nurses really want to attain "full professional recognition." But at the same time the meaning of "full professional" tends to be left in limbo.

Reluctance by nurses to make the changes necessary for nursing to be identified as a learned profession is implicit in many chapters throughout the book. Differences in proposed directions are multiple. Why is there delay in differentiating careers according to levels of preparation in nursing? Does this represent a commitment to "gradualism" or is it a subtle denial of a body of knowledge specific to nursing?

Today is often referred to as the age of the entrepreneur. A major societal shift is under way. Is nursing an autonomous field of endeavor or are nurses dependent on the power, profits, and political wishes of others? Traditionally this dependency has signified M.D.'s. However, today psychologists are seeking legislative authority to write orders for nurses. Who else would like to control nurses? Two hundred years ago James Madison (June 16, 1788) wrote, "I believe there are more instances of the abridgement of the freedom of the people by gradual and silent encroachments of those in power than by violent and sudden usurpation."

Hospital and medical doctor charges continue to exacerbate. The nature and quality of health care and of its providers are debatable. Nosophobia intensifies. Ethical and legal issues increase. Old world views are already out-dated. Space travel is expanding. What kinds of nurses are needed for the future? Who will the robots replace? New frontiers for nurses in space are on the horizon. If there is a shortage of nurses where is it? What kinds of nurses are in short supply?

These are but a few of the questions that come to mind as one peruses this volume. Chaska's summary focuses on a kaleidoscope view of the different scenarios emerging out of the book's contents. *Turning Points* provides a valuable compilation of thought-provoking prospects for nurses to consider, weigh, and determine appropriate action.

Enjoy!

Martha E. Rogers, ScD, RN, FAAN
Professor Emerita, New York University
New York, N.Y.
June 1, 1989

Contents

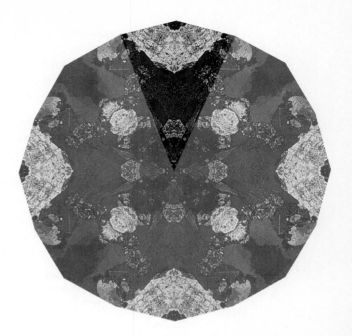

PART I
PROFESSIONALIZATION

The kaleidoscope offers a metaphor—the symmetry, brilliance, and ever-moving views for the world of the professions. Each turn of the disk brings a new image, renewed vision, and refreshment. In particular for nursing, each turn evolves into another as the profession takes shape within the changing mold of the professions. The design of perfect symmetry is unfolding.

The contributions in Part I of this volume show the emergence of nursing as a profession. Like the unpredictability yet order within a kaleidoscope, nursing's past is filled with the unexpected. In the first chapter Olga Maranjian Church sheds light on the historical beginnings that helped to shape and provide substance for the kaleidoscope of the evolving profession of nursing.

We cannot understand the workings and use of a kaleidoscope without knowing something of how it is created. So too we cannot appreciate the development of nursing into professional status without acknowledging the basic designs and facets of professions. Myrtle Aydelotte in Chapter 2 addresses the professionalization process of nursing. She particularly emphasizes the importance and role of power in achieving professional status.

Elaine Beletz aptly points out in Chapter 3 that professional status is just the beginning for nursing and nurses. The internalization and ongoing enactment of a professional subculture are essential for the empowerment of professionhood and the legitimization of nursing as a profession.

In Chapter 4 Marsha Fowler focuses on the interrelatedness of ethics, professions, and society. In so doing she highlights nursing's moral mandate as a profession. Having profes-

1

sional moral concerns raised to a conscious level, it is appropriate that Fowler's chapter be followed by one that illustrates legal aspects of professional status.

Thus, Ellen Murphy in Chapter 5 examines in a timely fashion the status of nurse autonomy in relation to legislatures, physicians, and employers. She offers suggestions for increasing autonomy, citing the employer-employee relationship as the primary obstacle to nurse autonomy.

Given that the linkages between legislation and professional status are acknowledged, nursing and nurses should appreciate their role and obligations in the development of health policy. Mary Wakefield in Chapter 6 delineates the process of formulating health policy. Strategies are offered on how nurses can help shape policy.

Margaret A. Newman in Chapter 7 offers further insight on professionalization of nursing and nurses. Emphasis is placed on defining the nursing paradigm that is directing nursing practice. She exhorts nursing to accept the challenge of articulating the contributions of the different types of nursing practitioners for a unified model of professional practice.

The professionalization section of the book is concluded with a focus on the socialization process into the profession. Rosemary Langston in Chapter 8 presents research findings supporting the conclusion that professional socialization differs according to the type of educational program.

Many questions remain to be addressed regarding professionhood, professionalization, the professional status of nursing, and the socialization process of nurses and nursing. Kaleidoscopes rely on the reflection of light rays from the mirrors to create multiple images. When you turn the disk, or change the angle or your view, those images change size and content. Kaleidoscopes reflect the unfolding growth of our inner beings and also of nursing. Nursing relies on the reflection of our inner selves and the heritage of our profession to evolve, create, and refresh. A new world perspective of nursing can be offered through the kaleidoscope metaphor. Where there were divisions, differences, and apparent disorder, there emerges integration, similarity, interrelatedness, wholeness, and fulfillment. Reflect on a new heart, a new spirit, a new perspective . . . turn and live!

1

Nursing's History:
What it was and what it was not

Olga Maranjian Church, Ph.D., R.N., F.A.A.N.

Throughout the history of nursing the word *professional* appears and reappears in documents that provide the investigator with a welcome paper trail (Crowder, 1985; Dean, 1983). Yet, there have been gaps between the rhetoric and the perceived reality inasmuch as the ideals and visions of nursing's status and domain as discussed by the leadership did not always match the popular image of the nurse or the limited realities of nursing practice and nursing education.

THE RHETORIC

During the late nineteenth and early twentieth century, a period referred to as the progressive era, reform-minded persons sought to transform society through their efforts toward improving educational opportunities, health and welfare, and working conditions. In response to society's unmet needs, some of nursing's early leaders were involved in many of the movements during this period, and contributed to important developments in child welfare, public health, and mental hygiene. For example, Lavinia Lloyd Dock, Lillian Wald, Margaret Sanger, and Euphemia Jane Taylor (Bullough, Church, & Stein, 1988) are well-known for their contributions in such reforms.

Dock maintained a lifelong commitment to wom-

en's rights and saw suffrage as the key to social status for all women. She was by far one of the more colorful pioneers in nursing's history. She carried banners as a suffragist, pacifist, and Marxist, and was arrested at least three times and jailed for her "outlandish" behavior. She lived and worked at the Henry Street Nurses' Settlement in New York for 20 years. She was the first nurse historian in the United States, and while doing her research discovered that the "special revolutionary feature of Miss Nightingale's plan for nurse-training has been to a single degree overlooked by commentators and even by nurses" (Dock & Stewart, 1938, p. 127). Dock felt that the Nightingale model for nursing education mandated that "the entire control of a nursing staff as to discipline and teaching, must be taken out of the hands of men and lodged in those of a woman, who must herself be a trained and competent nurse" (Dock & Stewart, 1938, p. 127).

Self-determination for women, nurses, and nursing was an overriding concern for Dock throughout her life. She was alone among nurses who publicly supported Margaret Sanger's efforts for voluntary motherhood. She praised Sanger for teaching poor, underprivileged, underserved women information that was available to the better educated women of privilege in society.

According to Ashley, "to the detriment of their

own growth as professional persons, nurses were among the most conservative of the conservatives" (1975, p. 1465). As an exception, Dock was considered deviant and she spoke of leaving nursing in order to devote full time to the suffrage issue. Both publicly and privately Dock campaigned and, in effect, did not really leave nursing as much as challenge it to join her in the larger concerns for women's rights. An articulate spokeswoman, she was determined to fight unfair male dominance not just in nursing but in society at large. In discussing the need for equality, in her correspondence with M. Adelaide Nutting, she wrote:

> I can't to save myself see why it should be different with women. [And] the proposition of absolute legal equality for all human beings is to me one that I can't deny or put aside. So I am cheerfully prepared to lose lots of my old friends. But I am used to that—you'd be surprised to know how unimportant it seems (Dock, date unknown).

In a document entitled *Letter to Nurses*, Dock (1923) appealed to the nursing community to support the Equal Rights amendment and solicited their membership in the Nurses' Council of the National Woman's Party. Annie W. Goodrich, a respected activist in her own right who later became the first Dean at the Yale University School of Nursing, joined Dock in this effort (Bullough et al., 1988). Goodrich was chair, and Dock vice-chair, of the Nurses' Council of the National Woman's Party at this time. In her appeal Dock informed the nurses of the need to remove all forms of subjection of women, and to support the amendment, which had been introduced into Congress by Senator Charles E. Curtis and in the House by Representative Daniel Anthony (a nephew of Susan B. Anthony). Dock concluded her request in the following manner:

> I believe that nurses as a whole will be in sympathy with the Equal Rights movement. Those who are imbued with faith in present welfare laws may consider that legislation planned for the conserving of the Public Health is bound to be more and more the aim of a community of free and equal citizens. This must be even more strongly emphasized in the future in regard to infancy and childhood and to ma-

ternity, which is now in some countries definitely recognized as service to the state and protected accordingly. To suggest that it must be otherwise in our country if equal right should be established by constitutional amendment seems an exaggerated fear (Dock, 1923).

Freedom to vote as part of the overall freedom of choice for women implied the basic freedom to develop and change in a changing world. For the most part, the prospect of such autonomy for those involved in nursing and nursing education continued to be a most provocative and elusive goal.

One such reformer was Lillian Wald, the founder of public health nursing and director of the Henry Street Nurses' Settlement, which she developed (Bullough et al., 1988). Her efforts resulted in establishing playgrounds where there were none, the concept of public health nursing, the Federal Children's Bureau, and school nurse programs. She was a pacifist, a suffragist, and a humanist. Before she died in 1940, she spoke of the changes in mental attitudes of the underprivileged. She observed that they no longer viewed themselves as the disinherited but felt entitled to certain standards of comfort and dignity.

Another reformer, Margaret Sanger—the leader of the movement for voluntary motherhood—was impressed by her own mother's premature death after having 11 children. The circumstances of her death spurred Sanger on in her lifelong pursuit of reproductive autonomy for women. Sanger also spent time in jail for what she believed, but ultimately lived to see her efforts succeed (Sicherman & Green, 1980).

Euphemia Jane Taylor was a visible advocate of a more inclusive approach to health (Bullough et al., 1988). She worked with Dr. Adolf Meyer, better known as the father of psychobiology, and was the first nursing director of the Henry Phipps Psychiatric Clinic at Johns Hopkins Medical Center in 1913. Taylor later became the second Dean of the Yale University School of Nursing. She was instrumental in attempts to integrate basic concepts from general and "mental" nursing for a more comprehensive knowledge base from which all nursing care should emanate.

The work of nurses such as these are regaining

some of the recognition due them by nurses today. However, one cannot hope to understand the reality as experienced by the individual by only looking to the rhetoric of the leadership. One must also look at the milieu, the context, the social-political-economic times out of which such leaders and their followers emerged.

Furthermore as nursing developed its foundation for practice, education, and research, it became obvious that nursing's development was complicated by certain historical imperatives. The gaps between the rhetoric of nursing's leaders and the reality as experienced by its practitioners might be explained by understanding some of the factors that influenced history. Leaders such as Mary Adelaide Nutting were faced with many challenges, as they sought to elevate educational standards from the apprenticeship system (Marshall, 1972). The women for the nursing work force previously developed out of apprenticeship systems. Nutting, among others, tried to change the status quo.

The historical imperatives (i.e., compelling factors) include

1. Gender-related issues and the ambiguity inherent in the role of women in society. Gender issues encompass the economic, political, social, and psychological impact of such ambiguity.
2. The enduring impact of religious and military influences as part of nursing's heritage, including altruistic traditions and the acceptance of the authority of a hierarchical order.
3. Nursing's fundamental misalliance with the medical ideology (i.e., disease orientation with cure as its goal). The alliance was, in part, due to the original dependent relationship nursing had with medicine as the nursing profession emerged.

To some extent these issues continue to influence and shape the rhetoric and reality of nursing education and practice today. The rhetoric of Nightingale's followers is consistent over time with regard to nursing's mission. The mission was perceived and presented by the leadership as "serving humanity." The following examples are illustrative of this point. Hildegard E. Peplau maintained that nursing's mission was "to manifest tenderness and to nurture human capacities and bring them to full fruition" (Peplau, 1964, p. 162). She saw this as basic to "developing nursing practice that fosters favorable changes in the living of troubled people" (1964, p. 154). Furthermore, Peplau urged nurses to be "using its findings from nursing research and making every possible effort to give all sick and troubled persons what they need in order to become whole and functioning to the full extent of their individual capabilities" (1964, p. 162).

Many years earlier, Mary Adelaide Nutting (1929) saw nurses as agents who would provide educational and preventive measures as paramount to their practice and preparation. For Nutting the importance of the university-based nursing school's influence on the nursing profession was yet to be realized. As she spoke of "the future" she praised the potential of such a "liberalizing movement" in nursing. The impact of the university on nursing education would be

> serving at once to strengthen, to energize, to enrich and to deliver it from some of the benumbing effects of continuous routine. . . .To the question therefore that may arise, how far can we go in these efforts to add the resources and powers of universities and other educational institutions to the opportunities and experience of the hospital to obtain for nurses freedom for educational development in their own field of work, I must answer unhesitatingly, just as far as possible. Believing as I do that universities, and all educational institutions, as well as hospitals, exist for the service of the people, I would see that service furthered by placing schools of nursing among the professional schools of the universities of this country and of other countries as far as existing conditions would make that relationship a practical wise measure. (Nutting, 1929, p. 903)

THE REALITY

Such was the rhetoric of the leadership as early as the first decade of the twentieth century, which provided the foundation for their divergence from the medical model ideology. However, the reality of apprenticeship education limited the possibilities for developing the educational programs and advancing the practice of nursing. Decision making in patient care and management was implicit in the rhetoric, yet the reality was that nursing's autonomy was short-lived and was outside of the institutions where most nurses worked. After World War I a major shift occurred from employment in the community to the hospital.

Special circumstances and conditions such as those found in public health programs, for example, the work of Mary Breckenridge (Bullough et al., 1988). In the Frontier Nursing Service and foothills of Kentucky, she sought to meet the health needs of a particular population. Breckenridge focused on midwifery, as a demonstration of what nursing could do when left unchallenged and unthwarted in efforts toward improved family care. She collected data and disseminated reports based on statistics, and was successful in raising funds and establishing national support for her experimental project. In her own words:

> The first demonstration in America of the use of nurse-midwives, under medical direction, to care for the lonely rural mother in rough country has now become a demonstration of use to countless rural people in isolated parts of the world (Quoted in Dammann, 1982, p. 103).

Although successful in Kentucky, her nursing model of responding to the health care needs of the nation remained isolated there. This too was the reality.

The prevailing medical or curative ideology would continue to limit the development of a scientifically and academically broader perspective for nursing practice and nursing education. Complicated by differences of viewpoint based on sex and discipline, as well as ideology, physicians—some sympathetic, others paternalistic, and many exploitive—continued to dominate the health care arena. Meanwhile, as hospitals became more acceptable and accessible to patients—with technology and medical care more effective—*graduate nurses* played a more visible part in the hospital work force. The transition from the community based practice of nursing through the 1920s to the move in the 1930s to insti-

tutionalized hospital care-taking included significant tradeoffs for nurses and nursing.

RELEVANCE: UNMET NEEDS AND UNMET EXPECTATIONS

By entering the male- and physician-dominated institution of the hospital, nurses and nursing formed an alliance with the medical system. Such an alliance supported the dominance of medicine, but also contributed to the development of better hospital care. At the same time, nursing became institutionalized in the process; for, the parameters of practice were far more limiting within the hospital than those that existed outside in the community. This alliance with medicine was the cost for employment security within the hospital walls. Ivan Illich has said, "All disease is a socially created reality. Its meaning and the response it has evoked have a history. The study of this history will make us understand the degree to which we are prisoners of the medical ideology" (Illich, 1976, pp. 162–163).

Whether nurses have been prisoners of the medical ideology of the past is a provocative issue. The historical record reveals nursing's early dependence on organized medicine, but one can also identify a mutual ambiguity and dependence of medicine on nursing. Furthermore, there is a detectable urgency with which early leaders sought to identify nursing as a separate discipline. Lavinia Dock advocated the separation between the medical and nursing spheres of authority as early as 1893. She spoke at the Colombian Exposition in Chicago, where nursing superintendents gathered together for the first time to discuss standards and ethics with regard to nursing education and practice. Yet the threat of animosity from organized medicine toward attempts at independence in nursing education and practice was effective as long as the nursing program remained dominated by them. Once nursing education programs found a firm footing in the educational mainstream of universities and colleges, nursing's vulnerability and dependent status were greatly diminished.

Findings from my research on the emergence of psychiatric nursing reveal the subjugation of nursing to "mixed messages." For example, Dr. Edward Cowles is credited with establishing the first psychiatric nursing education program at the McLean Asylum in Massachusetts in 1882. However, he was motivated by many purposes, the least of which was to benefit nursing education. He was straightforward in the use of women as nurses and emphasized the importance of acquiring the true asylum spirit in the process of "training" nurses. He asked:

> How shall we make a nurse that will be useful to the public and command its patronage; in other words, how shall we best subserve the grand purpose of all our work, the public good to which the general interest of the nurse is incidental and complemental and really a means to a greater good?" (Cowles, 1887, p. 183)

Cowles was proud to have been responsible for opening the "first formally organized training school within an institution for the insane in the world" (Cowles, 1887, p. 176). His view was that

> Attendants may attend the infirm and incurable but nurses attend the sick and the experience of recovery from illness is so common that the very idea of the presence of a nurse logically carries with it the other idea, that something is being done to promote recovery and that inspires hope and is curative" (Cowles, 1887, p. 176).

Cowles maintained that given these "natural capabilities for nurturance," women in their role as nurses provided great beneficial value to the inmates, who at this point were to be considered patients.

Within 10 years of opening the school for nurses, the asylum was officially renamed the McLean Hospital. Thus medicalization of the Asylum became a reality through establishing a school for nurses. This is precisely where the mission of nursing crystallizes—not so much to medicalize but to *humanize* the patient's experience. Although Cowles spoke favorably of Nightingale and her efforts in founding modern nursing, he avoided following her basic principle of training school autonomy in the establishment of the nurses' training program. He took pride in the fact that his hospital training program for nurses was part of the hospital organization itself

and independent of *outside* assistance. This was diametrically opposite to Nightingale's model!

Nursing's identity has been inextricably bound to the very word and notion of nurturance as well as to the "myth" that women exist to be mothers. According to Ashley (1975), this myth has fostered male dominance in society and "has been used as a means of urging nurses not to compete economically with men for monetary rewards in the health field" (Ashley, 1975 p. 1465).

The history of nursing is replete with such gender related consequences. Only within the second half of this century has the interplay of social reforms, such as the consumer movement, civil rights, the women's movement, and a concerned number of enlightened, proactive nurses, surfaced once again. Nurses have seized a variety of opportunities to *realign* their efforts to meet the needs not of the institutions or those who control them, but those of the clients or patients for whom they are committed to provide care.

According to Tomes (1984), the "socialization of nurses differed markedly from that of doctors. Historians and sociologists have used a model of professionalization based so exclusively on medicine that they have neglected the variations and alternatives evident in the development of other professions" (p. 467).

The resurgence of interest in nursing's history has been a welcome by-product of the women's studies movement, and as such has provided the nursing profession with an opportunity to develop fresh insights to old concerns. There has also been remarkable resurgence of interest in nursing as a profession brought on in part by the current severe nursing shortage, which by all accounts will become even more so. One prediction states that "by the end of this century . . . the demand for nurses will be double the supply" (Will, 1988, p. 80).

Nursing's history provides support for its ongoing mission to society. The prevailing wisdom, as one social critic has stated, is that "physicians are an episodic presence in the life of a patient. Nurses control the environment of healing. Assisting the rehabilitation of a stroke victim or monitoring and coping with chronic disease is essentially a nurse's not a physician's function" (Will, 1988, p. 80). Ultimately the future promise and direction for nursing will depend on its most basic mission, that is, the continual challenge to humanize the technological advances in treatment that our patients are subjected to and to renegotiate approaches in demonstrating our competence and compassion in responding to the human condition.

REFERENCES

Ashley, J. A. (1975). Nurses in American history: Nursing and feminism. *American Journal of Nursing, 75*, 1465.

Bullough, V. L., Church, O. M., & Stein, A. P. (Eds.). (1988). *American nursing: A biographical dictionary.* New York: Garland Publishers.

Cowles, E. (1887). Nursing reform for the insane. *American Journal of Insanity, 44*, 176–191.

Crowder, E. L. M. (1985). Historical perspectives of nursing's professionalism. *Occupational Health Nursing, 33*(4), 184–190.

Dammann, N. (1982). *A social history of the frontier nursing service.* Sun City, Arizona: Social Change Press.

Dean, D. J. (1983). The development of professional and political awareness in nursing. *Journal of Advanced Nursing, 8*(6), 535–539.

Dock, L. L. (Date unknown). *Letter to M. Adelaide Nutting from L. L. Dock.* Signed L.L.D. (Dear M.A.). Folder, M.A.N. File, Personal communication. New York Teachers College, Columbia University Archives. Unpublished.

Dock, L. L. (1923). *Letter to nurses.* Harrisburg, Pennsylvania. Author

Dock, L. L., & Stewart, I.M. (1938). A short history of nursing: *From the earliest times to the present day* (4th ed.). New York: G.P. Putnam's Sons.

Marshall, E. E. (1972). *Mary Adelaide Nutting: Pioneer of modern nursing.* Baltimore: The Johns Hopkins University Press.

Nutting, M. A. (1929, August). The future. Paper presented at the International Congress of Nurses, General Session, Ottowa, Canada.

Peplau, H. E. (1964). A personal challenge for immediate action. *In Facing up to changing responsibilities: An institute sponsored by the conference group on psychiatric nursing practice of the American Nurses' Association* (pp. 154–162). New York: American Nurses' Association.

Sicherman, B., & Green, C. H. (Eds.). (1980). *Notable American women the modern period: A biographical dictionary.* Cambridge: The Bellknap Press of Harvard University Press.

Tomes, N. (1984). Little world of our own: Pennsylvania Hospital Training School for Nurses, 1895–1907. In J. W. Leavitt (Ed.), *Women and Health in America: Historical Readings* (pp. 467–481). Madison, WI: University of Wisconsin Press.

Will, G. F. (1988). The dignity of nursing. *Newsweek, 111* (21), 80.

✳ EDITOR'S QUESTIONS FOR DISCUSSION ✳

Discuss the historical imperatives indicated by Church and the influence they have in nursing education and practice today. Trace the influence of the early leaders in nursing. Discuss how the medical or curative ideology limited the development of a scientific and academically broader perspective for nursing practice and education.

Discuss what is the mission of nursing. What evidence is there that history has provided support for its mission? What ideals and visions of nursing should be promoted? Provide examples of rhetoric used by nursing leaders today versus the realities of nursing education and practice. How can a nursing leader best provide leadership to promote ideals that are realistic? Provide strategies for how ideals can be promoted and developed to become reality.

2

The Evolving Profession:
The role of the professional organization

Myrtle K. Aydelotte, Ph.D., R.N., F.A.A.N.

Since 1939, a major concern in our society has been the trend toward the development of professional services, a result of the continued growth of technology and science. Both old and new occupations have contributed to that trend. The older, well-established professions, such as law and medicine, have developed new specialties, all of which are viewed as professional, and other occupations have pushed toward professionalization through specialization and other strategies (Hughes, 1971). Since the status of a profession has not yet been conferred upon nursing, nursing continues to evolve as a profession.

Professionalization is the process by which an occupation moves toward a special form of control called a profession (Aydelotte, 1982). A profession, in our society and worldwide as well, represents a special social class, a unique class in the division of labor. This social stratification is socially acceptable and provides for social mobility and social differentiation. A profession is a complex, organized occupation whose practitioners have engaged in a long training program geared toward the acquisition of exclusive knowledge, through which they gain monopoly of a service essential to or desired by society. This monopoly provides autonomy, public recognition, prestige, power, and authority for the practitioners of the profession. The knowledge and the re-

sultant features are accompanied by an element of occupational mystique, which is perceived as such by those they serve and others in society (Gruending, 1985).

Freidson (1986) stated that an important aspect of professional status is that specialized education is a prerequisite to employment in particular positions. Without the special education, a person would not be qualified for those positions. The profession, then, is a labor shelter, which closes out others who have not been privileged to acquire the education. Although some may see professions as harmful, monopolistic oligarchies, it can be argued that they represent a rational form of control of technology and exist for the common good. A profession stabilizes the esoteric services and creates within the profession itself a form of control over its practitioners. This is achieved by the development of a moral uniformity and a class ideology among practitioners, leading to an altruistic and collective orientation, a sense of social responsibility (Johnson, 1972).

Authors and researchers concerned with the study of the professions do not agree about the existence of an "ideal type" of profession, one portraying traits or attributes that must be present for an occupation to be called a profession. Barber proposed four essential attributes:

1. A high degree of generalized and systematic

knowledge culminating in exclusive knowledge.

2. A primary orientation to community interests rather than self-interest.

3. A high degree of self-control of behavior through a code of ethics internalized in the process of socialization and through voluntary association with other professionals. The association is organized and operated by the professionals alone.

4. A system of rewards, both honorary and monetary, that is primarily a set of symbols of work achievement. These rewards are ends in themselves, not means to some other end of individual self-interest (Cited in Johnson, 1972, p. 33).

Others have identified additional attributes of a profession. Included among these are the identification of the occupation as full-time commitment to a calling, existence of a formal association of members, autonomy to define one's own work, and the right to structure it without interference. Emphasized by others are the social service orientation, a unique body of knowledge, a cognitive rationality, and the development of trust in the provider by the recipient of the professional services (Greenwood, 1957; Hall, 1973; Hughes, 1971; Larson, 1977; Moore, 1970). The view of a profession as composed of select attributes has lost favor among those who study the professions. The current view is that the professions are occupations that exercise great power and influence in the wider social structure (Hall, 1982).

Regardless of how one defines a profession, the occupation of nursing continues to be viewed as semiprofessional. It continues to be listed in the *Occupational Outlook Handbook* (1987) as such, and in the collection of U.S. census data, nurses are not classified as professionals.

The difficulties encountered by nursing at this time in its press for professional status—that is, to gain the power that leads to recognition as a profession—lie in four problem areas. First, there is a limited body of knowledge that has been tested and identified as underlying nursing practice. Further, there are serious credibility gaps between the ideal prescriptive theory that is taught and the practical knowledge used by its practitioners. The knowledge base of nursing is weak (Conway, 1982). Second, the occupation continues to be made up of segmented work groups who have varying amounts of education, hold varying sets of values, and express varying concerns. There is a lack of a common pervasive ideology. There is no standard of education for entry into practice; consequently, there is no monopoly over the work itself. The collective is not strong because of these diversities. Third, the occupation possesses no common mode of thought in viewing its work. The use of the nursing process has become more procedural than that characterizing intellectual inquiry and diagnostic reasoning. Fourth, the educational base is not extensive enough to warrant professional status. Both the preprofessional education base and the professional education program are too short, when compared with programs preparing persons for the established professions. The knowledge base is not exclusive. In our society, exclusive knowledge is a source of power.

PROFESSIONAL ASSOCIATIONS

One of the major catalysts in the movement of an occupation toward achieving professional status is the organization of a voluntary association of the members of the occupation. The role of the voluntary organization in the evolution of an occupation into a profession is highly critical. The professional association "creates, sustains, and alters the official framework of professional activities" (Freidson, 1986, p. 185). Crowder (1985) pointed out that professional associations have their roots in the guild movement of the Middle Ages, during which craftsmen controlled who entered a guild and defined what kind of work was to be done plus who would be prepared to perform that work. The modern professional association is the major "formal means by which the interests of its members are pressed collectively and focused politically" (Freidson, 1986, p. 185). The intent is to gain a privileged position for the members of the occupation through persuasion and influence with an outside elite who controls prestige, power, status, and resources. The professional association desires to improve the status of its members and increase its power in relation to other occupations and professions.

Professional associations represent a collective held together by a common ideology, a common style of work, a shared mystique, and usually a technical language. In essence, a professional association is a form of private government, the leadership of which consists of an oligarchy (Larson, 1977; Moore, 1970). The large majority of the members grant consent for the conduct of association activities by apathy, for although the leadership of an association endorses participation by the members, it also fears it since too much participation will threaten their leadership. Professional associations are not democratic, but are characterized by social stratification within the organization itself. Through structural changes giving rise to decentralization, the leadership of the association dissipates and extends the oligarchy, leading to the development of some hierarchies in the organization that are more equal than others (Moore, 1970). Consequently strains may result between intellectuals and practitioners, and some status figures or the elite of the profession may choose not to participate in the association.

A professional organization carries out a set of basic functions: to act as a professional locus for its members, to serve educational functions, to regulate the quality of work performed by its members, and to serve the function of control (Cullen, 1978). These functions are implemented through a set of activities such as promotion of regulations and licensure, the offering of continuing education programs, credentialing of its members, conduct of public relations programs, the establishment of standards of the product (professional services) rendered by its members, and introduction of a code of ethics. The functions and the activities of the professional association are directed toward gaining power, through cultivating and controlling a market for the services offered by its members and controlling the behavior of its members. The intent of the professional association is the establishment of places for its members in the labor market that are complex, difficult, and exclusive, while making sure that the practitioners the association represents are legitimate and credentialed (Freidson, 1986).

POWER OF PROFESSIONAL ASSOCIATIONS

Professional associations exercise power through a number of channels. Through the use of councils and committees, the association makes decisions on the training of the practitioners. The power of these decisions is implemented through continuing education programs, examinations for credentialing, issuance of guidelines for quality assurance programs, and making pronouncements on educational standards (Cox, 1984). Professional associations also make use of a conscious manipulation of symbols, including language, to establish identification with the professionals. The selection of slogans, language, preparation of testimony, and interpretation of factual data are directed to build unity and a favorable picture of the profession as it is presented to the public. Efforts are directed toward standardization of services through setting of standards of education and standards for practice and delivery of services; codes of behavior; peer review mechanisms; and licensing.

Associations of the professions and semiprofessions serve to mediate with others to gain special recognition and prestige for their members. This is an attempt to secure a privileged position for the profession. The association, through its staff and volunteer leadership, selects an elite group to sponsor its efforts toward increasing the power and prestige of the occupation. As it lobbies the public and legislative elite, the association cannot stress too narrowly and manifestly self-interested goals and legislation. Maintaining public respect for the work of the occupation is essential. The problems associated with the work of the professional association relate significantly to obtaining public recognition, which must also be favorably disposed to the occupation. Thus a dilemma is created when an association seeks to place an item on the public agenda. The item must be socially acceptable and promote the welfare of the profession, and yet it must not appear as self-serving and selfish. The agenda item must relate the value of the work of the profession to the needs and values of society (Larson, 1977).

Other problems of power are inherent in the work of the professional association. The work entails implementing changes from the past activities of the profession. This change produces strains between the intellectuals in the profession and practitioners engaged in day-to-day effort. For the practitioner, professional concerns—the day-to-day bread and butter issues—come to supplant intellectual concerns. The prestige in the occupations that are aspiring recognition as professions goes to those whose careers are removed from practice, whereas in older professions this is not the case. Practitioners who have already defined themselves as professional in the more stringent terms set by the association leaders move in defense of upgrading the profession (Larson, 1977). Others are threatened, indifferent, or believe the change irrelevant. During the period of transition, a social distance develops between divergent groups. Those who are uncertain of their status experience pain and anger. The confrontation becomes a form of contest, in which the object of the confrontation is to gain a monopoly of the market especially important to those seeking the upgrading. Goode (1969) identified this conflict between the old-timers, the traditionalists, and the new who seek to upgrade the occupation by controlling education and the market. The group splits into subgroups and consensus is impossible to secure, creating problems within the association.

Freidson (1986) stated that there are serious limits of associations to speak forcefully and to exert power. He observed that many professional organizations tend to be federated, rather than centralized, and that as a result subgroups develop with different interests. Since there are few issues that unify members, it is difficult to obtain consensus among subgroups. Further, he observed that professional associations are not conspicuous in having easy access to congressional committees.

The power of professional associations is also limited in its ability to discipline individual members and to control the professional elite, who have high personal influence. These are the persons who offer expert advice to legislators and the executive branch at both the federal and the state level. What these elite professionals offer may be more valued by powerful persons than the official positions taken by the association.

POWER OF THE PROFESSIONAL NURSES' ASSOCIATION

Since its founding, the American Nurses' Association (ANA) has exerted its influence and pressed for recognition of nursing as a profession. Licensure has been obtained legally, recognizing that those successful in obtaining a state license may use the title *professional nurse*. State associations, however, have not been successful in increasing the educational requirement for licensure. Neither has the national association, except through state licensure, been successful in obtaining the exclusive right from society to fill all nursing positions with licensed persons.

A number of states have been successful in obtaining legislation, permitting reimbursement for credentialed nurses practicing as midwives, nurse practitioners, and nurse anesthetists. However, since the principle of substitution continues to be used by many institutions and since graduates of all three types of educational programs (associate, diploma, and baccalaureate) practice as staff nurses, nursing does not hold a true monopoly of the labor market. Faculty positions and nursing service leadership positions may require academic credentials, but the labor monopoly is by no means universally secure.

In the transition of an occupation to a profession, it is essential that the members hold special and exclusive knowledge essential to its practice. Currently, nursing is experiencing difficulty in achieving this essential ingredient. Since the position paper of 1965 was issued, the ANA has been pressing for the baccalaureate degree as the entry to practice professional nursing. At the present time, the ANA is one of ten organizations engaged in the implementation of the recommendations of the National Commission on Nursing. Under their efforts to differentiate between professional and technical nursing, the scope of practice of each and the educational preparation for each have been defined (National Commission on Nursing Implementation Project, 1987). The resolution of the basic problem—that is, who is a professional—has not been reached, since the design and determination of which positions will be filled exclusively by professional nurses remain ambiguous and as yet not fully tested. The accomplishment of this end will involve convincing nurses, employers, the public, and policy makers of the desirability of position differentiation and how that differentiation benefits the public.

The knowledge base for each type of graduate must be sufficiently differentiated so that the practice of each resides upon a different base and the exchange or substitution of one type of practitioner is not possible. The corpus of knowledge for the professional practitioner must be vastly different from the technical and contain far more exclusive knowledge than that which is provided today.

The National Commission on Nursing Implementation Project (NCNIP) is in itself an example of how the association is striving to gain power through coalition building. The influence of the governing board of the NCNIP is far-reaching, but it too is limited. The board has no official enforcement power. To achieve changes in education and roles requires action on the part of many bodies, such as schools of nursing, universities and colleges, accrediting agencies and bodies, and employing agencies. As Hall (1982) pointed out, the role of the professional associations is to influence the sources of control.

The ANA is attempting to increase its power through coalitions with other organizations, both those whose members are nurses and those who are not. To achieve power through coalition building the ANA has sought issues around which organizations can coalesce and has engaged in preparing nurses to become politically more active. The American Nurses' Association Political Action Committee has been highly involved in educating members of state nurses' associations in the use of political strategy and action. Few studies have been made of nurses and their political activities, but one study indicated that nurses are less involved in local and state political activities than are female teachers and female engineers (Hanley, 1987). This research also revealed that nurses in the study were members of fewer professional organizations than those in the other two professions.

A few nurses have been selected to the Institute of Medicine; others have received awards, honors, and honorary degrees; and still others have been elected or appointed to offices in other organizations or have gained positions in institutions and government. These nurses are among the professional elite who have achieved recognition and position by their own achievements or their own personal connections and influence. These persons, who may hold membership in the professional association, have the authority and right to express their own opinions and ideas. The ANA has no control over them, other than through peer pressure and through lobbying efforts by officers and others representing the official position of the ANA.

The ANA exerts power through its statements of practice, education, and service; its credentialing program; and the economic security program, the latter implemented primarily at the state association level. These activities influence decisions at the institutional level where practice and education are carried out, but the ANA has no enforcement power such as censoring or disciplining members, other nurses, or institutions. The accreditation or approval of educational programs is conducted by the National League for Nursing and state boards of nursing. Nursing service delivery is accredited or regulated by state agencies, Medicare and Medicaid, and the Joint Commission on the Accreditation of Hospitals. Licensing and practitioner discipline is conducted by the state boards of nursing. The ANA has no procedure for the review of the actions of individual nurses or restrictions that may result in censoring. At the state level, if the nurses of a unit are organized and represented by the state association, a strike may be called, but the issue on which the strike revolves must also have a sufficient degree of public support and understanding to be effective.

A number of authors have suggested ways by which the ANA can become more effective in its drive for professionalism (Capuzzi, 1980; Ezell, 1983; Rosenfeld, 1986; Santis, 1982; Speedy, 1987). Hall (1973) urged that professional associations examine where the association can exert influence if not control. Kalisch and Kalisch (1982) portrayed the influence of the ANA in legislative matters over the years and the importance of political acumen, timing, and the need to be proactive. Recently, the ANA has been successful in two major actions that were helpful in the movement toward professionalism. The establishment of the National Center for Research and the modified provision for community nursing organizations included in the Budget Reconciliation Act of 1987 are recent examples of its influence and the effectiveness of coalition building.

The role of the ANA in continuing education programs has been stressed by many (Peutz, 1985). The importance of accrediting these programs through state and national bodies of the ANA and through state boards of nursing is not minimized, but this is influence and power exerted by the ANA on the nursing community itself. The effect of continuing education programs is indirect, that is, as it effects the competency of the individual nurse. The same is true of the credentialing of nurses. The impact on the long-range goal—professionalization of the nursing occupation—is somewhat dispersed, though commendable. A more effective means would be the massive upgrading of the education of entrants to the occupation and socializing them as professionals. This end can be achieved through the continued use of the ANA's influence.

The power of the professional association in nursing is not unlike the power of all associations. It is limited. Hall (1982) stated that the power of an association is achieved through the use of influence with power brokers and groups. He urged the development of a strong collective, the building of coalitions around major issues, the limiting of goals, and maintenance of a sensitivity to the changing external environment. The achievement of power also requires the leadership of an association to be aware of the vulnerability of the practitioners, the nature of the controls on the profession, the sources of influence, and the identification of the power brokers. An association may be powerful, but its power stems from the power and influence of its leadership, the individual members, and the collective. The power

image the profession conveys to the public is a reflection of the self-concept held by these three groups.

REFERENCES

Aydelotte, M. K. (1982). Nursing: Societal discontent and professional change. In R. R. Wieczorek (Ed.), *Power, politics and policy in nursing* (pp. 121–137). New York: Springer.

Capuzzi, C. (1980). Power and interest groups: A study of ANA and AMA. *Nursing Outlook, 28,* 478–482.

Conway, M. E. (1982). Prescription for professionalization. In N. L. Chaska (Ed.), *The nursing profession: A time to speak* (pp. 29–37). New York: McGraw-Hill.

Cox, K. (1984). Decision making in a professional association. *Social Science Medicine, 19,* 1159–1165.

Crowder, E. L. M. (1985). Historical perspectives of nursing's professionalism. *Occupational Health Nursing, 33,* 184–190.

Cullen, J. B. (1978). *The structure of professionalism.* New York: Petrocelli Books.

Department of Labor, Bureau of Labor Statistics. (1987). *Occupational outlook handbook,* (1986/87 ed.). Washington, DC: U.S. Government Printing Office.

Ezell, A. S. (1983). Future social planning for nursing education and nursing practice organizations. In N. L. Chaska (Ed.), *The nursing profession: A time to speak* (pp. 764–777). New York: McGraw-Hill.

Freidson, E. (1986). *Professional powers: A study of the institutionalization of formal knowledge.* Chicago: University of Chicago Press.

Goode, W. J. (1969). The theoretical limits of professionalization. In A. Etzioni (Ed.), *The semiprofessions and their organization* (pp. 266–313). New York: Free Press.

Greenwood, E. (1957). Attributes of a profession. *Social Work, 2*(3), 45–55.

Gruending, D. L. (1985). Nursing theory: A vehicle of professionalization. *Journal of Advanced Nursing, 10,* 553–558.

Hall, C. M. (1973). Who controls the nursing profession?—The role of the professional association. *Nursing Times, 69*(23), 89–92.

Hall, R. H. (1982). The professions, employed professionals and the professional association. In the American Nurses' Association, *Professionalism and the empowerment of nursing.* Paper presented at the 53rd convention (pp. 1–15). Kansas City, MO: American Nurses' Association.

Hanley, B. E. (1987). Political participation: How do nurses compare with other professional women? *Nursing Economics, 5*(4), 179–185.

Hughes, E. C. (1971). *The sociological eye: Selected papers*. Chicago: Aldine-Atherton.

Johnson, T. J. (1972). *Professions and power*. London: MacMillan Press.

Kalisch, B. J., & Kalisch, P. A. (1982). *Politics of nursing*. Philadelphia: J. B. Lippincott.

Larson, M. S. (1977). *The rise of professionalism: A sociological analysis*. Berkeley-Los Angeles-London: University of Chicago Press.

Moore, W. E. (1970). *The professions: Roles and rules*. New York: Russell Sage Foundation.

National Commission on Nursing Implementation Project. (1987, November). *Conference papers from the National Conference*. San Diego.

Puetz, B. (1985). The role of the professional association in continuing education in nursing. *The Journal of Continuing Education in Nursing, 16*(3), 89–93.

Rosenfeld, P. (1986). Nursing and professionalization: On the road to recovery. *Nursing and Health Care, 7*(9), 484–488.

Santis, G. E. (1982). Power, tactics, and the professionalization process. *Nursing and Health Care, 3*(1), 14–24.

Speedy, S. (1987). Feminism and the professionalism of nursing. *Australian Journal of Advanced Nursing, 4*(2), 20–28.

✳ **EDITOR'S QUESTIONS FOR DISCUSSION** ✳

How does nursing exercise its power and influence in the wider social structure? How could it increase its power? Compare the points made by Aydelotte with those made by Beletz in Chapter 3. To what extent do they agree regarding the role and influence of power in nursing? How can the ANA more effectively use its power base? Discuss whether or not the ANA should have enforcement power over its members and, if so, how it might be obtained and used.

What strategies can be offered to socialize entrants into nursing as professionals? Discuss how the professional association of nursing has sustained and altered the official framework for professional activities. How and why do strains result within professional associations? What suggestions might be offered to reduce the strains and social stratification?

Discuss the extent you agree with Aydelotte concerning the four problem areas she cites as being obstacles in nursing's achieving professional status. Provide suggestions and strategies to resolve the obstacles. What factors have come into play that are promoting mobility options rather than defining education programs as terminal programs with terminal outcomes for a specific type of practice? Discuss the pros and cons of defining programs as terminal for a specific type of practice.

3

Professionalization—A License Is Not Enough

Elaine E. Beletz, Ed.D., R.N., F.A.A.N.

For nearly a century, nursing has engaged in an arduous pursuit and heroic struggle to achieve legitimization and recognition as a full profession. The emotional debate regarding nursing's professionalism continues. Students and practitioners ask: Is nursing a profession? Who is the professional nurse? The intent of this chapter is to examine both the attributes of a profession and the factors affecting perceptions of professional status.

BACKGROUND

The professions, as an occupational category, are at the apex of income, prestige, and power. Whether the society is highly industrialized or developing, the professions serve as an elite cadre of power and influence. Societal perceptions of professionals have been markedly influenced by European stereotypes. Carr-Saunders (1955) describes the older professions as learned—having possessed broad culture and comprehensive competence—and as being made up of influential members of society to whom leadership was granted. Espoused professional values included a liberal education; a dislike of competition, advertising, and profit; preference for independent practice and fee-for-service, rather than salaried institutional employment; and above all, reflected a belief

in the supremacy of service as a motivating force (Elliott, 1972).

The professions have retained a highly esteemed position in contemporary society. One's work identity implicitly references a person's ranking in the larger society with respect to appropriate occupational positions and work, socioeconomic class position, opportunities for class mobility, and ability to access those who have the power to mold policy (Becker & Carper, 1956). As a result, the professions who are at the top of the occupational hierarchy are perceived as having great power, prestige, and economic comfort. Therefore, the motivation in seeking professional status by an occupation involves a complex mix of goals.

PROFESSIONALIZATION

In today's world, the terms *profession* and *professional* are frequently misused and abused. The professional athlete is distinguished from the amateur by virtue of payment. Many occupations claim professionhood; numerous groups have achieved licensure, yet recognition of professional status may not have been accorded by the larger society. When an occupation seeks professional status, it engages in a dynamic process of professionalization that is associated with becoming congruent with the criteria of professionhood. Professionalism is an ideology intrinsic to professionalization. Vollmer and Mills (1966) suggest that when evaluating the professional status of occupations, it is more fruitful to view them, at a point in time, on a professionalization continuum with the ideal profession at one end and blue-collar occupations at the other. The distinction between professionals and nonprofessionals is quantitative and not necessarily qualitative. As an example, Etzioni (1969) and Reiss (1955) refer to nurses, social workers, and teachers as semiprofessionals. The rationale is that, when contrasted to recognized professions as law or medicine, these "semiprofessionals" have a shorter educational requirement, lower status, less established right to privileged communication, less of a specialized body of knowledge, and less autonomy. Further, the emphasis for these semiprofessionals is on precise technical skills and on knowledge of the basis for such skills, as opposed to theoretical study.

Is it important for society to have professions or for nursing to achieve professional status? A yes or no answer may be argued depending on one's philosophy. Some may view professionalization and the establishment of professions as a barrier to upward mobility and as the arbitrary creation of an elite within a classless society. On the other hand, society benefits through the ordering and categorizing of the increasing complexities of today's knowledge explosion. Professions provide society with an essential social service that affects the lives and safety of people. The particular domain of a profession is considered so special and mysterious that the layman could not practice it safely. As a result of the uniqueness of professional knowledge, society engages in a trust relationship and exchanges with the professional the recognition, status, and privileges of professionhood for the provision of excellence in services and unrestricted access to services.

CRITERIA OF PROFESSIONALIZATION

Numerous typologies, attributes, and criteria for judging groups on the professional continuum have been developed. According to Greenwood (1966), the distinguishing attributes of a profession include systematic theory, authority, community sanction, ethical codes, and a professional culture. Cullen (1978) compressed the criteria of 14 theorists and adds the following dimensions: complex occupation, self-employed, person oriented, altruistic service, lengthy educational preparation, system of organization, competence tested, licensed, high income, and high prestige. As professions have matured, each of these characteristics has become internalized in professional value systems and they have become the standards by which professionalizing occupations are judged. Many of the characteristics are reciprocally related and overlap. Selected traits are presented below to provide a more comprehensive understanding of the value system of the professions.

Expertise

Expertise is a composite of a knowledge base, gained through long years of study in an academic setting, and superior skill. It requires the mastery of intellectual material, derived through research, which leads to theory construction; the systematic body of knowledge on which professional practice is based is thereby established. Expertise is the primary distinguishing difference between professionals and nonprofessionals. Although earlier professionals' expertise was generalized to all areas of knowledge, in contemporary society the spectrum of influence of professionals has been narrowed to expertise and competence within their specific spheres.

Control and Autonomy

Licensure is one of the ways by which the social contract of trust between society and the profession is established. It benefits the public by protecting it from the unqualified, and it protects the professional's job territory by providing a monopoly over skill. Legal protection also enhances status by authenticating a profession. An occupation that has achieved licensure has attained a monopoly in the public's interest. The achievement of a license is viewed by many within a discipline as the ultimate rite of passage to professionhood. However, a license cannot be equated with full professional status. It should be noted that hairdressers, morticians, airline pilots, and nursing home administrators also hold licenses. Governments grant licenses to practice when the nature of a service is viewed as sufficiently complex to require a minimum amount of knowledge to protect the public from unqualified practice.

The ultimate privilege that government accords the professions is the ability to claim privileged communication and the right of confidentiality. It is a rare immunity and can be used by the law, medicine, and clergy. Other powers of regulation imparted to the professions include control over education, credentialing, scope of practice, establishment of standards, self-evaluation, and discipline.

Those aspiring to professionhood, as well as the recognized professions, have promulgated codes of ethics. It is through this mechanism that a profession establishes standards for self-regulation. This medium allows for the profession's commitment to society to become a matter of public record. The tenor of the code tends to be altruistic and service oriented, and the code incorporates behaviors pertaining to client, profession, and colleague relations. A necessary corollary of a code is cohesion and solidarity, without which implementation of the code's provisions and self-regulation will not be achievable.

Since the work of a profession incorporates a service which no other group can claim or perform, any supervisory attempt by laypersons is strongly resisted. Professional loyalties are to peers and to their profession. As such, there is an attempt to control practice in light of the discipline's own standards (Freidson, 1984). Strauss (1963) describes a professional as one bound by values and standards other than those of his or her employing organization, setting one's own rules, seeking to promote standards of excellence, and being evaluated and looking for approval from one's own professional peers.

The ideal situation in the traditional professional model is a person who is not a salaried employee. Yet, most professionals have always been salaried. Even the physician who has an independent practice may be considered a quasi-employee because of dependence on the hospital for patient care and referrals. This, in turn, subjects him or her to administrative rules. The conditional loyalty of the professional to his or her place of employment and emphasis on autonomy is at the crux of professional-bureaucratic conflict. Organizational employment is perceived as reducing autonomy and produces a resistance to bureaucratic rules. The essence of autonomy is for the professional to have almost complete control over what is done for the client (Hughes, 1963). Guy (1985), however, has concluded that bureaucracies and professionalism are not antithetic and that professionals meld their personal and professional goals with those of the organization. Under certain conditions, autonomy is always vulnerable, whether in a self or institutionally employed position. Examples are if market demand is low and there is overdependence on clients or if there is strong resistance by administrations to independent professional judgment.

Commitment and Investment

A person who chooses to be a professional has made a commitment to a subculture whose values, norms, and beliefs have an impact on one's lifestyle, behavior, and personality. Work is central to the life of a professional and occupies much of one's waking moments, whereby the sharp demarcation between work and leisure time almost disappears. The professional's work becomes the individual's life. Characteristically, intrinsic to professionalism is a commitment to a calling, the service ideal, and altruism.

The commitment to a calling incorporates all of the occupation's norms and standards as well as identification with professional peers and the profession as a collective (Moore, 1970). The established rules become an inclusive set of normative and behavioral expectations of loyalty and identification. Although many have interpreted the service and altruistic orientation to be an aversion to money, Moore (1970) defines the service orientation as requiring the professional to "perceive the needs of the individual, or collective clients, that are relevant to his competence and to attend to those needs by competent performance" (p. 6). A professional tends to be a perfectionist in his or her work and is internally motivated, and further the professional tends to give secondary importance to monetary considerations.

Obligations of a Professional

With privilege always comes obligation. The right to self-governance that society grants professionals also incurs attendant responsibilities. These responsibilities, as suggested by Moore (1970), include (a) preservation and enhancement of the image of one's profession; (b) adherence to standards of performance and conduct promulgated by the profession; (c) accountability for individual actions; (d) demonstrating respect for the public interest by exhibiting honorable public conduct; (e) participating in peer review and discipline; and (f) remaining competent by staying abreast of the latest developments in one's field. A more tacit obligation affects decision making. A professional is expected to use one's intellectual base, to be objective, and to adhere to the methods of the scientific, or other analytical model, when assessing problems and making decisions. Fiction is rejected for fact, as is fathom for substance.

Professional and Client or Community Interrelationship

The client seeks the services of a professional in the spirit of *credat emptor*—let the buyer (client) trust. A client seeks out the services of a professional and accepts those services on the professional's terms. Greenwood (1966) suggests that the authoritative air presented by the professional serves as the source of the client's faith that there is a potential for meeting his or her needs. Detachment, being impersonal, and preventing the relationship from becoming a personal one, beyond the professional setting, is recommended by Greenwood (1966). The rationale presented for this type of manner is to prevent the introduction of emotional bias in actions or advice, impairment of professional authority, and diminution of the professional's effectiveness. Within the ideology of private practice, the client is identified as an individual, such as a patient. Contemporary writers propose that the client may also be an employer, corporation, community, or membership. The professional and client trust interrelationship requires intense obligations to the client and a willingness to give unselfish service to the community.

Intraprofessional Relationships

The professional's bond with colleagues emanates from relationships established by shared mysteries of a common technical language, educational background, rites of passage, styles of work, attire, and a consciousness of being set apart and insisting on being set apart from other occupational categories (Moore, 1970). Colleague relationships are expected to be cooperative, equalitarian, and supportive vis-à-vis clientele and peers. It is assumed that the professional will refrain from any actions that jeopardize the authority of colleagues and it is also anticipated that colleagues will sustain one another when that authority is threatened. The strategy of mutual respect is the foundation of a profession's viability.

The structural embodiment of a professional community is a professional association. This vehicle serves as the collective identity, the body politic, and the voice of the profession to society, the profession, and all other publics with whom the profession interacts. The expectation of membership of the individual professional in the professional association is a requirement of professionalism.

Relations with Nonprofessionals

Professionals work with a cadre of occupational groups. Equality is not the norm. Pecking orders and caste systems develop. The professional will protect the exclusiveness of his or her domain, will seek to retain control at the higher echelons of the pecking order, and will employ any mechanism to prevent role confusion. Yet, there are components of the professional role that are so routine they can be safely delegated to an ancillary occupation. The purpose of the ancillary group is to facilitate the work of the professional and release the professional for more intellectual activities.

In economic theory the presence of substitutes, real or perceived, reduces power and bargaining position. If not strongly controlled by statute by requiring supervision and accountability to professionals, paraprofessionals can become sources of competition and jeopardize the professional status of the primary profession. Although professions try to control ancillary occupations, none seem to have attained total control (Moore, 1970).

Rewards

Altruistic calling notwithstanding, when investments are made, rewards are expected. The perceived return on investment provides for recruitment and inducement to stay in a profession. The reward system of professions includes prestige, titles, medals, prizes, leadership positions, and sufficient money to live the lifestyle expected of and consistent with being a professional. Money is a symbol of value, recognition, and importance. Kliengartner (1967) suggests that the economic objectives of professionals are to achieve levels of compensation reflective of knowledge and education as well as the job. In addition, professionals believe that superior remuneration and personal security are prerequisites for the dignity, status, and competence associated with professional rank.

When professionals become salaried, they lose the autonomy of establishing their wages and working conditions. A number of professionals have opted for collective bargaining. Whereas this strategy was one almost universally touted as being unprofessional, today it has been adopted to some degree by almost all salaried professions, except the clergy and the military. The major areas of contention between collective bargaining and professionalism are collective bargaining's association with blue-collar workers; its emphasis on the collectivity and equalitarianism, rather than individual achievement; and the potential of violating the duty to provide unrestricted access to services during a strike.

Prestige and Power

Economics is certainly the most concrete factor in determining prestige and power; however, prestige and power are also determined by people's perceptions, based on mind-sets created from values and norms collected over time. An occupation may have all the attributes of a profession and still may not be able to operate or be perceived as a profession. Ben David (1965) deduced that status is associated with factors inherent in either the nature of an occupation's service or the public view of it. Societal devaluation of female and domestic qualities is a corollary of public perceptions. Cullen (1978) affirms that, regardless of income, complexity of the service, and education, occupations have lower prestige if they remain physical. Physical demands are associated with the unpleasantness of manual labor, and therefore efforts to maximize prestige generally require allocation of the more physical aspect of an occupation to subordinates. Noteworthy is that, more than any other characteristic, the principal requirement for prestige is extensive education (Cullen, 1978).

Prestige is closely associated with the concept of power. The ability to influence and affect the direction of decisions in many arenas is greatly pursued. The growing preeminence of gaining power has resulted in the replacement of the classic professional characteristics with "power perspective" theories, which focus on occupational group power and its distribution in the larger society. Today's sociologists tend to view the "power perspective" as the most important variable in achieving full professionalization (Hall, 1982). However, power requires that one has resources or can obtain them. Within a resource context, one can argue that it is the characteristics of professionalism that provide the resources and power to permanently influence public perception. Power, especially when exercised only through numbers, requires constant application to have any impact, and even then, its effect may only be fleeting. Power tends to be elusive if one's foundation and substance are shallow.

Professional Culture and Social Class

Professional culture is an important component of professionalism. In a sense, professional culture constitutes the internal political dynamics of a discipline. It incorporates informal and formal networks, the language, symbols, norms, and beliefs of a profession. A professional culture seems to differentiate and create distance from the laity. Great symbolism is associated with occupational title and ideology. Characteristics are ascribed to the group, pertaining to its image, qualities, interests, and capabilities.

Professional cultural norms may be considered guides to behavior in interpersonal situations. Such norms affect schooling, clients, peers, career, dealing with controversy, and overall decorum. It is generally believed that the practitioner must adjust to the profession's subculture to achieve success. Expertise and proficiency in one's knowledge base is insufficient.

Professional culture may not always be in the mainstream of society. For example, the belief in the importance of performing an important public mission has assisted nursing in its endeavors to achieve professional recognition and an honorable image. Nevertheless, society values sophisticated technology, and if it does not accompany a missionary orientation, the missionary ideology is perceived as hurting rather than helping attempts at professionalization (Ben David, 1965).

A cultural difference that distinguishes the professions and the semiprofessions is an emphasis on a wholistic focus of service. Simpson and Simpson (1969) describe the prevalence of wholistic ideology (the desire to give service and relate to the whole person) among semiprofessionals. The "true" professional focuses on a task orientation, whereby the individual self-identifies specific expertise and skills possessed and renders them. Simpson and Simpson (1969) suggest that the attraction to semiprofessions appears to be emotions and beliefs in humanitarianism rather than intellectual mastery. Humanitarianism is distinguished from altruism, whereby, in the latter, rewards are derived from the exercise of skill rather than the response of the client.

The impact of societal culture and social class on attaining professional status is rarely discussed. One reason is that some occupations, as nursing, are considered an avenue of upward mobility for lower socioeconomic groups. Persons from occupations classified as semiprofessions tend to come from lower income families than do recognized professionals, whose roots tend to lie in professional, entepreneurial, and semiprofessional families. Nursing tends to be perceived as a first-generation career (Green, 1987). Discussion of class differences may be shunned by the professions because the nature of their work requires that services be provided to all people regardless of divisions of class, status, power, and interest (Elliott, 1972). However, stemming from immersion in professional culture, professionals are aware of the decorum, lifestyle, and symbols that are required because of professional identity and status. Society expects professionals to display moderate economic comfort, unquestionable respectability, monetary support of cultural interests, patronage of the arts, and support of charities and education (Moore, 1970).

There is an old saying that "water seeks its own level." People tend to form bonds when cultures, dreams, affinities, and experiences are similar. The elite strata of society have the power and influence to legitimize and raise the prestige of occupational groups. Major decisions affecting society and policy are influenced at country club affairs, socialite dinners, golf courses, and health clubs. One of the sources of medicine's power is its long alliance with societal elites (Hall, 1982). Informal access to those in power is essential for achieving prestige and power. Consistent with liberal backgrounds and ideologies, many groups aspiring to professionalism emphasize that their services are provided for the poor and disadvantaged. While this is necessary and laudable, it does not engender an image of desirability or affinity with those in society who can pay. Demand for service is a function of affluence (Moore, 1970), and attraction to the affluent may be a function of uniqueness. Professionalizing groups must seek out, become comfortable with, and market their services for the wealthy. It is an access route to professional recognition, class mobility, and power.

CONCLUSION

Is nursing a profession? After a century of struggle without an end in sight, it is essential that nursing take inventory by objectively contrasting its current status with the professional standards, ideologies, and cultural nuances presented. On the continuum of professionalization, qualitatively nursing and many individual nurses excel far beyond contemporary recognized professions in many areas. Quantitatively the road ahead is very long.

Nursing history demonstrates myriad efforts to

meet professional standards. The presence of a professional association, code of ethics, and achievement of a license are but a few of the successes. The license has always been viewed as the premier source of validation of professional status. Yet by itself, it is insufficient. What does society say? The legal system serves as a mirror of societal beliefs. Within a legal sense, the courts are split with respect to designating registered nurses as professionals. Segal (1985) asserts that the points of contention are (a) insufficient authority and prestige of the field and (b) absence of intense systematic educational preparation for entry. Ultimately, it would appear that although nursing is permeated with the ideas of professionalism, it has been little touched by its substance. Every profession in its early history has had to fight for recognition. There is a growing trend in nursing to either compromise or forego the traditional professional traits in favor of emphasizing strategies for attaining group power. Yet, one must consider that ideal values and norms do not become irrelevant because of failures to achieve them.

Several years ago while I was giving testimony before a legislative body, a legislator asked, in all sincerity, what was wrong with nurses spending their time doing required paperwork for third-party payors? I responded with the analogy that to utilize nurses in this way was the equivalent of mounting the Hope diamond in a tin setting. Just as the value of all precious gems increases when they closely conform to the standards of color, cut, clarity, and carat weight, so too nursing will achieve its dreams of full professionalization when it adheres to the hallmarks of excellence in professional criteria. Only then will nursing have demonstrated its willingness to meet the challenge of professionalization on society's terms.

REFERENCES

Becker, H. S., & Carper, J. (1956). The elements of an identification with an occupation. *American Sociological Review, 21,* 341–347.

Ben David, J. (1965). Professionals and unions in Israel. *Industrial Relations, 5,* 48–66.

Carr-Saunders, A. M. (1955). Metropolitan conditions and traditional professional relationships. In R. M. Fischer (Ed.), *The metropolis in modern life* (pp. 286–287). New York: Doubleday.

Cullen, J. B. (1978). *The structure of professionalism.* New York: Petrocelli Books.

Elliott, P. (1972). *The sociology of the professions.* New York: Herder & Herder.

Etzioni, A. (1969). *The semi-professions and their organization.* New York: Free Press.

Freidson, E. (1984). The changing nature of professional control. *The Annual Review of Sociology, 10,* 1–20.

Green, K. D. (1987). The educational "pipeline" in nursing. *Journal of Professional Nursing, 3,* 247–257.

Greenwood, E. (1966). Attributes of a profession. In H. M. Vollmer & D. L. Mills (Eds.), *Professionalization* (pp. 10–19). Englewood Cliffs, NJ: Prentice-Hall.

Guy, M. E. (1985). *Professionals in organizations debunking a myth.* New York: Praeger Publishers.

Hall, R. H. (1982). The professions, employed professionals and the professional association. In the American Nurses' Association, *Professionalism and the empowerment of nursing* Paper presented at the 53rd convention (pp. 1–15). Kansas City, MO: American Nurses' Association.

Hughes, E. C. (1963). Professions. Daedalus 92, 655–668.

Kliengartner, A. (1967). *Professional and salaried worker organization.* Madison, WI: University of Wisconsin Industrial Relations Institute.

Moore, W. E. (1970). *The professions: Roles and rules.* New York: Russell Sage Foundation.

Reiss, A. J. (1955). Occupational mobility of professional workers. *American Sociological Review, 20,* 693–700.

Segal, E. T. (1985). Is nursing a profession? *Nursing 85, 15,* 40–43.

Simpson, R. L., & Simpson, I. H. (1969). Women and bureaucracy in the semi-professions. In A. Etzioni (Ed.), The *semi-professions and their organization* (pp. 196–265). New York: Free Press.

Strauss, G. (1963). Professionalism and occupational associations. *Industrial Relations, 2,* 7–31.

Vollmer, H. M., & Mills, D. L. (1966). *Professionalization.* Englewood Cliffs, NJ: Prentice-Hall.

✳ EDITOR'S QUESTIONS FOR DISCUSSION ✳

Discuss the motivation of the profession of nursing in seeking professional status. How important is it for nursing to achieve professional status? To what extent does professional status become a barrier to upward mobility and create an elite class? How is the process of professionhood and professionalization in nursing the same or different? To what extent is expertise the primary difference between professionals and non-professionals? Discuss why a license cannot be equated with professionhood and professional status.

Discuss the factors that contribute to a professional-bureaucratic conflict. What strategies can be used in organizations to reduce that conflict? How can characteristics inherent to formal organizations be capitalized on to enhance professionalism and professional practice?

Discuss the pros and cons of work becoming the life of a professional. What type of behavioral expectations are associated with commitment? Should there be degrees of commitment held and shown by professionals and a profession? Discuss aspects of professionalism that can create or contribute to problems or conflicts for the professional. What strategies can be implemented by professionals to maintain a "balance" between their professional and personal life? How can a professional monitor his or her own professional growth, development, and actualization as a person?

Discuss the professional aspects of colleague relationships. How can competition and conflict best be supportive for collegial relationships rather than destructive? Discuss strategies for promoting relationships within the profession as a means for growth and development rather than escalation into conflict. How can conflict be resolved within the profession and between colleagues when it becomes an impediment for accomplishing goals?

Discuss the power perspective as being the most important variable in achieving full professionalization in nursing. Discuss effective and ineffective ways that nursing has used its power. Present strategies for a more effective use of power within the profession and for the profession. What trends indicate that nursing may be compromising professional traits in favor of strategies for obtaining group power?

How would one define the professional culture of nursing in terms of characteristics, norms, and behaviors? How do values relate to the development of culture within a profession such as nursing? Contrast the current status of nursing with regard to professional standards, ideologies, and culture nuances held by professions.

Social Ethics and Nursing

Marsha Fowler, Ph.D., R.N.

A profession's social ethics, the ethical critique of society and social policy, is influenced by the nature of the profession and its form of occupational control. Yet a profession's social ethics is not, as some would believe, entirely captive to its social context. What is the role of ethics vis-à-vis a profession? And what is the role of a profession vis-à-vis its ethics? If ethics, professions, and society are interrelated, what is the nature of that interrelatedness? The answers to these questions address the influence of nursing's moral identity, its moral mandate, and its professional and social ethics on both nursing and society.

THE ROLE OF ETHICS AND THE PROFESSIONS
Divergent Perspectives on Defining Professions

The role that can be envisioned for ethics in a profession depends in part on one's perspective on the analysis of professions. Discourse in the sociology of professions shows a clear divergence of opinion in the analysis of occupational groups as professions. Some see professions as unique social groupings that require "variant forms of analysis," differing from what is used to analyze other social groups (Johnson, 1972, p. 10). Thus, lists of attributes, or "trait definitions" of professions, are constructed to define those occupational groups that possess the requisite characteristics.

Trait definitions abound and form the backbone of many of the discussions of nursing-as-a-profession (Styles, 1982; Bixler & Bixler, 1959; Sleicher, 1981). They often focus on a core that includes (a) a well-defined body of knowledge, (b) specialized education and expertise based in higher education, (c) provision of a practical service, (d) existence of a professional association, (e) autonomy of practice, (f) profession-determined standards, (g) adumbration of a code of ethics, and (h) altruistic motivation (Flexner, 1915; Carr-Saunders & Wilson, 1933; Bixler & Bixler, 1959). Within a trait definition framework, whether or not an occupational group is to be regarded as a profession depends on its realization of the attributes specified. Ethics, in this approach, is a defining characteristic, yet may have no potency of its own.

The use of trait definitions is flawed (Johnson, 1972). Trait approaches assume that there are "true" professions and that they will demonstrate all of the essential core attributes. However, the attributes themselves are often an untidy aggregation of overlapping, arbitrarily chosen, or undifferentiated elements, lacking a unifying theoretical framework that explains their interrelationship. Trait theories tend empirically to generate a definition of a profession and then ascribe to it a normative rather than a descriptive status (Johnson, 1972).

Alternatively, functionalist models of professions stress the "functional value of professional activity for all groups and classes in society" (Johnson, 1972, p. 37). In functionalist models, there is no attempt to present an exhaustive list of 'traits'; rather the components of the model are limited to those elements which are said to have functional relevance for society as a whole or to the professional-client relationship." (Johnson, 1972, p. 23)

Although the emphasis is different in specifying "those elements," functional models bear some resemblance to trait definitions.

In functionalist models, professional ethics has social utility because it assures that the values of the profession are reinforced and displayed by individual practitioners and it constrains the negative effects that monopolization of practice may have for the consumer. In some respects, however, ethics in this sense potentially serves to reinforce group norms to the extent of prioritizing the good of the profession over the welfare of general society, or even of individual clients.

There are problems with functionalist models also. Chief among them is the fact that they are ahistorical and rationalistic, causally linking professional function to upward social mobility of the profession's members and social position. Such models have a false view of the power of expertise and rationality to affect society and fail to take account of nonrational social power relations that mitigate against social mobility (Johnson, 1972).

The trait and functionalist models' focus on the homogeneity of professions, on the upward social mobility of professionals, and on the elevated social stratification of the professions has served to avoid the economic, political, and social role of professions in society. There are two major perspectives on the relationship of professions to society which, in turn, produce differing perspectives on the role of ethics in the professions.

THE ROLE OF PROFESSIONS IN SOCIETY

The first view is that, in the general disintegration of society, the profession forms a moral community. Durkheim (1933) maintains that as society evolves ties become looser and morality less binding. Professions, then, as a part of that division of labor pro-

vide an altruistic moral community, which is self-policing, and serves to augment if not replace the increasingly loosened moral ties of society. The force of moral suasion and moral penalty restrains the individual from engaging in a wholesale pursuit of an egocentric ethics at the expense of the professional community, its clients, or society at large. However, the compelling evidence of political power-brokering, of the failure of self-policing, and of the failure of altruism among the "classical professions" in this society tends to mitigate against this theoretical view (Hatch, 1988; Knowles, 1977; Melosh, 1982; Ashley, 1976).

The second view of professions is substantially more cynical, and is perhaps more consistent with empirical evidence. This perspective maintains that professions are themselves specialized, monopolistic, power elites that serve their own ends of social dominance, further power, privilege, exclusive authority, suppression of competition, and a secured position, through the exploitation of a social need. Members of these communities possess a highly specialized but exceedingly narrow expertise, with a limited sense of moral responsibility (Veatch, 1972). Their moral responsibility is limited to their "piece of the action," and focuses on the expert production of their piece of social labor. Ethics becomes a matter of measuring the technical accuracy, excellence, precision, and perfection of that labor, rather than one of social conscience and altruism. Ethics can in this instance, as Stamey writes,

> become ideological rather than critical . . . Ethical reasoning . . . has served to validate and perpetuate the (unjustifiable) privileges of a limited segment of the human community." (Quoted in Deats, 1972, p. 39)

Both the trait and functionalist models attempt to resolve the problem of differential demonstration of traits or functional values through the concept of professionalization and professionalism. Variations among professions are a reflection of lesser or greater professionalization, rather than any true lack of homogeneity of characteristics among professional work groups. Ethics in either of these approaches may develop within an occupational group as it becomes more professionalized. Neither trait nor functionalist views come to grips with the tension between the profession-as-moral-community and profession-as-power-elite perspectives.

Johnson (1972) rejects professionalism and professionalization as an adequate explanation of professions. His emphasis is on the consequences of the social division of labor for the client-professional relationship and their influence on power relationships and occupational control. For Johnson, "a profession is not . . . an occupation, but a means of controlling an occupation (p. 45). His approach allows us to reconcile and explain the differing perspectives on the role of ethics in professions, although his view presents another sort of problem.

EFFECTS OF THE DIVISION OF SOCIAL LABOR

The chief effects of the social division of labor on the client-consumer/professional-producer relationship consist in social and economic dependence, social distance, and "indeterminacy," all of which are deeply interrelated (Johnson, 1972, p. 41). Social and economic dependence arises when the advancement of occupational specialization leads to a reduction in the knowledge or skill of the consumer; the more the occupational group becomes specialized, the more the consumer becomes "unspecialised" (p. 41) and dependent on the profession for the provision of goods or services he himself cannot produce. Social distance results. Where social distance is great there is greater potential for professional autonomy at the expense of the consumer. Social distance produces "a structure of uncertainty," or indeterminacy (Johnson, 1972, p. 41; Jamous & Peloille, 1970, p. 138). Indeterminacy produces a struggle for control and power. Those occupations that can control and emphasize indeterminacy

> control the system of evaluation, of sanction and control, impose their definition of the production(s) [of goods or services], have a tendency to exclude or place in a position of subordination those who could be brought by technical and scientific changes to redefine these productions. It is possible

to say that the system includes dominant members and dominated members. (Jamous & Peloille, 1970, p. 138)

In order to regulate the degree of uncertainty and the resultant levels of autonomy of a profession, and its potential for exploitation of the consumer, several institutionalized forms of occupational control "will arise to reduce the uncertainty. Power relationships will determine whether uncertainty is reduced at the expense of the producer or consumer" (Johnson, 1972, p. 41). One of those institutionalized forms of occupational control is "professionalism." Those occupations conventionally regarded as professions demonstrate differing forms of occupational control, thus accounting for their lack of homogeneity of attributes and functional value to society found in earlier forms of analysis of professions.

FORMS OF OCCUPATIONAL CONTROL

Collegiate control, of which professionalism is one form, is associated with a high level of uncertainty, great producer-consumer social distance, autonomous occupational control, and consumer dependence, and is often associated with the professions of law, medicine, and ministry. In this form of control, it is the producer who determines what consumer needs are and how they will be met. Professional associations exercise a degree of monopoly over production. In the collegiate form of control, "community-generated role-definitions and standards are maintained by a code of ethics and autonomous disciplinary procedures" (Johnson, p. 56). Here, the occupation may form a moral community, as Durkheim would envision, yet it may also become a power elite whose ethics are directed toward cementing the status and privileges of the profession.

In the patronage form of occupational control, the professional is subject to an individual or corporate patron, who defines the needs and how they will be met. Accounting and engineering are examples. Social distance benefits the patron, not the professional, and uncertainty is reduced in favor of the consumer. With regard to ethics, the authority of the patron reduces the clear function of ethics and autonomous disciplinary procedures. . . . Occupationally defined norms have under corporate patronage less significance than corporately defined expectations. Thus the scope of ethics is narrowed. (Johnson, 1972, p. 69)

The focus of ethics here is upon the technical adequacy and proficiency of the producer, vis-à-vis the consumer's needs and wishes. The professional is characterized by a very limited sense of ethical responsibility—limited to the harms or benefits that accrue to the patron (Johnson, 1972, p. 71).

The mediative form of occupational control is seen in situations where the state exercises authority over both the producer and consumer and defines the needs and ways in which they may be met; the state controls the content of practice. Consumers are defined by the state, and both consumer and producer choices are reduced. In this form of occupational control, "the clear-cut ethical prescriptions of professionalism which specify 'client' and colleague relationships are no longer entirely applicable" (Johnson, 1972, pp. 79, 82, 83).

In early approaches to the definition of professions, ethics plays the role of a defining characteristic, or a functional social value. Such approaches were unable to account for the tension between the view of a profession as a moral community versus the profession as a power elite. This tension is more effectively addressed by examining professions through their form of occupational control. These forms of occupational control, all of them evident within nursing, can account for the differences between and even within groups regarded as professions. They also serve to identify the crux of the differing opinions and observations of the role of ethics in relation to professions; occupational control influences the way in which ethics functions for occupational groups.

The collegiate model accords ethics a high status in its ability to construct a moral community, but a potentially negative status in its ability to function selfishly. The patronage model accords ethics little effect and, underneath, seems to assume little power for professional values and perhaps a fairly high degree of social disregard on the part of the patron. The mediative form of control fails to take into account the moral sensitivity that is demonstrated in state operations and the ability of the practitioner ethically to influence those operations. Indeed, ethics may in fact fail in all of these forms of occupational control. But not necessarily so. Social ethics, as a field within the broader discipline of ethics, holds out a different perspective and a greater hope for the force of ethics.

SOCIAL ETHICS

Structures of social power, whether their analysis proceeds from a focus on social ideas (e.g., jurisprudence), social relations (e.g., family or group associations), or the material conditions of society (e.g., technology and economic production), present but one set of variables in the preservation, rectification, or destruction of the moral ethos of society (Stackhouse, 1973). A second set of variables resides in the patterns of meaning and worth found in collective structures *and* personal and interpersonal relations, and cultural patterns. This is the set of variables that are neglected in any focus on ethics that looks only at power structures; such analyses are correct in their own domain, from their own perspective, but are necessarily incomplete. Although it is beyond the scope of this paper to pursue the interrelationship of the two sets of variables, it is important to say that the role of ethics for professions is not entirely constrained by the occupational control to which it is subject; the patterns of value and meaning are influenced, but not entirely determined, by factors such as social distance and indeterminacy. Ethics, as a part of the patterns of meaning and value of professionals, their professional groups, and the larger culture can influence those very power structures.

Social ethics, whether an individual or collective enterprise, is concerned with social criticism and social change. Winter (1966) defines social ethics as dealing with

issues of social order—the good, right, and ought in the organization of human communities and the shaping of social policies. Hence the subject matter of social ethics is moral rightness and goodness in the shaping of human society. (p. 215)

Social ethics performs several moral functions. First, it is possessed of a reformist bias that contends for change within a given community. Here, ethics seeks to bring the "is" into conformity with the "ought" in the workings of the group and its individual members, through critical self-reflection and evaluation. It cannot, however, accomplish this through a reliance solely on the power of rationality to effect change. Such a perspective has an exaggerated view of the world's plasticity and human power to reconstruct society. Social ethical critique must be joined with the second function of social ethics.

That function is to reaffirm the perspectives of the community as legitimate. This is often accomplished through "epidictic" (meaning "to show") discourse that

> sets out to increase the intensity of adherence to certain values, which might not be contested when considered on their own, but may nevertheless not prevail against other values that might come into conflict with them. (Perlman & Olbrechts-Tyteca, 1969, p. 51)

The function of epidictic moral discourse is to speak the values of the group, for and to the group, in order to "increase the intensity of adherence to values held in common by the audience and the speaker . . . mak[ing] use of dispositions already present in the audience" in order to induce action (Perlman & Olbrechts-Tyteca, 1969, pp. 52–53). Here, the two functions of social ethics work together to bring the "is" into conformity with the "ought" in the workings of the group and its individual members, through critical self-reflection and evaluation, and evocation of the ethical norms of the group, calling it to action.

The third function of social ethics is to represent the perspective of the community to the larger society (Perlman & Olbrechts-Tyteca, 1969). This function argues for changes in society itself, in accord with the moral norms that the profession holds. Social ethics, here, becomes in part a political act.

Nursing, as a community, as a profession, embraces a social ethics that reforms and reshapes the community, that evokes action in accord with its values, and that speaks its ethical perspectives to the larger society. Nursing's ethics is a social ethics.

NURSING AND SOCIAL ETHICS

Since its inception in this country, nursing has viewed itself as a moral endeavor. The 1896 articles of incorporation of the American Nurses' Association (ANA) identified the first objective of the Association as the establishment and maintenance of a code of ethics (American Society of Superintendents of Training Schools for Nurses, 1896). Goodrich captured the sense of nursing as a moral endeavor when she wrote: "So much is nursing of the essence of ethics that it is consistent to assert that the terms good and ethical as applied to nursing practice are synonymous" (1932, p. 5).

Despite its early concern for ethics as intrinsic to the nursing enterprise, there is compelling evidence that nursing shifted its focus to regard its ethics as partial confirmation of its status as a profession. The *Tentative Code* of 1940, written by the ANA Committee on Ethical Standards, begins with the statement that "nursing is a profession" and enumerates the "distinguishing characteristics of a profession" (ANA, 1940, p. 977). Nursing's ethics is, however, more than simply a pathognomonic professional attribute. It forms the very character of the nursing community, gives it meaning, and specifies its values.

The moral identity of nursing resides in its central moral motif, which is the ideal of service (Fowler, in press). That ideal is expressed through a number of metaphors that are specific to history and culture. The service ideal transcends nursing's history but is rooted in it, and today finds its expressions in notions of caring and advocacy as contemporary American metaphors for nursing, employed to realize the ideal of service (Fowler, in press). It is the ideal of service as the central moral core that, in part, distinguishes nursing ethics from medical ethics. (Although medicine "serves," initial research indicates that its central moral motif may be "mastery," an ideal that is closely aligned, as is service, with beneficence (Fowler, in press). Given the functions of social ethics, how does nursing live out an ethics of service-as-caring?

REFORM OF THE NURSING COMMUNITY

The first function of social ethics, that of reform within a community, is evident in nursing's history. Although there are numerous examples, one in particular stands out. Nursing had long held that "a truly professional nurse with broad social vision will have a sympathetic understanding of different creeds, nationalities, and races" (ANA, 1940, p. 977). If nursing's social ethics would not tolerate racial discrimination toward patients, it could not then condone it within the profession itself. In 1948, as a response to "concern[s] with the tensions, rifts, and cleavages between nurse groups of different origin, stemming from different peoples or races," ANA began an intergroup relations program (Flanagan, 1976, p. 166). That year, the ANA House of Delegates voted to "provide direct individual membership for black nurses restricted from membership in the state nurses' associations" (Flanagan, 1976, p. 166).

EPIDICTIC DISCOURSE IN NURSING

The epidictic function of ethics is evident in the speeches and writings of the profession's leaders and ethicists that evoke the ethical tradition of the nursing community. The *Suggested Code* of 1926 provides a clear example of the epidictic function of ethics, in its attempt to evoke the moral norms of the community in the face of competing values. It states:

> Heir throughout all the ages of those who have nurtured the young, the weak and the sick, the mother, the kindly neighbor, the knight on the battlefield, the nun and the deaconess within or without enclosing walls—nursing emerges as a profession from its historic setting . . . The most precious possession of this profession is the ideal of service extending even to the sacrifice of life itself. (ANA, 1926, p. 599)

The *Suggested Code* goes on to state that "the supreme responsibility of the nurse in relation to her profession is to keep alight that spiritual flame which

has illuminated the work of the great nurses of all time" (ANA, 1926, pp. 600–601). It is this commingling of ethical past, present, and future that reaffirms the perspectives of the community to its members, individually and collectively, and provokes action in concert with the values expressed by the profession.

NURSING'S ETHICS AND SOCIAL REFORM

Nursing's social ethics extends beyond those whom the community serves directly. It also speaks nursing's values to society at large to induce it to change. Stackhouse writes that

> Ethical analysis takes place in order to approve and strengthen those institutions or aspects of a sector of the social system that sustain the moral community, and in order to criticize, transform, or undermine those institutions or aspects of the social system that destroy such possibilities. (1973, p. 185)

How does nursing criticize and transform society in accord with the values of the profession? It does so both indirectly, through documents such as the *Code* and directly through political action.

The *Code for Nurses*, 1976, states in the interpretive statements of the eleventh provision:

> Quality health care is mandated as a right to all citizens. Availability and accessibility to quality health services for all citizens require collaborative planning by health providers and consumers at both the local and national level; . . . nurses have a responsibility to help ensure that citizens' rights to health care are met. (ANA, 1976, p. 19)

In the 1985 revision of the interpretive statements, as a social critique, that same passage becomes:

> The availability and accessibility of high quality health services to all people require collaborative planning at the local, state, national, and international levels that respects the interdependence of health professionals and clients in health care systems; . . . nurses have an obligation to promote equitable access to nursing and health care for all people. (ANA, 1985, p. 16)

Equitable access to health and nursing care for all persons, not only for citizens, is for this profession no idle ideal. Nursing moves from the values articulated in the *Code for Nurses* into the political arena, and fights for the realization of the profession's values in the delivery of health care.

One example of the political implementation of nursing's ethical concerns for high quality and equitable access to health care (including public education, research, and treatment) is evident in a 1988 issue of ANA's *Capital Update*. The lead article discusses "AIDS Legislation." It states:

> The AIDS Research and Information Act, [sic] S. 1220, was approved by the Senate after two days of intensive debate regarding several controversial amendments. . . . Senator Hatch urged his colleagues not to attach extraneous amendments to the bill. Hatch's plea reflected ANA's letter to the full Senate requesting support for S. 1220. ANA urged the Senate not to delay the research and education programs in the bill with debate on issues such as mandatory reporting and testing. (ANA, 1988, p. 1)

This is a rather specific example of nursing's action upon its values. A second less direct example can be seen in ANA's *Social Policy Statement* (1980). The statement consciously links nursing's social concerns with political action. It states that

> Public and political determinations are being made in five major areas, in each of which nursing has leadership responsibilities. 1. Organization, delivery, and financing of health care . . . 2. Continuing development of health resources . . . 3. Provision for the public health through use of preventive and environmental measures . . . 4. Development of new knowledge . . . 5. Health care planning as a matter of national policy. . . . In these and other areas, public determinations find expression through political processes . . . The political process . . . can be and is used to shape public perceptions of needs, and thus to create public demands. At best, such use of the political process is made out of impartial concerns for the public good. At worst, it occurs for the advancement of vested interests, with the public good being of lesser or no concern. For nursing, the public good must be the overriding concern. (ANA, 1980, pp. 3–4)

The public good frames nursing's activity in the public-political arena.

CONCLUSION

It is clear that, for the profession of nursing, ethics is not simply an attribute that proves it to be a profession. Neither is it simply an element of functional social value. Nor does it blindly preserve the community of nursing as an end in itself to the detriment or harm of those whom nursing serves. And whatever form of occupational control nursing takes, its ethics are not entirely dominated by structures of power. Nursing's ethics transcends definitions, functional value, and structure. Nursing's ethics supports the nursing community's ethical tradition, maintaining it while judging it. From the moral core of that tradition, the profession speaks its ethics into the social context that both legitimates and shapes nursing. But nursing's ethics is not captive to that context; its ethics also informs and shapes society.

REFERENCES

American Nurses' Association. (1926). A suggested code. *American Journal of Nursing, 26,* 599–601.

_____. (1940). A tentative code. *American Journal of Nursing, 40,* 977–980.

_____. (1976). *Code for nurses with interpretive statements.* Kansas City, MO: Author.

_____. (1980). *Nursing: A social policy statement.* Kansas City, MO: Author.

_____. (1985). *Code for nurses with interpretive statements.* Kansas City, MO: Author.

_____. (1988). ANA Senate approves AIDS legislation. *Capital Update, 6,* 1.

American Society of Superintendents of Training Schools for Nurses. (1896). *Proceedings of convention.* Harrisburg, PA: Harrisburg Publishing.

Ashley, J. A. (1976). *Hospitals, paternalism, and the role of the nurse.* New York: Teachers College.

Bixler, G. K., & Bixler, R. W. (1959). The professional status of nursing. *American Journal of Nursing, 59,* 1142–1146.

Carr-Saunders, A. M., & Wilson, P. A. (1933). *The professions.* Oxford: Clarendon Press.

Deats, P., Jr. (Ed.) (1972). The quest for a social ethic.

Toward a discipline of social ethics. Boston: Boston University Press.

Durkheim, E. (1933). *The division of labor in society*. (G. Simpson, Trans.). New York: The Macmillan Company.

Flanagan, L. (1976). *One strong voice*. Kansas City, MO: American Nurses' Association.

Flexner, A. (1915). Is social work a profession? *School and Society, 1*, 901–911.

Fowler, M. D. M. (in press). *Nursing's Ethics*. Philadelphia: J. B. Lippincott.

Goodrich, A. W. (1932). *The social and ethical significance of nursing*. New Haven, CT: Yale University Press.

Hatch, N. O. (1988). *The professions in American history*. Notre Dame, IN: University of Notre Dame Press.

Jamous, H, & Peloille, B. (1970). Professions or self-perpetuating systems? Changes in the French university–hospital system. In J. A. Jackson, (Ed.), *Professions and professionalization* (pp. 109–152). Cambridge, MA: Cambridge University Press.

Johnson, T. (1972). *Professions and power*. London: Macmillan.

Knowles, J. H. (1977). *Doing better and feeling worse: Health in the United States*. New York: W. W. Norton.

Melosh, B. (1982). *The physician's hand*. Philadelphia: Temple University Press.

Perlman, C., & Olbrechts-Tyteca, L. (1969). *The new rhetoric: A treatise on argumentation*. Notre Dame, IN: University of Notre Dame Press.

Sleicher, M. N. (1981). Nursing is not a profession. *American Journal of Nursing, 81*, 186–192.

Stackhouse, M. L. (1973). Ethics: Social and Christian. *Andover Newton Quarterly, 13*, 173–191.

Styles, M. M. (1982). *On nursing: Toward a new endowment*. St. Louis: C. V. Mosby.

Veatch, R. M. (1972). Models for ethical medicine in a revolutionary age. *Hastings Center Report, 2* (3), 5–7.

Winter, G. (1966). *Elements for a social ethic: The role of social science in public policy*. New York: Macmillan.

✳ EDITOR'S QUESTIONS FOR DISCUSSION ✳

How do the trait and functionalist models attempt to resolve the problem of different values through the concept of professionalism? Discuss the implications for nursing of the social distance that may result between the client and the professional. How does social distance really benefit the patron and not the professional with uncertainty being reduced in favor of the consumer? To what extent do you believe that nurses and nursing determine what the consumer's needs are rather than determining from the consumer what they believe their needs are?

What is the difference between viewing nursing as a profession in the moral community rather than as a profession in the power elite? How can the ethics of professionals as part of the pattern of meaning and value influence power structures? Provide some examples in nursing of the three moral functions of social ethics.

5

The Legal Perspective of Nurse Autonomy

Ellen K. Murphy, J.D., M.S., R.N., F.A.A.N.

Law and nursing, like all other elements in society, interact. Both shape and are shaped by the other, as well as by the other elements in society. Through statutes and court decisions, the legal system directly shapes what nurses are required, permitted, and prohibited to do. Likewise, within the context of a representative democracy, such as that in the United States, nurses can use legal mechanisms to expand their sphere of autonomous function.

Although no authoritative definition of a profession has been broadly accepted (Monnig, 1978), autonomy is generally recognized as an essential attribute of a profession (Etzioni, 1969). An examination of the status of nursing autonomy as presently recognized in statutes and case law (to the extent "the law" exists), reveals that nurses are regarded as both autonomous professionals and as subject to outside control. This chapter uses statutory and case law examples to illustrate nurses' interrelationship with three sources of outside control: legislatures, physicians, and employers.

STATUTORY AND CASE LAW PERSPECTIVES ON NURSE AUTONOMY
Statutes and Relationships with Legislatures

Independent professional licensure is frequently cited as evidence of nursing's autonomy (e.g., Kelly,

1981, pp. 163–165). Nurses have been relatively successful at achieving legal recognition of nurse autonomy through the legislative process. The passage of the first nurse registration act by North Carolina in 1903 notably predated women's suffrage. Similar successes have continued through passage of the first mandatory practice act in New York to the more recent efforts to secure independent prescriptive and other "expanded role" authority. Indeed nurses' relative success in licensure may have resulted in an overreliance on the legislative process to achieve professional goals. By seeking goals through the legislative process, nursing submits itself to that process, which by design enables input and influence from other groups as well as the legislature, in determining the scope of nursing practice. Three examples of the profession's present reliance on the legislature are expanded practice, payment, and entry into practice.

Evolving practice

Some nurses have looked to changes in the states' nurse practice acts to allow practice in nurse practitioner or other expanded practice roles. Rather than regard legal silence as permissive (one can do X as long as the law does not say one cannot do X), some nurses consider statutory silence as restrictive (one cannot do X unless the law says one may). These nurses have worked very hard to get express recognition of expanded role functions enumerated in states' statutes that license nurse practice.

Specificity in the statute is not without its costs. Specifically worded statutes tend to freeze the status quo rather than accommodate evolving roles.

Specific statutes that "laundry list" permitted actions invite the argument that unless the action is listed, it is prohibited; or if certain enumerated acts are permitted for one group of nurse specialists, they are prohibited to another group unless also enumerated. Statutes that expressly identify prohibited actions are even more problematic to evolving practice. For example, the wording in the ANA's Model Practice Act of 1955 that nursing practice did not include "acts of diagnosis or prescription of therapeutic or corrective measures" (American Nurses' Association, 1959, p. 39) was codified in many states' nurse practice acts. This express prohibition precipitated no small amount of distress to the evolution of the concept of nursing diagnosis as an integral part of nursing practice.

These situations also require nursing to return to the legislature for statutory language changes as practice changes. Every return to the legislature to codify evolving practice requires submission of nursing practice issues to nonnurse groups: to the legislators and to the lobbyists for other groups.

The Florida Nurse Practice Act (1981) is an example of a specifically worded statute that expressly recognizes the role of the nurse practitioner and lists permitted functions for practitioners. The statute, as passed in 1979, defined eight distinct categories of advanced practice: nurse anesthetist, nurse midwife, family nurse practitioner, family planning nurse practitioner, geriatric nurse practitioner, pediatric nurse practitioner, adult primary care nurse practitioner, and clinical specialist in psychiatric mental health nursing, and it provided for other categories as might have been determined by the Board of Nursing. In addition to these categories, the statute delineated selected advanced practice functions such as initiate immunizations, manage selected medical problems, provide family planning services, initiate treatments and medications, and alter dosages within established protocol. However, not all such functions were listed under each category. For

example, adult primary nurse practitioners could "monitor and manage patients with stable chronic disease," whereas this function was not listed under geriatric nurse practitioners. This construction supported an argument that geriatric nurse practitioners apparently could not do so, a result clearly contrary to their actual practice.

The Florida practice act was amended in 1986 (Florida Nurse Practice Act, 1988). The amended statute has collapsed advanced nurse practice categories to three: nurse anesthetist, nurse midwife, and advanced nurse practitioner. It retains more specificity than most nurse practice acts, but it is much less specific than in 1979. The change is both noteworthy and not unpredictable.

A different approach to language in practice acts is to avoid grants of specific permission and to use broader language to guide rather than dictate the practice of nursing. The Missouri Nurse Practice Act (1975) is an example of such an approach. Rather than defining nursing in terms of delineated acts that nurses may perform, the Missouri statute defines professional nursing in broad language and makes no reference to nurse practitioners or identified expanded role functions. Lack of specific reference results in uncertainty. No doubt, Florida family planning nurse practitioners were initially more comfortable that family planning services was a legally recognized component of nursing practice than were Missouri nurses. The Missouri nurse practice act did not even include the words "nurse practitioner," let alone family planning services. However, Missouri nurses have received the more expansive grant of autonomy. This was proved when the Missouri Supreme Court interpreted the Missouri statute to recognize the overlapping functions of nursing and medicine. The interpretation also included the functions of nurse practitioners as within the scope of nursing practice under the statute without restricting the evolution of nonnurse practitioner practice (*Sermchief v. Gonzales*, 1983). This case was brought by the clinic where the nurses practiced to enjoin any charge of the unauthorized practice of medicine against them.

The cost of the more permissive statute was nurses' ability: (1) to tolerate legal ambiguity; (2) to not let lack of specific permission deter the development of their practice in accordance with sound professional principles; and (3) to be prepared to litigate their position if needed. These three abilities must be fostered within the profession to promote the continued evolution of autonomous practice without unnecessary legislative interference.

Payment issues

Nurses have also looked to legislated solutions to payment problems. Nurses have sought statutorily mandated payment for nursing services plans even when no legislative barrier to payment existed. Most states had no prohibition against private third-party payment to nurses; those payors had just chosen not to do so, whether because of inertia, resistance from other providers, or failure to be convinced it was within their best fiscal interests to do so. Thus the political expenditure to mandate payment might be questioned. However, Congress and legislatures directly controls whose services get paid from public funds. In this regard, legislative efforts may be entirely well placed. This is especially true in view of the fact that private payors frequently adopt payment plans initiated in the public sector.

The point here is not to discontinue or diminish legislative activity on payment issues, but to realize it is not the only approach, nor should all efforts be devoted to achieving payment in the legislative arena. Rather, nurses need a more comprehensive strategy that includes the private sector to accept payment to nurses on its own merits, good business. To rely solely on the legislature is to allow the legislature total control of payment issues. Thus any favorable legislated payment decision is subject to reversal in future legislative sessions.

Entry into practice

Entry is an example of seeking legislated resolution of what should ideally be an autonomous, internal issue. Legislators can read these attempts as requests by nurses to do for nurses what nurses are not autonomous (professional) enough to do for themselves. Sometimes legislation must be used to effect a change that cannot be made through use of other social or market forces; more frequently legal changes reflect changes already made. The need to use legislation to effect the change rather than to reflect a change effectuated by the profession in the marketplace will require the expenditure of significantly more political capital. Along with pursuing legislation to modify entry requirements, nurses must continue to develop the marketplace preference for the baccalaureate-prepared nurse.

Recommendation

Use of the legislative process is a tacit admission that the group resorting to use of this external power source lacks the inherent autonomy to otherwise achieve its aims. This is not to say it should not be used. To the contrary: legislation is an avenue available, amenable, and with a history of effective use by nurses to achieve autonomy. The message here is (a) that nurses avoid looking to legislators as permission grantors for what should be nursing decisions; (b) that legislation be part of a larger strategy rather than the only strategy; and (c) that nurses be aware that the use of the legislative process is not without its own costs in reduced autonomy and expended political capital.

Case Law Perspective on Relationship with Other Providers

Case law decisions also reflect legal recognition of nurse autonomy. Cases involving a perspective on the relative autonomy of nurses in nurse-physician and nurse-employer relationships are presented in this section. Although nurses have long regarded their relationships with physicians as a primary threat to their achieving autonomy, case law analysis shows that it is the nurse-employer, not the nurse-physician, relationship that is likely to prevent full legal recognition of nurse autonomy.

Nurse-physician relationship

One approach to analyzing court recognition of nurse autonomy relative to physicians is examining cases involving liability for malpractice. Cases where nurses are found not liable pursuant to following physician's orders evidence nonautonomous, dependent function. Cases where nurses are found liable despite following physician's orders or for failure to act in the absence of physician's orders evidence a legal requirement of independent, autonomous function.

Traditionally "when a nurse acts under the orders of a private physician in matters involving professional skill and decision, she is absolved for liability for her acts" (*Buzan v. Mercy Hospital*, 1967, p. 13). Nurses are protected from liability when they follow the orders of the attending physician unless the nurse knows the physician's orders are "so clearly contradicted by normal practice that ordinary prudence requires inquiry into their correctness" (*Killeen v. Reinhardt*, 1979, p. 177). However, the fact that nurses act in accordance with the orders of the patient's physician does not excuse them from using their independent judgment (Murphy, 1987). As stated by a Florida appellate court:

> We agree that a nurse acting under the direction and orders of a physician in matters involving medical professional judgment is absolved from liability for the acts performed, absent independent negligence upon the part of the nurse, and absent a performance of those acts or duties a nurse is called on to perform at a level of performance below which is expected of a similarly qualified nurse. (*Drew v. Knowles*, 1987, p. 396)

Legal recognition of the requirement that nurses exercise independent judgment is not new. A 1958 California court decided it was insufficient for a nurse to tell the physician on three different occasions that a postpartal patient was bleeding too much. The physician indicated that bleeding was normal. The nurse ceased to monitor blood pressure, pulse, and respirations. However, she continued to monitor the rate of blood loss. She testified that she did not call the physician for the fourth time to express her concern about the patient's bleeding because "he would not have come anyhow" (p. 316). The court refused to accept this decision making as being that of a reasonable and prudent nurse (*Goff v. Doctors General Hospital*, 1958). A 1967 Kentucky court upheld a finding of liability against two nurses for injuries sustained in a fall when the nurses forced a protesting patient to get out of bed and walk

pursuant to the physician's order. The court found that the fact the patient was being ambulated in accordance with her physician's order did not excuse the nurses from their duty to use proper care for her safety (*Arnold v. James Haggin Memorial Hospital*, 1967).

The oft-quoted *Darling v. Charleston Community Hospital* (1966) held that nurses have a duty to inform the attending physician of a patient's untoward condition. If the physician fails to act, nurses must advise hospital authorities so appropriate action can be taken.

Courts are increasingly recognizing nurses' affirmative duty to act to protect the patient from physician negligence—not only a recognition but a requirement—of and for nurse autonomy. In a 1987 New Jersey case, the jury was allowed to find a nursing supervisor negligent for failure to act—when the actions of the staff nurse (who was not found negligent) were insufficient to protect the patient—when a physician performed a femoral cutdown on a 1130 g baby. The staff nurse assessed that the physician had placed the cutdown in an artery, not a vein. She brought this to the attention of the physician. The physician responded that she did not know what she was talking about. Despite the staff nurse's alerting the physician to the baby's blanched extremity, pulsing blood return on the "intravenous" line, and repeated requests to "please come back and look at it," he replied there was no need to do so. The staff nurse notified her supervisor who only told her to talk to that same physician. The supervisor apparently took no further action nor involved any other physician. The leg eventually required amputation at the hip (*Edwards v. Our Lady of Lourdes Hospital*, 1987).

In a Florida case, *Cedars of Lebanon v. Silva* (1985), perioperative nurses were liable for their failure to call a code in a timely manner when a patient arrested in the operating room. Apparently, the anesthesiologist who was present had not accurately placed or adequately maintained the endotracheal tube. Of particular interest in this case is the fact that the surgeon was not found liable, even though she admitted she "panicked" and fled the room to seek help. Similarly in a California case, the perioperative nurse's absence from her patient's operating room during the patient's emergence from anesthesia was not excused by the fact that the surgeon had already left and ordered the nurse to assist him in another room (*Czubinsky v. Doctors Hospital*, 1983).

Indiana nurses were found liable in 1982 for their failure to take action to protect the patient when the physicians failed to change the patient's endotracheal tube for over 5 days. The patient incurred tracheal necrosis (*Poor Sisters of St. Francis v. Catron*, 1982).

Summary

Because all the above cases arose in the procedural posture of negligence cases, and because negligence cases require provable injury as a necessary element, the more autonomous nursing functions such as client teaching and support (less likely to cause physical injury) have not received similar court review. The review of court cases provides only a legal review of only a small segment of nursing practice.

Analysis of these admittedly limited negligence cases reveals court confusion regarding nurse autonomy. While nurses continue to be considered subject to the control of the physician, they are also required to be independent decision makers. Superficially, these positions appear mutually incompatible, but may in fact reflect nursing's social status as a profession with evolving autonomy.

Case Law and the Nurse Employee-Employer Relationship

Despite these gains in recognition of autonomy in the nurse-physician relationship, similar recognition in the nurse-employer relationship is not evident. Under long-standing principles of employer-employee law, the employer has the highly protected right to control the employee. Only very strong public policy considerations override this right for "at-will" employees. At-will employees are those unprotected by an employment contract. Most nurses presently function as employees. Unless governed by an individual employment contract or a collective bargaining agreement, most are at-will employees. The right of the employer to control the nurse is of course

the antithesis of nurse autonomy unless the employer is also a nurse.

The right of the employer to control the employee is so strong that this right apparently even overcomes any independent responsibility of the nurse conferred or arguably required by nurse practice acts. A line of cases beginning in 1978 reveals a pattern most disturbing to notions of nurse autonomy.

In 1978, one of the first reported cases that upheld employer discipline of nurses involved the discharge of a head nurse for failure to cooperate with staffing reductions which, in the opinion of the head nurse, compromised patient safety. The nurse unsuccessfully argued that the Colorado Nurse Practice Act required her to act in the interests of patient safety (*Lampe v. Presbyterian Medical Center*, 1978).

A New Mexico nurse's suit against his employer for wrongful discharge was similarly unsuccessful. The nurse plaintiff in this case had refused to float to a unit where he felt incompetent to perform safe care. He maintained that the principles embodied in the New Mexico Nurse Practice Act mandated his refusal. The court did not agree. In its decision, the New Mexico Supreme Court noted that the nurse had been presented with the opportunity for orientation to the floors where he might "float" in the future to overcome his feeling of incompetence:

> This was done in deference to his ethical scruples, yet [he] refused to find out whether he could ever become comfortable with floating. Because he declined in deference to his scruples, he cannot now complain that he was fired for following them. (*Francis v. Memorial General Hospital*, 1986, p. 855)

A New Jersey nurse sued her employer to challenge her discharge for failure to administer kidney dialysis to a terminally ill double amputee. On previous occasions when the nurse had administered the dialysis, the patient suffered cardiac arrest and severe internal hemorrhaging. The nurse believed that dialysis was only causing the patient additional complications and her refusals to dialyze was justified by her adherence to the *Code for Nurses*. The court disagreed that the *Code* promulgated by the

American Nurses' Association was a statement of sufficient public policy to overcome the employer's right to discipline or discharge an at-will employee (*Warthen v. Toms River Community Memorial Hospital*, 1985).

An even more disturbing situation is described in *Free v. Holy Cross Hospital* (1987). The nurse had been on duty as evening supervisor when one of the patients was arrested for possession of a handgun. The nurse was informed that an order had been given to transfer the patient to another facility. The police officer guarding the patient told the nurse that because bond was being posted for the patient, the patient would not be accepted at the other facility, and the patient would be returned to the transferring hospital. The nurse relayed this information to the hospital's chief of security who told her that the patient was to be removed from the hospital "even if removal required forcibly putting the patient in a wheel chair and leaving her in a public park" (p. 1189). The nurse then discussed the matter by telephone with the hospital vice-president who shouted and used profanity in telling the nurse it was he who had given the order to remove the patient. The nurse then notified her immediate supervisor, who told her to contact the patient's physician. The physician opposed the transfer and ordered that the patient should remain at the hospital if bond was posted. The nurse then visited the patient's room, checked her condition, and attempted to calm her. While so occupied, she received a phone call telling her to report to the vice-president's office, which she did. She was advised her conduct was insubordinate and her employment was immediately terminated.

In her suit against the employer, the nurse alleged that the hospital discharged her for insubordination because, as an act of conscience, she refused to evict a bedridden patient from the hospital. This refusal was based on her ethical duty as a registered nurse to not engage in dishonorable, unethical, or unprofessional conduct of a character likely to harm the public as mandated by the Illinois Nursing Act. The Illinois court decided the nurse did not have a claim under the Illinois Right of Conscience Act since that act only protected refusal to perform services as they relate to religious beliefs, not ethical concerns. The court did allow that she might have a claim for breach of contract in that the employee handbook provided for discharge for "Just Cause," although the handbook reserved management's right to immediate discharge for insubordination (*Free v. Holy Cross Hospital*, 1987, p. 1191).

Presently, a school nurse is appealing her discharge for her refusal to comply with, and her attempts to change, a school district policy that included dispensing medications to pupils from unlabeled containers. Her discharge was upheld at the trial court level and is now on appeal to the tenth circuit (*Johnson v. Independent School District*, 1988).

While nurses' interpretations of their responsibilities under the nurse practice act have not been deemed sufficiently strong public policy reasons to protect a nurse from discharge for failure to follow an employer's directive, the following of the nurse's interpretation of an employer's directive is also insufficient to protect nurses from discipline for failure to meet their responsibilities under the nurse practice act. An emergency care nurse's license was suspended for 1 year for "unprofessional and dishonorable conduct likely to injure the public" (*Lunsford v. Board of Nurse Examiners*, 1983, p. 394). She instructed the friend of a person who presented complaints of chest pains radiating into his arms to drive him to another hospital 24 miles away. The patient died of a myocardial infarction en route. Although she admitted she had suspected cardiac involvement, the nurse claimed that she was following a strongly worded—although handwritten—memorandum that threatened termination of nurses who admitted patients who did not have a family doctor at the facility (*Floyd v. Willacy County Hospital District*, 1986).

Nurses may occasionally be successful in suits against employers for wrongful discharge. A nurse anesthetist successfully established that she was terminated for her refusal to perjure herself as a witness in the malpractice trial of a staff anesthesiologist. The court quoted with approval a California court's statement that perjury is a felony and "to hold that one's continued employment could be made contingent upon his commission of a felonious act at the instance of his employer would be to encourage criminal conduct" (*Sides v. Duke Hospital*, 1985, p. 825).

It is evident that in order to be successful at challenging employer discipline or discharge for a nursing act deemed undesirable by the employer, the nurse will have to show very strong public policy reasons to overcome the employer's right to discharge. Sufficient reasons include (a) the refusal to commit a felony; (b) the exercise of some other heavily protected right, such as the right to vote or serving on jury duty; or (c) a specific statutory right. Citation of nurse practice acts or codes of ethics or ethical concerns have not been found sufficient to defend nurses' practice decisions from employer control.

Summary

These cases indicate that any autonomy rendered under the state nurse practice act's requirements that the nurse deliver safe care, or ethical concerns regarding the efficacy of participation in a treatment, can be overcome by the employer's clear legal right to direct the activities of the employee. The right of the employer to control the employee prevails regardless of the "professional" status of the employee. It is small solace that physicians too are losing their autonomy as they increasingly find themselves as employees with the reorganization of health care financing and Health Maintenance Organization (HMO) models.

If nurses wish to practice with greater autonomy, with less control by nonnurses, it is imperative that nurses develop alternatives to functioning as at-will employees. Examples of alternatives include independent contractual models for individual nurses or for groups of nurses in nurse-managed business associations. In addition, true shared governance or professional practice models, and strengthened nurse manager roles must be implemented in facilities where nurses continue to function as employees.

CONCLUSION

Nurses find themselves at a variety of turning points with regard to legal recognition of their professional autonomy. Unlike Frost's (1967) roads diverging in a yellow wood, the choices are not dichotomous ones. Nurses should look not for one alternate route, but to several possible and emerging patterns of options. Increasing legal recognition can be pursued through the legislative process, but legislation cannot be effectively pursued to the exclusion of the marketplace. Nurses must remain vigilant of complementary practices with physicians that can compromise autonomy, but also realize that case law and the marketplace are combining to reduce physician autonomy. Finally, nurses must develop alternatives to the greatest threat to the continued evolution of nurse autonomy—the employer-employee relationship.

REFERENCES

American Nurses' Association. (1959). *Functions, standards and qualifications for practice*. New York: Author.

Arnold v. James Haggin Memorial Hospital, 415 S.W.2d 844 (Ken. App. 1967).

Buzan v. Mercy Hospital, Inc., 203 So.2d 11 (Fla. App 1967).

Cedars of Lebanon v. Silva, 476 So. 2d 696 (Fla. App. 1985).

Czubinsky v. Doctors Hospital, 188 Cal. Rptr. 685 (Cal. App. 1983).

Darling v. Charleston Community Hospital, 211 N.E.2d (Ill. 1965); Cert. denied 383 U.S. 946 (1966).

Drew v. Knowles et al., 511 So. 2d 393 (Fla. App. 1987).

Edwards v. Our Lady of Lourdes Hospital et. al., 526 A.2d 242 (N.J. Super. A.D. 1987).

Etzioni, A. (1969). *The semi-professions and their organization: Teachers, nurses and social workers*. New York: Free Press.

Florida Nurse Practice Act, Fla. Stats. Ann. 464.012 (1981).

Florida Nurse Practice Act, Fla. Stats. Ann. 464.012 (West Cumm. 1988).

Floyd v. Willacy County Hospital District, 706 S.W.2d 731 (Tex. App. 1986).

Francis v. Memorial General Hospital, 726 P.2d 852 (N.M. 1986).

Free v. Holy Cross Hospital, 505 N.E.2d 1188 (Ill. App. 1987).

Frost, R. (1967). The road not taken. In E. C. Lathen (Ed.), *The poetry of Robert Frost* (p. 105). New York: Holt, Rinehart & Winston.

Goff v. Doctors General Hospital, 166 C.A.2d 314 (1958).

Johnson v. Independent School District No. 3 of Tulsa, Oklahoma et. al., Case No. 86-2755. Cited in *Inside TAANA 1988: 1*, 1–3 (available from The American Association of Nurse Attorneys).

Kelly, L. Y. (1981). *Dimensions of professional nursing.* New York: Macmillan.

Killeen v. Reinhardt, 419 N.Y.S.2d 175 (App. Div. 1979) citing Toth v. Community, 22 N.Y.2d, 255; 239 N.E.2d 368 (1968).

Lampe v. Presbyterian Medical Center, 590 P.2d 513 (Colo. App. 1978).

Lunsford v. Board of Nurse Examiners, 648 S.W.2d 391 (Tex. App. 1983).

Missouri Nurse Practice Act, Mo. Ann. Stat. 335.016 (Vernon Cum. 1988).

Monnig, G. M. (1978). Professionalism of nurses and physicians. In N. L. Chaska (Ed.), *The nursing profession—views through the mist* (pp. 35–49). New York: McGraw-Hill.

Murphy, E. K. (1987). The professional status of nursing: A view from the courts. *Nursing Outlook 35* (1)12–15.

Poor Sisters of St. Francis v. Catron, 435 N.E. 305 (Ct. App. Ind. 1982).

Sermchief v. Gonzales, 660 S.W.2d 683 (Mo. 1983).

Sides v. Duke Hospital, 328 S.E. 818 (N.C. App. 1985) citing Peterman v. International Brotherhood, etc., 344 P.2d 25, 27 (1959).

Warthen v. Toms River Community Memorial Hospital, 488 A.2d 229 (N.J. Super. A.D. 1985) pet. den. 501 A.2d 926 (N.J. 1985).

✴ EDITOR'S QUESTIONS FOR DISCUSSION ✴

Provide examples as to how statutes freeze the status quo rather than accomodate evolving roles. Discuss the strategies that might be utilized to provide for private third-party payment to nurses for their services. How can the profession of nursing affect change in the marketplace for demands of service and the type of graduates needed from academic programs?

Provide examples in nursing practice where nurses in performing dependent functions might be protected from liability and in completing independent functions may not be excused from liability. Indicate and discuss examples where the autonomous and dependent nursing roles may be incompatible in regard to legal liability. To what extent is legal incompatibility between the dependent, interdependent, and independent roles of nursing a reflection of nursing's social status? From this chapter, what implications exist for the content expressed by Lyon in Chapter 34 concerning the autonomous practice of nursing?

What are the implications in this chapter regarding Pettengill's (Chapter 54) discussion of the at-will employee? Discuss the ethical ramifications of the examples cited in this chapter and the principles presented in the chapters by Flynn and Davis (Chapter 39), and Brown and Davis (Chapter 38). To what extent would you agree or disagree that the American Nurses' Association Code for Nurses is a sufficient statement of policy to overcome the employer's rights to discipline an at-will employee? How can one reconcile the statements made by Murphy regarding employer control and the defense of nurse practice decisions as outlined and advocated by Flynn, Brown, and Davis (Chapters 38 and 39)? Discuss the strategies and means by which shared governance and professional practice models can be a means for decreasing control of at-will employees.

6

The Nursing Profession and Federal Health Policy:
A view from within

Mary K. Wakefield, Ph.D., R.N.

Health care delivery systems are consuming more of everything; more dollars, more technological resources, and in some cases more health professionals. Despite the current and projected fiscal constraints in the United States, ranging from a bulging federal deficit to strapped state economies, health care in this country manifests an appetite out of control. This trend has tremendous implications for the nation's economy as the health sector increasingly draws larger percentages of the gross national product. One of the many consequences of this phenomenon is that fewer resources will be available for producing services and goods in other economic sectors as health care delivery absorbs more labor and capital (Pearson, 1987).

The insatiable appetite of the health care system has increasingly attracted the attention of the media, consumers, and government at local, state, and national levels. Along with focusing more attention on growing health care costs, both the public and private sectors have begun to exert effort toward redirecting and containing this tremendous consumption. Concomitantly, questions are raised concerning the quantity and quality of the products purchased at this high cost. Accusations have been made that an oversupply of services are available for select groups, while for millions of people health care is marginal or simply nonexistent. Consequently, the form and substance of health care delivery is under scrutiny, in some cases at a seemingly microevaluation level. A search for solutions to issues of cost, balanced against demands for quality and accessibility, predominate discussions about health care in federal as well as other arenas.

With federal level policymakers expanding their focus on health care problems, it is imperative that nurses acquire adequate knowledge about both the health issues being considered and the process by which these issues are generated, analyzed, and affected. This knowledge is essential because as the outcomes of changing health policy are implemented, they will increasingly affect both consumers and providers of nursing care over the next decade. Consequently nurses cannot afford to be illiterate in health policy. The purpose of this chapter then is threefold. First, selected issues predicted to dominate federal health policy are identified. Second, a brief overview of the structure in which federal health policy decisions are made is provided. Finally, strategies that can be employed by nurses to shape facets of federal level health policy are presented.

PIVOTAL ISSUES THAT WILL DRIVE THE FEDERAL HEALTH AGENDA

On the threshold of the 1990s, health concerns engaging congressional attention are both diverse and complex. A kaleidoscope of issues demanding federal level consideration is highlighted here. They include health care costs, rationing resources, aging and related demands on health care services and research, shifts in child health, effects of increased numbers of poor and uninsured, and changes in health care delivery systems. Highlights of these issues provide insight into the reasons congressional attention and action are increasingly focused on health care.

Health Care Costs and Resource Allocation

The United States spends more money on its health care system than any other country. The amount of money expended, and its distribution, are fundamental considerations. These characteristics reflect both the financial commitment extended to health care as well as the related funding priorities.

The expenditure for all health spending in 1987 in the United States reached $498.9 billion and it is expected to reach a phenomenal $1.5 trillion in 2000 (Sorian, 1988; Pearson, 1987). In 1987, 41% of all health expenditures emanated from public sources such as Medicare and Medicaid, while 59% originated from private sources including private health insurance.

Federal spending for health care now exceeds 10% of the federal budget. Accompanying this federal level increase is a projected decline in the state and local portion of all health funding. Over 90% of federal health care dollars are spent to fund the Medicare and Medicaid programs. Hospital care and physician services receive the majority of funds across all federal health care programs. Hospital care, for example, absorbed 39% of total health spending in 1987. For purposes of comparison, in 1965 hospital care expenditures were $13.9 billion compared with $193.5 billion spent in 1987 (Sorian, 1988). The increasing scrutiny Congress devotes to seemingly unbridled health care costs is easily understood when figures such as these are considered.

Health care costs, coupled with the federal budget deficit, reflect a growth in health spending that is rapidly outstripping the nation's ability to purchase unlimited health care services. This unequal equation has served as a major catalyst for budget-driven decision making as opposed to need-based decisions for federally funded health programs. According to most forecasts, this trend will continue to worsen (Pearson, 1987). In view of increasing fiscal constraints applied to health care, nurses need to anticipate potential outcomes and actively shape them.

One positive result of efforts to restrain health care costs has already begun to develop. That is, closer scrutiny is being applied to health programs receiving federal dollars. For example, increasing attention is devoted to improving the efficiency of health care services. Efforts to decrease cost are evident in the federal government's attempts to eliminate unnecessary or poor-quality services and unjustified high charges for health services. This is reflected in congressional initiatives such as the Prospective Payment System (PPS), which has resulted in moving consumers through inpatient care more quickly in order to keep costs down. Although the system is not flawless, it is generally more efficient than the reimbursement system it replaced. This improvement has led to the recent consideration of applying PPS to home health and other services. Efforts to curb costs are evident in federal efforts to empower and fine-tune peer review organizations, in order to minimize Medicare payments for inappropriate services and eliminate inflated payments for a number of physician-provided procedures. A greater premium will be placed on ideas, personnel, and technology that present as less expensive alternatives without diminishing quality.

In the process of checking health care costs, both deliberate and unintended efforts to ration health resources have materialized (Kosterlitz, 1987). With a finite federal bank account, not all of the purchases one wishes to make can be implemented. Therefore, decisions have to be made regarding which health care services are essential and cost-effective and how these services can be dispensed in an equitable manner. Money spent to support neonatal intensive care for one infant may be money unavailable to support prenatal care for 30 uninsured pregnant women. Funds directed toward pharmaceutical treatment to extend the lives of AIDS patients may be funding unavailable for preventive education or for research aimed at finding a cure. Perhaps the choices for federal level policymakers have never been so difficult. Demographics, technology, and new diseases contribute to the pressure to debate these ethical issues and ultimately arrive at decisions, debates and decisions in which nursing should play a part.

In considering distribution of selected health resources, policymakers and others must wrestle with probing questions regarding how to most effectively allocate resources in order to optimize the health of society (Evans, 1983). What types of services are available or unavailable to which strata of the population? What gaps in essential services exist or are predicted to develop? To what extent do factors such as geographical locale, employment status, and other variables influence access to and quality of care? How should limited resources be allocated between rural and urban dwellers, between young and old, and for the poor and the uninsured (Demkovich, 1987)? As the federal government supports research, development, and utilization of new technology aimed at preserving and extending quantity of life, are there concomitant improvements in the quality of life (Health Care Financing Special Report, 1987)? The crux of the health care resource allocation issue was poignantly presented in a television documentary, "Who Lives, Who Dies," when the narrator stated:

> It is a cruel irony that some patients receive useless care they don't want while others cannot get care they . . . need. It's time to . . . face the way we ration . . . care, [and] sort out . . . priorities that determine who lives, who dies. (Reinhardt, 1987)

Unless our country is willing to forego massive spending in areas such as defense or citizens are willing to shoulder significantly higher taxes, new choices will be inevitable. The notion that the United States should be a font of unlimited health care is, for all practical purposes, a nonissue. Nurses and other health professionals have an obligation to enter into a partnership with policymakers so that visceral decisions are not made within a "first come—only served" system. Rather, a comprehensive, sensitive approach to meting out resources should be orchestrated. If nursing, with its unique perspective, abdicates responsibility in this arena because of the inherent complexity and difficulty of the issues needing to be addressed, a tremendous disservice is afforded consumers of health care.

Trends in Health Care Needs of Selected Populations

Demographic and socioeconomic trends are brought to the attention of Congress because of the important insight provided regarding future demands on the health care system. The stimulus-response interaction of demography and policy change can be exemplified by considering the aging of the United States population. The increasing number of Americans over age 65 will directly affect federal level programs including big-ticket demands for payments and services from Social Security and Medicare (Robinson, 1982). A related response is also evident in the commitment of more federal funds to gerontological education.

With a rapidly increasing older population, especially in the 85 and older category, chronic illnesses frequently associated with the aging process will serve as a substantial challenge for the health care system over the next decade and beyond. With the exorbitant cost of diseases like Alzheimer's, it will be incumbent on the federal government to support health care professionals as they explore the physical and cognitive functioning of this expanding population segment (Ginzberg, 1985). To avoid paying large sums of money for extensive care, the federal government will probably continue to invest in research geared toward eliminating or minimizing the effects of Alzheimer's disease and other debilitating, older-onset diseases. One saving may be replaced by another cost. While some chronic illnesses are on the verge of cure, such as diabetes, other disabilities will become manifest because of therapies available today that were virtually nonexistent even 10 years ago. Consequently, rehabilitation services may assume a more central role in the health care system as persons with chronic health problems survive normal and near-normal life spans. These changes have and will continue to prompt a redirection of federal resources.

At the other end of the age continuum, developing trends are also placing demands on the federal government. For example, immunizations of preschool children are declining (Johnson, 1987). Between 1980 and 1985, the proportion of 1- to 4-year-olds who did not receive polio vaccines rose by 40% for all races and 80% for nonwhite children. In addition, an increase in infants inadequately immunized against diphtheria, pertussis, and tetanus occurred along with a rise in the number of reported cases of measles, mumps, and pertussis (Johnson, 1987). Related to the changing health status of some children, recent census data indicate that whereas the poverty rate for children in 1969 was 14%, it has increased to 20% in 1986. In contrast, the poverty rate for the aged was 25% in 1969 and has decreased to 12% in 1986 (Burke, 1988). These and other negative trends will likely evoke additional federal level response as various advocacy organizations, including those of nursing, bring the needs of the nation's children to the steps of the Capitol.

Even with the wealth of population and related health status data available today, mismanagement of resources still occurs and related phenomena are difficult to control. For example, a substantial oversupply of hospital beds along with a surplus of physicians exists in numerous areas of the country. Yet many of the poor and 35 to 37 million uninsured, one third of whom are children under the age of 16 (Reinhardt, 1987), are unable to access adequate health care in a timely fashion or are denied it entirely (Reinhardt, 1986). Uninsured, poor patients have frequently been dumped from hospitals unwilling to absorb the cost of their care. The federal government has attempted to diminish this practice through the initiation of related penalties. Yet with Medicaid gaps, the poor and uninsured will place heavy financial burdens on the hospitals that serve

them. In contrast to their insured counterparts who tend to obtain care when they first need it, the uninsured enter the health care system in a considerably more debilitated state. Consequently, the poor and uninsured frequently require more expensive acute restorative care to remediate exacerbated health problems. Reinhardt (1987) proposes that in the current health care system, the best the poor uninsured can hope for is critical care. Health promotion, prevention, and care for common health problems needing intervention are simply not available to this population.

Reinhardt (1987) suggests that the general news media fail to call sufficient attention to the problems that exist in our health care delivery system. As a result, solutions are not actively pursued. Perhaps nurses and other health care professionals could ponder the same question. That is, are providers working with these underserved populations, or cognizant of their health needs, also guilty of failing to call federal attention and propose solutions to the problems associated with accessing adequate health care?

Transitions in the Health Care Delivery System

Similar to changes in the health characteristics of selected populations, the nation's health care delivery system is also in transition. For example, it is predicted that even in the presence of both an aging population and a population of poor and uninsured who are unable to access adequate care, hospital admissions will be 10% to 15% lower in 1995 than they are now (Blendon, 1986). Blendon underscores the significance of this decline by indicating that this decrease could result in between 100,000 and 200,000 empty beds by 1995, which equals approximately 1000 empty average-sized hospitals. Furthermore, certain transitions in health care delivery systems are being encouraged by the federal government. Selected incentives are and will continue to be offered to encourage a more competitive market through structures such as Health Maintenance Organizations (HMOs), Preferred Provider Organizations (PPOs), Medicare Insured Groups (MIGs), and other yet to be developed systems. The implications of this predicted trend are far-reaching, influencing types of professional practice available, consumer access to health care, and even the economy of many communities.

Reflecting on the issues presented, a case can readily be made for increasing health care resources. Additional resources could be allocated to virtually all age-groups for a host of pathologies, as well as to persons with selected socioeconomic backgrounds. The questions about how to allocate limited resources and what policy directions can best address these needs remain to be answered. These complex issues demand knowledge of the process used to influence health policy and they call out for the best thinking available from every health discipline, including nursing.

AN OVERVIEW OF THE FEDERAL LEGISLATIVE PROCESS

Just as health care is a complex phenomenon with its own language, so too the legislative process can appear somewhat complicated. Knowledge of core characteristics of the legislative process is necessary in order to interact with congressional offices. An overview of salient aspects of the process is presented here.

Ideas expressed by constituents and organizations are often the genesis for new legislation. For example, individual nurses may wish to have federal funding for demonstration grants directed toward the exploration of alternative health care delivery systems in rural areas. Such an idea would be shared with one or more members of the nurse's congressional delegation through written correspondence or meetings. In addition, the idea would be conveyed to the congressional member's legislative assistant responsible for health issues. Similarly, professional nursing organizations approach congressional members and their staff to consider drafting bills designed to address particular concerns. Nursing organizations frequently focus on members who have a particular interest in the issue and who serve on the committee that will ultimately have jurisdiction over the bill.

Once a senator or representative drafts a bill, incorporating the ideas expressed, it is introduced in the respective chamber and is subsequently referred to the committee(s) that has (have) jurisdiction over the content of the bill. While nurses may wish to ask their congressional delegation to vote for a bill that has been introduced, support should be requested even earlier. It is useful to ask legislative members to cosponsor a bill that will be or has been introduced but has not yet come to the floor for a vote. Cosponsorship indicates commitment and a large number of cosponsors can enhance the likelihood of a bill's moving through Congress.

There are two general categories of committees in both the House and Senate that are responsible for considering bills. One committee type is responsible for authorizing government programs and the other type of committee is responsible for appropriating money to support these authorized programs. Generally, a program is authorized first and then, in separate legislation, money to support the program is appropriated. Therefore, while a bill to authorize spending money to explore strategies for minimizing the nursing shortage may pass the Congress and be signed into law, it is impotent until additional legislation is passed that appropriates money to carry out the provisions of the authorizing bill.

The authorizing committees for most health legislation are the Senate Labor and Human Resources Committee, the House Energy and Commerce Committee, and the House Ways and Means Committee. Although there are many authorizing committees that have jurisdiction over various programs such as agriculture, defense, or health, there is just one appropriating committee in each chamber. Each appropriations committee, however, has a number of subcommittees with responsibility for different programs. Most of the federally funded discretionary health programs are appropriated money through the Senate and House Appropriations Subcommittees for Labor, Health and Human Services and Education. To illustrate the authorization and appropriation process, while the National Center for Nursing Research was authorized in 1986, nurses now need to focus their efforts each year toward obtaining adequate funding for the Center through the appropriations committees.

Another characteristic of most federal programs is reauthorization that occurs at various intervals, often from 3 to 5 years. For example, the Nursing Education Act, which includes all of the programs carried out through the Division of Nursing, was most recently reauthorized in 1988. Considerable attention is focused on reauthorization because significant programmatic changes can be made more expeditiously while the program is being reviewed for reauthorization.

Recognizing the role that selected committees and subcommittees play in reviewing and shaping bills, the importance of knowing the many committee assignments of one's congressional delegation should be clear. Committee assignments often determine the issues with which House and Senate members will be most involved and can be most influential. Furthermore, as Woodrow Wilson (1885/1967) stated, "it is not far from the truth to say that Congress in session is Congress on public exhibition, while Congress in its committee rooms is Congress at work (p. 69)." Members with health care committee assignments are in a strategic position to influence the content and viability of the bills considered by their respective committees. These congressional members typically have more direct influence over authorization and appropriations for selected federal health programs. Committee members are also important because committees almost always determine which bills will actually come to the floor for a vote. If a bill is not moving out of a committee, nurses who have members of their delegation serving on that committee can request their assistance in obtaining action on the bill.

Prior to a committee sending an authorizing or appropriating bill to the full House or Senate, committee hearings are frequently held to allow input into the provisions of the proposed legislation. Usually arranged by their professional organizations, nurses frequently testify at relevant congressional hearings. This is an important opportunity because testimony becomes a part of public record, and nurses who testify have an opportunity to speak directly to the committee members.

After the hearings, the committee meets to consider and recommend changes in the bill, a process referred to as the "mark up." If there are provisions that nurses believe should be added or deleted prior to a bill going to the full House or Senate for a vote, recommendations should be made known to committee members prior to the mark up. Changes are usually much easier to accomplish in a relatively small committee than through amendments introduced on the Senate or House floor.

Once the bill has been forwarded to the full House or Senate, it is typically up to the Majority Leader to determine when and if it will be considered on the floor. After the chamber votes on the bill as forwarded by the respective committee, it is then sent to the other chamber. The other chamber may ignore the bill and work on similar legislation that it is developing, or it may pass the bill in its original form as sent from the initiating chamber. Or, after having been received, the bill may be sent to the appropriate committee for evaluation and eventually returned to the full chamber for a vote ("How A Bill Becomes Law," 1984).

After similar bills are passed by each chamber, a conference committee is formed consisting of members from both chambers. The conference committee is primarily composed of members from the committees of jurisdiction, and the purpose of their work is to eliminate differences in the bills. Because of the significant role it plays, the conference committee has sometimes been referred to as the third house of Congress. Since the two chambers frequently pass different versions of a bill, members of the conference committee are obliged to negotiate the differences. While members of this committee are not supposed to insert new provisions, such activities are not uncommon. It is important to know whether any member of a nurse's congressional delegation is serving on the conference committee because of the significant changes that can still be made in the final version of the bill. That is, provisions included in one version of the bill may be more acceptable than provisions included in the other bill. Once the majority of committee members have signed the conference report, the report is sent back to both the House and Senate for a final vote. With passage at this point, the bill is then forwarded to the White House.

After the legislation is signed by the President, it is forwarded to the federal agency that has jurisdiction over that legislation. For example, if a bill allows Medicare reimbursement to nurses, regulations to implement that bill would come from the Health Care Financing Administration, which has jurisdiction over Medicare payment methods. The federal agency is obligated to write regulations that accurately reflect the intent of the new law.

As can be seen, there are a number of entry points in the process where nurses can attempt to influence legislative outcomes. In addition to individual efforts, many nursing organizations, on behalf of their members, employ health policy analysts and lobbyists to draft, track, and evaluate legislative proposals. Considering the magnitude of federal health care issues, it is apparent that nurses can influence the health care of individuals, families, and communities on a vastly greater plane by means of health policy than through virtually any other function. It is also clear that involvement in policy formation is not only desirable, it is imperative.

STRATEGIES FOR INFLUENCING POLICY

Nurses can effectively make their views known to Congress through two different vehicles. First, individual nurses can establish ongoing working relationships with congressional offices, and second, through membership in professional associations, nurses are able to influence health care policy. The significance of these channels and strategies to optimize their effectiveness are presented here.

In making contact with congressional members, working relationships should also be established with the legislative assistants who handle the congressional members' health issues. Grupenhoff (1986) has stated that this group of aides exercises considerable influence in shaping the attitudes and opinions of congressional members on health issues.

When communicating with members and staff, either through writing or personal meetings, it is important for nurses to indicate their own educational background and expertise relevant to the issues they are presenting. Also, holding an office in a statewide or national nursing organization is pertinent if the views expressed are representative of organization members. Financial implications of the proposal should be delineated, and the extent to which constituents would be affected should be identified. Additionally, accurate facts should be offered and the actions requested of the member identified.

While appointments can be arranged to take place in Washington, D.C., meetings with legislators and their staff can effectively occur in the state, often over weekends, or during congressional recess periods. In addition to considering in state meetings with the congressional member and Washington-based legislative assistants, staff in the member's state offices can also be contacted. Local staff are often an underutilized vehicle for communicating information to congressional members.

To assist the legislator or staff person to focus on issues of concern to nurses, it can be helpful to arrange visits to schools or health care settings so that the legislative member or assistant can observe a situation firsthand and also meet with other interested individuals. Lobbying from a coalition stance is effective and indicating that the views presented are shared by others is important. In general, personal interactions with the legislator and staff often make stronger impressions than reading concerns expressed in a letter.

The format of a meeting should include presenting the issue and then allocating time to answer questions. A typical appointment lasts from 10 to 20 minutes, and brevity also characterizes correspondence. Because of the tremendous volume of mail and the related time constraints of the members and their staff, letters to congressional offices should be very concise. In addition to expressing concerns over an issue or recommending a position on a particular bill, correspondence is also effective in conveying appreciation for votes on particular issues. Knowing that a particular vote or stand on an issue was well received by constituents is beneficial to legislative members.

Regardless of the method used to communicate with congressional offices, many contacts should be made in relation to the legislative timetable. If, for example, support is being solicited for funding of a program, interaction early in the appropriations process that is maintained by mail or telephone is important. Single-shot efforts to influence action are not nearly as effective in producing a desired response as ongoing communication.

In addition to individual nurses' interacting with the congressional delegation, significant strides in influencing policy are frequently made when representatives of national nursing organizations develop ongoing relationships with congressional offices. The American Nurses' Association, the American Association of Colleges of Nursing, and other specialty organizations have developed strong and effective working relationships with many offices on Capitol Hill. Policy analysts from nursing organizations spend considerable time educating legislative assistants, congressional members, and others on nursing and health issues. Nursing organization representatives draft legislation, provide statistics and other information requested by congressional offices, identify and assist nurses to testify at hearings, and evaluate proposed legislation, in all of these activities sharing their perceptions with staff and congressional members.

Nursing organizations that have committed time and resources to shape health policy provide an immeasurable service to their members, other nurses, and health care consumers. Without the investment made by professional nursing associations to commit expertise to influence policy, both nursing and consumer health care would be adversely affected. The extent to which this investment can be made is contingent on the continued and expanding support of nursing organization membership; thus, it is an activity dependent on the support of all nurses. Views shared by groups of people are typically more motivating to congressional members than single voices. When a nursing organization representative states that the position presented is supported by hundreds, thousands, or even a million nurses, it is often difficult for congressional members to ignore the position.

In conclusion, the health issues that Congress is and will continue to grapple with are complex and far-reaching. It is absolutely imperative that the nursing profession and individual nurses use their expertise to assist Congress in developing health-related policy. To accomplish that objective, nurses must make their views known on health issues individually and also capitalize on and support the structures that are available to nurses collectively through their professional associations.

REFERENCES

Blendon, R. (1986). Health policy choices for the 1990's. *Issues in Science and Technology, 2*(4), 65–73.

Burke, V. (1988). *Welfare* (Congressional Research Service Issue Brief No. IB87007). Washington, DC: Government Printing Office.

Demkovich, L. (Ed.). (1987). *Death and Dignity Life Sustaining Treatments* (George Washington University Issue Brief No. 484). Washington DC: George Washington University.

Evans, R. (1983). Health care technology and the inevitability of resource allocation and rationing decisions. *Journal of the American Medical Association, 249*(16), 2208–2219.

Ginzberg, E. (1985). *Directions for policy*. Totowa, NJ: Rowman and Allenheld Publishers.

Grupenhoff J. (1986, May). Profiles of congressional health legislature aids. *Newsletter*. Bethesda, MD: Grupenhoff, Maldonado, & Fenninger, Inc.

Health Care Financing Special Report. (1987). *Findings from the National Kidney Dialysis and Kidney Transplantation Study*. Washington DC: U.S. Department of Health and Human Services.

How a Bill Becomes Law. (1984). *Guide to current American Government*. Washington, DC: The Congressional Quarterly.

Johnson, K. (1987). *Who is watching our children's health? The immunization status of American children*. Washington, DC: Children's Defense Fund.

Kosterlitz, J. (1987). Are we curbing costs? *National Journal, 19*(2), 69–72.

Pearson, C. (1987). National health expenditures, 1986–2000. *Health Care Financing Review, 8*(4), 1–36.

Reinhardt, U. (1986). An American paradox. *Health Progress, 67*(9), 42–46.

Reinhardt, U. (1987). [Film] *Who lives, who dies*. New York: Public Policy Productions.

Robinson, W. (1982). Analyzing the impact of demography on social programs. In *The impact of demographic changes on social programs* (Committee Report for the

Joint Economic Committee, Congress of the United States). Washington, DC: Government Printing Office.

Sorian, R. (Ed.). (1988). *Medicine and health*. Washington DC: McGraw-Hill.

Wilson, W. (1967). *Congressional government*. Reprinted by Meridian Press: Oklahoma City, OK. (Original work published 1885).

✳ EDITOR'S QUESTIONS FOR DISCUSSION ✳

How can nurses anticipate potential outcomes of fiscal constraints in health care and help shape desirable outcomes? Provide strategies by which health care services may be provided more efficiently. Suggest models for nursing care delivery of services in which resources could be used more efficiently. Discuss the basis by which choices might be made concerning federal money that might be allocated for treatment, education, and research by policymakers. How can nursing play a definite role in the decision-making process regarding the allocation of funds for health care?

Discuss the legislative process for funding areas of concern to nursing, such as demonstration projects for providing health care services by nurses; funding for nursing centers for practice, education, and research; and funding for education programs, such as through the Nursing Education Act, and undergraduate, graduate, and postgraduate programs. How can the planning of new programs be a stimulus for inclusion of programs or additional funding in the reauthorization of the Nursing Education Act? Discuss who in your state and nursing organization is most knowledgeable regarding the analysis of legislative proposals, health policy, and outcomes of law pertaining to health care. Discuss the advantages and disadvantages of various methods for developing and maintaining legislative contacts to influence action in health care. Indicate some specific strategies by which nurses can increase their involvement in health policy formation in your district and state.

Define from your perspective what is health policy. Provide some specific strategies as to how nurses can make their views known on health issues and influence health policy through their professional associations. Track a proposal for funding of a nursing program through the legislative process from the inception of the idea, through the various committees and subcommittees, and the congregational delegation that might be pertinent to approach and become involved with. Provide examples whereby your nursing organization might be more effective in influencing the development of health policy. What particular services has the American Nurses' Association provided to nurses in general in relation to their involvement with the development of health policy?

7

Professionalism:
Myth or reality

Margaret A. Newman, Ph.D., R.N., F.A.A.N.

Have we as nurses deluded ourselves regarding our professionalism? We call ourselves professionals and interminably defend the development of our profession. Yet at the present time, we are still largely unsuccessful in actualizing a distinction between professional nursing and its technical counterpart. We have the mission, knowledge, and commitment for a vital professional service to society. Why then is it not a reality?

A professional relationship involves a direct connection in the form of an informal contract between the professional and the client for an identifiable service in a particular area of expertise. It is not bound by place or time. It requires knowledgeable judgment in a specific area. The client makes the ultimate decision whether or not the relationship occurs and is maintained.

A technical role involves the performance of repetitive tasks prescribed by and under the surveillance of a professional authority. The performance of these tasks requires specific knowledge and judgment. The place and time of the performance of these tasks is determined by the professional or institutional authority. Persons performing these tasks are readily exchangeable.

The law defining professional nursing incorporates a dependent function, the ultimate authority for which rests with the medical profession. Medical technology comprises the major portion of the practice of nursing in hospitals. Observation of the work of hospital nurses reveals primarily the performance of delegated medical treatments and observations with little or no *specific nursing* connection to the patients.

This was not always so. In the early history of nursing, nurses functioned relatively independently in direct relationships to individuals regardless of whether or not the individual had a diagnosed disease. Increasingly, however, nursing became more dependent on medical authority and hospitals for its practice. The momentum of our recent history has been to widen the dependent path by expanding the performance of tasks aimed at the diagnosis and treatment of disease (Orlando, 1987).

As I talk to nurses about their current practice (Newman & Autio, 1986), I am forced to conclude that the fulfillment of a professional role in nursing is largely a myth. Schlotfeldt (1987) too concludes that "nursing remains essentially an other-directed and controlled occupation, rather than a self-directed profession."

A MATTER OF PARADIGM

Bruner (1986) suggests that myth serves as a substitute or filter for experience. Nurses who are committed to taking good care of patients and who work

49

hard and are skilled in what they do are convinced that they are functioning as professionals, in spite of the fact that their work more clearly fits the definition of technical practice. These attributes—human compassion, dedication, and technical expertise—are *essential but not sufficient* to characterize the whole of nursing professional practice. We have debated the issue of professional vis-á-vis technical for at least a quarter of a century, with little resolution. Recently I realized with astonishing clarity that the issue is not primarily one of professional versus technical! The issue is one of *different paradigms of practice:* person-oriented care in contradistinction to disease-oriented care.

An editorial by Mary Mallison (1987) called for a recognition of the need for different types of practitioners with different types of education and for both types of practitioners to respect the abilities of the other. A reasonable exhortation. Why haven't we been able to accomplish it? In order to do so we need to recognize that the barrier to valuing the role and education of each other is the fact that the different roles and educational programs emphasize different paradigms, *different world views*. The predominant practice perspective derives from the paradigm of health as the absence of disease, a paradigm in which the "battle" against disease is uppermost and the practice mode is one of dominance and control. The person-oriented health paradigm, espoused by the nursing profession, places personal meaning and quality of life at the forefront and requires a practice mode of collaboration and mutuality. When one is viewing the world from one side, it is difficult to imagine, much less value, the view from the other side.

Schlotfeldt (1987) sees "the perspective within which nurses view their world of work and inquiry" as crucial to the future of nursing. She points out that we are agreed that nursing's mission is the optimizing of persons' health. But there is where the agreement ends: Is this mission for all persons or just for those being treated for medical problems?

Divergent views on this issue indicate different paradigms of health.[1] And different paradigms of health require different types of technology. If the institution is ruled by the medical paradigm, activities within that paradigm are the ones that will be honored and rewarded. Nurses functioning primarily in the medical model are operating in the currently more powerful paradigm; those functioning primarily in the nursing model are addressing concerns that are viewed as nonessential extras by the prevailing paradigm. The "anti-education" bias that Mallison (1987) refers to among practicing nurses is more a function of conflicting paradigms than of educational status. If it is important that nursing concern itself with both paradigms, then at least we should know what paradigm directs the practice.

Nursing roles within the hierarchy of medically oriented institutions are under the authority of medicine and the institutional administration. In the past, some of the professional priorities of nursing were integrated in this role. The current emphasis on cost-effectiveness within institutions dominated by the medical paradigm accentuates the priority of the medical regimen in the delivery of care, and nursing practice within this system is diminished as nursing priorities fall by the wayside.

AN OPPORTUNITY TO ACTUALIZE PROFESSIONAL NURSING

The authority of a profession lies in its knowledge. The professional role requires *a direct relationship with the client on an ongoing basis*. It permits relative autonomy in decision making based on the knowledge of the professional discipline.

The nursing void created by dominance of the medical model is making room for a new nursing practitioner[2] who is responsible directly to patients for coordinating their continuing care wherever they might be—in the hospital, at home, or in other health care sites. The functions of this nurse are not new, but the designated position makes it possible to actualize the essence of nursing in a direct connec-

---

[1]For further discussion of the two major prevailing paradigms of health, see Chapter 30.

[2]This position has been referred to alternately as a patient care coordinator, continuing care coordinator, and case manager. Although the case manager title has gained more recognition, the term *case* connotes an impersonal approach and the term *manager* connotes one-sided dominance, both of which meanings are antithetical to the person-centered collaborative approach of the nursing paradigm.

tion to clients on an ongoing basis, regardless of setting, for as long as the client has a need for nursing care—a truly professional role that stems from the nursing paradigm.

The impetus for this continuing care role is the realization, both public and professional, of today's general lack of personalized care and the tremendous gap in patients' ability to care for themselves after hospitalization. Expanding hospital corporate structures now include the full spectrum of health care services, with increasing emphasis on home and ambulatory care; this expanded structure makes it possible to employ nurses in positions that span the various care settings. Private insurance companies have moved ahead to provide reimbursement of long-term care, and governmental support will probably not be far behind. Professionally educated nurses are well prepared to relate to clients in ways consistent with the emerging paradigm of health and to collaborate with clients and other health professionals in the coordination of their care.

There is a common stereotype of technology as inhuman and concerned primarily with machines and techniques. This is the stereotype that nurses tend to reject. A more illuminating view of technology is stated by Eisler (1987) as "the use of both tools or techniques *and our bodies and mind to achieve human-defined goals*" (p. 55). The emphasis here is on human. This definition has meaning for nursing technology as we interact with clients on a human-to-human level and use ourselves as well as the knowledge and techniques at our disposal to assist clients in their health-related goals. A paradigm shift toward a collaborative model of practice based on person-centered patterns of health *is occurring*, and when it establishes itself as the prevailing paradigm, medical technology will assume its place as an alternative within the whole, rather than as the primary focus. A shift in paradigm does not discard the old knowledge; it transforms it by viewing it from another perspective. If we are clear on the perspective of the nursing paradigm, we can transform medical technology within the larger context of nursing.

We are at a turning point in the development of our profession. During the early first phase of our development, the knowledge of our practice was derived through intuition and qualities of human car-

ing. As we moved into the second stage, the medical paradigm dominated the education of nurses. The emphasis was on knowledge about disease, its recognition, and treatment. Emphasis was on finding out what was wrong and taking action to remedy the situation. The responsibility for performance of a large aspect of medical technology was delegated to and accepted by nursing. At the same time, nursing educators recognized the importance of knowledge about health per se and about patients as persons. In the current stage, as the transition to a person-oriented health curriculum takes priority, we are faced with conflict because the practice world is still dominated by the medical paradigm, and we are uncertain how the transformation will take place.

UNITED DIVERSITY

We need to unite as a profession. We have bemoaned the confusion inherent in the statement that "a nurse is a nurse is a nurse." Now is the time to recognize the core of nursing in the various roles that nurses perform. Nurses have a perspective on health that is important and have a responsibility to society to be involved in the planning and coordinating of the continuing care of individuals and their families. Nurses need also to be involved in the direct day-to-day care, which incorporates medical and nursing technology. Nurses need to be involved in the organization and implementation of this care wherever it occurs. But the same nurse cannot do it all. One nurse plans and coordinates on a continuing long-term basis; another nurse organizes and coordinates the care in immediate short-term settings; and another nurse provides the day-to-day direct care in both institutional and home settings. The execution of these three roles requires different types of expertise and different educational preparation. There is some consensus that the coordinator role, which spans institutions and settings, requires master's level preparation; the organizer/supervisor role within a specific setting, a baccalaureate degree; and the direct care provider, an associate degree (Stull, Pinkerton, Primm, Smeltzer, & Walker, 1986).

In the past we have practiced an all-or-nothing approach in handling these responsibilities. Now we need to recognize the essentials of each of the above roles and the aspects that can be performed more effectively by each. This approach involves delegation, not in the traditional sense from top to bottom, but in the sense of shared and differentiated responsibility.

There is great dissatisfaction with the old system of health care and a need to burst into a new organization. Transformation will involve moving from a dominator model to a partnership model. The practice of nursing is not, as Mechanic and Aiken (1986) so ably put it, "the soft underbelly" of medicine but the mind and heart that makes transformation of the health experience possible.

CONCLUSION

Nursing practice is riddled with the problem of mixed paradigms. The predominant paradigm, health as absence of disease, is embraced by the medical model and incorporates characteristics of a paradigm of patriarchy such as dominance, power, efficiency, and control. The nursing model embraces a paradigm of dynamic patterning of relationships. It incorporates the feminine principles of caring, cooperation, collaboration, and mutuality. Nursing has been caught in a catch-22 situation. We have been mesmerized by the myth of professionalism in the status quo and have allowed our energy to be dissipated both in support of and opposition to the medical paradigm. It is time to recognize the values and directives of the nursing paradigm and move into the reality of our professional responsibility.

REFERENCES

Bruner, J. (1986). *Actual minds, possible worlds*. Cambridge: Harvard University Press.

Eisler, R. (1987). The chalice and the blade: Technology at the turning point. *International Synergy*, 2(1), 54–63.

Mallison, M. (1987). Must we be divided by degree? *American Journal of Nursing*, 87, 763.

Newman, M., & Autio, S. (1986). *Nursing in a prospective payment system health care environment*. Minneapolis: University of Minnesota School of Nursing.

Mechanic, D., & Aiken, L. H. (1986). Social science, medicine and health policy. In L. H. Aiken & D. Mechanic (Eds.), *Applications of social science to clinical medicine and health policy*. New Brunswick, NJ: Rutgers University Press.

Orlando, I. J. (1987). Nursing in the 21st century: Alternate paths. *Journal of Advanced Nursing*, 12, 405–412.

Schlotfeldt, R. M. (1987). Resolution of issues: An imperative for creating nursing's future. *Journal of Professional Nursing*, 3, 136–142.

Stull, M. K., Pinkerton, S., Primm, P., Smeltzer, C., & Walker, M. K. (1986). Entry into practice roundtable. *Current Concepts in Nursing*, 1(1), 2–7, 10–12.

✳ **EDITOR'S QUESTIONS FOR DISCUSSION** ✳

How do nurses view their world of work in inquiry? What effect does using different and multiple paradigms in education programs have on professional practice? To what extent is there an emphasis in nursing education on wellness-oriented care versus disease-oriented care? How can it be determined which nursing paradigm is directing professional practice? How can a nursing paradigm of health be used to direct the care of someone who is ill? Is functionability actually a paradigm concept that belongs to the general medical model paradigm of health as the absence of disease? What models might be more meaningful to nursing than a paradigm of dynamic patterning of relationships?

What are the implications for professional practice in differentiating specific roles and outcomes for graduates of different education programs? Should the nursing role be defined first and then the curriculum and education program planned for specific role preparation or vice versa? Or should education programs be planned and determined by the setting where the care may be provided or the type of care needed, such as inpatient and outpatient, or long-term, acute, or hospice care?

8

Comparative Effects of Baccalaureate and Associate Degree Educational Programs on the Professional Socialization of Nursing Students

Rosemary A. Langston, Ph.D., R.N.

In professional nursing the issue of differential socialization is currently a major vexation. Nursing is attempting to delineate the professional and nonprofessional levels of nursing practice and to restructure educational programs accordingly. Aspiring nurses can now enter the nursing profession through diploma, associate degree, or baccalaureate programs. Baccalaureate programs are purported to prepare a professional nurse, while associate degree programs and diploma programs are said to prepare a technical nurse. Yet consumers, lawmakers, academic leaders, and nurses themselves have not been able to distinguish graduates from various education programs (Chamings & Teevan, 1979; Michelmore, 1977; Watson, 1986). The state of confusion emphasizes the problem within the profession and the need for continued studies to identify empirical differences among the various types of nursing programs.

LITERATURE REVIEW

With different educational programs for aspiring nurses, an important question is: Which program results in greater professional socialization for its graduates? "Professional socialization is the process by which a person acquires the knowledge, skills, and sense of occupational identity characteristic of a professional [and] involves the internalization of the values and norms of a professional group" (Jacox, 1973, p. 10).

Autonomy and patient advocacy are two attributes that are considered essential to the professional nursing role (Watts & O'Leary, 1980). Both attributes are in line with national proposals that recommend professional licensure for graduates of baccalaureate programs (Mundinger, 1980). The two concepts, independence for nurses and independence for patients, are tied together according to

Pankratz and Pankratz (1974). It is assumed that nurses can be more valuable to the patient if they can use their autonomous role to serve as the patient's advocate.

Attitudes toward nursing practice reflect the socialization process that has occurred in nursing education (Watson, 1986). Research findings on comparisons of professional attitudes and personal characteristics among students of various programs have been inconclusive. In similar studies, Thomas (1978) found that professional orientation scores did not differ significantly from program to program; however, Lynn (1979) found that associate degree students held a more traditional view of nursing than did baccalaureate students. When leadership was explored in terms of autonomy, senior students in both baccalaureate and associate degree programs showed a similar degree of autonomy (Meleis & Farrell, 1974). Contrasting results were obtained in a study conducted by Murray and Morris (1982). In that investigation, the Pankratz Nursing Questionnaire was used to compare the degree of autonomy among 224 senior nursing students in a diploma, an associate degree, and a baccalaureate program. The researchers found that baccalaureate seniors scored significantly higher on all dimensions of nursing autonomy than associate degree seniors.

Grant (1979) reported that younger, clinically inexperienced nurses had increased attitudes toward autonomy. On the other hand, Meleis and Farrell (1974) attributed the greater feeling of autonomy among associate degree senior students to the fact that these students were older. Pankratz and Pankratz (1974) indicated that years of education was associated with increased attitudes of independence in the nurse role. Jones (1976) and Thomas (1978) found that demographic variables indirectly influenced role conceptions with regard to choice of program.

PURPOSE OF STUDY

The purpose of this study was to determine the effect of socialization processes in two modes of nursing education. Specifically, the purpose was to determine whether female students from baccalaureate and associate degree nursing programs incline significantly in attitudes toward independence versus dependence in the nurse role. A second purpose was to identify differences between students on selected demographic data.

HYPOTHESIS

The hypothesis was that senior nursing students in baccalaureate programs would score significantly higher on scales measuring nursing autonomy, patients' rights, and rejection of traditional role limits than would associate degree senior students, taking into account relevant demographic data.

METHOD
The Instrument

Data were collected by use of a questionnaire, which included a demographic section and attitude scales. Demographic variables included age, years attended college, highest degree held, licensure, type of licensure: registered nurse (RN) or licensed practical nurse (LPN), and years worked in nursing. These demographics were associated with professional socialization in the literature (Grant, 1979; Jones, 1976; Meleis & Farrell, 1974; Pankratz & Pankratz, 1974; Thomas, 1978).

The attitude scales developed by Pankratz and Pankratz (1974) comprised the second section of the questionnaire. The Nursing Autonomy Scale measures the degree of initiative that nurses feel comfortable in taking and the flexibility they feel is appropriate in the nurse role. For example: "Patients in a hospital have a right to select the type of treatments or care they wish." The Patients' Rights Scale assesses a nurse's attitudes on how much patients should be told about their care plan and the extent of patient responsibility. For example: "I believe a patient has a right to have all his questions answered for him." The Rejection of Traditional Role Limits Scale evaluates the level of a nurse's active involvement in a patient's personal matters and the decisions relevant to the patient's treatment plan. For example: "I have fulfilled my responsibility when I report a condition to a physician." Respondents were asked to rate each item on level of agreement using a 5-point Likert-type scale ranging from Strongly Agree (5) to Strongly Disagree (1).

Pankratz and Pankratz (1974) established construct validity and internal consistency (Cronbach alpha) of the scales. The alpha computed on non-standardized scores for each of the scales was .93 for nursing autonomy, .81 for patients' rights, and .81 for rejection of traditional role limits. The alpha also computed by the investigator for each scale with the total student sample was .81 for nursing autonomy, .78 for patients' rights, and .76 for rejection of traditional role limits.

Setting and Sample

A convenience sample was obtained consisting of female nursing students in the last year of the respective registered nurse preparation programs in one Midwestern state. To obtain the most representative sample possible, five baccalaureate and five associate degree programs were selected from three geographical areas that contain at least one baccalaureate and one associate degree nursing program. All baccalaureate programs were 4 years in length (typically 2 years of liberal arts and 2 years of nursing), while the associate degree programs were approximately 2 years in length (typically 1 year of liberal arts and 1 year of nursing).

A total number of 634 female nursing students were available. Eighty-one percent of the students participated in the study—80% of the baccalaureate and 83% of the associate degree students. The resulting sample consisted of 224 baccalaureate and 291 associate degree nursing students.

FINDINGS
Student Characteristics

Age: Associate degree students were significantly older ($M = 26.0$) than baccalaureate students ($M = 24.3$), t (513) $= 2.96$, $p <.000$.

Years attended college: There was a significant difference between programs on the number of years attended college, χ^2 (4, $N = 515$) $= 203.26$, $p <.000$. All of the baccalaureate ($n = 224$) and

72% ($n = 211$) of the associate degree students had 3 or more years of college.

Licensure: There was a significant difference between programs on number of previously licensed students, χ^2 (1, $N = 515$) $= 6.03$, $p <.025$. Of those licensed ($n = 96$), 13.8% ($n = 31$) were in baccalaureate and 22.3% ($n = 65$) were in associate degree programs.

Type of licensure: There was a significant difference between programs on type of licensure held by students, χ^2 (2, $N = 515$) $= 91.64$, $p <.001$. All 65 of the associate degree graduates were licensed as LPNs, while one baccalaureate graduate was licensed as an LPN. Ninety percent ($n = 28$) of the licensed baccalaureates were licensed as RNs; 6.5% ($n = 2$) had been licensed as LPNs before obtaining education to become RNs.

Highest degree held: There was no significant difference between programs on highest degree held, χ^2 (2, $N = 515$) $= 91.64$, $p = .103$. Proportionally, almost twice as many associate degree students as baccalaureates already held one associate degree (13.8%; 7.6%). Almost as many associate degree students (5.9%) as baccalaureates (6.7%) held a bachelor's degree in another field.

Nursing experience: There was no significant difference in nursing experience between program types. The mean number of years for baccalaureate students was 8.3; for associate degree students, the mean number of years was 7.03, t (94) $= 1.96$, $p = .232$.

Nursing Autonomy, Patients' Rights, and Rejection of Traditional Role Limits
Analysis of Scale Scores by Program

Table 8-1 shows baccalaureate students on the average scored higher than associate degree students on all scales. The largest difference between mean scores was for nursing autonomy. The smallest difference was for patients' rights.

Additional testing revealed that baccalaureate students scored significantly higher on nursing autonomy than did associate degree students, t (513) $= 13.31$, $p <000$. The same pattern of significantly higher scores for baccalaureate degree students was

TABLE 8-1

Means and standard deviations of students' scores on all scales by program

PROGRAM		NURSING AUTONOMY	PATIENTS' RIGHTS	REJECTION OF TRADITIONAL ROLE LIMITS
Baccalaureate	Mean	96.2	62.4	55.4
n = 224	SD	8.2	4.4	3.9
Associate	Mean	85.9	59.6	50.9
n = 291	SD	9.0	4.6	4.7
Total sample	Mean	90.4	60.9	52.9
n = 515	SD	10.1	5.0	4.9

SD, Standard deviation.

found for patients' rights, t (513) = 6.81, p <.000, and for rejection of traditional role limits, t (513) = 11.29, p <.000.

Program effect after adjusting for relevant demographics

Although there were significant differences between the programs on each scale, there were also significant differences in certain background data of students in the two different programs. To determine whether observed differences were due to program type, a further analysis was conducted on the data. Analysis of covariance (ANCOVA) was used to control for selected demographics (covariates)—age, years attended college, licensure, type of licensure (RN and LPN), and years of nursing experience. Eta, the generalized correlation coefficient, was generated to describe the amount of variability attributable to various covariates and to the actual program on independence in the nurse role.

For nursing autonomy, the overall effect of covariates was significant and accounted for 14% of variation of nursing autonomy scores (Table 8-2). When the covariates were considered individually, all but age had a significant effect on variation of nursing autonomy scores. However, even after taking into account the effect of covariates, the effect of program was still significant, accounting for 13% of variation. The mean scale scores adjusted for relevant covariates were 95.6 for baccalaureate and 86.4 for associate degree programs (See Table 8-5).

In relation to patients' rights, the overall effect of covariates was also significant (Table 8-3). Covari-

TABLE 8-2

Analysis of covariance of nursing autonomy by program adjusted for relevant covariates

SOURCE OF VARIATION	df	F	P VALUE
Covariates	5	19.519	.001*
Age	1	2.532	.112
Years attended college	1	59.085	.001*
Licensed	1	18.497	.001*
Type of licensure	1	9.897	.002*
Years worked in nursing	1	5.120	.024*
Main effects			
Program	1	93.524	.001*
Explained	6	31.853	.001*
Residual	507		
TOTAL	513		

*Significant at the .05 level.

ates accounted for 4.9% of variation. When the covariates were considered individually, only years attended college had a significant effect on variation in patients' rights scores. Again, even after taking into account the effect of covariates, the program effect was significant, accounting for 5.5% of the variation in patients' rights scores. The mean scale scores adjusted for relevant covariates were 62.4 for baccalaureate and 59.7 for associate degree programs (see Table 8-5).

For rejection of traditional role limits scores, the overall effect of covariates was significant (Table 8-4). All covariates accounted for 11% of variation. When the covariates were considered individually,

TABLE 8-3

Analysis of covariance of patients' rights by program adjusted for relevant covariates

SOURCE OF VARIATION	df	F	p VALUE
Covariates	5	5.490	.001*
Age	1	.157	.692
Years attended college	1	15.209	.001*
Licensed	1	3.711	.055
Type of licensure	1	1.258	.263
Years worked in nursing	1	3.022	.083
Main effects			
Program	1	31.313	.001*
Explained	6	9.794	.001*
Residual	507		
TOTAL	513		

*Significant at the .05 level.

TABLE 8-4

Analysis of covariance of rejection of traditional role limits by program adjusted for relevant covariates

SOURCE OF VARIATION	df	F	p VALUE
Covariates	5	14.336	.001*
Age	1	3.685	.055
Years attended college	1	49.577	.001*
Licensed	1	7.242	.007*
Type of licensure	1	3.110	.078
Years worked in nursing	1	8.158	.004*
Main effects			
Program	1	68.980	.001*
Explained	6	23.444	.001*
Residual	507		
TOTAL	513		

*Significant at the .05 level.

all but age and type of licensure had a significant effect. The effect of program was significant, taking into account the effect of relevant demographics. Program accounted for 11% of variability of rejection of traditional role limits scores. The mean scale scores adjusted for relevant covariates were 55.1 for

TABLE 8-5

Means scale scores adjusted for relevant covariates by program

PROGRAM	NURSING AUTONOMY	PATIENTS' RIGHTS	REJECTION OF TRADITIONAL ROLE LIMITS
Baccalau- reate	95.6 (96.2)*	62.4 (62.4)	55.1 (55.4)
Associate	86.4 (85.9)	59.7 (59.6)	51.1 (50.9)
GRAND MEAN	90.4 (90.4)	60.9 (60.9)	52.9 (52.9)

*Note: Means in parentheses are the unadjusted mean scale scores for comparison.

baccalaureate and 51.1 for associate degree programs (Table 8-5).

DISCUSSION

From the results of this study one can conclude that socialization tends to occur differently according to type of educational program. Students enter a nursing program with individual differences, and these differences are important in terms of attitudes on independence in the nurse role. In addition, students who select themselves into baccalaureate and associate degree nursing programs differ in certain background factors. Even after taking into account all of these initial differences, the program socialization effect is still substantial, with the baccalaureate program providing greater professional socialization for its students. The baccalaureate student is prepared to function in an autonomous, independent role, while the associate degree student is taught a traditional pattern for providing care.

The results of this study support the findings of Murray and Morris (1982) and help to strengthen generalization of findings to other populations. However, the findings in this study that only years attended college had a significant effect on amount of variation on patients' rights scores, together with small variation accounted for by program on this scale, suggest that attitudes on patients' rights are more influenced by individual differences. These findings were also reported by Gliebe (1977), who concluded that professional socialization may have less of an effect on patients' rights attitudes. Another possibility is that the scale in these studies did not adequately tap patients' rights attitudes. Additional formal research needs to be conducted before any conclusions can be drawn about findings related to patients' rights.

REFERENCES

Chamings, P. A., & Teevan, J. (1979). Comparison of expected competencies of baccalaureate and associate degree graduates in nursing. *Image, 11*, 16-2.

Gliebe, W. (1977). Faculty consensus as a socializing agent in professional education. *Nursing Research, 26*, 428–431.

Grant, C. (1979). Attitudes concerning nurse autonomy in relation to the physician in the hospital setting: A comparative study of the attitudes of graduates. *Dissertation Abstracts International, 40*, 3094B. (University Microfilms No. 80-00, 857)

Jacox, A. (1973). Professional socialization of nurses. In N. Chaska (Ed.), *The Nursing Profession* (pp. 10–20). New York: McGraw-Hill.

Jones, S. L. (1976). Socialization versus selection factors as sources of student definition of the nurse role. *International Journal of Nursing Studies, 13*, 135–138.

Lynn, M. R. (1979). The professional socialization of nursing students: A comparison based on types of educational programs. *Dissertation Abstracts International, 40*, 5017A. (University Microfilms No. 80-05, 474)

Meleis, A., & Farrell K. (1974). Operation concern: A study of senior nursing students in three nursing programs. *Nursing Research, 23*, 461–468.

Michelmore, E. (1977). Distinguishing between AD and BS education. *Nursing Outlook, 25*, 506–510.

Mundinger, M. (1980). *Autonomy in Nursing*. Germantown, MD: Aspen.

Murray, L. M., & Morris, D. R. (1982). Professional autonomy among senior nursing students in diploma, associate degree, and baccalaureate nursing programs. *Nursing Research, 31*, 311–313.

Pankratz, L., & Pankratz, D. (1974). Nursing autonomy and patients' rights: Development of a nursing attitude scale. *Journal of Health and Social Behavior, 15*, 211–216.

Thomas, J. (1978). Professional socialization of students in four types of nursing education programs. *Dissertation Abstracts International, 39*, 5966A. (University Microfilms No. 79-07, 801)

Watson, A. B. (1986). Professional socialization of the registered nurse. In W. L. Holzemer (Ed.), *Review of Research in Nursing Education I* (Publications No. 15-2170, pp. 41-71). New York: National League for Nursing.

Watts, V., & O'Leary, J. (1980). Ten components of primary nursing. *Nursing Dimensions, 7*, 90–103.

✳ EDITOR'S QUESTIONS FOR DISCUSSION ✳

Define the main issues of concern to the nursing profession regarding the similarities and differences between associate degree and baccalaureate programs. Discuss why it is that autonomy is a highly valued attribute of a professional and a profession. Provide specific examples of strategies that can be used to increase the development of autonomy in nursing students, whether associate degree or baccalaureate students. Are there different degrees of autonomy that should be developed for professional practice? If so, how can a student be socialized for appropriate autonomous practice? Discuss what may be the most important factors related to developing autonomy within a nursing program.

Discuss the strengths and limitations of this study. What other research designs or methods might be used to address the research question? Under what conditions may the findings have implications for the professionalization of nursing? Suggest what some implications might be.

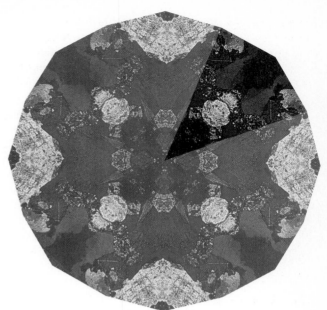

PART II
NURSING EDUCATION

The kaleidoscope works as a unique type of viewing tube. The loose bits of colored glass or such objects as pieces of dried flowers, seashells, sequins, and beads are so placed that by shaking or rotating the cylinder the "bits and pieces" are reflected in an endless variety of patterns. Nursing education can be viewed from multiple perspectives, each showing a different pattern. Indeed some persons may refer to nursing education as a "constantly changing set of colors" or a "series of changing phases or events." It helps to note that the kaleidoscope "memories" fall in and out until the right picture is framed.

The chapters selected for this section reflect many prisms through which to view nursing education. In the first chapter of this section, Chapter 9, Elaine Beletz characterizes the political dynamics of the education for entry into professional nursing conflict as being similar to a civil war. She suggests that the failure to resolve the issue may be an indication that nursing does not wish to achieve full professional status.

Mary Rapson follows in Chapter 10 with a discussion of why educational mobility opportunities must be provided if entry-into-practice issues are to be solved. Five educational models designed for mobility of the registered nurse are discussed. Recommendations are made for future planning and national articulation.

In Chapter 11 Mary Mundt addresses salient issues related to clinical learning experiences for nursing students. The content is relevant for all types of undergraduate programs.

Mary Duffy in Chapter 12 initiates a focus on the factors that are influencing a demand for new educational models to prepare future professional nurses. She poses new models for consideration.

The first Doctor of Nursing (ND) program is described by Joyce Fitzpatrick and Doris Modly in Chapter 13. This program was the major initiative to establish postbaccalaureate education as a model for entry into professional practice.

Jean Watson and Em Bevis in Chapter 14 highlight an alternative approach to nursing education and postbaccalaureate nursing models. The science of human caring for nursing is being advanced.

Mariah Snyder in Chapter 15 grapples with the issues of specialization in nursing, such as the delineation of program levels for certain types of specialization. She further suggests that frameworks for organizing specialization areas in nursing would assist nursing to define its scope of practice and to develop its body of knowledge.

Elizabeth Lenz examines in Chapter 16 doctoral programs in nursing, the curricular diversity that exists, and differences between programs offering professional and academic doctorates. The development of limited numbers of substantive specialties within a program is encouraged.

In Chapter 17 William Holzemer introduces criteria for the evaluation of quality in graduate education. A strategy to synthesize evaluation approaches is offered.

An intercultural perspective as the basis for a common ground in international nursing education is advanced by Donna Jensen and Carol Lindeman in Chapter 18. Communication, collaboration, and sharing are mandated between countries to meet health goals for all.

The increasing emphasis on international nursing and the obligations of the more developed countries to assist those that are less advanced is further evident in Chapter 19 by Estelle Rosenblum. What may appear as the end products, outcomes, or education ending in some countries could be viewed as the beginning and continuing of nursing education in others.

Although nursing education is a commonplace subject, it is an immensely complex one. Something of this complexity can be seen in the variety of chapter selections. There are viewpoints with which the reader will heartily agree. Other comments, or suggestions may be disconcerting, startle, or amaze the reader. Discussion may be required before the points come clearly into focus in all of their brilliance.

Some of the pieces or facets within the kaleidoscope may be "old friends" as nursing education goes through various turns and turning points. And with each turn, the pieces may take on a fresh meaning. With each turn also comes new ideas, questions, emphases, and programs about which educators, practitioners, and researchers should be aware. The total collection in this section shows that nursing education is a fascinating and dynamic field.

The "Red Herrings" of the Entry Issue

Elaine E. Beletz, Ed.D., R.N., F.A.A.N.

Amerian society can be described as upwardly mobile and increasingly educated, professionalizing, and materialistic. Evident since antiquity, education is the key to unlocking the doors of power, prestige, and money; it likewise is the passport for achieving a preeminent place in shaping the direction of the future. Nursing has been a professionalizing occupation for nearly a century. Despite these efforts and the knowledge of the importance of education in society, nursing has failed to elevate and standardize its educational system. The current status of education and progress toward professional nursing is discussed in this chapter. Also covered are related issues that serve as "red herrings"—issues that divert attention from the basic need to establish the baccalaureate degree for entry.

An educated person forms part of society's elite. According to *Webster's Ninth New Collegiate Dictionary (Mish, 1988)*, an elite is a group or part of a group regarded as the finest, most distinguished, and most powerful. Intellect and education are intrinsic to professionalism. Society expects professions and their members to be learned.

STANDARDIZING NURSING'S EDUCATIONAL ENTRY LEVEL
Overview

Nursing has a peculiar mélange of educational entry routes to professional nursing practice. Hospital diploma, 2-year community college, 4-year baccalaureate degree, generic master's and doctoral programs, and external degree programs that do not require physical attendance in a classroom purport to prepare professional nurses. No profession can or would claim so diverse an educational product.

Numerous studies (Brown, 1948; Goldmark, 1923; Lysaught, 1970; Nutting, cited in Kelly, 1981; U.S. Public Health Service, 1963) called for the movement of nursing education out of hospitals and the establishment of the baccalaureate in nursing as the minimum professional credential. The lack of significant progress toward this goal may have resulted from the absence of extensive support and action by both nursing and society.

In the early sixties, the progressive efforts of several nursing leaders resulted in the educational issue being brought to the foreground of nursing's national professional association and its state constituents. In 1965, the American Nurses' Association (ANA) published *Educational Preparation for Nurse Practitioners and Associates to Nurses—A Position Paper*. This document challenged nursing to achieve professional legitimization by calling for the establishment of the baccalaureate in nursing as the educational level for professional nursing and the associate degree for technical nursing practice. It also suggested that practical nurse programs be replaced with programs in junior and community colleges. The intense reaction and controversy generated by this position paper has never quieted.

Some state nurses' associations moved more quickly than the ANA. For example, in 1974, the voting body of the New York State Nurses' Association (NYSNA) approved a motion establishing both organizational position and intent to seek legislative enactment of the baccalaureate. In the spring of 1976, NYSNA was the first state nurses' association to introduce legislation, called the "1985 Proposal," which sought implementation of the elevated educational standards by 1985. This author was the president of NYSNA in 1976. The 1978 ANA House of Delegates adopted the 1985 Proposal. Although no state nurses' association was able to achieve legislative implementation by 1985, the 1985 ANA House of Delegates unanimously reaffirmed the position.

At the 1985 ANA annual meeting, titling was the major issue being discussed. "Registered nurse" was accepted for the professional nurse and the choice of "associate nurse" was made from an array of 17 potential titles for the technical nurse. In 1986, the ANA House of Delegates approved the concept of grandfathering currently licensed nurses into the new titles. Thereby, licensed practical nurses would become associate nurses, and since the title registered nurse was retained for the professional nurse, grandfathering would not be necessary, since currently licensed registered nurses would keep their title.

As of December 1986, all of the 53 ANA members had taken positions supporting elevation of educational standards for the two categories of nursing (ANA, 1986). However, approximately half of the state associations acted on the question of titling. Registered nurse is one of the most widely accepted titles for the professional nurse category. Titling for the technical nurse has yielded such varied responses as licensed practical nurse, associate nurse, registered nurse technologist, and registered nurse

associate. Grandfathering, as a concept, has been supported by 25 state nurses' associations, with 22 specifically supporting grandfathering of practical nurses into the technical nurse category of nursing practice. Approximately 20 state nurses' associations have developed specific plans to prepare legislation or revisions in rules and regulations of nurse practice acts within the next 5 years. Planning and laying the groundwork for implementation of the baccalaureate is occurring in many of the other state associations. Opposition to the proposed changes continues to be strong and widespread.

Approaches taken to implement entry are as varied as the states and in some instances undermine the accepted standards for professions. Three states have had legislation passed that thwarts advancement on the educational issues. North Dakota is the first state to have achieved the upgrading of educational qualifications in 1986 by changing its rules and regulations (North Dakota Board of Nursing, 1987). Although North Dakota establishes a precedent, it is a small state and it is dubious whether its success will be of sufficient impetus for it to cause a chain reaction in the other 49 states.

The state of Maryland's movement in the area of entry emanates from the work of its Governor's commission on nursing issues and proposals of the Maryland State Board of Examiners of Nurses (1984). Essentially, Maryland's proposals would require professional nurses to take an additional examination, beyond the national board, to practice professional nursing. Further, the proposed definition for professional practice is based on functional job categories such as teaching, administration, nursing in community health settings, and so on. In October 1984, the Florida Nurses' Association passed a resolution patterned after Maryland's, which also supported a variety of routes to initial licensure as well as requiring two examinations for the professional nursing license ("Titling," 1984).

An ANA news release in April 1986, acknowledges Maine as "the first state to adopt legislation to standardize educational requirements for two levels of practice" (ANA, 1986). However, the legislation only calls for the establishment of a study group on nurse supply and educational accessibility. The group is to report to the legislature by January 1990, at which time it is anticipated that legislation would be introduced requiring the elevated standards for the two categories of nursing practice. The Maine legislation does not guarantee that a future legislative body will mandate the baccalaureate degree for professional nursing. The only substantive viable victory will be one where a legislature clearly passes entry legislation.

THE "RED HERRINGS"

In recent years because of the stated acceptance of two categories of nurse, each with its own educational base in collegiate settings, some nursing leaders have concluded that the entry issue is no longer an issue. Styles (1985) suggests that the entry-into-practice issue is one of titling and licensure, whereas the problem of entry into practice incorporates manpower supply. However, within the framework of classic models of professionalism, the entry-into-practice issue may be more of a failure to recognize the substance of professionalism, as well as a manifestation of competition for students, status, and prestige.

Titling

The heated debate over titling emanates from the symbolic meanings associated with titles. What one is called relates to personal identity, group identification, and characteristics ascribed to the title by society. "Registered nurse" is the societally recognized title for the professional component of nursing, whereas the title "practical nurse" tends to be of lesser status and prestige. Exclusive control over title is a concomitant of the professional's exclusive control of the knowledge base. One of the stated missions of a coalition of resistance groups to entry is to retain the registered nurse license, title, and scope of practice for associate degree and diploma graduates ("Newscaps," 1987). The adoption of the title "associate nurse" by the ANA was a compromise. The nuance of the new title was that the new technical nursing practitioner would be different from the current practical nurse. Ultimately, the argument over titling represents an intransigence in the nursing community of not accepting differences between technical and professional roles.

Scope of Practice

An occupation that has been granted professional status is given control over the entire scope of practice. Even when ancillary workers are recognized, they remain accountable to and dependent on the professional practitioner for direction. In an attempt to ease tensions for entry, the ANA developed a new scope of practice for the occupation of nursing (ANA, 1987). As a single scope of practice, it may be perceived as having blurred demarcations between technical and professional practice. Clear accountability to the professional is absent. Rather, technical nurses' accountability is to practicing within guidelines of policies, procedures, and protocols established by professional nurses. This appears to provide for discretionary judgment on the part of the technical nurse and promotes the potential for down-substitution (replacement of professional practitioners by nonprofessional personnel) once guidelines are developed. A scope of practice for any professional is one characterized by independence and discretionary judgment. Educators of future technical graduates wish to retain the independence of the registered nurse. Scope of practice is a major point of negotiation for resolution of the entry issue (Heller, 1986).

Licensure

Compromises in several states tend to support multiple routes to initial licensure and the requirement of additional examinations for the professional practitioner. This approach suggests that technical practice is the foundation of professional practice; the consequence is creation of another avenue of diminishing the exclusive control over the knowledge base by the professional. Many nursing leaders believe that the examinations that the two categories of nurses take should continue to be separate and distinct, with the technical examination testing competence on activities that professional nursing decides may be safely delegated. Proposals for changing nurse practice acts, which attempt to define professional practice in terms of employment roles, denigrates the dignity of client practice, which is the diagnosis and treatment of all patients with actual or potential health problems.

Competencies

An emphasis on identifying distinguishing competencies between the technical and professional practitioner has resulted from the rivalry regarding who is the better practitioner. Wilensky (1964) points out "that we can know how to discriminate a complex pattern of things without being able to specify by what features we discriminate it" (p. 149). Particularizing the professional role invites criticism, debate, vulnerability, and in all likelihood, quick displacement. A true profession has the right to determine its minimal educational level without having to carve itself up.

Educational Articulation

One of the approaches suggested for resolving the entry problem is through educational articulation, whereby associate degree education becomes the first 2 years of a baccalaureate nursing program. Some educators believe that core knowledges are the same for both programs. Although some of the required knowledge taught in professional schools may not be used in daily practice, the public will rank professions on the basis of how much learning is demanded (Goode, 1969). The entry point for recognized professions is generally beyond the baccalaureate. To allow 2-year graduates to qualify for admission to licensure for professional nursing would establish entry at less than the nationally recognized standards for professional education. To assume a common core knowledge is to suggest an apprenticeship model of education. In addition, the focus, orientation, and expectations differ in professional and technical education. The real issue embedded in educational articulation may be continued viability of the 2-year program.

Membership in the Professional Association

Among the negotiated issues and compromises offered to attain support for entry is the allowance of membership in the professional association for current practical nurses and future "associate nurses." Action supporting this proposal was taken at the 1987 ANA House of Delegates. There are many nurses who believe that this compromise will change the nature of ANA and its constituents to an occupational rather than a professional association. This issue suggests that, despite espousals of acceptance of technical practice for the associate degree nurse, the technical practitioner is to be accorded professional rights and privileges. The lack of acceptance of role differences can only serve to deprofessionalize the professional. Society tends to judge an occupation by its least common denominator.

Career Mobility and Economics

Important to entering a profession is the gaining of access to the variety of career paths available. In education, as well as administrative positions in major urban hospitals, the minimum of a baccalaureate becomes a qualifying credential. Entry level positions are available to all registered nurses regardless of educational preparation, although a number of prestigious hospitals and public health settings have indicated preference for baccalaureate graduates as staff nurses. Link (1987), however, has identified that nurses with baccalaureate and associate degrees, with similar years of experience, are equally likely to be head nurses, nurse specialists, or administrators.

In regard to return on investment, the associate degree nurse earned less per hour than the diploma nurse, and baccalaureate nurses earned 78¢ more per hour than the associate degree nurse or $1400 more per year (Link, 1987). Greater significant returns are achieved with the master's degree. At the entry practice level, there appears to be little economic incentive for an additional 2 years of education beyond the associate degree. It seems evident that neither the health care industry, nursing administrations, nor bargaining representatives of nurses have sought or have been successful in concretely valuing the baccalaureate graduate. In American society, value frequently translates into dollars. Arguments advanced by the opposition, about the restrictiveness of the baccalaureate degree for career opportunities are not borne out by the findings on career mobility and the negligible economic difference between the graduates. It is obvious that institutional needs of maintaining low labor costs and nursing's penchant for equalitarianism undermine incentives for the baccalaureate. In addition, wages will continue to remain low until there is a uniform product.

Nursing Shortages

Once again the health care industry is facing shortages in nurse supply to meet demand. This shortage differs from previous ones in that the decline in nursing school enrollment portends a marked inability to increase graduate nurse supply. Competition from formerly male-dominated fields, poor return on investment, and low prestige, status, and economic incentive are forcing nursing out of the competition for students.

Nursing was listed as one of the worst careers for women in 1986 (Konrad, 1986). Years ago, because of the limited opportunities available to women, nursing could attract students in the top 10% of their high school graduating classes. Current Scholastic Aptitude Test (SAT) scores of nursing students are lower than the national average and are below those of their peers in other disciplines in the same school, and the gap is widening ("News," 1986). Two-year college students are less able academically than their peers in 4-year colleges (Green, 1987). The impact of lower academic ability in the practice arena has yet to be investigated or discussed. Nursing has never enjoyed an image of providing for intellectual challenge, and the current situation reinforces this perception. The nursing shortage is being used by the opponents of entry to prevent implementation of entry standards. The focus is once again on increasing supply. Yet the model used by the recognized professions is to restrict supply in order to elevate income and prestige.

Driscoll (1980) compares nurses to migrant workers. She suggests that they are accorded the same treatment as migrants in American society—made unattractive and powerless by keeping them dumb, down, and dispersed. In the final analysis the red herrings discussed above serve the same purpose.

STATUS OF ENTRY'S POLITICAL DYNAMICS

Since its inception, the entry dilemma has been a game of politics, an expression of power, and an internal devastation of nursing. It is a civil war. To understand its continuance, the agendas of the proponents and antagonists are presented below.

The Proponents

The source of motivation for those seeking to advance nursing professionalism has been a strong belief in the compelling rightness of the cause. The passion with which this belief is held has outweighed the almost overwhelming odds. Welch (1984) analyzed the national behavioral trends. She concluded that within the nursing community there is a prevalence of boredom with the entry issue that has led to the emergence of crippling patterns of avoidance, acquiescence, and accommodation.

Nurses have always had a history of avoidance of adversarial and confrontation situations. The approach is not to alienate anyone, not to offend anyone, and to keep channels of communication open. While these approaches are appropriate for certain situations, they become benign when strength is needed. The state nurses' associations are in the forefront of the struggle and have borne the consequences in terms of reduced membership and revenue.

Within a narrow framework, the group with the most to gain—deans, directors, and faculty of baccalaureate programs—have been conspicuously absent from the front lines. While certainly some educators have been activists, the organized groups to which educators belong have delivered little but rhetoric. There have not been efforts to organize politically faculty, students, alumni, parents, colleagues in other departments, college presidents, and boards of trustees. Yet a continuous visible outpouring of support from these groups, coupled with their prestige and numerical weight, would only have a positive influence on legislators. At times it appears as if faculty in baccalaureate programs do not perceive the threat, perhaps view such activities as beneath them, or consider their involvement as educationally inappropriate. How much of a threat, however, does one need when enrollment is down, schools are closing, and the goals of nursing are in jeopardy of annihilation?

In general, most licensed registered nurses are in a state of anomie with the issue. Among the activists, fatigue and disillusionment are overwhelming. Among the leaders, the intent of achieving peace at any price threatens to negate any significant progress.

The Opposition

The opposition comprises a loose amalgam of organizations representing associate degree faculty, practical nurse faculty, community college presidents, minority nurse group organizations, traditional unions, and individual supporters attracted to these groups. Earlier, the issue was described as nursing's internal civil war. As reported in *The Chronicle of Higher Education* (Heller, 1986), community colleges perceive the efforts to implement the baccalaureate as a plan to diminish the careers of their graduates and as a means of crippling the health care system. Community college activists were quoted as saying, "They've declared war and we're going to beat them on the battlefield wherever it is," and as having vowed a state-by-state attack (Heller, 1986). Most opposition groups tend to be effective because they are small and fanatical in achieving their purposes. Driscoll (1980) has described the opposition as being cleverly orchestrated, vicious, and hysterical.

The opposition's bottom line is to retain current title, independent scopes of practice, and all professional prequisites for the technical practitioner. Although this approach has been the stated agenda, more subtle goals and feelings may represent the true agenda. The underlying issues are program viability, competition for funds and students, and faculty job security. Krainovich and Mitchell (1976) cite the threatened feelings of associate degree faculty regarding potential closing of programs and job loss. Other aspects reported include perceptions of diminished self-esteem, image, and status in being associated with teaching in practical nurse or technical nursing programs. Moreover, many faculties in community colleges do not have the doctoral credentials required for senior college positions. Therefore, they might not be able to continue teaching or command current salaries if their programs closed.

The involvement of community college presidents probably reflects the need to maintain nursing programs to augment declining student enrollment. Educational funding is often linked to student enrollment or numbers of degrees granted. Union agendas traditionally seek to eliminate "elitist" barriers, such as licenses and educational credentials. Of course, joining with the opposition assists in the union's organizing efforts to boost reduced memberships. The tactics used by the opposition, although in some instances velvet-gloved, are political in orientation and designed to demoralize. Such activities intimidate and subjugate the proponents of nursing professionalism and the baccalaureate degree for entry.

CONCLUSION

For nearly eight decades, nursing has been challenged to professionalize its educational requirements. Although significant advancement has occurred since 1965, it still appears that progress on this issue is under siege. The hostage status of nursing's professional adulthood will remain unrelieved by ransom because the price demanded violates society's accepted standards of professionalism. Society has not indicated a desire or willingness to renegotiate its educational criteria for full professional recognition. Constructive negotiations can only occur when there is not infringement of basic principles.

After so long, it is understandable that supporters of the baccalaureate degree are morally offended and ethically outraged by the pervasive antiintellectualism and antieducationalism endemic to nursing. Moore (1970) states, "We regard it as extremely improbable that technically trained persons with less than the equivalent of the American baccalaureate degree could manage to achieve the higher relative positions in any scale of professionalism" (p. 13). Therefore, one must conclude that the entry issue, in and of itself, is the greatest of red herrings. The conflict serves to cover up that nursing does not want to be a profession. It is absurd to consider self-governance, control of practice, and creation of standards until a uniform product is developed. Nursing has to show society that it is willing to earn professional rights.

The fork in the road has never been more evident than at present. Nursing will either become a working class occupation or develop as a profession as defined in the sociopolitical sense. Although obtaining understanding and support from the entire nursing body politic would minimize obstacles to progress, nursing cannot afford to wait until everyone has been convinced. Professional nursing will have to mobilize from the depths of anomie and passivity. It will have to employ all effective means necessary to achieve the reasonable goal of the baccalaureate as the entry requirement for professional nursing practice. Else, nursing will have to take credit for assisting those forces which seek to keep it at a subprofessional level.

REFERENCES

American Nurses' Association (ANA). (1965). *Educational preparation for nurse practitioners and associates to nurses—a position paper*. Kansas City, MO: Author.

American Nurses' Association (ANA). (1986, April 14). *News release: Maine legislation standardizes nursing education*. Kansas City, MO: Author.

American Nurses' Association (ANA). (1986). *Report to ANA board of directors on analysis of progress toward implementation of ANA's goals on education for nursing practice*. Kansas City, MO: Author.

American Nurses' Association (ANA). (1987). *The scope of nursing practice*. Kansas City, MO: Author.

Brown, E. L. (1948). *Nursing for the future, a report prepared for the National Nursing Council*. New York: Russell Sage Foundation.

Driscoll, V. M. (1980). Remedies for a troubled health care system. *Journal of the New York State Nurses' Association, 11*, 15–22.

Goldmark, J. (1923). *Nursing and nursing education in the United States: Report of the Committee for the Study of Nursing Education*. New York: Macmillan.

Goode, W. J. (1969). The theoretical limits of professionalization. In A. Etzioni (Ed.), *The semi-professions and their organization* (pp. 266–313). New York: Free Press.

Green, K. C. (1987). The education "pipeline" in nursing. *The Journal of Professional Nursing, 4*, 247–257.

Heller, S. (1986, April 23). Two year colleges prepare for battle over nursing programs. *The Chronicle of Higher Education*, p. 3.

Kelly, L. Y. (1981). *Dimensions of professional nursing* (4th ed., pp. 216–217). New York: Macmillan.

Konrad, W. (1986, July). The 25 hottest careers of 1986. *Working Women*, pp. 65–73.

Krainovich, B., & Mitchell, C. A. (1976). The associate degree nursing faculty and the resolution on entry into professional practice. *The Journal of the New York State Nurses' Association, 7*, 8–11.

Link, C. (1987). What does a B.S. degree buy? An economist's view. *The American Journal of Nursing, 87*, 1621–1630.

Lysaught, J. P. (1970). *An abstract for action report of the National Commission for the Study of Nursing and Nursing Education*. New York: McGraw-Hill.

Maryland State Board of Examiners of Nurses. (1984). *Interim report #2—preparation for a separate examination for graduates of baccalaureate nursing education programs*. Annapolis: Author.

Mish, F. C. (Editor-in-Chief). (1988). *Webster's ninth new collegiate dictionary*. Springfield, MA: Merriam-Webster.

Moore, W. E. (1970). *The professions: Roles and rules*. New York: Russell Sage Foundation.

News: Educators worried by decline in SAT scores for students seeking careers in nursing. (1986). *The American Journal of Nursing, 86*, 1179, 1188.

Newscaps: ADNs, LPNs, diploma RNs unite on entry issue. (1987). *The American Journal of Nursing, 87*, 1368.

North Dakota Board of Nursing. (1987, January 9). *News release*. Bismarck: Author.

Styles, M. M. (1985). Keynote address: Taking the tide. *The Journal of the New York State Nurses' Association, 16*, 9–17.

Titling and licensure of registered nurses in Florida (1984, October 3). Resolution adopted by Florida Nurses' Association House of Delegates. Unpublished mimeographed manuscript.

U.S. Public Health Service. (1963). *Toward quality in nursing: Needs and goals, report of the Surgeon General's consultant group in nursing*. Washington, DC: U.S. Government Printing Office.

Welch, C. A. (1984). Keynote address. *Journal of the New York State Nurses' Association, 15*, 8–17.

Wilensky, H. L. (1964). The professionalization of everyone? *The American Journal of Sociology, 70*, 137–158.

✳ EDITOR'S QUESTIONS FOR DISCUSSION ✳

Discuss the issues involved with upgrading educational standards for professional practice in the various states. To what extent would you agree that the entry-into-practice issue is a failure to recognize the substance of professionalism and not one of titling and licensure? Discuss the symbolism related or pertaining to titles in nursing and how it pertains to various nursing roles.

What are the similarities and differences between the perspectives of Beletz and Newman (as shown in Chapter 7)? As suggested by Newman, should the framework for one's practice distinguish whether one is professionally practicing nursing rather than using the so-called distinctions between technical and professional practice? Discuss the issues involved in defining professional practice in terms of employment roles rather than nurse practice acts. Is technical practice a foundation for professional practice, or is there a separate knowledge base required distinct from technical practice for professional practice? Discuss strategies by which rivalry and conflict can be reduced regarding identifying distinctions between technical and professional practice and the inherent competencies expected for each level of practice.

Define what areas of nursing practice are not sufficiently controlled by the profession. How can the scope of practice be a major point of negotiation for resolution of the entry issue? To what extent can educational articulation between programs be a base for resolving the entry problem? What assumptions exist for articulation of programs regarding the socialization process, development of competencies, and knowledge for professional practice?

What types of nursing care services are being requested predominantly by the public? If the public is not aware of a need for nursing services or care, on what basis does nursing have the right to indicate that nursing services and care are needed? Is it a care need if the public does not recognize it as a need?

How can the lack of acceptance of role differences within the profession serve to deprofessionalize the professional? How does society show that it tends to judge nursing functions and nursing roles by its "least common denominator" as suggested by Beletz? Do you agree that the conflict regarding the entry issue serves to cover up that nursing does not want to be a profession? If it is true that nursing is in a state of anomie and passivity, how can nursing be mobilized to achieve any goals? Present and discuss strategies that might be effective means for mobilizing professional nursing into effective action regarding the entry issue and also the professionalization of nursing.

10

Educational Mobility:
The right of passage for the R.N.

Mary Fry Rapson, Ph.D., R.N.

The concept of accessible educational mobility for registered nurses has been fraught with controversy within the profession for years. Nurses from associate degree and diploma programs and their employers have repeatedly expressed their concerns to legislators and educators, describing the tortuous pathways that were required to obtain a baccalaureate degree. To complicate the situation, nursing experts radically disagree about registered nurses' "right" to pursue a professional degree. Some educators believe that all accelerated baccalaureate programs for the RN are suspect and should not exist. Other nurse academicians assert that there is a core of nursing knowledge shared by all levels of nursing. Advocators of this concept think that the preferred pathway for every nurse should first be attainment of a technical degree. Thus those RNs choosing professional education should pursue a baccalaureate degree in nursing only after first achieving an AD degree and taking the NCLEX (National Council Licensure Examination) examination. The controversy is viewed differently by each party involved and their perceptions and solutions depend more on politics of articulation than on facts, universal theories, curricular concepts, or outcome evaluation. What is the basis of these opposing viewpoints? What are the advantages or disadvantages of educational mobility for registered nurses? Why is the nursing community so resistant to a universal educational model for the RN?

POLITICS OF ARTICULATION

The decision to articulate (or not to articulate) upper division (baccalaureate [BS]) programs with lower division (associate degree [AD] or diploma) programs is basically a curricular design issue. The issue is not based on meticulously researched articulation theory. It is clearly a struggle between educational access of individuals versus quality control of nursing programs. Because there are no nationally standardized competencies expected of the two levels of nursing education, articulation models are based on professional judgments, group values, and many unvalidated assumptions. Thus, achieving a satisfactory articulation decision frequently involves negotiation of conflicts concerning territoriality, goals, missions, beliefs, and institutional or program survival. Acceptable solutions usually require change and compromise that is tolerable for both the proponents and the opponents of articulation.

Opponents

The opponents of articulation state that professional nursing education cannot and should not be directly or indirectly articulated with AD or diploma programs (Kramer, 1981; Montag, 1980). Those educators with this philosophy argue that the associate degree programs were originated by Montag with assumptions that this level of education was technical and terminal. Their perception is that AD and diploma competencies, curricular content, emphases, and teaching methods are so different from those of baccalaureate programs that the quality and integrity of the latter are compromised when an attempt is made to articulate the two levels. Another view held by many educators is that upper division nursing (obtained in the junior and senior years) is the only appropriate foundation for graduate studies. It is further argued that RN students must be resocialized and must be taught to reconceptualize, as they learn the required content in the baccalaureate program. This undesirable sequencing of concepts and experiences complicates learning for the RNs, thereby creating unnecessary stress and anxiety. Also, nursing educators are concerned that the proliferation of RN to BSN programs may contribute to underselling, undermining, and underrating basic baccalaureate programs. Their idea of the worst case scenario is that these programs might be responsible for the demise of traditionally sequenced generic nursing education.

Short-Term Plan

Some educators advocate a radical articulation plan that would be short-term only. This plan would be instituted for 5 to 10 years to assist RNs in obtaining advanced degrees. At the end of this period, permanent closure of RN student admissions is supported. Nurses could only obtain their baccalaureate degree by progressing through traditional generic programs with no advanced placement options. Those who support this option want to encourage basic nursing baccalaureate education and discourage a permanent two plus two articulation model. The danger inherent in this approach is that a temporary educational program is often difficult to dismantle as a result of pressure from involved interest groups. Also, implementation of this philosophy would cause a hardship for many registered nurses who could not

obtain their basic nursing education through the traditional baccalaureate pathway. Many students are restricted in their educational options by geography, limited finances, family responsibilities, and other barriers. Philosophically this option violates the National League for Nursing's position statement on educational mobility, which states that "individuals who wish to change career goals should have educational opportunities to advance from one type of nursing practice to another" (NLN, 1982, p. 1).

Proponents

Other experts believe that opportunity for educational mobility for the RN is an essential factor for successful implementation of two levels of practice (Southern Regional Education Board, 1982a). Many national and state commissions, task forces, and professional organizations have advocated the concept of articulation between lower and upper division nursing programs. Also, because registered nurses represent a powerful political constituency, educational mobility has been legislated or mandated in some states, that is, California, Arkansas, and Maryland. In anticipation of change in practice requirements, access to baccalaureate education seems to be universally demanded. The majority of RNs in the United States do not have a baccalaureate degree. Thus, their educational mobility is imperative if the profession is to remain vital in the future. Not educating RNs who wish to return to school could be expensive indeed, given the present large exodus of skilled but frustrated people from nursing.

Forces internal and external to nursing are creating changes in attitude about the RN's entitlement to educational mobility. Sufficient numbers of baccalaureate nurse graduates are not being produced and applications for basic nursing programs are at an all-time low ("BSN Enrollments," 1987). Educators who were once against the concept of integrating RN students with basic nursing students have willingly recruited the registered nurse, nontraditional, mature, or second-degree student to fill their empty enrollment spaces. Under these circumstances, resources normally allotted to the generic student are being reallocated to the registered nurse. However, if generic applications return to normal, philosophical decisions will have to be made concerning where to budget scarce resources, to basic BSN education, RN-to-BSN education, or to both programs.

Many successful models have been implemented nationally which have demonstrated that articulation between the two levels of nursing works well when appropriate validation of previous learning is implemented (Rapson, 1987; Little & Brian; 1982, Searight, 1976). Legitimate strategies have been developed to document achievement of required competencies from lower division nursing programs without undue obstacles to the student and without jeopardizing the integrity and diversity of baccalaureate programs.

VALIDATION OF PREVIOUS LEARNING FOR ADVANCED PLACEMENT

Validating the depth and breadth of each prospective student's previous education is usually a significant hurdle to advanced placement for RNs in the United States. Assessment for credit granting or transfer presents a particularly difficult dilemma when nurses have graduated from diploma schools that have awarded little or no credit for nursing and general education courses. Compounding the problem is that some RNs have taken courses, such as integrated science or psychology for nurses, which are not usually transferable to baccalaureate programs. In addition, many students have been educated using the "medical model" and baccalaureate educators are uncertain where to place the applicant in an "integrated" curriculum. Finally, numerous registered nurses believe they should not have to prove their competencies because they have graduated from approved programs and are successfully working in health care agencies.

The position of the NLN and other national accrediting bodies and standard setting organizations is that previous education must be comparable in quality and substance as that of the basic baccalaureate nursing programs. The Council of Baccalaureate and Higher Degree Programs of NLN has stated that they "heartily endorse and support the granting of credit by the use of examination and/or other validating mechanisms which are designed to assess knowledge and skill gained previously" (NLN, 1975, p. 1). However, this organization was not supportive of the concept of blanket credit for nursing courses. The rationale for this position is: (a) that it is impossible to know accurately where the student is beginning in the curriculum unless previous learning is evaluated, and (b) that the student must prove that her or his nursing knowledge is equivalent to a portion of the upper level nursing courses required for the baccalaureate degree.

Although there has been no standardization regarding credit granting, admission, progression, and graduation criteria for RNs, several methods have been accepted by the profession for validating previous learning. The techniques are advanced placement examinations (either teacher-prepared or standardized), course-by-course transfer, competency testing of clinical performance, and compilation of professional portfolios. The methods have all proved to be effective strategies and are used by different schools to meet the specific needs of their students, curricula, and program. Credit granted to R.N.'s for their previous lower division nursing education courses usually amounts to one-half of their general education requirements (approximately 30 credits) plus one-half of their nursing requirements (approximately 30 credits) for the baccalaureate degree.

Arlton and Miller (1987) surveyed all NLN accredited baccalaureate nursing programs in the winter of 1986 concerning their advanced placement policies. They ascertained that 95% of the respondent programs granted academic credit for prior learning to the RN requirement. The challenge examination (including theory and clinical) was the most frequently used method. Course-by-course transfer from a lower division (usually AD institutions) with a grade of C or better was the second most frequently used method. A few programs reported use of professional portfolios for validation purposes.

Although the methods may be deemed appropriate by nursing educators, many registered nurses have been discouraged from obtaining a baccalaureate degree because of the advanced placement policies. In particular, they perceive the challenge examinations to be a financial and psychological barrier that is insurmountable even with counseling, syllabi, and tutoring. In addition, the documentation required of a professional portfolio is very time-consuming for both the student and the faculty evaluators. For many programs, clinical performance examinations are prohibitive because of time and financial constraints. In addition, opponents of validation procedures argue that there is a limited availability of reliable and valid measurement instruments to assess previous classroom and experiential learning. Finally, the process involved in granting academic credit is frequently expensive in terms of counseling, time, and commitment for both the student and the nursing program.

NURSING EDUCATIONAL MODELS FOR THE RN

To pursue a baccalaureate degree, registered nurses can choose from a variety of educational models ranging from advanced placement in a generic program to receipt of an external BSN degree. In this section, five options are discussed, identifying basic strengths and weaknesses of each from the perspective of both nursing programs and potential students.

Advanced Placement in a Generic Program

The generic program comprises approximately 2 years of arts and science courses and 2 years of upper division nursing courses. The "normal" participant in this model is the 18-year-old traditional student, who has entered the baccalaureate program after high school, and has progressed directly through the sequenced curriculum. RNs usually complete their general education requirements before they apply for entrance to the upper division nursing major within the generic program. They have also received advanced standing through direct transfer or an acceptable validation process. This arrangement customarily requires the nurse to spend only 1 year in residence in the baccalaureate nursing major. Some-

times the student is required to take a bridge course, which facilitates socialization into the professional nursing role, and teaches new concepts that will be used throughout their senior year.

The positive aspects of the RN student's participation in the generic program is that the nurse is socialized with and receives the same education as the basic student. In addition, this approach does not require expansion or large allocations of new resources to teach the RN.

There are several disadvantages to this model. The RN student usually has unique characteristics which differ significantly from that of the generic student. The former tends to be older, mature, more experienced, and in a different life stage than her or his younger counterpart. Also, they often encounter many stressors such as marriage, children, jobs, divorces, and back-to-school syndrome. In addition, they may have a need to attend school part-time, which often is not allowed in generic programs. RN students learn best in an environment that is flexible, includes counseling, and is based on adult learning principles. These educational parameters are not necessarily appropriate for the generic student.

Dynamics between the two types of students may be very complex. The generic student can be intimidated by RNs who possess superior clinical and experiential skills. Conversely, basic students may conceptualize and adapt to an integrated curriculum faster than their nurse peers. As RNs are being socialized into the professional nursing role, their anxiety frequently causes indignation about their learning experiences. This anger of the RN may have a detrimental effect on the vulnerable basic student. In addition, when the nurse is placed in the generic program, it is difficult to prevent duplication of some previous learning experiences or requirements. Nurses can be very resentful about this repetition. Positively, integration of the two groups of students can expand the depth and breadth of knowledge and skills obtained by all involved. Meeting the complicated needs of RN and generic students can be both frustrating and rewarding to faculty who teach them concurrently.

Advanced Standing in Separate RN Tracks

RN only or second-step baccalaureate programs in nursing offer 2 years of study and grant credit for the nursing education obtained in AD or diploma programs. This model can take two forms: (a) the student follows completion of the technical education with fulfillment of liberal arts prerequisites and completion of the upper division nursing courses; and (b) the student combines liberal arts courses with nursing courses in each year of the program. The curriculum objectives must be the same as that of generic programs but teaching methodology, clinical experiences, and other parameters may differ according to the individual needs of RN students. This educational model usually strives to use adult learning theories, to build on unique backgrounds of individuals, and to be flexible, accessible, and available to the RN. These programs have proliferated rapidly over the last several years (Southern Regional Education Board, 1982b).

RN students usually prefer this model because they are being educated with other students with the same needs and characteristics that they possess. Usually unnecessary duplication has been eliminated and enrichment courses are frequently offered for students who have rich backgrounds in clinical specialty areas. However, there is a tendency to expect a higher level of performance from the RN in the separate track than is demanded of them in the generic program. Additionally this design requires a separate allocation of resources that might not be available to many schools of nursing during periods of economic retrenchment and decreased enrollments. Finally, faculty must be selected carefully because teaching RN students requires broad-based clinical and educational expertise.

Outreach Programs

Many RN students have been deterred from obtaining their baccalaureate degree because of geographical barriers. Outreach programs increase access by delivering baccalaureate offerings or complete BSN programs to the RN at sites other than the main campus of a college or university. Courses have been offered at regional satellite sites of universities, community colleges, citizenry centers, libraries, temporary facilities, and high schools. The Illinois (State) Board of Higher Education has a policy requiring that baccalaureate completion programs be located within a 40-mile radius of diploma and AD nursing programs (Forni, 1986). The University of Maryland has provided six outreach sites for RN students. From 1985 to 1988, student enrollments in the latter have increased from 20 to over 200 students. This increase demonstrates the current need and popularity of outreach programs.

These programs are very difficult and expensive to deliver. In many regions, enrollments are small, usually around 20 students. A variable that further complicates planning of these offerings is the fact that only about 10% of those expressing interest will eventually enroll in the program. Another disadvantage is that students are deprived of the opportunity to be enriched by a campus environment with a variety of students and teachers. Faculty involved in this model must be very committed because they frequently travel long distances, coordinate and teach the offerings, counsel the students, and market the program. However, the big advantage to the outreach effort is the gratitude of nurses in underserved communities who get their BSN. A significant increase in the educational level of nursing in these areas is also a notable outcome.

External Degree Programs

The New York Regents External Degree Nursing Program (REX) has combined elements of independent study, competency-based testing, and adult learning theory as a basis for its NLN-accredited BSN degree. This model appeals to RN students who are highly self-motivated, clinically experienced, and geographically bound. The process of learning in the program is totally individualized and the student is responsible for documenting achievement of the required competencies. REX is concerned only with the assessment process and not the instructional process. The content required in this model is equivalent to that of the conventional programs, although methods of meeting objectives are different. Students do not necessarily have to attend conventional classrooms. Seekers of the REX degree must document attainment of required knowledge and clinical competence through transfer credit, or through rigorous theory and performance examinations.

General education credits may be earned entirely through proficiency examinations taken at 200 different American College Testing-Proficiency Examination Program sites. The nursing major is divided into cognitive and performance examinations. The nursing cognitive requirements may be satisfied by passing five nationally standardized written examinations or by using coursework from other BSN programs. The performance examinations must be taken at one of five designated assessment centers developed by the REX program. REX was once considered an extreme departure from conventional educational practice. However, data from evaluation studies and pressures now occurring within the profession and society have made this model a desirable alternative for capable, motivated nurses. At the very least, many of the examinations or methodology used while developing these tests have implications for use in traditional programs for assessing previous learning.

While external degree programs offer a viable alternative to RNs, they are not without problems. Not every student is suited to this type of education because some prefer a structured learning situation that provides them with guidance and supervised practice. Even self-disciplined students may lack the sophistication to assume responsibility and accountability for their own learning. Also, expenses can be significant for the REX candidate because they must defray costs of travel and lodging at the test site and pay substantial fees for examinations. In addition, some traditionalists within nursing have been slow to accept this concept as a legitimate educational alternative.

Statewide Nursing Articulation Models

Several states (Maryland, Minnesota, North Dakota, California, Florida, New Mexico, Texas, Utah, Missouri, and others) have established statewide articulation plans that allow the RN to transfer to BSN programs or to obtain full credit for work completed at lower level schools (Zusy, 1986; Ehrat, 1981). One notable example is Maryland's Statewide Nursing Articulation Model, which involves 5 publicly supported BSN, 14 AD, and 5 diploma nursing programs. This design was developed by a statewide committee (Governor's Task Force) and was mandated by the Governor in 1985. Students must meet the admission requirements for the individual BSN programs but three entry pathways are available for the RN, each involving a different validation procedure, as discussed below.

Option 1: advanced placement examinations. All diploma and AD graduates may take advanced placement examinations for assessment of both nursing (up to 30 credits) and general education courses (up to 30 credits). This option has been a popular one for many years especially for those planning graduate education and those wanting to eliminate hours of classroom time. However, for many students, this pathway presents a formidable barrier because of test anxiety.

Option 2: transition courses. Diploma and AD graduates who completed their programs before September 1979 or graduated from out-of-state schools, may take three transition (or bridge) courses. These courses are designed to assess previous learning and update current knowledge in three areas: (a) scientific concepts; (b) social science and humanities concepts; and (c) nursing concepts. These noncredit courses require 45 hours of classroom time. After completion of all three transition offerings, RNs can receive 60 credits for previous general education and nursing coursework. This second pathway was designed for a temporary period of time and was originally scheduled to be discontinued in September 1989. In 1988, the period for offering these transition courses was extended to 1994. The transition courses have been received enthusiastically by the nursing community, especially by those intimidated by examinations.

Option 3: direct transfer of course credits. Using this option, the RN can transfer 30 nursing credits as well as a maximum of 40 general education courses from lower division schools. It is available for those who have graduated from Maryland nursing programs after September 1979. The lower division schools had to receive approval for direct transfer of credits by meeting criteria established by the Validation Committee. This evaluation ensured that a sending institution had incorporated critical didactic and clinical learning experiences in its curriculum that were equivalent to the junior year nursing courses in BSN programs. This pathway involved validation of programs rather than assessment of prior learning of individuals.

This model has met the unique needs of individual RNs, has radically increased numbers of nurses returning to school, and has protected the quality and integrity of individual schools within Maryland. It has not negatively affected the status of accreditation of the participating schools. In addition, two of the three remaining private BSN programs are considering voluntarily adopting the model. This plan has wide applicability for other regions of the country.

RECOMMENDATIONS FOR EDUCATIONAL MOBILITY FOR THE FUTURE

If entry-into-practice standards are to be legislated, viable routes to achievement of the BSN degree must be established in each state. These statewide or regional plans should be based on a *national* articulation policy, which protects the quality and integrity of both sending and receiving institutions, as well as provides fair, equitable educational access by RNs. Factors to be considered for statewide planning are institutional purposes, variability, and resources; student demand and number of available enrollment spaces; validating procedures to be used; financial implications; effects on faculty and curriculum; need for outreach sites; interagency collaboration necessary; and ramifications of decisions on program accreditation.

Research and evaluative studies should be done to measure the exact outcomes of existing or future models. The question needs to be addressed: Is there a difference in academic performance among nurses who choose different validating pathways to enter BSN programs? Regional or national articula-

tion decisions should be based on research data and not upon professional hunches alone.

A national computerized data base should be established. Information on all participating lower and upper division nursing programs, that is, admission requirements, contents of curriculum, and validating procedures used, should be available from one source to assist students in choosing programs and to make appropriate transfer decisions. Also access to this data base could expedite articulation decisions by receiving institutions. In addition, a computerized national test bank with standardized questions for advanced placement examinations could be maintained. Finally, information on methodology, validity, and reliability of a variety of validation procedures could be housed in this national nursing computer center.

The profession should plan carefully to ensure that generic education is not jeopardized as RN-to-BSN educational opportunities proliferate. Collaboration should be prevalent among all institutions so that students will be assured of entering the educational pathway that is the most "legitimate" option for them, generic or two-plus-two. At no time should the two-plus-two program be marketed as preferable for the freshman student unless barriers such as finances, location, family stressors, and the like are intervening. It is time that nursing's shared interests provide impetus for a unified, cohesive strategy for educational mobility for registered nurses while solidifying generic programs as the preferred route for professional practice in the United States.

REFERENCES

Arlton, D. M., & Miller, M. E. (1987). RN to BSN: Advanced placement policies. *Nurse Educator, 12*(6), 11–14.

BSN enrollments are falling at a faster rate: AACN finds biggest losses in generic students. (1987). *American Journal of Nursing, 87*(2), 529.

Ehrat, K. S. (1981). Educational/career mobility: Antecedent of change. *Nursing and Health Care, 2*(11), 487–490.

Forni, P. R. (1986). Changing needs of society and the response of nursing education. *Journal of Nursing Education, 25*(6), 258–260.

Kramer, M. (1981). Philosophical foundation of baccalaureate nursing education. *Nursing Outlook, 29*(4), 224–228.

Little, M., & Brian, S. (1982). The challengers, interactors and mainstreamers: Second step education and nursing roles. *Nursing Research, 31*(4), 239–244.

Montag, M. L. (1980). Looking back: Associate degree education in perspective. *Nursing Outlook, 28*(4), 248–250.

National League for Nursing (NLN). Council of Baccalaureate and Higher Degree Programs. (1975). *Utilization of blanket credit for nurses enrolling in baccalaureate degree programs*. New York: Author.

National League for Nursing (NLN). (1982). *Position statement on educational mobility* ([Statement approved by the Board of Directors] Publication No. 11-1892). New York: Author.

Rapson, M. F. (1987). *Collaboration for articulation: RN to BSN*. New York: National League for Nursing.

Searight, M. W. (1976). *The second step, baccalaureate education for registered nurses*. Philadelphia: F. A. Davis.

Southern Regional Education Board. (1982a). *Pathways to practice, RN education: The basic issues*. Atlanta: Author.

Southern Regional Education Board. (1982b). *Pathways to practice: Types of RN programs*. Atlanta: Author.

Zusy, M. L. (1986). RN to BSN: Fitting the pieces together. *Nursing Outlook, 7*(4), 394–397.

✳ EDITOR'S QUESTIONS FOR DISCUSSION ✳

What are the unvalidated assumptions alluded to by Rapson concerning articulation models in nursing education? Discuss the extent that the content, skills taught, competencies expected, and teaching methods differ in the diploma, AD, and BSN programs. Essentially, what does an RN student gain and what benefit comes from a "completion" or articulation program? What challenges and new learning experiences exist in completion programs for the RN student? Discuss strategies for increasing as a positive experience the professional development and growth of RN students in articulation programs. How would implementation of a short-term plan for articulation programs as outlined by Rapson cause hardship for RNs? Should RN students have to demonstrate their competencies before being placed in advanced programs, if they have graduated from an NLN-accredited program? How can anger and frustration be effectively resolved for RN students who have negative feelings and beliefs regarding the need to complete an articulation-type program or advanced placement type of program? Discuss the advantages and disadvantages of each articulation model as presented by Rapson. Essentially, what is the difference between the advanced standing and basic articulation two-plus-two programs? Of all the options, which model do you perceive to be the best and why? How do the statewide nursing articulation programs differ from advanced placement in generic programs? What effect does the acceptance of blanket credits have on quality control in education programs? How can a university appeal to lower division schools to have their courses and programs reviewed for validation?

How appropriate are the education parameters as outlined for the RN student also appropriate for the generic student? What are the advantages and disadvantages of the basic generic program? What presocialization into nursing should be planned and occur for the generic student before their enrolling in upper division clinical courses in nursing?

Discuss a possible national articulation policy that might be implemented to protect quality and yet provide access for RNs to earn a degree. Propose and design an evaluation study for the five proposed models and the three options within the statewide articulation model. How, where, and by whom should a national computerized data base on nursing education programs be kept, monitored, and evaluated? Discuss the pros and cons of the data base being affiliated with NLN activities.

11

Organizing Clinical Learning Experiences in the Baccalaureate Nursing Curriculum

Mary H. Mundt, Ph.D., R.N.

The education of professional nurses for generalist practice is a complex challenge for nurse educators. The work of curriculum development demands clarity of vision and sensitivity to social and professional change. This chapter addresses one of the essential aspects of curriculum work—the organization of clinical learning experiences in the baccalaureate nursing curriculum. A major thesis presented is that curriculum work is a value-based activity. It is proposed that the manner in which experiences are organized and presented to students is a value statement about the profession and its relationship to society. In exploring this, three criteria for developing clinical learning experiences are proposed, and four specific issues related to the organization of clinical learning are discussed. Finally, a conceptual framework is suggested to guide curriculum work in this area.

BACKGROUND AND DEFINITIONS

Clinical learning experiences are defined as the totality of directed learning activity in which a student engages in professional practice with clients (Haukenes & Mundt, 1983). This definition implies real-life, face-to-face contact with clients, as op-posed to the clinical laboratory experiences that are simulated and preparatory for working with clients. Clinical learning situations present the student with opportunities to utilize knowledge and skills in professional decision making and problem solving. A major aim of the educational program is to prepare competent practitioners who will engage in responsible practice in the community.

Clinical learning has always been an important part of nursing education, as in the tradition of other professional groups. This form of learning is common to physicians, lawyers, social workers, psychologists, teachers, ministers, and others who engage in professional practice (Boley, 1977; Howey & Gardner, 1983; Warner, 1976). A major purpose of professional education is to expose students to the work of the profession and assist them in adopting professional ideologies and behaviors. This is accomplished by providing students contact with clients of the profession, work settings, and other professionals.

CHANGES IN NURSING EDUCATION

Nursing education has evolved from an apprenticeship system organized around the medical model to an academic system organized around nursing models. The effect of this evolution is seen in educational thought about the nature of clinical learning (Christy, 1980). Traditionally, nursing courses were titled Pediatrics, Obstetrics, Medical-Surgical Nursing, and Psychiatric Nursing, in accordance with the medical specialties. Public Health Nursing was the only nonmedical model course included in the baccalaureate nursing curriculum, and its philosophical and practice roots developed from a community-based public health model.

Because of the strong tradition of hospital-based education, most clinical experiences have occurred in acute care inpatient hospital settings. As a consequence, an ideology has prevailed in nursing that preparation for acute care hospital practice is the most valued outcome of the educational program. In addition, instructional patterns in clinical learning have maintained a model derived from hospital-based instruction, with one faculty supervising a group of students on a single unit for a block of time.

One of the current instructional problems facing faculty is the changing nature of the acute care hospital, with limited admissions, decreased inpatient stays, and increased acuteness of conditions of patients who are hospitalized. These changes make the client mix available for student experiences in hospitals more limited. An increasing portion of clients' health care experience is occurring prior to and after hospitalization. The tremendous growth in ambulatory services, including surgery, and home care creates a need for different patterns of clinical experiences and potentially different patterns of student-instructor supervision.

Despite these changes, a recent survey by the American Association of Colleges of Nursing (1986b) reported that inpatient hospital settings continue to predominate as sites for clinical experiences. In an earlier survey of a national random sample of generic baccalaureate programs, Mundt (1984) found that 76% of clinical courses analyzed used inpatient hospitals for clinical learning experiences. There have been frequent reports in the nursing literature of the use of "nontraditional" settings for clinical learning experiences, for example, pris-

ons, day-care centers, occupational health settings, and summer camps. These alternative experiences, however, do not appear to have significantly changed the organization of clinical learning experiences at the baccalaureate level.

WHAT CONSTITUTES A GOOD CLINICAL LEARNING EXPERIENCE?

A fundamental question needing exploration prior to selecting and organizing clinical learning experiences is what constitutes a good experience? This question can be answered using three very broad criteria: social, curricular, and instructional. These criteria are ordered to indicate the levels of decision making that must guide the selection of appropriate experiences.

First, a good clinical learning experience is one that makes a social statement about the nature of the profession's relationship to those it serves. This includes legal parameters for practice, as well as the social responsiveness of the profession to clients and consumer groups. This primary responsibility of the profession to clients is often clouded for nursing students through the haze of organizational needs of the institutions that employ nurses. For example, the rapid changes occurring in health care are primarily reimbursement driven, and frequently the client is shifted in and out of systems in a fragmented fashion, without total attention to needs for nursing and other services. This is especially true in cases of early discharge from hospitals and fragmented interface with home care services. Often students experience the clinical learning of powerlessness and hopelessness and do not see active leadership of nursing in advocating for clients within the system. I propose that the articulation of the social policy context of client needs and nursing's response to these needs should be an active responsibility of faculty designing and organizing clinical learning experiences. The implications of this proposal are that faculty need to be knowledgeable and skilled in handling change and contributing to policy development.

This attention to social policy in clinical learning experiences does not mean that beginning students are expected to be radical change agents, but rather that they emerge with an understanding of their responsibilities to the protection of clients in a changing health care system—a commitment to never leave a patient without supportive resources. A new sense of faculty and students working together in a clinical setting to influence positively the care received by clients should be the emerging instructional mode. In *Thriving on Chaos*, Peters (1987) encourages managers and others to engage themselves actively in the challenge of dealing proactively with a chaotic system, rather than passively responding in a survival mode to massive change. This spirit is very appropriate learning in clinical nursing—to deal responsibly with change as it occurs, rather than reacting to the effects of change.

Second, a good clinical learning experience is philosophically consistent with the aims of the curriculum. In a study of clinical learning experiences in baccalaureate nursing education, I conducted a content analysis of the philosophy and program objectives document from 62 generic baccalaureate schools of nursing. The philosophy documents supported a conceptualization of generalist preparation in nursing as preparation to care for individuals, families, and communities with primary, secondary, and tertiary health care needs in a variety of settings (Mundt, 1984). This finding is consistent with the recently developed *Essentials of College and University Education for Professional Nursing (1986a)* by the American Association of Colleges of Nursing (AACN). In this document the professional nurse completing educational preparation at the baccalaureate level is described as one who "provides nursing care to individuals, families, groups, and communities along a continuum of health, illness, and disability in multiple settings" (p. 9).

While the philosophical agreement among programs seems high, there is less agreement about how this aim should be translated into a workable educational plan. There is not a clear picture of what this "generalist" practitioner looks like or what should be expected of her or him as a beginning practitioner. The challenge to educate a professional who is competent in practice across a variety of settings and levels of client need often seems impossible in an undergraduate program without a structured internship. In addition, the gap between education and service continues to exist. There is a lack of a working consensus on what to expect from the new graduate in depth of knowledge and skill.

Faculty involved in curriculum work should develop a master clinical plan demonstrating how the philosophical aims of the curriculum will be carried out through clinical learning experiences. This plan should include answers to these questions: Where are students encountering clients with different levels of health need, and what are the settings where clients with these needs are appropriately found?

The third criterion of a good clinical learning experience is that it should be well matched to the learning needs of the student and the instructional aims of a particular course. According to this criterion, a clinical experience should reflect adequate exposure to the client population and to the nursing roles in interacting with a particular population. The clinical instructor should be competent in both clinical practice and clinical teaching and able to direct the student's learning positively.

In each experience, the student should be challenged to analyze the social context of the setting and client health needs, how each experience relates to the overall clinical plan, and how each experience relates to the student's individual progress in the generalist preparation. A positive outcome of a well-planned set of clinical experiences in the professional curriculum is students who can articulate the experience they have had, the level of proficiency they have achieved, and an active plan for continued clinical development.

CHALLENGES IN DESIGNING CLINICAL LEARNING EXPERIENCES

Based on the previous discussion of criteria for clinical learning experiences, it is evident that faculty must carefully consider the curriculum organization of these experiences and meaningfully portray a clinical plan to students. Having a plan that is sensitive to social, curricular, and instructional criteria will guide faculty in systematic selection of experiences across the curriculum. Additionally, such a plan will assist faculty in describing clinical preparation of students to agencies and others in the community. In fact, the way in which the plan is written and presented may also be a social statement about the role of nursing in a changing health care system.

The realities of doing curriculum work are always present. It appears that several questions and issues are recurring themes as faculty meet to plan the clinical portion of the curriculum. Four frequently debated questions are identified and briefly discussed here. The questions are:

1. How should nursing specialties be represented within a generalist model?
2. What are essential clinical experiences that all students should have in the baccalaureate program?
3. How should clinical learning be sequenced?
4. How should rapid changes in a fluctuating health care marketplace be incorporated into the nursing curriculum?

These questions represent rather classic concerns of curriculum: the structure of the discipline and its knowledge, the scope and sequence of learning experiences, and the integration of new knowledge into the educational program.

In responding to the first question, it should be noted that most faculty come from a specialty background and bring personal and professional biases to the curriculum. Faculty prepared in specialty areas have intensely debated the nature of settings, populations, and experiences thought to be essential for preparing the professional nurse. The need for specialty groups to have visibility for specific content and experiences has sometimes caused great conflict in the "integrated" curriculum. At times attempts at integration have resulted in minicourses reflecting specialty content put together with an "integrated" title.

The real charge to faculty who are developing a plan for educating the professional nurse is to clarify the generic aspects of nursing practice, regardless of setting or specialty. The AACN (1986a) document on the essential components of professional nursing education presents such a generic approach.

The second question relates to the scope of the clinical experiences and whether or not all students need to have exactly the same experiences. This is an extremely important question. For example, if the focus of the clinical learning is primary health care needs of clients, does it matter if the clients are older adults, children, or pregnant women? What level of responsibility is there to see that all students have experiences with all age-groups in all levels of health need? One approach is to group clinical experiences that present students with similar learning opportunities even though they are with different populations. In this situation, a student may have an experience within the group of clinical experiences but it may not be exactly like the experiences of another student.

The third question relates to sequencing of clinical experiences and involves the debate over what should come first in the clinical learning plan. One major issue related to this question is the determination of what is simple and what is complex in nursing practice. Specifically, what are the most appropriate clinical learning experiences for the beginning learner and how can clinical experiences best build on one another? I have heard arguments from faculty in all specialty areas that their area of clinical practice was too complex for the beginning student, and there was little agreement on where the first clinical learning experiences should occur.

Sequencing of experiences is also related to the social policy context of clinical learning discussed earlier. It is important for faculty to consider the value statements made to students in the organization of clinical learning experiences. For example, does placement of initial clinical experiences in community-based settings dealing with underserved populations make a different value statement than initial experiences in, perhaps, a nursing home or an acute care hospital. Both the sequencing and the proportional distribution of experiences in the curriculum will have an influence on students. The rationale for the sequencing of clinical learning experiences should be made explicit in the plan for clinical learning experiences.

Finally, the question of how to integrate new knowledge and changes in the health care system is of immediate concern to nursing faculty. There are two areas of rapid change that I think exhibit this particular problem: one is the rapid expansion of home care, and second is the tremendous growth in ambulatory surgery.

The massive expansion in home care, as a result of changing reimbursement systems and cost containment efforts, has introduced high-tech care to the home. The preparation of professional nurses for community-based care at levels of increased acuteness of patients' conditions presents a new challenge to clinical preparation. This pattern of care requires a merger of acute care experiences and a community health framework. Does this trend demand a rethinking of the organization of clinical learning experiences presently in the curriculum? Further, does it imply that all students should have more extensive exposure to home care in the baccalaureate curriculum?

The second area of change, ambulatory surgery, is closely tied to the move toward home care. The American Hospital Association (1986) reports that close to 40% of all surgical procedures can now be safely performed on an outpatient basis, and it is predicted that up to 60% of surgeries will eventually be performed in ambulatory settings. What implication does this have for clinical learning experiences? Should this change be incorporated into the overall clinical plan? There needs to be some agreement about when a trend or change is important enough to effect the overall clinical plan.

These issues point to the need for a periodic assessment of the clinical experience plan and the assumptions made by faculty in designing it. Faculty must again be sensitive to social policy context of changes in the health care system and assure that changes in the clinical plan reflect responses to changing patient needs, not simply responses to pressures from institutions that employ nurses to meet their crisis needs.

A final comment is related to the need for faculty to engage in futurist thinking as they develop a plan for student clinical learning experiences. While incorporating changes in clinical learning experiences to accommodate where clients find themselves in the health care system, faculty should engage in creative thinking about alternative nursing practice arrangements. Issues of faculty practice and the development of nurse-managed centers should be incorporated into the planning process.

CONCEPTUAL FRAMEWORK FOR ORGANIZING CLINICAL LEARNING EXPERIENCES

A conceptual model is proposed to facilitate curriculum work in developing a plan for clinical learning experiences. This framework draws upon the previous discussion of criteria for clinical learning experiences and should assist faculty in dealing with the issues of generalist clinical knowledge, its scope and sequence, and the incorporation of changes in practice into the curriculum plan. The model outlines the approach to be followed in designing a plan for clinical learning experiences, as well as identifies essential groups of variables to be considered in designing clinical experiences (Fig. 11-1).

The fundamental assumption of the model is that curriculum work is a value-based activity and the products of curriculum work form a value statement. Having acknowledged this fundamental assumption, faculty need to make explicit the value framework of the professional curriculum. This is especially important as it relates to the socialization of neophyte professionals and the relationship of the profession to society. The professional nursing curriculum is derived from these broader statements of professional values, and one of the ways these values are communicated to students is through clinical learning experiences.

Because the design of clinical learning experiences implies a relationship between the role and function of the nurse, client populations, and settings, these three variables are identified as core planning points in the model. The overall clinical plan must clearly specify the generic nursing practice focus, which includes the phenomena of nursing practice as "human responses to actual and potential health problems" (American Nurses' Association, 1980, p. 9). This nursing care focus then needs to be integrated with appropriate client populations according to the variables of age (across the life span),

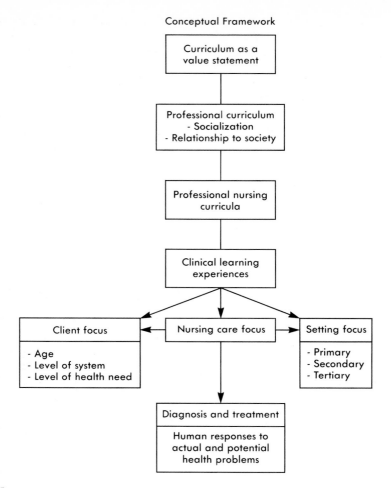

Conceptual Framework

Curriculum as a
value statement

Professional curriculum
- Socialization
- Relationship to society

Professional nursing
curricula

Clinical learning
experiences

Client focus

- Age
- Level of system
- Level of health need

Nursing care focus

Setting focus

- Primary
- Secondary
- Tertiary

Diagnosis and treatment

Human responses to
actual and potential
health problems

FIGURE 11-1

Conceptual framework for organizing clinical learning experiences.

level of system (individual, family, group, and community), and level of health need (primary, secondary, and tertiary). Both nursing and client foci need to be matched with appropriate settings (primary, secondary, and tertiary) that reflect where client populations are found and where meaningful instructional experiences can be obtained.

In conclusion, the incorporation of this model into the curriculum planning process will assist faculty to develop a clear, written plan for the organization of clinical learning experiences in the baccalaureate curriculum. The availability of the plan should aid in the curriculum orientation of faculty, students, and the community. In addition, a well-developed plan for clinical learning experiences will aid in curriculum evaluation.

REFERENCES

American Association of Colleges of Nursing. (1986a). *Essentials of college and university education for professional nursing (final report)*. Washington, DC: Author.

American Association of Colleges of Nursing. (1986b). *Generic baccalaureate nursing data project (1983–1986) (summary report)*. Washington, DC: Author.

American Hospital Association. (1986). *Outreach*, 7(2), 1–2.

American Nurses' Association. (1980). *Nursing: A social policy statement*. Kansas City, MO: Author.

Boley, B. A. (Ed.). (1977). *Crossfire in professional education: Students, the professions, and society*. New York: Pergamon Press.

Christy, T. E. (1980). Clinical practice as a function of nursing education. *Nursing Outlook*, *28*, 493–497.

Haukenes, E., & Mundt, M. H. (1983). The selection of clinical learning experiences in the nursing curriculum. *Journal of Nursing Education*, *22*, 372–375.

Howey, K. R., & Gardner, W. E. (1983). *The education of teachers*. New York: Longman.

Mundt, M. H. (1984). *The conceptualization and organization of clinical learning experiences in the baccalaureate nursing curriculum*. Unpublished doctoral dissertation, Marquette University, Milwaukee, WI.

Peters, T. (1987). *Thriving on chaos*. New York: Alfred A. Knopf.

Warner, A. R. (Ed.). (1976). *Clinical experiences and clinical practice in professional education*. Washington, DC: Monograph, Fund for the Improvement of Post-Secondary Education. (ERIC Document, Reproduction Service No. EO 123-209).

✳ EDITOR'S QUESTIONS FOR DISCUSSION ✳

How can nursing students best be prepared for professional nursing practice through clinical experiences offered in programs? What constitutes a "good experience" clinically for students? What are the contributing factors for a good experience? What are the settings and experiences most appropriate for nursing students? Suggest strategies for resolving the basic questions raised by Mundt regarding the design of clinical experiences. What clinical experiences should all students have? Discuss the pros and cons of providing specialty-type or specialty discipline–specific clinical experiences with limited generalist experiences versus only all generalist-type clinical experiences? Discuss the rationale and strategies for organizing clinical experiences.

Discuss strategies by which clinical instructors can provide active leadership for professional nursing practice in the clinical setting. When students are gaining experience in the clinical setting, how can a stronger social statement be made there regarding the potential for the professional practice of nursing? How can instructors in a clinical setting be the primary role models for students' socialization to professional values, attitudes, behaviors, and practices of the profession?

12

Needed: New Models for Professional Nursing Education

Mary E. Duffy, Ph.D., R.N.

Since the beginning of time, human beings have dealt with paradox. Nurse educators are no exception. Professional nursing currently sits on the horns of a dilemma. Societal needs require more and better prepared professional nurses. At the same time, the student applicant pool to nursing programs is shrinking and the cost of nursing education is escalating (Mundinger, 1988). Will better marketing strategies designed to improve nursing's public image and to attract new and different types of students help to solve this problem? Or is the problem more deep-rooted? Are we trying to pour new wine into worn-out wineskins?

This last question hits at the heart of this paper: What type of professional nursing education will meet society's future needs? According to forecasters, three major factors will shape future lifestyles: demographic shifts, changes in family patterns, and technology. They will have an enormous impact on education in general and nursing education in particular.

SOCIETAL FACTORS AFFECTING THE NURSING PROFESSION
Demographic Shifts

Demographically, the school-age population will continue its decline in size from 32% in 1980 to 28% in the year 2000 (Cetron, 1985). At the same time, the median age of the population continues to rise from 30.6 years in 1982 to 36.3 years by 2000.

The proportion of older Americans is also rising. Americans 65 years and above currently comprise over 12% of the population. By 2000, this number will be closer to 17%. Today's 3:2 ratio of older women to older men will shift. Futurists project that the stresses of the workplace will affect women's health, narrowing the age margin between men and women in the 55-plus age-group. The fastest-growing group in the population will be Americans 85 years and older. Their numbers will double by the year 2000; by 2050, 1 in 29 Americans will be over 85 years old.

Minorities, most notably Hispanics, make up 22% of new entrants into the labor force. By the year 2000, minorities will make up a larger voting block than unions. Women's political power will increase, and migration to the Sun Belt will continue. Young Americans in particular will move South and West because that is where most new jobs will be created.

Changes in the Family

Family roles will continue to change. By the end of the century, almost 70% of women between the ages of 25 and 44 years will be employed. Fathers will take over more responsibility for their children. The birth rate will continue to fall for all groups of women, including minorities, who will have fewer children as they move up the economic ladder. Although futurists anticipate that divorce rates will level off in the future as a result of longer life spans, at least one divorce for most Americans will be common.

More people will work at home because of the availability of advanced technology. Families will have opportunities to spend more time together. For some, this may bring family members closer together. For others, it could create increased stress and tension. The need for child care, home management, and care for the chronically ill and the aged will become increasingly important in the next century (Cetron, 1985).

Technology

Cable television and personal computers will be prime forces in people's lives in the future. As more people gain access to cable television, they will choose from a variety of subscription services. For example, people will be able to purchase general and individually tailored information packages for self-care and reminders for daily treatments and integrated diet—exercise—stress reduction advice. "Hospitals-on-the-wrist" will provide practitioners long-distance monitoring of patients' conditions. Microchip health records that contain a person's ongoing health history will improve continuity of care among health care providers (Milio, 1986).

Most American workers will use a computer at work; the majority of homes will have at least one computer. Futurists predict that older Americans and disabled Americans will be able to communicate with their health care providers, order groceries, and conduct many business transactions without leaving home. Computers will permit them to monitor and regulate their own health and illness at home. People will become their own primary practitioners, having access to their own records, laboratory and drug information, and medical knowledge and equipment (Lutz, 1985). Disabled and older Americans will be in positions to lead self-sufficient lives for a longer period of time than currently (Cetron, 1985).

HEALTH CARE NEEDS OF THE FUTURE

The impact of these societal shifts has already touched nursing. Along with other health professions, nursing stands at a critical junction. The direction chosen will determine where, and whether, nursing will fit into a dramatically altered health care delivery system (Felton, 1986).

According to Bezold and Carlson (1986), nine major factors will shape nursing's future:

1. Institutionalization for acute care will decrease, acute care hospitals' services will expand, and changes will occur on where nurses work.
2. Consumers will change, having increased knowledge of and participation in their own health care, decreased trust in organizations and governments, increased questioning of health care costs and delivery systems, and an interest in health behavior and promotion.
3. Better prepared nurses will be in leadership positions and will influence and reshape the future of nursing and health care delivery.
4. Lifestyles will change.
5. Demographic changes, particularly the aging and chronically ill, will create greater needs for nursing care.
6. There will be greater need for an all-professional staff because of an increase in acuity of illness, and the need to reduce cost and to improve efficiency in hospitals.
7. More effective preparation of the professional nurse with a baccalaureate or higher degree will be needed because of the higher demand for professional skills.
8. Increased entrepreneurial activity will occur in health care, some of which may be initiated by nurses.
9. Legislative and regulatory changes may alter the power and authority of nurses.

HIGHER AND PROFESSIONAL EDUCATION: STATE OF THE ART

Sakalys and Watson (1985) recently reviewed six significant and influential published reports assessing the quality of higher education and professional education in the United States. These were *The Paideia Proposal: An Educational Manifesto* (Adler, 1982); "Needed: A New Way To Train Doctors," Harvard Magazine (Bok, 1984); *Physicians for the Twenty-First Century; The GPEP Report* (1984); *Involvement in Learning: Realizing the Potential of American Higher Education* (1984); *To Reclaim A Legacy* (Bennett, 1984); and *Integrity in the College Curriculum: A Report to the Academic Community* (Association of American Colleges, 1985). They note a number of strikingly similar recommendations for improving the quality of American education:

1. Restore the central nature of the liberal arts in postsecondary and professional education.
2. Increase curricular structure and coherence.
3. Increase emphasis on intellectual skills, such as analysis, problem solving, and critical thinking.
4. Increase emphasis on mastery of basic principles rather than specific facts.
5. Increase emphasis on fundamental attitudes and values.
6. Increase emphasis on lifelong learning.
7. Decrease specialization at the undergraduate level.
8. Increase emphasis on broad and rigorous baccalaureate education prior to professional preparation.

Each report voices concern about the excessively vocational and narrow nature of professional education and the erosion of liberal education. Sakalys and Watson (1986) believe that basic nursing education needs restructuring. The professional nurse of the future must have a different type of educational preparation than is currently available. The baccalaureate degree is no longer adequate in light of the expanding body of knowledge about the rapidly changing, complex demands of nursing practice and the health care delivery system. It should serve as a prerequisite to professional nursing education.

Nurses of the future should be educated to be mature, competent, independent learners possessing the values, attitudes, knowledge, and intellectual skills needed to question current practices and to be directly accountable to clients and society (Sakalys & Watson, 1985). Nursing education's emphasis on science and technology has produced narrow practitioners ill-prepared for the changing demands and complexities of health care demanded by society. Liberal education in nursing is rudimentary; the professional component is mostly training (Sakalys & Watson, 1986).

What kind of education should prepare the professional nurse of tomorrow? Clearly, it should not take place at the baccalaureate level. Evidence is increasing that postbaccalaureate education for nursing is the wave of the future. Then the baccalaureate degree will truly become generalist preparation for all health care disciplines. Nontraditional education will become the norm rather than the exception. Cooperative educational endeavors and problem-focused professional education will be more common.

POSTBACCALAUREATE PROFESSIONAL NURSING EDUCATION

All professions involved in caring for people begin their professional preparation at the postbaccalaureate level, except for nursing. Styles (1982) believes that nursing has created this state of affairs by trying to incorporate our 3-year diploma and 2-year associate degree heritage into an awkward professional model. She calls for a new model of education: the postbaccalaureate degree as the first professional degree in nursing. Conway-Welch (1986) echoes this sentiment. She writes that nursing, a professional discipline, can benefit from the trials and tribulations of other professional groups who have seen that professional education must build on a postbaccalaureate base. Several postbaccalaureate nursing program models currently exist in the United States: the nurse doctorate (ND) program; generic master's program; and the registered nurse−to−master's degree program.

The Nursing Doctorate

The ND program was formally conceptualized and begun at the Frances Payne Bolton School of Nursing at Case Western Reserve University in 1979. The first class of candidates had previously completed undergraduate study in a wide variety of academic programs. As of June 1985, this 3-academic-year program had produced 96 graduates (Lutz & Schlotfeldt, 1985).

The ND curriculum has three phases. Phase 1, 34 weeks long, consists of considerable nursing science, artistry, history, and philosophy. This type of learning helps students develop an appropriate concept of professional practice before they assume any practice responsibilities (Lutz & Schlotfeldt, p. 141). Phase 2, 54 weeks in length, focuses on providing students varied practice opportunities in many health care settings with skilled nurse practitioner mentors. These practice opportunities foster students' development of independent nursing judgments. Phase 3, 14 weeks, consists of two parts. Part 1 focuses on helping students take more personal responsibility for their own learning. Accordingly, students themselves design learning experiences in nursing areas of interest under the guidance of nursing mentors. Part 2, the culmination of their clinical experience, provides students with opportunities to increase competence and confidence in working with groups of clients and collaborating with other health care professionals. Upon completion of the program, the majority of graduates assume positions in acute care settings at salaries higher than those granted to BSN graduates.

The goals of the ND program do not differ much from the goals of present-day baccalaureate nursing education. What is different, however, is the students' educational preparation: all are baccalaureate graduates prior to entering the program. They bring with them backgrounds rich in liberal arts and sciences on admission to the ND program. It seems reasonable to expect that their professional education would be qualitatively different than that of current baccalaureate graduates (Duffy, 1987).

Generic and RN—to—Master's Degree Programs

The term *generic* when applied to nursing education, commonly refers to any program that prepares students for entry into professional practice. This means that master's programs admitting nonnurses are generic programs irrespective of whether they provide basic or advanced education (Forni, 1987). The schools of nursing at The University of Tennessee at Knoxville, Pace University (New York), and Yale University (Connecticut) offer generic programs. In addition, a growing number of professional schools of nursing have implemented master's programs for RNs who hold bachelor's degrees in other fields or who have graduated from National League for Nursing (NLN)—accredited associate degree and diploma nursing programs. Some of these schools are The University of Tennessee at Knoxville, Yale University, Pace University of Illinois, Adelphi University, Case Western Reserve University, Wayne State University, Seton Hall University, the University of Illinois, the University of Massachusetts at Amherst, and the University of Iowa. As of 1988, the University of Rochester and The University of Texas Health Science Center at Houston offer programs for clinically experienced RNs who wish to earn a master's degree. These, and other schools contemplating such programs, are futuristic in their thinking and in the forefront of professional nursing education. They epitomize what Conway-Welch (1986) believes professional nursing needs: liberal education in the arts, sciences, and humanities that addresses, on the graduate level, the four functional areas of knowledge—teaching, research, practice, and administration.

NONTRADITIONAL NURSING EDUCATION

Traditional education, including nursing, is dead of self-inflicted wounds. Rigidity, inefficiency, stagnation, myopic vision, exalting form over substance, and lack of creativity were the instruments of death (Mitchell, 1987). Nontraditional nursing education will be the norm rather than the exception. For over 20 years, nontraditional educators have used their vision, knowledge, expertise, and research to provide education for people living in a technologically driven, information-service society. Using the principles of adult education (Brookfield, 1986) and the needs of today's and tomorrow's college students, nontraditional educators are grounded in a new paradigm of learning. The focus is on how to learn, knowing concepts and context, being autonomous and flexible, and applying ideas to real problems. It emphasizes complementariety between abstract formulations and real world experimentation and experience to develop new insights and deal with societal change (Mitchell, 1987; Association of American Colleges, 1985; Ferguson, 1980).

The most notable nontraditional nursing education model is the Regents College Degrees Nursing Programs (RCDNP) of the University of the State of New York (Lenburg, 1984a). The RCDNP NLN-accredited nursing programs have been in existence over 12 years. They provide competency-based associate and baccalaureate degree educational alternatives for adult learners (Lenburg, 1984b). In recent years, several colleges and universities have formed partnerships with RCDNP for several reasons, which include increasing assessment options for their own degree students, assisting nontraditional students through making courses available, and generating other sources of revenue. Strong supporting research evidence of the quality of nontraditional education is accumulating (Mitchell, 1987).

COOPERATIVE EDUCATION

Cooperative education, not new to the American higher education community, was introduced in 1906 at the University of Cincinnati. This form of experiential education exhibited slow growth until after World War II. By the midseventies, approximately 370 institutions had started cooperative programs in a variety of disciplines (Collins, 1976). Cooperative education is commonly defined as integrating classroom study with practical, on-the-job experience. Cooperative program students have specific periods of attendance at the particular college alternated with specific periods of employment. This alternate work-study program has many names: internship, field experience, off-campus period, professional practice program, extramural term, interval and interlude. Collins (1976) cites several institutional side benefits of formal cooperative education programs. Such programs reduce the isolationism of the institution; make better use of the college's physical plant; create rapport with the local community; provide reality-based experiences for the classroom; stimulate student recruiting; provide facilities and equipment (such as laboratory equipment) that the institution cannot usually afford; increase the employability of the graduate; and aid the institution's fund-raising activities by providing linkages with potential donors.

The major types of cooperative programs are known as mandatory, optional, and selective. *Mandatory programs* have been totally adopted as the keystone of the institution's educational thrust. Approximately 10% of senior colleges and universities and 9% of junior colleges have mandatory programs. Antioch College, Drexel University, Northeastern University, and Wilberforce University are wholly committed to mandatory programs. The University of Cincinnati, the University of Detroit, and the Rochester Institute of Technology have some mandatory programs within several of their colleges.

Optional programs, the most popular type of cooperative education, are offered as choices to students who may wish to benefit from a work-study experience while at college. About 51% of baccalaureate-degree granting institutions and 58% of 2-year colleges operate such programs. Optional programs may involve only a small number of students in some institutions and may exist only in particular departments or colleges within the university. The third type, *selective programs*, is a form of optional program. It usually involves enrolling cooperative students on the basis of academic performance. To qualify, a student must have and maintain a specified grade-point average throughout the educational experience.

Two patterns of cooperative arrangements exist within cooperative education: the *alternate plan* and the *parallel plan* (Ross & Marriner, 1985). In the alternate plan, the baccalaureate educational experience extends about 5 years, with students alternating periods of full-time study and full-time work for as long as 6 months at a stretch. Usually students begin the program with a period of concentrated study prior to work. This provides a firm theoretical foundation for their practice. Under this plan, students can immerse themselves completely in either work or study for a specific period of time.

In contrast, the parallel plan involves concurrent part-time study and part-time work relevant to the student's level of education and professional goals. It looks more similar to traditional baccalaureate nursing education. The advantages of this plan are that it promotes direct interaction between work and study experiences; results in fewer problems with sequencing courses; permits students a continuous relationship with employers; allows for continuity of projects and work assignments; and provides stable part-time workers for employers.

The parallel plan has some drawbacks. It can occur only if the educational unit and the work setting are within commuting distance. In addition, the concurrent nature of the work-study experience may produce burnout in students trying to juggle half-time study loads and half-time work loads. There may also be conflicts with class and work schedules. Also employers may not find it economically feasible to employ part-time persons. In summary, students in this plan may find that the burden of simultaneous study and work may cause excessive strain on their already crowded lives (Ross & Marriner, 1985).

Nursing has only a few cooperative education programs. Northeastern University in Boston is the most well known. Most innovative cooperative education programs exist in liberal arts colleges that have a tradition for experimentation. Much employment focuses on areas of social concern, urban problems, and the betterment of humanity. Students from many disciplines find employment in government agencies, educational institutions, physical and mental health institutions, and business and industry.

Many future nursing students will be older, having to pay for their own education thus necessitating part-time study, or may be changing careers. Cooperative educational approaches offer much as an alternative enterprise to attract and retain these students. Cooperative education would permit students

to earn an income while attending school; assist students' adjustment to professional practice realities; and pave the way for employment after graduation. Nursing already utilizes the method of combining work and study in actual practice settings. Developing a cooperative nursing educational option would pose fewer difficulties in nursing education than in other disciplines (Duffy, 1987).

PROBLEM-FOCUSED PROFESSIONAL EDUCATION

Problem-focused learning (Neufeld & Chong, 1984) is a professional educational approach that represents a clear alternative to traditional subject- or content-based education. Students become involved with defining, analyzing, and managing problems. They acquire the competencies needed to deliver effective, efficient, and humane services to clients. Problem-focused learning is not new. It has often been used as a teaching strategy in higher education, but its widespread use in professional education has been limited. The case, or problem-focused, method, pioneered by the Harvard Business School, bridges the gap between the classroom and the reality of practice (Christensen, 1981). In the beginning, Harvard faculty invited businessmen to the school to discuss their company's problems. Later, case researchers went into the field to observe and then write up problem situations. In nursing education, the problem-focused, or case method, technique has been used in many ways, but no nursing curriculum has used this method as its major base. The same exists in medical education, with one exception.

In the early seventies, McMaster University, in Hamilton, Ontario, Canada, used the problem-focused approach as the base for its medical (MD) program curriculum. The founding members of the McMaster program committed themselves to providing students with access to patients and their problems. They believed that packaged problems, called problem boxes, would complement students' contacts with actual or simulated patients (Barrows & Mitchell, 1975, 1980). The entire medical school curriculum was constructed on the study of a series of clinical cases or problems (Neufeld & Barrows, 1974).

Recent research findings on clinical reasoning processes shed positive insights on the usefulness of a problem-focused approach. This line of reasoning assumes the physician's task is ultimately to identify, analyze, and manage or solve patients' medical problems effectively, efficiently, and compassionately. Dealing with health and illness problems is the crux of the matter. Therefore, problem situations are the logical basis for designing a medical curriculum (Neufeld & Chong, 1984). Findings of Elstein, Shulmann, and Sprafka (1978) and of Barrows, Norman, Neufeld, and Feightner (1982) support this rationale. They found that physicians facing a clinical challenge exhibit a markedly consistent pattern of thinking. They find most of the important information within the first 10 minutes of clinical assessment. They spend the remaining time collecting confirmation data, building a case for the initial problem-formulation, developing rapport with the client, and gathering information to be used in developing a plan of investigation and management. Similarly, medical students, very early in their education, have clinical reasoning patterns remarkably similar to seasoned clinicians. They too generate hypotheses early in the clinical interaction, and collect further data to support them. The key difference between the two groups lies in the quality and accuracy of the hypotheses, which are dependent on the person's knowledge and experience.

Nursing education is very similar to medical education. Both disciplines prepare practitioners to diagnose and treat problems of health and illness. Thus a logical conclusion is that nursing education curricula could benefit greatly from a problem-focused, rather than a content-based, approach. The McMaster educational program may be a very useful model for nursing education to appraise.

The key features of the McMaster problem-focused curriculum are analysis of problems as the main method for acquiring and applying information; fostering independent student learning; and using small groups as the principal educational forum. The 33-month program consists of a series of multidisciplinary curriculum units, several elective blocks,

and a 1-year clerkship or internship. There are no discipline-specific courses. Students learn basic sciences within the context of clinical cases. Students do not take examinations. Evaluation is informal and continuous, done in tutorial groups and supplemented by students' performance in a variety of individual problem-focused exercises. The admissions process is rigorous. Students whose learning habits are compatible with the philosophy of the program, who demonstrate both academic ability and desirable personal qualities, are admitted. The operation of the program is entrusted to a program committee, rather than to departments or disciplines.

The McMaster program has graduated about 1000 physicians. They enter academic or research positions at a rate higher than the Canadian national average. Their attrition rate is low (less than 1%). Supervisors in postgraduate training view McMaster graduates very favorably; and graduates surveyed at 2 and 5 years after graduation are generally supportive of the program's approach to learning (Neufeld & Chong, 1984).

An important goal in the problem-focused learning approach is developing critical appraisal skills in students. Critical-appraisal guidelines and materials are an integral part of the basic analysis of health problems. The McMaster faculty define their major educational challenge as the creation of an efficient and comprehensive curriculum that prepares the practicing physician of the future for a career of lifelong learning. The major challenge for their students is to acquire a critical ability to identify, analyze, and manage clinical problems in order to provide effective, efficient, and humane patient care (Neufeld & Chong, 1984).

FUTURISTIC PROFESSIONAL NURSING CURRICULA

The present structure of professional nursing education at the undergraduate level is clearly deficient and unable to prepare professional nurses of the future. Nurse educators cannot bury their heads in the sand and naively assume that the future will take care of itself. Strategic planning using futuristic projections about societal and health care changes and current knowledge must form the base of our deliberations. The four areas described in this chapter (postbaccalaureate professional nursing education, nontraditional nursing education, cooperative education, and problem-focused curricula) represent some viable alternatives to current nursing educational practices. Each model has the potential to resolve some of the problems that we, as nurse educators, will experience in the near future.

Consider thoughtfully the eight recommendations previously presented for improving the quality of higher education and professional education (Sakalys & Watson, 1986). If nursing faculty decided to adopt just two of the proposed models, many recommendations would be addressed. Moving to postbaccalaureate professional nursing education would provide future professional nurses with a sound, humanistic, and broad, general liberal arts base. This would result in greater emphasis on basic human values; decrease specialization at the undergraduate level; and provide broad and rigorous baccalaureate education prior to professional preparation. In addition, if a problem-focused rather than a content-specific curriculum were used, future nurse professionals would develop greater problem-solving and critical thinking skills. Graduates would be masters of basic principles, rather than specific facts, and possess the process skills needed to be lifelong learners in an information-oriented, service-driven society. In addition, using nontraditional approaches including cooperative educational models would provide many types of students with quality and cost-effective education.

We in nursing education stand at a crossroad. What direction we choose will determine where, and whether, the nursing profession will fit into a dramatically altered future. We need to understand, insofar as possible, the trends that affect American society. Using this knowledge, we will be better able to make changes in nursing education. Nursing faculty have access to the knowledge, experience, and power to shape nursing education. Change is needed now so that future professional nurses will have the requisite knowledge and skills to meet societal health care needs in a world very different from the one we now know.

REFERENCES

Adler, M. J. (1982). *The Paideia proposal: An educational manifesto*. New York: Macmillan.

Association of American Colleges. (1985). *Integrity in the college curriculum: A report to the academic community*. Washington, DC: Author.

Barrows, H. S., & Mitchell, D. L. M. (1975). An innovative course in undergraduate neuroscience: Experiments in problem based learning with 'problem boxes'. *British Journal of Medical Education*, 9(4), 223–230.

Barrows, H. S., Norman, G. R., Neufeld, V. R., & Feightner, J. W. (1982). The clinical reasoning of randomly selected physicians in general medical practice. *Clinical and Investigative Medicine*, 5(1), 49–55.

Barrows, H. S., & Tamblyn, R. M. (1980). *Problem-based learning: An approach to medical education*. New York: Springer Publishing.

Bennett, W. J. (1984). *To reclaim a legacy*. Washington, DC: National Endowment for the Humanities.

Bezold, C., & Carlson, R. (1986). Nursing in the 21st century. *Journal of Professional Nursing*, 2(7), 69–71.

Bok, D. (1984). Needed: A new way to train doctors. *Harvard Magazine*, 85(3), 32–71.

Brookfield, S. D. (1986). *Understanding and facilitating adult learning*. San Francisco: Jossey-Bass.

Cetron, M. J. (1985). *Schools of the future: How American business and education can cooperate to save our schools*. New York: McGraw-Hill.

Christensen, C. R. (1981). *Teaching by the case method*. Boston: Division of Research, Harvard Business School.

Collins, S. B. (1976). Cooperative education and internships—college. In Goodman, S. E. (Ed.) *Handbook of contemporary education* (pp. 585–590). New York: R. R. Bowker Co.

Conway-Welch, C. (1986). School sets sights on bold innovations. *Nursing & Health Care*, 7(1), 21–25.

Duffy, M. E. (1987). Innovation as a survival strategy. In *Patterns in nursing: Strategic planning for nursing education* (Publication No. 15-2179, pp. 47–70). New York: National League for Nursing.

Elstein, A. S., Shulmann, L. S., & Sprafka, S. A. (1978). *Medical problem-solving: An analysis of clinical reasoning*. Cambridge: Harvard University Press.

Felton, G. (1986). Harnassing today's trends to guide nursing's future. *Nursing & Health Care*, 7(4), 211–213.

Ferguson, M. (1980). *The aquarian conspiracy: Personal and social transformation in the 1980s*. Boston: Houghton Mifflin.

Forni, P. R. (1987). Nursing's diverse master's programs: The state of the art. *Nursing & Health Care, 8*(2), 70–75.

Involvement in learning: Realizing the potential of American higher education. (1984). Washington, DC: National Institute of Education.

Lenburg, C. B. (1984a). Preparation for professionalism through Regents external degrees. *Nursing & Health Care, 5*(6), 319–325.

Lenburg, C. B. (1984b). An update on the Regents external degree program. *Nursing Outlook, 32*(6), 250–254.

Lutz, E. M., & Schlotfeldt, R. M. (1985). Pioneering a new approach to professional education. *Nursing Outlook, 33*(3), 139–143.

Lutz, L. (1985). Computers and health care. In C. Bezold, (ed.), *Pharmacy in the 21st century* (pp. 13–21). Alexandria, Va: Institute for Alternative Futures.

Milio, N. (1986). Telematics in the future of health care delivery: Implications for nursing. *Journal of Professional Nursing, 2*(1), 39–50.

Mitchell, C. A. (1987). Future view: Non-traditional education as the norm. In *Patterns in nursing: Strategic planning for nursing education* (Publication No. 15-2179, pp. 71–89). New York: National League for Nursing.

Mundinger, M. O. (1988). Three-dimensional nursing: New partnerships between service and education. *Journal of Professional Nursing, 4*(2), 10–16.

Neufeld, V. R., & Barrows, H. S. (1974). McMaster philosophy: An approach to medical education. *Journal of Medical Education, 49*(11), 1040–1050.

Neufeld, V., & Chong, J. P. (1984). Problem-based professional education in medicine. In S. Goodlad (Ed.), *Education for the professions—Quis custodiet. . . . ?* (pp. 249–256). Surrey, England: SRHE & NFER-Nelson.

Physicians for the twenty-first century: The GPEP report. (1984). Washington, DC: Association of American Medical Colleges.

Ross, S., & Marriner, A. (1985). Cooperative education: Experienced-based learning. *Nursing Outlook, 33*(4), 177–180.

Sakalys, J. A., & Watson, J. (1985). New directions in higher education: A review of trends. *Journal of Professional Nursing, 1*(5), 293–299.

Sakalys, J. A., & Watson, J. (1986). Professional education: Post-baccalaureate education for professional nursing. *Journal of Professional Nursing, 2*(2), 91–97.

Styles, M. (1982). *On nursing: Toward a new endowment.* St. Louis: C. V. Mosby.

✳ EDITOR'S QUESTIONS FOR DISCUSSION ✳

What are the implications for nursing programs in the recommendations made in the six reports reviewed by Sakalys and Watson? Discuss the positive and negative aspects of the RN-to-master's program. What is the difference in program content, goals, objectives, and outcomes between the generic master's program and "bypass" master's programs for RNs who hold baccalaureate degrees in other fields, or have an AD or diploma in nursing but do not have a nursing baccalaureate degree? What hallowed assumptions regarding nursing education are ignored in using nontraditional nursing education models for programs?

Discuss the applications of problem-focused learning as a professional education approach for nursing. Indicate the strengths and limitations of each of the approaches and models proposed by Duffy. What evidence exists that supports consideration of the models? How can a potential nursing student, or consumer, be accurately informed of the differences in the programs, projected outcomes, and settings for practice?

Compare this chapter with those written by Fitzpatrick and Modly (Chapter 13), Watson and Bevis (Chapter 14), and Conway-Welch (Chapter 65). How similar are their views and suggestions? Should there be consistency and, if so, to what degree regarding the content taught in various nursing programs, such as for the associate, baccalaureate, or master's degree? Discuss an effective process for bringing about change in nursing education through program evaluation. Propose a method and process for evaluating a program.

13

The First Doctor of Nursing (ND) Program

Joyce J. Fitzpatrick, Ph.D., F.A.A.N.
Doris M. Modly, Ph.D., R.N.

The Frances Payne Bolton School of Nursing of Case Western Reserve University has been an acknowledged leader among the schools of nursing in this country since 1923 and has consistently been a pacesetter for nursing education and practice. Early in the 1970s, the faculty of the Bolton School under the visionary leadership of Rozella Schlotfeldt began discussions and deliberations about an innovative program: the Doctor of Nursing (ND), a professional doctorate, as the entry level educational preparation for professional nursing. The purpose of this chapter is to describe the first doctor of nursing program in the United States as developed and implemented at the Bolton School in the late 1970s and the 1980s.

PROFESSIONAL EDUCATION FOR NURSES

In 1977, the American Nurses' Association Commission on Nursing Education recognized the concept of the professional doctorate as the first professional degree in nursing (Fitzpatrick, 1986). Though still quite controversial, there is a support within the discipline for postbaccalaureate entry-level education for professional nursing practice (Carter, 1988; Fitzpatrick, 1988; Schraeder, 1988; Watson, 1988). The question of the professional doctorate as preparation for basic nursing practice is, however, complicated by several factors within the profession, for example, the general lack of clarity in the purpose of and distinction among the other doctoral programs in nursing, the PhD, the DNS, and the DNSc; and a lack of consensus about what constitutes "professional" education in nursing in general.

The primary characteristic proposed for professional education is that it exists to serve a societal need and that it is based on a firm liberal arts background, a body of specialized knowledge, and the code of values and ethics on which the profession is based. Considering the ethical and moral components of professional behavior for which professional education provides a foundation, educators are continuously exploring how to best educate and socialize students for professional practice. Explorations of these issues led the faculty of the Frances Payne Bolton School of Nursing to the establishment of a postbaccalaureate basic nursing education program, the first ND program.

CONCEPTUAL AND PRACTICAL RATIONALE FOR THE PROGRAM

Schlotfeldt explicated the rationale for postbaccalaureate professional education for nurses in her classic paper, "The Professional Doctorate: Rationale and Characteristics," published in *Nursing*

Outlook in the fall of 1978. Schlotfeldt based her rationale for the ND on the thesis that, "if nursing is to become a full-fledged professional discipline, then its practitioners need a full-fledged professional program of study with entry at the post-baccalaureate level" (Schlotfeldt, 1978, p. 302).

The conceptualization of the nature of human beings and the nature of nursing as a scientific discipline provided the foundation for the development of the ND program. The basic argument proposed by Schlotfeldt was that of nursing's scientific responsibility to focus on holistic understandings of human health. Concerns with aspects of implementation of the professional nursing role, including issues of collaborative health care, practice, and status, and the strongly identified need to advance both nursing education and professional nursing practice, provided the impetus to develop this educational program.

One of the compelling arguments of a practical nature was that it was not appropriate to educate persons with baccalaureate degrees in other disciplines, who were interested in pursuing a career in nursing, in programs offering less than graduate level education. At the time that the doctor of nursing program was initiated, one-third of the baccalaureate students enrolled in the basic educational program at the Bolton School had a baccalaureate degree in another discipline; this convinced the faculty of the feasibility of offering a postbaccalaureate for professional study in nursing.

The resources of the Bolton School of Nursing and of Case Western Reserve University were thought to be an appropriate setting for experimentation with such a novel and timely program. The faculty described the leadership role that was assumed by the Bolton School of Nursing as based on the following (Frances Payne Bolton School of Nursing, 1978, p. 6):

1. Heritage and reputation for innovative leadership;
2. Commitment to the concept of the professional doctorate and careful deliberation of the potential for program implementation;
3. Responsibility of a private, independent university that encouraged innovation, empha-

sized research, and provided for graduate study in a variety of disciplines;
4. Role as an integral part of a health sciences complex in which inter-preprofessional collaboration and respect were valued and nurtured;
5. Support from significant leaders in nursing education to develop the pioneer doctor of nursing program;
6. Success in developing interinstitutional relationships with a clinical learning setting, whereby the School accepted responsibility for quality controls relative to nursing practice and nursing research;
7. Experience in teaching college graduates and recognition of the need for change to better utilize their prior education;
8. Awareness of the increasing competition for college graduates by targeted educational programs designed within nursing.

HISTORICAL OVERVIEW

The professional doctorate as the entry level educational preparation for professional nursing was revolutionary at the time of its introduction in the late 1970s. In 1972, there were only seven doctoral programs in nursing in the country, three offering the PhD, or research doctorate; three offering clinical doctorates for advanced specialty practice, the DNS or DNSc; and one offering an EdD. An understanding of doctoral preparation for nurses and doctoral education within nursing was minimal. In the early 1970s fewer than 500 nurses with any kind of doctoral preparation could be identified. Additionally the great debate regarding basic levels of nursing education, which notably is still present in the profession, was paramount at that time (Fitzpatrick, 1986).

A formal document describing the new doctor of nursing (ND) program was prepared by the faculty of the Bolton School in 1978. The document contained the program philosophy, conceptualization, curriculum, content, and program objectives developed by the faculty. Formal approvals for the program implementation were obtained from the Faculty Senate and Board of Trustees of Case Western Reserve University, the Ohio Board of Regents, and the Board of Nursing Education and Nurse Registration. In the fall of 1979, the first class of 43 students matriculated and began the 3-year course of study. Program design and implementation proceeded simultaneously, as faculty and students realized the revolutionary nature of the conceptualization of nursing and the new approach to nursing education.

Changes in the patterns of health care delivery systems and in education influenced further program development. A national nursing shortage, a decrease in applications and enrollments into university based programs, and plans for changes in funding of health care, all effected how the program and how graduates of the program were perceived by the service sector and by the consumers.

The graduation of this first class of 34 students in the ND program, nevertheless, marked a significant milestone for the profession of nursing. A reassessment and program evaluation was instituted after the first class's graduation. During the evaluation process it was learned that nurses, as well as other health care providers, did not understand the goals of the program or the nursing expertise of the program graduates. This led to efforts to educate more fully the nursing community and the community at large about the program and its objectives. Following a thorough evaluation funded by the Cleveland Foundation, curriculum revisions were instituted to develop the program's focus as a professional doctorate. The curriculum has evolved over the 10 years since it has been implemented. Thus it has been difficult to measure the impact of curricular content on graduates' practice proficiencies.

THE CURRICULUM

During the 10 years of its existence, the curriculum of the ND program has been revised based on continuous faculty and student input through an ongoing evaluation process. A major change was implemented following the graduation of the class of 1985, based on data of the evaluation study of the graduates of the first classes (Fitzpatrick, Boyle, & Anderson, 1986). The discussion of the curriculum that follows reflects the structure and content of the curriculum as instituted initially, and the characteristics of the curriculum following this major change.

The course of study in the first ND program was 3 academic years. Students were expected to complete successfully all coursework for graduation; the curriculum did not include a predetermined number of required credit hours. The first year was focused on mastery of basic knowledge essential for the practice of nursing. The goal for students within this first level was to conceptualize the professional art and science of nursing before they were expected to assume responsibility for the practice of nursing (Lutz & Schlotfeldt, 1985). Emphasis was placed on the development of a nursing perspective and knowledge about human health and health-seeking behaviors of persons, groups, and communities. Students explored the practical and theoretical frameworks that formed the basis for nursing practice. Students synthesized their knowledge as they observed the efforts of individuals, groups, and communities to attain, maintain, and regain health. They also were introduced to variables that influence these processes. Students learned nursing strategies that affect health-seeking behaviors of individuals, groups, and communities, and nursing actions congruent with the defined strategies.

Within this first level, students had opportunities to observe individuals, including actual and potential patients. These patient-based experiences facilitated students' learning about the essence of being human, growing and developing over the life span, and seeking and maintaining health. These learning experiences provided an opportunity to integrate the relationship between the science, the art, and the personal way of knowing in nursing. Concepts basic to understanding ethical ways of knowing were interwoven as human development over the life span was discussed. The study of interpersonal skills was introduced early to allow students time to master communication skills and develop interpersonal competencies. Students' psychomotor skills were enhanced through their study and practice of assessment skills. Students were encouraged to integrate the various concepts and skills and "to conceptualize nursing as a field of professional study and professional practice different from technical training" (Lutz & Schlotfeldt, 1985, p. 142).

Learning experiences on the second level included the extension of clinical experiences and the use of nursing interventions with persons in various patient populations. Clinical learning opportunities during the second level were varied and extensive to facilitate students' becoming skillful in devising nursing strategies designed to assist patients' attaining of optimal levels of functioning. Students were encouraged to ask significant questions about observed phenomena and clinical data. They were also led to inquire into the nature of nursing practice from legal and ethical orientations (Lutz & Schlotfeldt, 1985).

The notion that nurses must be self-directed in enhancing their knowledge and skills throughout their careers led to the inclusion of a learning opportunity for third level students that was student-designed and based on each student's particular interest. Students selected one or a combination of a focused clinical practice, a phenomenon of concern to nursing, and/or the study of the function of a health care agency. These experiences resulted in writing and presentation of a scholarly paper based on a theme that emerged during the experience. The culminating clinical experience of the third level provided students the opportunity to increase their confidence in providing nursing care. Students had opportunities to learn to delegate, supervise, and evaluate work performed by other care providers. The ND curriculum, as it evolved during the first 5 years, provided learners the opportunity to acquire an understanding of the scientific and theoretical bases of nursing practice and sufficient skills to enter general practice (Lutz & Schlotfeldt, 1985).

Curriculum revisions were implemented in 1985 to develop further the program focus as a professional doctorate. Changes were instituted so that priorities of clinical practice, clinical inquiry, and professionalism were evident.

The revised ND program of study also was designed as three academic years in length. The first level is focused on basic nursing knowledge and skills, with emphasis on the development of a nursing perspective and knowledge about human health.

Students explore the practical and theoretical frameworks that form the bases for practice. Students are introduced to well-client populations in a variety of settings, as well as to patients in acute care clinical settings. The second level is planned to build on the basic professional nursing foundation introduced on the first level. Learning experiences on the second level include the extension of clinical experiences and the use of nursing interventions with persons in various patient populations.

Students participate in beginning courses on nursing theory and nursing research with other beginning graduate (MSN) students in the School of Nursing, and with students in other professions (law, medicine, social work) in a multidisciplinary course in professional ethics. The culminating experience on the second level includes the clinical practicum experiences that provide students with concentrated clinical opportunities to integrate fully the skills and knowledge necessary for professional nursing practice.

The third level is focused on development of knowledge and skills for advanced clinical nursing practice. This level includes an opportunity for students to select from one of four focal areas for concentrated clinical practice. Areas represented include acute care, parent/child/family, community health/mental health, and long-term care/aging. Further, students extend their emphasis on a clinical evaluation project that is formally presented as a major project of the professional education. As this component of the program continues to be strengthened, it is expected that through these clinical studies students and faculty will make significant contributions to the clinical nursing literature and to clinical nursing practice. During the third year, the student is introduced to major content in health policy and planning and information systems and management.

CHARACTERISTICS OF THE GRADUATE

Graduates of the ND program are expected to initiate a range of opportunities for their professional practice. Furthermore, the program prepares individuals with the knowledge, skills, and values for clinical practice, clinical scholarship, and for a professional career. As a clinically competent practitioner of nursing, faculty expect the graduate to be proficient in professional nursing skills; engage in autonomous, collaborative health care practice; display interpersonal competence; assume a leadership role in nursing; demonstrate the ability to manage health systems and resources; and practice at an advanced level in a selected area.

As clinical scholars, graduates are expected to use theoretical and empirical knowledge; know and apply the process of theoretical thinking; pursue and test concepts, models, and theories; use and explicate the rationale and data for clinical nursing decisions; analyze critically nursing phenomena and evaluate clinical situations; and study systematically a selected area to advance practice in that area. As professionals, graduates are expected to be ethical in decision making, display professional values, and assume responsibility for their own learning and professional growth. As health care professionals, graduates are expected to understand the management of information and systems, analyze systems to implement change, and influence health policy and planning.

The ND program is characterized by educational depth and an emphasis on inquiry and collaboration in patient care, hallmarks of other health professions. The faculty believe that the strong undergraduate educational preparation that the student brings, plus the comprehensive professional and clinical course of study of nursing offered through the ND program, enables graduates to function effectively as professional nurses and partners with other professionals in the provision of quality health care.

PROFILE OF GRADUATES

Over the 9 years since the inception of the ND program, 278 students have matriculated for study in the ND program at the Bolton School. Seven classes graduated from 1979 to 1988. There are currently 200 ND graduates practicing nursing. A longitudinal study initiated to track all graduates of the program continues to be in progress. Results of a shorter, 3-year Cleveland Foundation–funded evalu-

ation project were reported by Fitzpatrick, Boyle and Anderson (1986). Generally the study results indicated a strong professional career commitment among ND graduates, persons who consistently describe themselves as leaders and as professionals. The majority of graduates assumed clinical practice positions immediately after graduation, and they addressed their need for attaining additional clinical experience as one of the primary motivating factors in selecting these first positions. Many graduates reported strong and continued interest in advancing their education through continuing education or by acquiring clinical specialization or depth in research. Employment flexibility and mobility were evident among these early program graduates; both lateral and hierarchical position changes were evident. Further, ND graduates expressed a desire to explore nontraditional practice settings and nursing practice roles.

Preliminary findings of the evaluation study revealed departures in the career and professional paths of ND graduates. ND graduates seem to progress more rapidly and inspire more nontraditional roles and higher educational goals than BSN graduates (Fitzpatrick, Boyle, & Anderson, 1986). This might be a reflection of a different socialization to professional nursing as well as a reflection of curricular content. The uniqueness of the program, however, also leads to selection of those applicants who are risk takers, innovators, and highly motivated individuals. ND students bring a more extensive background of work and educational experience to their professional education resulting in more varied outcomes.

CURRENT STUDENTS

During the 1987/88 academic year there were 47 students enrolled in the ND program. Forty-one were women, six were men, and two were from minority groups. The average age was 24.8 years, with a range from 20 to 48 years. The students have come from 13 different states: Ohio, Pennsylvania, and New York were most strongly represented. Students received their undergraduate educations from 39 different colleges and universities. Five students have master's degrees with advanced degrees in sports medicine, wildlife management, nutrition, and history. Undergraduate degrees include majors in the life sciences, social sciences, mathematics, humanities, and business. The profile of students enrolled during the 1987/88 academic year at the Bolton School was no different from student profiles of previous classes. ND students can be characterized as diverse, with a wide range of educational and varied life experiences. Students in the ND program continue to challenge both their teachers and fellow students to become "colleagues in learning" (Lutz & Schlotfeldt, 1985, p. 140).

FUTURE DIRECTIONS

The focus for further development of the ND program will be a continued strengthening of the program of study. Program development is planned to lead to an even clearer distinction between ND graduates and graduates of other educational programs. Important dimensions of the ND graduate that will guide all future aspects of program development are competency in both clinical practice and inquiry, and a commitment to the discipline through individual and collective professional action.

In preparing graduates with clinical expertise, the clinical emphasis has become the content focus of the program. At the present time four focal areas are described: acute care, long-term care and aging, parent/child/family, and community health. Clinical strength will be achieved by further enhancing the model of professional education. The model of placement of students in one-to-one clinical preceptorships will be expanded. The preceptors are expert clinicians, members of the clinical faculty who serve as clinical role models.

Competence in scientific inquiry will be achieved through a strong focus on clinical scholarship. Models of faculty practice with strong clinical and evaluation components have already been implemented and will be further expanded. Planned integration of administration, scientific, and educational computer-based activities is a priority for future program development; these changes will be influential in the development of ND students. An emphasis on inter-

disciplinary education, and collaboration at the basic science level, as well as in clinical practice, will be further strengthened. In all these learning opportunities there will be an emphasis on building on the students' prior learning experiences. Program flexibility, with opportunities to choose supplementary learning experiences congruent with students' career goals, will be promoted.

Professional socialization, the third major expected outcome, will be enhanced through various professional activities to provide students the opportunity to internalize their professional role and to understand professional nursing "not only to be part of their professional identity but touch all aspects of their lives and beings" (Fitzpatrick, 1986, p. 19). Collective commitment to the profession will enable ND graduates to provide necessary leadership for the profession.

A collective consciousness among ND graduates based on an appreciation of their knowledge base, values, and commitment to the discipline has been evident among graduates; this outcome characteristic is expected to be even stronger with future graduates. They will create a critical mass necessary to influence the profession's advancement and acceptance of postbaccalaureate doctoral education in nursing. The ND program has been planned to educate professional practitioners who are reflective in their practice. These are professionals who will rise to the "unprecedented requirement for adaptability" (Brooks, cited in Schön, 1983, p. 15) essential for all professional practitioners in the 21st Century. The ND program at Case Western Reserve University represents the first step in the transformation of Schlotfeldt's visionary concept of preservice doctoral education in nursing into a reality.

REFERENCES

Carter, M. A. (1988). The professional doctorate as an entry level into practice. *Perspectives in nursing 1987–1989* (pp. 49–52). New York: National League for Nursing.

Fitzpatrick, J. J. (1986). *The N.D. program: Integration of past and future*. Cleveland, OH: Frances Payne Bolton School of Nursing, Case Western Reserve University.

Fitzpatrick, J. J. (1988). The professional doctorate as an

entry level into clinical practice. *Perspectives in nursing* (pp. 53–56). New York: National League for Nursing.

Fitzpatrick, J. J., Boyle, K. K., & Anderson, R. M. (1986). The N.D. (doctor of nursing) program: Preliminary evaluation of the graduates. *Journal of Professional Nursing, 2*(6), 365-372.

Frances Payne Bolton School of Nursing. (1978). *A new program at Frances Payne Bolton School of Nursing, Case Western Reserve University: Doctor of nursing.* Cleveland: Author.

Lutz, E. M., & Schlotfeldt, R. M. (1985). Pioneering a new approach to professional education. *Nursing Outlook, 33*(3), 139–143.

Schlotfeldt, R. M. (1978). The professional doctorate: Rationale and characteristics. *Nursing Outlook, 26*(5), 302–311.

Schön, D. (1983). *The reflective practitioner.* New York: Basic Books.

Schraeder, B. D. (1988). Entry level graduate education in nursing: Master of science programs. *Perspectives in Nursing 1987–1989* (pp. 33–39). New York: National League for Nursing.

Watson, J. (1988). The professional doctorate as an entry level into practice. *Perspectives in Nursing 1987–1989* (pp. 41–47). New York: National League for Nursing.

✳ EDITOR'S QUESTIONS FOR DISCUSSION ✳

How can graduate level nursing education be presented in the ND program, as it was originally designed and intended, when the students have no previous nursing knowledge or content? How can a person practice at an advanced level in a selected area of nursing practice without prior understanding and experience about the totality of nursing practice? What evidence is there regarding the minimum in type and amount of clinical content and experiences that is essential for professional practice?

If the graduates of ND programs are expected to practice at an advanced level in a selected area, what evidence exists regarding their employment and the type of nursing positions that they choose? What are the critical issues that need to be addressed regarding ND programs? To what extent is the present-day ND program similar to the "bypass" (baccalaureate) master's program at Vanderbilt University, the University of Colorado, and Rush University? What are the advantages and disadvantages of each of those programs and models? How similar was the original content and curriculum plan in the ND program of the first 3 years to the current content being offered in baccalaureate nursing programs? What future direction would you suggest for the generic baccalaureate, the ND, and "bypass" (baccalaureate) master's programs in nursing? Indicate rationale and evidence for your beliefs and suggestions.

14

Nursing Education:
Coming of age for a new age

Jean Watson, Ph.D., R.N., F.A.A.N.
Em Olivia Bevis, M.A., R.N., F.A.A.N.

Life had a different shape; it had new branches and some of the old branches were dead. It had followed the constant pattern of discard and growth that all lives follow. Things had passed, new things had come.

(Markham, 1983, p. 197)

Nursing is growing up. Old things must pass, be discarded; new things must come, if nursing is to come fully of age for a new age. As complex technology becomes an increasingly larger part of health care, the patient is in danger of being dehumanized. The proliferation of scientific knowledge has necessitated accommodation of much new scientific content in nursing and other health professional curricula—at the expense of attention to values, ethics, and the knowledge, understanding, and practices—that are associated with subjective health and human caring experiences. The result is a state of educational disequilibrium. This affects the ability of the nurse and other health professionals to engage in critical thinking and inquiry, while dealing with the human, technological, and scientific complexities of health care. However, there is emerging agreement that the institutional, scientific, technological orientation of today's educational and health delivery systems cannot be sustained into the 21st century. The inevitable conclu-

sion is that nursing education derived from and perpetuating these systems will graduate health professionals ill-equipped to meet the challenges they will face. Thus the morality, efficiency, efficacy, and economics of health care in general are being critically examined, as are the effectiveness and appropriateness of professional educational structures and processes.

A NEW MORALITY OF HEALTH, HEALING, AND HUMAN CARING

The medical-scientific technological enterprise that has dominated American health care (and nursing practice) in modern time represents an outdated morality, and now lacks the expertise or skills to meet the health care needs of a population that is increasingly aged, chronically ill, poor, and without access to reimbursed health and human caring services (Moccia, 1988). The new morality now called for is linked to the advancement of nursing as a human science focusing on scholarship, research, and practice of the art and science of human caring, health, and healing. Such a notion is tied to caring as a moral ideal in a human science and practice model that acknowledges the interconnections among persons, and between humans and nature, through caring, health, and healing. Such ideals of human science and caring are rooted in receptivity, intersubjectivity, relatedness, and human responsiveness (Noddings, 1984), rather than separation, distancing, control, or manipulation.

A more radical thesis, now brought on by the impact of the old morality of extremism of science and technology, is that American medicine is moving out of an era where curing is dominant into an era where *caring* must take precedence (Callahan, 1987). Such thinking posits caring as not only a moral ideal and unifying goal for nursing but an end in and of itself (Watson, 1985; Gadow, 1988). In this new morality–human science framework proposed by Watson (1985) and Gadow (1988), the relationship between curing and caring, between treatment and healing, between disease and health, becomes inverted, thereby designating knowledgeable human caring as the highest form of commitment to patients. Further, this focus designates health and healing (or peaceful death) and caring processes as morally, scientifically, and socially respectable places where nurse professionals can live. In this framework, knowledgeable human caring becomes the ethical principle and human science standard by which medical curing and technological knowledge and interventions are measured (Gadow, 1988).

Such a gestalt shift requires a radical transformation, a new world view of the nature of the health care system, the nurse's role in the system, and certainly the nature of nursing education. Such a future calls out for leaders in nursing education and practice to establish nursing as a full health and human caring profession in order to respond to the new morality, to redefine the possibilities—to acknowledge that to do otherwise, now that a new light falls on our trouble, is unbearable (Sartre, 1956).

One starting point to redefine the possibilities for the future lies in a different view of the nursing profession and a new model of nursing education. Re-

definition of both is necessary if nursing is to come of age for the new age.

REVOLUTION IN NURSING EDUCATION

In 1987 the National League for Nursing sponsored a nursing educator conference entitled "Curriculum Development Revolution" (NLN, 1988). The conference was a strategic historical moment marking the beginning of the new age in nursing curricula. The NLN conference emphasized that the nursing profession must not only restructure its educational format, but also its standardized behavioral approach to teaching and learning.

The behavioral-driven curriculum model currently in use is a training model, not an educational one. Students are still largely trained to be entry-level employees for a bureaucratic system in which curing and technology take precedence.

Baccalaureate nursing educators include intellectual goals such as critical thinking, analysis, judgment, integration, and synthesis in their curriculum framework. However, such goals are rarely accomplished because of the objective-task-oriented educational format, time constraints, and socialization in the traditional medical paradigm. As Allen put it:

> Our schooling practices exemplify and actively encourage future nurses to adopt values and behaviors that minimize their ability to engage in critical reflection. We actively seek experts to convey current "knowledge" of specialties rather than emphasizing disagreement . . .including conflicts and how to think. . . . We often regard schooling issues as being technical—the best means to create a certain set of behaviors—rather than practical—the creation of conditions for critical reflection and argumentation. (1985, p. 64)

The kinds of persons who must be educated for the new age in nursing and health care are those who can accept the ambiguities of the modern medical and health care world. This is a complex world, in which there are no certainties, nor any easy and clear solutions; a world in which everyday judgments are fraught with ethical and moral dilemmas that require daily reevaluation of our most basic ideas about human life. The nurse we seek is a compassionate scholar-clinician. This is a truly educated nurse with a professionalism that arises out of a firm base of liberal arts and humanities that has equal status with the sciences. Current nursing education is incomplete and inadequate at programmatic, pedagogical, and curricular levels.

CRITIQUE OF INSTITUTIONALIZED TYLER CURRICULUM

An even greater problem than the amount and content of education is the restrictive curricular model that dominates nursing education pedagogy and nursing's professional thinking alike. The model impedes the carrying out of its societal and scholarly mission. Since the mid-1950s the Tyler-type curriculum development models have governed nursing curriculum through institutionalization in the state approval and national accreditation criteria. Only recently have educators begun to critique the Tylerian models, to understand their legacy, and to seek alternatives. Nursing educational practices are being freed from the constraints of behaviorism and rigid behavioral objectives. The deficiencies of the behaviorist models of curriculum development parallel the outmoded morality. One cannot change without the other; in order for the new morality to be effective, it must be pervasive. It must not only address the axiology, but the epistemology, ontologies, metaphysics, and praxis issues of nursing. The behaviorist model and its familial empiricism have influenced not only the Tyler-type curriculum development models, but dictated most of nursing's other cherished elements: (a) the sanctioned modes of inquiry, (b) competency-based evaluation, (c) nursing diagnoses, and (d) the stylized, linear-type, problem-solving format that masquerades as "nursing process."

REDEFINING CURRICULUM

Since it is the behaviorist educational paradigm that has pervaded nursing philosophy, research, and practice, it is in the educational paradigm that we must find a passage to transform the health care system and nursing's role in that system. To do this, several educational issues must be addressed:

1. Curriculum must be viewed not as a plan that lists behavioral objectives as its primary focus as in the past, but as those transactions that take place among teachers and students, and among students and students, so that learning occurs. Lectures alone do not provide opportunities for engagement. When curriculum is defined this way, the teaching methods become the key to the curriculum.

2. Since educative learning for professional nursing practice demands more than the prescribed training of behavioral objective–structured curricula, faculty must change their role. Faculty must change from those who give information, prescribe the lecture content, "regulate the outer phenomenon," and control the educational setting, to those who are experts in learning and content, helping novice learners find their way into the "deeper structures" of the discipline in order to see the patterns, meanings, assumptions, and implications of the content (Stenhouse, 1975, p. 91).

3. Nurse educators in the new age must have as their ultimate goal the graduation of mature, compassionate, scholar-clinicians in health and human caring. Only then will nursing make the transition from employee vocational status to professional status. The question arises, can this be done in the traditional 4-year academic period allotted to "professional" education?

REDEFINING NURSE AND NURSING: THE NURSE AS EDUCATED PERSON AND FULLY EDUCATED HEALTH AND HUMAN CARING PROFESSIONAL

If nursing is to come of age, the educational structure of nursing for a new age must be transformed. Basic to understanding human health and the caring process are areas of study that are uniquely human. The national *Essentials* document of the American Association of Colleges of Nursing

(AACN) identified basic fields of study for nursing students that are both particularistic, such as psychology, sociology, anthropology, and biology, as well as those fields that are not, such as music, language, art, history, and literature. In addition, it has been acknowledged that nurses must understand and deal with human caring values and ethics, moral judgments, political systems, religion, and spirituality, as well as mathematics and philosophy (AACN, 1986).

Sakalys and Watson (1985) reviewed the numerous national studies and reports over the past several years: *The Paideia Proposal* (Adler, 1980); *The President's Report to the Harvard Board of Overseers* (Bok, 1984); *Physicians for the Twenty-First Century* (AAMC, 1984); National Institute of Education Report on Conditions of Excellence in American Higher Education (1984); National Endowment of Humanities Report on the State of Learning in Humanities in Higher Education (Bennett, 1984); and the Association of American Colleges Report on Redefining the Meaning and Purpose of Baccalaureate Degrees (AAC, 1985). They summarized all study recommendations as having commonalities relevant to nursing, including restoration of the centrality of the liberal arts; decreased specialization at the undergraduate level; and increased emphasis on curricular structure and coherence, intellectual skills such as analytical thinking, problem solving, and critical thinking, mastery of principles rather than specific facts, fundamental attitudes, and values; lifelong learning, and broad and rigorous baccalaureate education prior to professional education (Sakalys & Watson, 1985).

The human science morality of health and human caring in postbaccalaureate nursing education is emphasized in the AACN *Essentials* document which recommended redirecting the nursing curricula for professional nursing "so the graduate will exhibit qualities of mind and character that are necessary to live a free and fulfilling life, act in the public interest, locally and globally, and contribute to health care improvements and the nursing profession" (AACN, 1986, p. 4).

As Carter (1988) points out, of all the professional practitioners in the U.S. health care system, "The one field that has the most all-encompassing practice has the lowest level of educational attainment. In pharmacy, medicine, and dentistry, practitioners begin their professional practice at the doctoral level" (p. 51). If nursing is to take itself seriously as a profession and respond to a new morality for a new age, then its educational and practice mission to society must change. Consistent with all higher education reports and directions, as well as nursing studies, a full professional program that values an educated person and professional calls for a postbaccalaureate education. Sakalys and Watson (1986) concluded that the broad base required for both cannot be learned without a number of years of college level study. This professional education should build on a broad liberal educational base and merit a doctor of nursing degree (ND). Moreover, such an educational structure parallels all other major health disciplines (medicine, dentistry, and pharmacy) and affords nurses the opportunity to interact as mature colleagues and peers with the other professionals.

A POSTBACCALAUREATE NURSING DOCTORATE IN HEALTH AND HUMAN CARING

The doctorate as the first professional degree, within a full academic framework, equivalent to the MD, was proposed by Schlotfeldt and developed at Case Western Reserve University in 1978 (Schlotfeldt, 1978). She identified two persistent flaws in baccalaureate nursing programs, which our position addresses: the technical emphasis in the curricula (on the order of a training model), wherein students are required to learn to do—prior to or concurrent with learning to know. (We propose that students learn how to learn from faculty who are expert learners rather than from faculty who are mere imparters of information). The second problem Schlotfeldt identified, which continues as a deficiency, is faculty's lack of responsibility for quality control over the clinical practice world.

Schlotfeldt has continued to point out the widespread inadequacies of the body of knowledge currently being taught in the baccalaureate nursing programs—inadequacies in conceptualizations of nursing, in the structure of nursing knowledge, and in the preparation for scholarship. Specifically, she cited as problems: (a) having to provide both the liberal and the professional education in a 4-year time span; (b) denying nursing's social mission of preserving, restoring, and promoting human health by focusing on diagnosis and treatment of illness; (c) allowing wide latitude among programs in the development and offering of professional knowledge basic to the practice of nursing; and (d) failing to socialize the student to the role of the scholarly practitioner who seeks answers through systematic inquiry (Schlotfeldt, 1985; Forni & Welch, 1987). We further support Grace (1982) who asserted that a parallel professional doctoral pattern designated to prepare the expert practitioner and teacher of nursing should be considered.

ND IN HEALTH AND HUMAN CARING: A MANDATE FOR THE FUTURE

The indicators, in the literature and in the reality of nursing in today's world, clearly show that if nursing is not to be relegated to the role of technician in the health care scene—it must move to the academic professional practice model. No other model will enable nursing to address the changing needs in society, in education, and in professional nursing, allowing nursing to come of age both educationally and professionally. Within such a model several new considerations must come into play. One is emphasizing the uniqueness of nursing with its concern for health and human caring as essential to curing and technology. Another is a humanitarian—human science—liberal educational paradigm (rather than a biomedical science—Tylerian-training model) for both pedagogy and professional practice. A third is the practice-based education necessary to practice discipline, and the fourth is promotion of a new social order in the health care system that accommodates the nurse as the human caring and health expert.

Postbaccalaureate ND preparation for profes-

sional nursing is already an emerging model in nursing education. Both Case Western Reserve and Rush Universities offer the ND at this time and several other universities have it under consideration or are actually developing it. New programs will benefit from the pioneering effort of Case Western; however, the newer programs must be designed to have a more expanded human science focus in the area of human caring knowledge and practices, and must employ liberating—educative teaching—learning methods. These things are not yet commonly part of standard nursing curricula.

For the past few decades, nursing has been clarifying and revising its ethics, theories, and research base to formulate more responsive modalities for health and human caring. During the past 20 years the increasing involvement of nurses in primary care has brought about an expanded view of nursing practice. This, among other features already mentioned, has highlighted the escalating disparity between the nature of nursing as a practice discipline and the amount of time allotted practice in curricula. The present overloaded baccalaureate educational system has been modeled inappropriately on nonnursing-practice disciplines, such as history and English. As a result, a new pattern of professional education is urgently needed and being demanded. A program pattern is emerging that builds on a humanitarian—human science paradigm of health and human caring. It is welded in a practice-based curriculum of postbaccalaureate professional nursing education that builds on the humanities and social sciences along with the biomedical sciences. This can be accomplished by simultaneously restructuring education and scholarly practice in a joint partnership with collaborating clinical agencies.

In light of new societal directions and of changing medical and nursing science and practice, it is timely and appropriate to initiate postbaccalaureate professional doctoral degrees for nursing. Nursing educators today are confronted with the need to reexamine the prospective values, content, pedagogies, and structure needed for professional education and practice in the year 2000 and beyond. The planning and progress of nursing's future cannot be guided by the simple criterion of the numbers of nurses graduated in order to respond to nursing shortages. Professional nurse educators must also address concerns of quality care and social responsiveness. Given nursing education's current status and needs for the future, nursing leaders and major schools of nursing have the responsibility to take a pacesetting position in fashioning appropriate curricula for the 21st century. A nursing doctorate model in health and human caring within the humanitarian–human science paradigm is one way to come of age for a new age, to reach beyond what is not yet, and to redefine nursing's possibilities for a new professional destiny.

REFERENCES

Adler, M. J. (1982). *The Paideia proposal: An educational manifesto*. (On behalf of the members of the Paideia Group.) New York: Macmillan.

Allen, D. (1985). Nursing research and social control: Alternative models of science that emphasize understanding and emancipation. *Image, 17*(2), 58–64.

American Association of Colleges of Nursing (AACN). (1986). *Essentials of college and university education for professional nursing: Final report*. Washington, DC: Author.

Association of American Colleges (AAC). (1985). *Integrity in the college curriculum: A report to the academic community* (Committee report on the AAC's project on redefining the meaning and purpose of baccalaureate degrees; Mark H. Curtis, Chairman). Washington, DC: Author.

Association of American Medical Colleges (AAMC). (1984). *Physicians for the twenty-first century: The GREP report* (Report of the panel on the general professional education of the physician and college preparation; Steven Muller, Chairman). Washington, DC: Author.

Bennett, W. J. (1984). *To reclaim a legacy* (Report of the study group on the state of learning in the humanities in higher education). Washington, DC: National Endowment for the Humanities.

Bok, D. (1984, May–June). Needed: A new way to train doctors (In The President's Report to the Harvard Board of Overseers for 1982–83). *Harvard Magazine*, pp. 32–71.

Callahan, D. (1987). *Setting limits: Medical goals in an aging society*. New York: Simon & Schuster.

Carter, M. (1988). The professional doctorate as an entry level into practice. In *Perspectives in Nursing, 1987–1989* (pp. 49–52). New York: National League for Nursing (NLN).

Forni, P., & Welch, M. (1987). The professional versus the academic model: A dilemma for nursing education. *Journal of Professional Nursing, 3*(5), 291–297.

Gadow, S. (1988). Covenant without cure: Letting go and holding on in chronic illness. In J. Watson & M. A. Ray (Eds.), *The ethics of care and the ethics of cure: Synthesis in chronicity* (pp. 5–14). New York: National League for Nursing.

Grace, H. (1982). Building nursing knowledge: The current state of doctoral education in nursing. In J. J. Fitzpatrick (Compiler), *Proceedings of the Sixth National Forum on Doctoral Education in Nursing* (pp. 1–14). Cleveland: Case Western Reserve University School of Nursing.

Markham, B. (1983). *West with the night*. San Francisco: North Point Press.

Moccia, P. (1988). The fault line: Social activism and caring. *Nursing Outlook, 36*(1), 30–33.

National Institute of Education. (1984). *Involvement in learning: Realizing the potential of American higher education* (Report of the study group on the conditions of excellence in American higher education; Kenneth P. Mortimer, Chairman). Washington, DC: Author.

National League for Nursing (NLN). (1988). *Curriculum revolution: Mandate for change*. New York: Author.

Noddings, N. (1984). *Caring: A feminine approach to ethics and moral development*. Berkeley: University of California Press.

Sakalys, J., & Watson, J. (1985). New directions in higher education: A review of trends. *Journal of Professional Nursing, 1*, 293–299.

Sakalys, J., & Watson, J. (1986). Professional education: Postbaccalaureate education for professional nursing. *Journal of Professional Nursing, 2*(2), 91–97.

Sartre, J. P. (1956). *Being and nothingness*. New York: Washington Square Press.

Schlotfeldt, R. (1978). The professional doctorate: Rationale and characteristics. *Nursing Outlook, 26*(5), 302–311.

Schlotfeldt, R. (1985). Lessons from past can help nursing reach its goals. (Editorial). *The American Nurse, 17*(2), 4, 18.

Stenhouse, L. (1975). *An introduction to curriculum research and development*. London: Heinemann Educational Books.

Watson, J. (1985). *Nursing: Human science and human care*. Norwalk, CT: Appleton-Century-Crofts.

✳   **EDITOR'S QUESTIONS FOR DISCUSSION**   ✳

Discuss nursing as a human science of caring. What are the assumptions and issues that must be addressed to develop nursing as a science of caring? Does the academic professional practice model mean that professional nurses should have a baccalaureate degree in the arts or sciences prior to obtaining a knowledge base of their discipline? Suggest variations of the academic professional model. What are alternatives to the postbaccalaureate professional doctoral degree? How is the nursing content offered in an ND degree program different from that offered in graduate education and for a postmaster's doctoral degree? What is the difference in the nursing content and position or role preparation in an ND program, and that in a baccalaureate nursing program, or a "bypass" (baccalaureate) master's nursing program?

Suggest or make recommendations for how the human science focus can be developed in curriculum for the knowledge and practice of human caring. Propose content for undergraduate nursing programs that could be included in a humanitarian–human science–liberal education paradigm that would be different from the standard biomedical science–Tylerian-training model for pedagogy and professional practice. Discuss examples of teaching methods that can be used to promote interactions between teachers and students, as suggested by the authors.

15

Specialization in Nursing:
Logic or chaos

Mariah Snyder, Ph.D., R.N., F.A.A.N.

OVERVIEW

Specialization is a narrowing of the focus of concern within a discipline or profession. According to the American Nurses' Association's *Nursing: A Social Policy Statement* (1980), specialization is a mark of the advancement of a profession or discipline. Much diversity is found in the types of specialization that exist in nursing. In most instances, however, that specialization focuses on the delivery of nursing care and not areas of concentration for development of knowledge within the discipline. Congruency between the categories used for designating practice realms and the areas of knowledge development in the discipline is lacking.

Traditionally specialization has prepared nurses for functional roles, with administration and education being the initial roles offered in educational institutions. A third functional area of specialization, clinical specialist, was introduced in the late 1940s. This necessitated that the program of study be expanded to include content on the specific patient population for whom the nurses were being prepared to provide advanced nursing care. Since the inception of the clinical specialist role, many areas of specialization within this role have evolved. However, it is difficult to determine an overriding framework for categorizing these areas of study offered in master's programs. This is so because body systems, diseases or conditions, developmental levels, places where care is delivered, and, occasionally, nursing phenomena are all designated as areas for specialization.

The emergence of doctoral programs in nursing has added to the diversity of specialization in nursing. Areas of study are equally diverse as those existing in master's programs, with functional areas, body systems, and nursing phenomena listed as areas for possible study in doctoral programs (National League for Nursing, 1985). Designating areas of specialization according to nursing phenomena, which would seem very appropriate for doctoral education, has not been widely adopted.

Ways in which specialization can arise within a profession are delineated in *Nursing: A Social Policy Statement* (American Nurses' Association, 1980). These are:

> The amount and complexity of knowledge necessitates that some members give particular attention to delimited practice areas.
> Members seek greater depth of understanding of phenomena related to a specific area of practice.
> Public attention and funding focus attention on an area that has not previously been of concern.

Complexity of services in an area demands that new knowledge be developed.

Professionals seek ways to expand their scope of knowledge and practice.

All of the above have contributed to the types of specialization found in nursing. The knowledge and technology explosion in health care has necessitated that groups of nurses focus on particular patient populations, so that they may obtain an in-depth grasp of the nursing needs of these patients. Critical care nursing and related subspecialties are examples of specialization arising from the introduction of complex technology in patient care. Initiation of diagnosis related groups (DRGs) altered the delivery of health care; the acuteness of condition of patients requiring care in their homes prompted the development of home health care specialists.

Current attention to acquired immunodeficiency syndrome (AIDS) will probably result in funding for educational programs that will prepare specialists to care for patients with this disease. Other major health care problems for which specialty programs have been established include gerontology and oncology. Additionally nurses have identified areas requiring knowledge development, such as human responses to events disruptive to health and health promotion; a few education programs that allow nurses to specialize in these areas have been developed. Since no one mechanism has served as the basis for the development of specialist programs, the result is a marked diversity in how specialization is conceptualized.

This diversity in specialization has had both positive and negative consequences for nursing. On the positive side, areas of specialization provide evidence of nursing's response to societal health care needs (McKevitt, 1986); for example, graduates of gerontology specialist programs have made significant contributions to the health of the elderly. Then, too, collaborative relationships with other professions have been furthered by clinical specialists, with advanced knowledge and skill in a particular area of practice, interacting with colleagues concerning care issues. Additionally the increase in research articles in specialty nursing journals reflects the identification of practice problems by clinical specialists and the seeking of solutions for improving nursing care. On the negative side, specialization according to diseases or conditions and functional roles has mitigated against nurses looking for commonalities of concern to nursing and has hampered the development of the body of nursing knowledge that could serve as a basis for nursing practice. Focus on preparation for functional roles directs emphasis on function rather than on the content of practice. Finally specialization has occurred on many educational levels within nursing, and it is difficult to identify the knowledge base of the person who purports to be a specialist. This creates problems in communication both within the profession and with the public.

Before looking at specialization at the master's and doctoral levels in nursing, several questions are posed for the reader to consider. What is the nature of the current specialization in nursing? Does any framework for organizing specialization in nursing emerge from the current manner in which specialties are defined? Can a framework for specialization be developed that would be meaningful in the practice realm and in the organization of nursing knowledge?

SPECIALIZATION AT THE MASTER'S LEVEL

Preparation for specialization in nursing practice has largely been conceptualized as occurring at the master's level. Early specialization occurred in the functional areas of administration and education, with specialization in clinical areas (clinical specialist) and practice settings (practitioner) being introduced much later. Many programs continue to offer specialization in the traditional functional areas of administration and education. Several programs require students to select a clinical area of specialization, in addition to the functional roles of administration and education.

Psychiatric—mental health nursing, medical-surgical nursing, and pediatrics were the initial areas for clinical specialization. Because clinical specialists were initially prepared to function in hospital settings, the areas of specialization emanated from how hospital units were organized. As the size and number of specialty programs increased, subspecialty areas developed with much diversity found in titles attached to these areas. Williamson (1983) identified 130 titles designating areas of specialization in nursing. Subspecialties, particularly in medical-surgical nursing, have emerged according to disease entities: cardiovascular, neuroscience, diabetes, nephrology, oncology, and respiratory are some of the commonly found subspecialties.

Some categories of specialization are focused on where the health care is delivered. Community health nursing is the most commonly known area of specialization that is based on place of practice. More recently, specialty programs in occupational health, home health care, hospice, rural health, and school nursing have appeared. Cary (1986) identified case manager of patient services, client advocate, community coordinator, and health promoter as new areas in which advanced nurse specialists are needed to assure continuity of care.

Human development levels are also used for designating areas of specialization within nursing. Programs in nursing care of newborns, children, adololescents, adults (sometimes broken into early, middle, and late), and elderly exist. Subspecialties within these have been formed, such as mental health nursing for adolescents.

The development of nurse practitioner programs in the late 1960s added another means for specialization at the master's level. Practitioner programs originated in response to a need for health care for particular populations who were deemed underserved because of physician shortages. Nurse practitioners are prepared largely to function in clinics and community settings. Specialization within the nurse practitioner role has been focused on phases of human development, with gerontology, adult, children, and midwifery being the commonly found specialties.

The differences that have existed between nurse practitioners and clinical nurse specialists are beginning to blur. Several authors have described roles that nurse practitioners have assumed in hospital settings (Ahrens & Norris, 1983; McCarty, 1986; Silver, Murphy, & Gitterman, 1984). The functions delineated by these authors for the role of the nurse practitioner are similar to those performed by clinical specialists. Nurses prepared in clinical specialist programs are functioning outside of the hospital, in sites such as home health care agencies and nurse-operated clinics. As federal funding for practitioner programs has diminished, educational programs are focusing more attention on ways in which clinical specialist and nurse practitioner programs can be combined. McCarty (1986) suggested calling the graduate of a combined program a "specialist in nursing" (p. 24).

Recently discussions have occurred regarding the plausibility of specialization in highly refined subspeciality areas of nursing. Declining federal monies for discrete specialty programs has prompted nursing education to consider alternative means for preparing advanced nurse specialists. A need for advanced practice specialists who have a broad foundation in certain areas of nursing practice has been identified (Reed & Hoffman, 1986; Welch, 1987). This advanced generalist would engage in a comprehensive approach to health care and be concerned with holistic health concerns. Having a broader foundation for practice would also provide the graduate with more options for practice; knowledge and expertise to function in several areas of practice will enable the person to function more readily in another area, when the current specialty in which the nurse is practicing disappears. Preparing generalists at the master's level is a break from traditional thinking in nursing that holds that generalist preparation occurs at the baccalaureate level and education for the specialist role takes place in a master's program.

Several nurses have questioned whether specialization, particularly for the role of clinical specialist, is possible at the master's level because of the large amount of knowledge and expertise needed to carry out this role (Andreoli, 1987; Bergesen, 1971). The length of master's programs in nursing vary from 9 to 28 months (Sills, 1983), with approximately one-third of the programs requiring 2 full academic years for completion (Feild, 1983). Thus the foundation that students receive for specialization varies greatly. Andreoli (1987) and Snyder (in press, 1989) recommend that specialization for clinical practice be at the doctoral level in doctor of nursing science programs. Graduates would be prepared to not only identify clinical nursing problems, but also engage in the research needed to find solutions for the problem. Such a change could have a profound effect on the delivery of nursing care.

SPECIALIZATION AT THE DOCTORAL LEVEL

Two main types of programs in doctoral education exist: doctor of philosophy and doctor of nursing science. Of the 35 doctoral programs in existence in 1985, 7 offered a DNS degree, 25 offered the PhD degree, 1 school offered both, and 1 offered the EdD degree (NLN, 1985). Despite the stated theoretical differences between the PhD and DNS degrees, nursing has not clearly differentiated the expectations for graduates of the two types of programs. In my review of the areas of study listed in the National League for Nursing's *Doctoral Programs in Nursing* (1985) no prominent feature that would differentiate one type of program from the other could be distinguished.

Considerable diversity in the areas of study (specialization) offered in doctoral education exists. Areas of study listed in *Doctoral Programs in Nursing* (NLN, 1985) include role development in administration (nursing services and educational programs) and in nursing education; clinical areas, such as medical-surgical, pediatrics, and psychiatric−mental health nursing; broad areas, such as nursing science, theory development, and nursing research; and specific nursing phenomena. No one framework for identifying specialization at the doctoral level emerged from the offerings currently listed.

Preparation for the role of researcher is paramount in doctoral education, with several programs listing research as an area of specialization (NLN, 1985). Although program descriptions rarely provide direction on the nature of areas in which research specialization occurs at that school, categorization of doctoral dissertations supplies indicators of these areas. Loomis (1985) examined dissertation titles and abstracts from doctoral programs in nursing; she found that the majority (78.4%) of the dissertation

abstracts were concerned with clinical nursing research, while 21.6% explored social issues in nursing. Categories developed by Loomis (1985), in her analysis of types of clinical nursing research, were actual/potential health problems, human response systems, and clinical decision making. Major units used in classifying dissertations on social issues were professional policy issues, unit of analysis, and social decision making. Loomis (1985) noted that each doctoral program appears to "specialize" in types of research conducted. She further observed that a major factor determining the topics explored in a particular program is the research expertise of faculty members at specific schools.

DIRECTIONS FOR THE FUTURE

A classification system for specialization in nursing does not emerge from the areas of study listed for master's and doctoral programs (NLN, 1985; NLN, 1986). Specialization for specific functional roles is evident at both the master's and doctoral levels, but using functional roles as a basis for classifying specialization does not encompass all offerings, particularly some doctoral offerings. Distinctions are not clearly delineated between the expertise possessed by persons prepared for the same functional role, such as administrator, at the master's and doctoral levels. Although advanced education for functional roles is needed, specialization that focuses solely on roles does little to further the body of nursing knowledge that is the basis for practice.

A number of structures for the organization of nursing knowledge have been proposed (Aydelotte, 1987; Donaldson and Crowley, 1978; McKay, 1977). Aydelotte (1987) suggests dividing the delivery of health care into four branches: health promotion, health education, self-help, and health evaluation branch; chronic disease management branch; trauma and critical illness branch; and frail elderly, physical limited elderly, and dying branch. These categories are similar to the divisions used at the National Center for Nursing Research (Merritt, 1986). The Center's divisions are health promotion and disease prevention, acute and chronic illness, and systems delivery. A major benefit from using

Aydelotte's proposed areas is that they are readily understood by the public and apply to clients across health care settings. Welch (1987) supports the use of these four categories for areas of specialization in nursing, for they allow nurses to have broader areas of specialization and thus enable nurses to function more effectively in the health care system. A major drawback to the use of this framework, however, is that nursing phenomena are not identified. Further, distinguishing between areas of concern in the four areas may be difficult; for example, persons with chronic illnesses and the frail elderly may have very similar nursing problems.

Nursing diagnoses and nursing interventions are two other taxonomies that are being developed in nursing (McLane, 1987; Snyder, 1987). Both of these, however, are in the developmental stage. Although specialization related to some of the nursing diagnoses would be feasible, meaningful specialization would best be thought of in terms of the nine human response patterns that serve as the major category headings for the organization of nursing diagnoses. These patterns are (a) exchanging, (b) communicating, (c) relating, (d) valuing, (e) choosing, (f) moving, (g) perceiving, (h) knowing, and (i) feeling. Using nursing interventions for areas of specialization is feasible for the practice realm, although interventions do not encompass all areas of concern to nursing. Specialization could be in terms of interventions such as stress management techniques or cognitive strategies. Nursing diagnoses and nursing interventions are not focused on a specific care setting or disease entity, but rather are directed at problems that fall within the scope of nursing.

Another structure to consider as a framework for specialization is a taxonomy of human responses for which nursing interventions would be appropriate. A number of responses are elaborated in *Nursing: A Social Policy Statement* (ANA, 1980). Responses include self-care limitations, impaired functioning in areas such as rest and sleep, pain, emotional problems, distortion of symbolic functions, deficiencies in decision making, self-image changes, dysfunctional perceptual orientations to time, strains related to life processes, and problematic affiliative relationships (ANA, 1980, p. 10). The list provides exam-ples of human responses of concern to nursing and is not meant to be comprehensive in scope. Carrieri, Lindsey, and West (1986) note other responses of concern to nursing; responses identified include anorexia, fatigue, ischemia, and alterations in consciousness. Areas of study in several doctoral programs are specified in terms of human responses.

Utilizing a common framework for specialization would assist nursing to define more clearly areas of study in graduate education, in addition to helping define the scope of nursing. Differentiation of expectations regarding research expertise for graduates of doctoral and master's programs has been developed (ANA, 1981). Further delineation of expectations for other role functions of nurses prepared at the master's and doctoral levels is needed. Greater clarity on the expertise for the two levels will assist educational programs in revamping existing specialty programs.

The necessity for an overriding framework for specialization in nursing can be argued. However, the enormous diversity in the types of specialty programs that currently exist is confusing for nurses and the public. A framework would assist the public in understanding the nature and scope of nursing practice, assist prospective students in selecting a program that fits their interests, help to clarify graduate education, and most importantly, contribute to the development of the body of nursing knowledge, which would ultimately improve patient care.

Because nursing is developing its body of knowledge and is also part of a dynamic health care system and society, the framework would be continually evolving. New specialties will emerge as the knowledge in the discipline of nursing develops. Likewise, nursing must be responsive to new health care problems and to changes in the delivery of health care and prepare practitioners who will provide expert nursing care. However, determination of a general framework for specialization in nursing that is usable in the practice realm and also for organizing nursing knowledge would provide guidance to educational programs in developing areas of specialization. Such a framework would also facilitate the transfer of research findings into the practice realm.

REFERENCES

Ahrens, W., & Norris, B. (1983). Expanded roles in critical care: Nurse practitioner or clinical specialist? *Dimensions of Critical Care Nursing, 2,* 98–100.

Andreoli, K. G. (1987). Specialization and graduate curriculum: Finding the fit. *Nursing & Health Care, 7,* 65–69.

American Nurses' Association (ANA). (1980). *Nursing: A social policy statement.* Kansas City, MO: Author.

American Nurses' Association (ANA). (1981). *Guidelines for the investigative functions of nurses.* Kansas City, MO: Author.

Aydelotte, M. K. (1987). Nursing's preferred future. *Nursing Outlook, 35,* 114–120.

Bergesen, B. (1971). Preparation for clinical specialization. *Journal of Nursing Education, 10,* 21–26.

Carrieri, V. K., Lindsey, A. M., & West, C. M. (1986). *Pathophysiological phenomena in nursing: Human responses to illness.* Philadelphia: W. B. Saunders.

Cary, A. (1986). Specialization without walls: Community-based nursing. In *Patterns in specialization: Challenge to the curriculum* (Publication No. 15-2154, pp. 257–269). New York: National League for Nursing.

Donaldson, S. K., and Crowley, D. M. (1978). The discipline of nursing. *Nursing Outlook, 26,* 113–120.

Feild, L. (1983). Current trends in education and implications for the future. In A. Hamric & J. Spross (Eds.), *The clinical nurse specialist in theory and practice* (pp. 237–256). New York: Grune & Stratton.

Loomis, M. E. (1985). An analysis of dissertation abstracts and titles: 1976–1982. *Nursing Research, 34,* 113–119.

McCarty, P. (1986). NPs, clinical specialists share nursing's cutting edge. *The American Nurse, 19,* 24.

McKay, R. P. (1977). Discussion: discipline of nursing—syntactical structure and relation with other disciplines and the profession of nursing. In M. V. Batey (Ed.), *Communicating nursing research: Optimizing environments for health: Nursing's unique perspective, Volume 10* (pp. 23–30). Boulder, CO: Western Interstate Commission for Higher Education.

McKevitt, R. K. (1986). Trends in master's education in nursing. *Journal of Professional Nursing, 2,* 225–233.

McLane, A. (Ed.) (1987). *Classification of nursing diagnoses.* St. Louis: C. V. Mosby.

Merritt, D. H. (1986). The National Center for Nursing Research. *Image, 18,* 84–85.

National League for Nursing (NLN). (1985). *Doctoral programs in nursing* (Publication No. 15-1448). New York: Author.

National League for Nursing (NLN). (1986). *Master's education in nursing: Route to opportunities in contemporary nursing* (Publication No. 15-1312). New York: Author.

Reed, S. B., & Hoffman, S. E. (1986). The enigma of graduate nursing education: Advanced generalist? specialist? *Nursing & Health Care, 7,* 43–49.

Sills, G. M. (1983). The role and function of the clinical nurse specialist. In N. Chaska (Ed.), *The nursing profession: A time to speak* (pp. 563–579). New York: McGraw-Hill.

Silver, H. K., Murphy, M. A., & Gitterman, B. A. (1984). The hospital nurse practitioner in pediatrics. *American Journal of Diseases of Children, 138,* 237–239.

Snyder, M. (1987, August). *Nursing interventions: Essential or irrelevant?* Paper presented at the University of Wisconsin–Eau Claire, Eau Claire, WI.

Snyder, M. (1989). Educational preparation of the CNS. In A. Hamric, & J. Spross (Eds.), *The clinical nurse specialist in theory and practice* (325-342). New York: Grune & Stratton.

Welch, C. C. (1987). A window of opportunity. *Nursing Outlook, 35,* 282–284.

Williamson, J. A. (1983). Master's education: A need for nomenclature. *Image, 15,* 99–101.

✳ EDITOR'S QUESTIONS FOR DISCUSSION ✳

Discuss the extent to which master's level preparation is a generalist preparation rather than a specialist preparation. Discuss the extent to which specialization according to disease conditions and functional roles have inhibited nurses from looking at commonalities of concern to nursing, as well as hindered the development of nursing knowledge for nursing practice? To what extent does using the term functional role imply that a specialized knowledge base is not required nor inherent in specific nursing roles such as nurse administrators, nurse education, clinical specialist, and nurse practitioner?

Suggest a framework or frameworks for specialization that might be developed that would be meaningful both for nursing practice and the development of nursing knowledge. What should be the criteria to determine whether or not a nursing program should develop a major area of concentration in a specialty area? How should the area, level of specialization, and content be determined in a graduate program? What should be the areas and level(s) of specialization offered in doctoral programs, and why? How might focus and content be different in doctoral programs from those in master's programs for areas of specialization such as critical care and gerontological nursing? What implications are there in Snyder's chapter concerning content addressed by Lenz (Chapter 16)?

Indicate some mechanisms and strategies for developing specialist-type programs, and the rationale, level of content, and outcomes for such programs. What is the most effective process for faculty in developing a new major within a specialized area of content to maintain a unified curriculum? Discuss the preparation of nurse practitioners and clinical nurse specialists in relation to Chapter 43 by Whitney, and Chapter 41 by Yasko and Dudjak. Defend your belief on whether or not the clinical nurse specialist and nurse practitioner content and role should be combined as one area of specialization. Should a global framework for specialization in nursing be developed for doctoral programs?

16

Doctoral Education:
Present views, future directions

Elizabeth R. Lenz, Ph.D., R.N., F.A.A.N.

After a decade of unprecedented increase in the number of doctoral programs in nursing, the doctorate is firmly established as the discipline's terminal degree. The early difficulties encountered in justifing the legitimacy of and need for doctoral programs in nursing have evolved into issues concerning their nature, quality, future directions, and ultimate impact. Some of the key issues confronting planners, deliverers, and consumers that have potential impact on future graduate nursing education are discussed. Particular attention is given to the degree of diversity that exists among and within programs, including appraisal of how much is considered desirable. The discussion is limited to post-entry-level doctoral education.

GROWTH

Perhaps the most remarkable feature of doctoral nursing education has been its growth and expansion. Between 1977 and 1987, the number of doctoral programs in schools of nursing increased 156%, from 18 to 46. During essentially the same period the number of annual graduations nearly tripled, growing from 59 in 1977 to 229 in 1986 (American Association of Colleges of Nursing, 1987a; Styles, 1987). As many as 40 more programs are currently being planned.

Although these data are welcome indicators that the need for increased numbers of doctorally prepared nurses is being addressed, cautionary notes have been sounded about the effects of too-rapid acceleration. There is concern that schools of nursing may prematurely initiate programs in their eagerness to enjoy some of the pride, prestige, and challenge associated with offering a doctoral program. A major potential problem is that schools may enter the arena of doctoral education without an adequate resource base of qualified faculty, support facilities and services, and funding to assure quality. For example, in a document to guide doctoral program planning in the southern United States, it was recommended as a program prerequisite that there be a core of 5 to 10 faculty who are not only doctorally prepared, but also have previous experience with conducting research, procuring grants, and guiding dissertation research (McPheeters, 1985). Amos (1985) suggested that in order to provide a quality doctoral program, a school should have at least two or three ongoing major research projects in which to involve students. It is questionable whether all existing programs meet these criteria and whether faculty resources can be developed quickly enough to meet the requirements of new and expanding programs.

Rapid quantitative growth has accentuated emphasis on defining, attaining, monitoring, and preserving quality in doctoral nursing education. Traditionally this has been the domain of the degree-granting institution (Downs, 1988). Some recent activities suggest growing interest in moving quality control beyond the institution to national or regional levels. For example, a national invitational conference was sponsored jointly by the Division of Nursing, (U.S.D.H.H.S), and the American Association of Colleges of Nursing (AACN) in 1985 to generate consensually agreed-on indicators of program quality (AACN, 1987b; Jamann, 1985). The indicators are sufficiently comprehensive to provide guidance for self-assessment, external review, and standard setting. They address faculty qualifications and activities, programs of study and core curricular elements, learning resources, student qualifications and policies, the research environment and infrastructure, and elements to be included in program evaluation.

Regional activity is exemplified by the Southern Regional Education Board's sponsorship of cost studies, a planning document (McPheeters, 1985), and a graduate education task force (Kelley and Stullenbarger, 1987). The outputs of these activities include not only data that can be used for planning purposes, but also some specific guidelines and recommendations for future policy. Some of the latter are controversial. For example, it was suggested that priority be placed on increasing enrollment in existing programs, rather than on opening new ones. In light of current growth-generated concerns and quality-oriented activities, it is not surprising that questions are increasingly being raised about whether professional accreditation should be expanded to include doctoral programs, and if so, which organization should be responsible (Spero, 1987; Styles, 1987).

ENROLLMENT PATTERNS: PART-TIME STUDY

Consistent with graduate nursing education as a whole, there has been an increasing trend toward part-time study in recent years, with part-time students now outnumbering full-time students (Styles, 1987). Full-time enrollees continue to represent a sizable minority overall and in some programs constitute the majority or entirety of the student body; however, there is considerable market pressure on schools to expand part-time study opportunities.

Although a few doctoral programs were designed primarily for part-time students, questions have been raised about how well most programs, particularly those designed for full-time study, are accommodating part-time students. One relatively recent response by several schools to the market demand for part-time study has been to develop summer options that are designed for students with academic appointments. Another has been to schedule classes in late afternoon or evening time slots, or to consolidate them on one day a week or on weekends. These solutions are not without problems for the institution; they place a considerable burden on faculty, often require hiring temporary supplementary faculty at considerable cost, and may compromise the schedules and learning experiences of the full-time enrollees. Part-time students not only spend up to three times longer completing their programs of study, but also may receive a less than optimal educational experience. Their periods of study are often episodic, learning experiences may lack continuity, prolonged and intensive mentorship experiences are virtually precluded, and there is often limited opportunity for contact with faculty and peers for support and mutual learning. Noting these problems, participants at the joint conference on doctoral program quality recommended that part-time students be assisted and encouraged toward full-time status (Jamann, 1985). A possible consequence of institutional pressure toward full-time study is that students may attempt simultaneously to work and study full time, at best a stressful and difficult situation that is not conducive to learning.

The trend toward part-time study has created a dilemma for the programs that were designed and structured primarily for the full-time student. The predicament is whether to hold to the "ideal" full-time pattern that is deemed optimal for socializing researchers, at the risk of losing out in market competition; or whether to adjust course sequences and learning experiences to accommodate part-time students, at the risk of compromising or having to redefine the desired product. Considerations in reaching a position on the issue include the philosophical stance of the faculty regarding the nature of education and the teaching-learning process, the purposes and goals of the program, availability of faculty and financial resources to support full-time students, and the program's current market position and anticipated competition. A decision to allow or encourage part-time study should carry with it a commitment to attempt to assure peer and faculty support and to provide adequate mechanisms and opportunities for socialization into the researcher or advanced clinician role.

DIVERSITY IN DOCTORAL NURSING EDUCATION

Certainly doctoral nursing programs are not all alike. There are striking differences, for example, in enrollment (from under 5 to over 350) (AACN, 1987a) and in credit requirements (from 0 to over 70 postmaster's semester credits). Particularly at a time when quality is being questioned and accreditation suggested, questions need to be raised about the extent to which diversity is and should continue to be characteristic of doctoral nursing education. To what extent does and should a common core of content exist in all programs in the discipline? With how much consistency are specialty areas defined? How much diversity exists and is desirable within programs?

Program Type: Differentiation by Degree

One of the most frequently discussed bases for program differentiation is the type of degree offered. There have been repeated admonitions to clarify and effect distinctions between programs offering the two major types of doctoral degrees: the academic and the professional doctorate (Downs, 1978; Grace, 1983). Recent empirical evidence suggests that there remain more similarities than differences between programs offering the two types of degrees (Murphy, 1985). Snyder-Halpern (1986) found that both types supported purposes aimed toward preparing teachers and applied researchers; however, preparation of clinicians was more likely to be a stated purpose of professional degree programs, and

preparation of pure researchers a key purpose only of the PhD programs. Professional degree programs were more likely to emphasize communicating research findings. She concluded that although the two types of programs were similar in most respects, the differences observed were consistent with the characteristics of the two types of degrees, and that these differences suggested "the presence of diversity within the profession's emerging doctoral degree structure" (p. 365).

Review of printed materials describing 29 of the 46 existing doctoral programs and phone interviews with 12 doctoral program directors (3 in each of the 4 major regions) revealed that the professional programs were more likely than the PhD programs to include clinical and role courses and practica and to require courses in nursing issues and policy. The PhD programs tended to provide greater depth in statistics and research methods and were more likely to include a research residency or practicum and research projects additional to the dissertation. That some differences are becoming apparent is a step forward in lessening the confusion that potential students and employers of graduates have been experiencing. To the extent that the two types of programs are actually producing different products, the current preponderance of PhD (33) over professional degree programs (12) may be resulting in underproduction of graduates with an applied focus and competencies that are relevant to designing and evaluating improved, innovative, cost-effective care (Andreoli, 1987). It is consistent with nursing school administrators' preferences for PhD program graduates to fill faculty positions (Lenz & Morton, 1988).

Diversity in Required Core Content

A common pattern in doctoral programs is to designate a core of content that makes up 25% to 85% of the curriculum and is required of all students. There seem to be several content areas—primarily metatheory, research methods, and nursing theories and conceptual frameworks—that are common to virtually all doctoral programs (Beare, Gray, & Ptak, 1981). The AACN "Position Statement" (1987b) recommended that programs of study include the following content areas, but not necessarily in formal coursework (p. 72):

1. History and philosophy and their relation to the development of knowledge
2. Existing substantive nursing knowledge
3. Theory construction
4. Critical analysis of social, ethical, and political issues of importance to the discipline
5. Research designs, methods, and techniques appropriate to the level of doctoral study
6. Data management, tools, and technology
7. Student research opportunities

Published materials and verbal information regarding 34 of the current doctoral programs were reviewed to determine the extent to which the recommended topics are included in required courses. Admittedly, examining only course requirements underrepresented the actual extent of content inclusion because some programs have no specified course or credit requirements, others designate some of the content areas as optional, and others may include content areas in courses without identifying them in either the titles or descriptions. The content elements most consistently required in over 75% of the programs were quantitative methods (in 32 programs), statistics (26), and nursing theory analysis and construction (31, of which 17 require content in theory construction). Half (16) of the programs required courses in philosophy. Fewer required courses in issue analysis (12), concept analysis and formulation (13), and history (4). As noted earlier in the discussion of type of degree, professional degree curricula were much more likely to include clinical and role course requirements. Whereas all of the professional programs examined required either clinical or role courses or both, only 25% of the PhD programs had these requirements.

The requirement that cognate courses or a minor field of study be taken in a related discipline is variable, undoubtedly influenced not only by the faculty's stance about the degree of nursing's interdependence with other basic and applied disciplines, but also by institutional requirements, norms, and politics. Of the programs whose curricula were examined, over half (20) included a cognate or nonnursing minor as a required component. Several of the program directors interviewed indicated that ability to engage in interdisciplinary study was a real strength of their programs and consistent with patterns in their universities. Although most allowed the student to choose the discipline(s) that best complements her or his chosen specialty, two programs involved specified dual majors, and a third specified the cognate discipline in which students must study.

Specialties

Unlike many disciplines whose subspecialties are defined relatively consistently across educational programs and practice settings, nursing is currently organizing its knowledge domain and identifying its specialties in many different ways. The diversity is even more apparent at the doctoral level than at the master's program level. Many schools have retained the medical-model scheme and terminology at the master's level, but have crossed traditional lines in defining (or alternatively leaving undefined) specialties within their doctoral programs. Specialties are a particularly interesting aspect of program diversity because they generally reflect the areas of substantive content that are being emphasized within a given program. It is common, but not universal, that one or two courses must be taken by all students choosing a given specialty; alternatively, the specialty may be developed solely through elective and cognate courses. Much of the curriculum's research-based, discipline-specific content, including middle-range theories and nursing research findings, tends to be included in specialty courses.

Of the existing programs 11 (24%) listed specialties with medical-model specifications (National League for Nursing, 1987). Perhaps because of their closer link to the practice arena in which specialties are most easily communicated in medical-model terminology, professional degree programs were more likely than PhD programs to list medical-model specialties. Functional roles, particularly administration, seem to be experiencing a resurgence, being listed as possible specialties in nearly half of the programs (20). Noteworthy is that four professional degree programs limited their offerings to functional role areas.

Among the other schemes used to divide the domain of the discipline into doctoral program subspecialties were developmental/life process stages (3); focal systems or populations, that is, individual, family, community, environment, organizations (6); disciplinary perspectives, that is, psychosocial, physiological (2); levels of prevention (2); and other schemes representing the unique perspective or research interests of a given faculty group (6). In a majority of the programs examined in detail, these alternatives to the medical-model approach did not parallel the departmental structure.

In 14 programs, more commonly those offering the academic doctorate, subspecialties were not differentiated. Rather, students were said to major in nursing research, nursing science, or clinical nursing research. Directors of several programs without subspecialties indicated that the advantage of such an approach is that it (a) promotes flexibility, (b) encourages students to cross traditional or departmental boundaries in defining their research foci, (c) allows them to take full advantage of faculty expertise, and (d) allows the evolving phenomena of nursing, rather than a preexisting structure, to dictate program content. On the other hand, it may be difficult to communicate to prospective students and others those substantive areas in which the program and its graduates are particularly strong.

There is a growing tendency in several programs without specialties to begin to identify possible emphasis areas within the broader domain, in which in-depth study will be available through courses and experience with faculty scholars. Ideally these areas reflect faculty strengths and the topics being investigated in clusters of faculty research projects. This approach helps provide some common foci for student recruitment and content development, while being sufficiently flexible to accommodate changes in faculty composition and research funding. Federal funding has been instrumental in helping schools with doctoral programs develop such emphasis areas. For example, the Division of Nursing's (U.S.D.H.H.S.) Nursing Research Emphasis Grants were designed to promote faculty research in specified emphasis areas, and Institutional National Research Service Awards, funded by the National Institutes of Health, can be used to support predoctoral and postdoctoral study in areas of departmental and interdepartmental strength.

Within-Program Diversity

One of the difficult questions facing doctoral programs is how much internal diversity in specialty foci and students' patterns of study is desirable and manageable. In part, the extent of within-program diversity is determined by the degree to which designated specialty areas define and delimit program content and the substantive interests of the students admitted. Two very different positions are being taken within existing programs. One is that specialties should be identified on the basis of faculty strengths, then content developed and students recruited and admitted accordingly. Students whose research interests and goals do not match the identified specialty areas may be denied admission, irrespective of their academic qualifications. This approach, which limits within-program diversity, allows efficient use of resources; it also provides student access to the faculty expertise and research opportunities needed to develop depth of knowledge. However, well-qualified students may be turned away, or those with innovative ideas may be dissuaded from pursuing them if they depart from program foci.

Another position is that students should be free to structure and define their own specialty areas and should not be constrained by a preexisting specialty structure. Specialized content is obtained by means of independent study experiences and existing courses in nursing or other departments. Elective courses are developed and offered when warranted by sufficient student interest in a given topic. Experts to guide the student, if not available on the nursing faculty, are located in other departments or institutions. This looser approach, while maximizing responsiveness to unique student needs and fostering creativity, places heavy demands on both student and faculty and may result in program content being process-oriented. It is an approach that fosters within-program diversity, too much of which may have the disadvantage of compelling faculty to take responsibility for substantive areas with which they are only marginally familiar. A possible compromise position assumed by several schools has been to publicize and inform clearly prospective and incoming students about the areas in which the program has particular strength, yet offer admission to some outstanding students whose research interests have only a marginal fit. Students often redefine their interest areas as they are exposed to new ideas, or they modify them after matriculation to match better program strengths.

Another source of within-program diversity is derived from students' goals and motives for pursuing doctoral education. Within the discipline, there is currently considerable variation. At one extreme are students who view the doctorate as the first step on a new career trajectory that is likely to include not only doctoral, but also postdoctoral education. These persons are likely to terminate job commitments and devote full-time effort to study and research. Often willing and able to move, they examine several programs and ultimately select the one whose focus and strengths best match their personal and professional interests and goals. At the other extreme are students who view the doctorate strictly as a credential that needs to be obtained in order to keep or upgrade a current job. These persons do not anticipate altering an established career to accommodate doctoral study; thus they prefer to remain in a given geographical area and to schedule doctoral study around job commitments that are given higher priority. Most students are, of course, between these two admittedly stereotypical and overstated extremes. Neither pattern is inherently preferable, since persons embark on doctoral education at very different points in their lives and careers, for different reasons, and with different goals. Certainly the needs of the two extreme types of students differ, and problems arise when there is a lack of fit among faculty expectations, program design, and student needs. It is questionable that a given program can optimize the learning of both types of students simultaneously.

FUTURE TRENDS

Diversity has long been a desired characteristic of doctoral nursing education. According to Jamann (1985):

> Diversity in types of programs offered, in emphasis or focus of content, in funding mechanisms, and in research efforts was, and is, recognized as a strength in the development of the science and professional of nursing. (p. 91)

Despite some limited consistency in core content, there is currently considerable diversity among programs in the core elements included, as well as in the subspecialties offered. Moreover, differential patterns are beginning to emerge between academic and professional degree programs. It seems appropriate that there be a few consensually agreed-on areas of knowledge that every nurse with a terminal degree in the discipline should be expected to have mastered; otherwise the degree lacks meaning within and outside nursing. These "essential" components can and should change over time as the discipline evolves. It seems equally appropriate that the degree being offered, the philosophy of a school's faculty about the nature of nursing knowledge and inquiry, the specific research interests and areas of expertise of the faculty, and students' interests and goals should influence the relative emphasis placed on core content elements. Given pervasive concerns among doctoral educators about limiting program flexibility and innovation (Spero, 1987), it is reasonable to expect that the current level of diversity in core content will be maintained.

The array of subspecialty foci of the existing doctoral programs also reflects a high degree of diversity and creativity. Current specialties, particularly in PhD programs, seem to reflect either the way in which a particular faculty group conceptualizes nursing or the expertise and research activities of individuals or clusters within the faculty; no single model is pervasive. That there is diversity in specialties offered by different programs seems to be a strength that should continue to be encouraged. Since doctoral programs are generally considered to be a national resource, it is reasonable that there should be some "division of labor" among them, whereby schools can tailor their offerings to their unique strengths without having to provide comprehensive coverage of the discipline. Diversity among doctoral programs has the advantage of allowing limits to be placed on within-program diversity without compromising the discipline as a whole.

Given the faculty and other resources available to them, it is and will remain desirable for schools to examine and consider limiting the diversity within their doctoral programs. Program scope, for example, should be limited to the specialty or emphasis areas in which quality learning experiences can be assured. The increasing trend toward part-time study will require programs to reexamine their objectives and identify target audiences of students that they can serve most effectively. Such a stance is difficult to take, given market demands, but has potential to encourage an unprecedented degree of intrainstitutional ferment and interinstitutional cooperation.

It has been predicted that a rapid increase in the number of doctoral programs will continue and that "a multiplicity of programs will continue to exist and thrive" (Forni, 1987, p. 70). Such growth will undoubtedly continue to stimulate efforts to assure quality. Whatever means are chosen to do so must permit doctoral education to exhibit the diversity, flexibility, and innovation that ultimately will serve to enrich the profession.

REFERENCES

American Association of Colleges of Nursing (AACN). (1987a). *IDS ranking report*. Unpublished report.

American Association of Colleges of Nursing (AACN). (1987b). Position statement: Indicators of quality in doctoral programs in nursing. *Journal of Professional Nursing, 3*(1), 72–74.

Amos, L. K. (1985). Issues in doctoral preparation in nursing: Current perspectives and future directions. *Journal of Professional Nursing, 1*(2), 101–108.

Andreoli, K. (1987). Specialization and graduate curricula: Finding the fit. *Nursing and Health Care, 8*(2), 65–69.

Beare, P. G., Gray, C. J., & Ptak, H. F. (1981). Doctoral curricula in nursing. *Nursing Outlook, 29*, 311–316.

Downs, F. S. (1978). Doctoral education in nursing: Future directions. *Nursing Outlook, 26*, 56–61.

Downs, F. S. (1988). Doctoral education: Our claim to the future. *Nursing Outlook, 36*, 18–20.

Forni, P. R. (1987). Models for doctoral programs: First professional degree or terminal degree? In S. E. Hart (Ed.), *Issues in graduate nursing education* (Publication No. 18-2196, pp. 45–73). New York: National League for Nursing.

Grace, H. K. (1983). Doctoral education in nursing: Dilemmas and directions. In N. L. Chaska (Ed.), *The nursing profession: A time to speak* (pp. 146–155). New York: McGraw-Hill.

Jamann, J. S. (1985). Proceedings of doctoral programs in nursing: Consensus for quality. *Journal of Professional Nursing, 1*, 90–121.

Kelley, J., & Stullenbarger, E. (1987, October). *Current considerations about future directions for graduate nursing education in the South*. Presented at the Southern Council on Collegiate Education in Nursing annual meeting, Atlanta, GA.

Lenz, E. R., & Morton, P. G. (1988). Non-nurse faculty in schools of nursing. *Nursing Outlook, 36*, 182–185.

McPheeters, H. L. (1985). *Planning for doctoral nursing education in the South*. Atlanta: Southern Regional Education Board.

Murphy, J. F. (1985). Doctoral education of nurses: Historical development, programs and graduates. In H. H. Werley & J. J. Fitzpatrick (Eds.), *Annual review of nursing research* (Vol. 3, pp. 171–189). New York: Springer Publishing Co.

National League for Nursing. (1987). *Doctoral programs in nursing 1986–1987*. New York: Author.

Snyder-Halpern, R. (1986). Doctoral programs in nursing: An examination of curriculum similarities and differences. *Journal of Nursing Education, 25*(9), 350–365.

Spero, J. R. (1987). Specialized accreditation of doctoral programs in nursing: To be or not to be. In S. E. Hart (Ed.), *Issues in graduate nursing education* (pp. 75–88). New York: National League for Nursing.

Styles, M. M. (1987). History as a strategy for shaping educational policy. *Proceedings of the 1987 National Forum on Doctoral Education in Nursing* (pp. 1–11). Pittsburgh: University of Pittsburgh.

✳ EDITOR'S QUESTIONS FOR DISCUSSION ✳

What criteria would you suggest to determine whether or not a doctoral program should be initiated? Discuss the advantages and disadvantages of full-time summer option programs for doctoral students. Provide strategies for resolving some of the difficulties involved in summer option programs. Discuss the implications and challenges that need to be addressed regarding part-time study for doctoral students. Indicate strategies to resolve the issues. Indicate specific mechanisms for socialization of doctoral students into the researcher or advanced clinician role.

Suggest strategies or mechanisms for providing quality control within and among doctoral programs in nursing. Should doctoral programs be accredited and, if so, by whom? How can ongoing evaluation of doctoral programs be conducted by individual schools?

Discuss whether there should be "core" content in all doctoral programs and what should be considered core. To what extent should students be free to structure and define their own doctoral program content and specialty area, or be directed by defined requirements? What are the advantages and disadvantages of cognate course requirements, and interdisciplinary types of course content and experiences in doctoral programs? Discuss the pros and cons of differentiating subspecialty areas of concentration in doctoral programs in terms of developing nursing as a science and as an area for professional practice.

What might be some criteria that can be suggested for resolution of the diversity versus specialty dilemma suggested by Lenz? Discuss the implications in Snyder's chapter (Chapter 15) for doctoral programs. Compare the views held by Snyder and Lenz. Discuss the positive and negative consequences for nursing of diversity and specialization within one doctoral program and between various types of doctoral programs.

What should be the primary determinants of the content defined, developed, and offered in doctoral programs? What are the implications of Deets's chapter (Chapter 20) for the development of nursing knowledge and doctoral programs? To what extent should there be consensus on the identification of nursing phenomena and the areas of concern for nursing in the development of doctoral programs and nursing knowledge? Discuss the implications for guiding doctoral programs, the development of nursing as a science, knowledge development, and professional practice using as three conceptual bases nursing's metaparadigm, clinical nursing content, and nursing diagnosis or taxonomy. Propose content appropriate to each conceptual base that might be developed as curriculum in doctoral programs. Propose strategies to implement a doctoral curriculum using one of the three conceptual bases. Defend your belief and choice on why a doctoral program should use one base more than another. Discuss and suggest research questions that might be addressed and research methods for each of the three conceptual bases.

Discuss the possibilities and implications of the divisional areas within the National Center for Nursing Research being the basis for the development of specialized areas of content and knowledge development in doctoral programs. What are the advantages and limitations of developing and utilizing a specific framework, focus of research, and content for each doctoral program? Discuss various strategies by which the research expertise of faculty members could be shared between schools for the development of stronger doctoral programs. Should doctoral dissertations be required in all doctoral programs and for all major areas of concentration? Suggest criteria for doctoral dissertations.

17

Evaluating Excellence in Graduate Nursing Education

William L. Holzemer, Ph.D., R.N., F.A.A.N.

This chapter discusses excellence of graduate nursing education by combining issues of quality, criteria and standards, and evaluation for both master's and doctoral programs. After a discussion of the concepts of standards, criteria, and program evaluation, three sets of criteria are examined for commonalities. These include those proposed by the National League for Nursing (NLN, 1983), American Association of Colleges of Nursing (AACN) (Jamann, 1985), and indicators proposed from the 1979 and 1984 evaluation of quality of nursing doctoral programs (Holzemer, 1987).

QUALITY EDUCATION

The academic nursing community has been examining various issues relating to doctoral education over the past several years. However, few have synthesized the many concerned voices regarding quality of graduate nursing education. Those with concerns about doctoral education mostly express fear of opening too many programs with too few qualified faculty (Leininger, 1985). Others have focused on the process of program evaluation. Some suggest that traditional methods of evaluating excellence in higher education, such as productivity measures, fail to capture the environment of these programs (Downs, 1988; Murphy, 1985). Others would argue

that excellence can be assessed by examining the contribution of doctoral dissertations to knowledge development (Leininger & Glittenberg, 1984).

In addition to these concerns, leaders recognize two further issues that confront quality graduate nursing education. One, there is awareness that a single nursing organization may attempt to be recognized as the one and only accrediting agency for doctoral education and that such an organization may be controlled by nurse educators unfamiliar with doctoral education. Two, leaders in nursing doctoral education recognize the early developmental status of programs of nursing research and the need for additional resources for these programs. They are also aware that these programs are being judged during their developmental period by graduate councils using criteria appropriate for well-established disciplines. This chapter proposes a national evaluation strategy to address these issues.

APPRAISAL OF CONCERNS

These concerns, identified above, have some validity. However, they do not appear to recognize higher education's history of having developed several strategies to assess excellence. Fox (1985), who quoted Mandell (1977) about scholarly productivity, may somewhat lessen the profession's worry about the proliferation of doctoral programs in nursing. Mandell (1977) wrote that the doctoral dissertation is the first and last scholarly activity of over one half of American academics. Some nursing doctoral program faculty, like faculty from all other disciplines in higher education, qualify for this normative position, yet the evidence suggests that most nursing faculty in doctoral programs are highly productive.

When nursing leaders express their concerns for the failure to assess the environment of nursing doctoral education, one wonders how carefully they have reviewed published literature. For example, study findings have reported valid and reliable measures of the environment as well as significant relationships between the quality of the environment of doctoral nursing programs and scholarly productivity, both at the program and individual level (Holzemer & Chambers, 1986, 1988).

When doctoral dissertation research is defined as the state of the art of a discipline's science, the discipline is in crisis. Excessive faculty energy is often directed to multiple student dissertation topics. These consume and fragment faculty time, and time spent by faculty on their own research has been significantly correlated with scholarship (Holzemer & Chambers, 1986). When faculty recognize this possibly unwise use of their time, they are quick to require that doctoral students select areas of study from faculty ongoing programs of research.

Recognizing the traditional models established for support of programs of research, the National Center for Nursing Research, National Institutes of Health, is now supporting institutional training grants as well as individual National Research Service Awards (NRSAs). This change in funding for nursing graduate education will help foster faculty programs of research, rather than fragmented individual student research.

As faculty begin to focus on students' doctoral studies in areas that complement their own programs of research, they quickly lose motivation to participate in master's theses. May and Holzemer (1985) documented that none of the 28 doctoral programs surveyed in 1984 required an MS thesis for admission. Those developing doctoral programs may wish to examine carefully dropping the thesis requirement

for master's level students as a mechanism to free faculty time for research and scholarly inquiry.

CRITERIA AND STANDARDS

Donabedian (1982) wrote, "All judgments of quality arise from the use of criteria and standards, even though these may not be openly avowed" (p. 19). He struggled with the definitions in his classic work, *Explorations in Quality Assessment and Monitoring*. Criteria were defined as "phenomena that one counts or measures in order to assess the quality" (p. 8). Standards were defined as the precise count or quantity that specifies an adequate, acceptable, or optimal level of quality; and these standards often imply general rules that indicate what quality is. An example of a criterion for faculty scholarship might be that faculty disseminate their research. The standard might be that each faculty member publish at least one peer-refereed article every 2 years.

The National League for Nursing (NLN) uses the term *criteria* in the title of their well-known publication, *Criteria for the Evaluation of Baccalaureate and Higher Degree Programs in Nursing* (NLN, 1983). These criteria define the components of higher education that are important to assess when examining the quality of baccalaureate and master's level programs. The NLN's use of the term *criteria* is consistent with Donabedian's definition as well as that of the Joint Committee (1981). If the criteria are well written, the standard may be implicitly stated as well. To illustrate this point, examine the NLN's (1983) criteria 4 under section I, Structure and Governance:

> 4. The program is administered by a nurse educator who holds a minimum of a baccalaureate in nursing and an earned doctoral degree and has experience in baccalaureate and/or higher degree programs in nursing. (p. 3)

This criterion identifies the phenomenon of interest, mainly the educational preparation of the administrative leader of a program, and specifies the level of the leader's education. The level of required education is a standard for judging the fulfillment of this criterion.

In 1981, the Joint Committee on Standards for Educational Evaluation reached consensus on definitions of criteria and standards (Joint Committee on Standards, 1981). Although these definitions were proposed by Holzemer (1982) for the evaluation of quality in graduate nursing education, they were not utilized in the development of AACN's criteria. Because nursing is familiar with quality assurance literature, which continues to use the terms *criteria* and *standards* interchangeably, nursing educators may not wish to force such narrow definitions.

It is difficult to formulate standards for many phenomena of interest to graduate nursing education. Although it is challenging to develop standards for concepts such as mentorship, most disciplines simply interview faculty and students and formulate standards in a way similar to the procedure reported for nursing by Holzemer (1986). He provided opportunities for leaders in nursing doctoral education to add survey items to a national questionnaire. Then, results for scale scores as well as additional items were reported for each school plotted against the performance of all doctoral programs combined. Individual programs tended to view their scores as having met "the standard" if they scored greater than one standard deviation below the groups' performance. The standard, therefore, was defined in a norm-referenced or statistical manner.

COMPARISONS OF THREE SETS OF CRITERIA

It is common to group the criteria for the evaluation of graduate nursing education. Three sets have been offered in the literature (see Table 17-1), and a proposed synthesis is presented (see box, Combined evaluation assessment). There is consensus about the importance of faculty, although the AACN chose to separate faculty qualifications from faculty research. The proposed model combines faculty qualifications with research activity. There was consensus about the importance of the program of study or the curriculum.

The NLN categories do not include a section on students because criteria related to students were felt to be covered under policies and curriculum for

TABLE 17-1

Comparison of three systems for categorizing criteria for evaluation of quality graduate nursing education

JAMANN (1985) OR AACN	NLN (1983)	HOLZEMER (1982)
Faculty qualifications	Structure and	Faculty
Program of study	governance	Program
Educational resources	Material resources	Students
Students	Policies	Resources
Research	Faculty	
Evaluation of the	Curriculum	
program	Evaluation	

Combined evaluation assessment model for quality graduate nursing education

Categories of
  criteria

Faculty
Program of study
Students   Structure→Process→ Outcomes
Policies
Resources

---

baccalaureate and master's programs. However, at the doctoral level it appears important to include a section on students. Only NLN included a section on policies. Because the focus of this chapter is on graduate nursing education and because there is a potential for the development of stand-alone, graduate-degree-granting institutions, inclusion of the policies category seems warranted here.

The resources category is included in all three sets of criteria groupings, although the referents are somewhat different. AACN refers to educational resources, NLN to material resources, and Holzemer simply to resources. Resources has been included as a category with the recognition that although faculty, students, and the program of study are types of resources, as a category it refers to educational and material resources.

Both the AACN and NLN systems include a category on evaluation. The criteria proposed by AACN are better conceptualized as indicators of individual standards and may not warrant a separate category. For example, AACN includes a criterion for documenting alumni accomplishments. Although this criterion refers to information that is important to collect, it is more consistent to classify the data as an outcome indicator for students. NLN's use of evaluation as a category for criteria is better placed in the category policies under structure. A program should have a policy to conduct systematic, ongoing evaluation. Therefore, no separate category for evaluation has been suggested.

TRADITIONAL SYSTEMS EVALUATION MODEL

The next challenge in developing a coherent view for the evaluation of graduate education in nursing would be to develop lists of individual criteria for each of the five categories organized around the traditional systems evaluation model for quality assurance (see box, Combined evaluation assessment). This model includes three time dimensions: structure, process, and outcomes (Donabedian, 1982; Holzemer, 1982). Definitions for these terms are paraphrased from Donabedian's work (1982, p. 6) on definitions of quality and criteria for the assessment of care. *Structure* refers to the resources used in the provision of education. *Process* refers to the activities that constitute education. *Outcomes* are the consequences of the educational activities as presented in the boxed data. It is beyond this chapter to develop data schemes for the categories of criteria. To illustrate this recommendation a beginning attempt has been made to synthesize and organize criteria for faculty.

SYNTHESIS OF CRITERIA

First, the proposed faculty criteria from AACN, NLN, and Holzemer have been listed (see Table 17-2) and these criteria have been synthesized (see box, Faculty criteria synthesized). The AACN's criteria listed in their section "Research" (Jamann, 1985) were not reviewed because they include criteria appropriate for categories other than faculty.

Faculty criteria synthesized and presented by Donabedian's evaluation model

Structure

1. Faculty have doctoral degrees with a core who have doctorates in nursing.
2. Expertise in curriculum and evaluation, instructional design, information technology, and research support activities are available.

Process

3. Faculty maintain their expertise and engagement in research, teaching, service, and clinical practice.
4. Faculty serve as mentors for students.

Outcomes

5. Faculty scholarship is disseminated and peer-reviewed.
6. Faculty contribute to professional activities and community service.

It is easy to edit and synthesize criteria when working alone with the opportunity to make decisions in isolation. However, having served on the NLN Baccalaureate and Higher Degree Executive Committee's Subcommittee on Accreditation criteria review during the 1980–1982 biennium (resulting in the fifth edition of the criteria), this author is painfully aware of the difficulty of accomplishing the task of criteria development collectively. However, there is significant overlap and redundancy among these criteria, and it would benefit the profession to find a mechanism to synthesize them into a manageable few.

Once consensus has been reached on specific criteria for the five areas outlined in the box on p. 124, empirical indicators must be developed that are valid and reliable (Holzemer, 1986). In recent years, nursing doctoral programs participated in two national studies of the quality indicators, and the data from the 1984 study is used to illustrate indicators for the proposed criterion 5 under faculty, "Faculty scholarship is disseminated and peer reviewed."

TABLE 17-2
Comparison of criteria for faculty of graduate nursing education programs

CRITERIA	CATEGORY
Jamann (1985) or AACN	
• Members should be actively engaged in continuing research related to the program of study in which doctoral students participate.	Process
• Members should hold graduate school appointments, if appropriate, at the university.	Structure
• Members should include a core of nurse faculty members holding earned doctoral degrees in nursing.	Structure
• Faculty research or knowledge development should take place in the context of the history and philosophy of science and lead to a better understanding of the phenomena of nursing.	Outcomes
• Publication of research and scholarly activity that disseminates new knowledge and perspectives should be subject to peer review.	Outcomes
• Faculty mentors should socialize the students into a career of stimulating and satisfying excellence of inquiry and service.	Process
NLN (1983)	
• The size, academic and experimental qualifications, and diversity of backgrounds of the faculty are appropriate to meet program goals.	Structure
• Faculty members hold as a minimum qualification a master's degree appropriate to their areas of responsibility.	Structure
• A majority of faculty members teaching graduate courses hold earned doctorates.	Structure
• Faculty members have and maintain expertise in their areas of teaching responsibility.	Process
• There is expertise within the faculty in curriculum development and evaluation, instructional design, and research.	Structure
• Faculty endeavors include participation in scholarly and professional activities, and community service consistent with the mission(s) of the parent institution and the goals of the program.	Outcomes
Holzemer (1982)	
1. Preparation and background	Structure
2. Research activity and productivity	Process and outcomes

The study (Holzemer, 1987) provided each of the 25 participating programs with a confidential report, plotting their program results against the average results for all 25 programs. The potential use of this data set as indicators for self-evaluation is presented in Table 17-3. Six separate indicators for criterion 5 are presented along with comparative data from the participating programs. The 1984 data set provides valid and reliable indicators for most of the five cat-egories of criteria that can be organized by structure, process, and outcome (Chambers & Holzemer, 1988).

Although it is clear that the data presented for indicators in Table 17-3 are norm-referenced, they can be extremely helpful in defining the parameters of excellence regarding faculty scholarship. There is no clearer indication of the scientific merit of scholarship than peer review. Two of these indicators rep-

TABLE 17-3

Example of indicators for criterion 5: faculty scholarship is disseminated and peer reviewed

INDICATOR	PROGRAM LEVEL DATA (N = 23 FACULTY)	NORM DATA* (N = 25 PROGRAMS: N = 289 FACULTY)		
	M	M	SD	RANGE
Process				
Scale† 2. Scholarly Excellence (1 = minimum, 4 = maximum)	3.62	3.24	0.37	2.16–3.73
Scale 15. Percent Time Faculty Engaged in Research Activity	63%	50%	0.12	17%–67%
Outcome				
Number of Publications				
Professional articles and book chapters for entire career	22	15	NA	4–40
Total publications for entire career	27	20	17.6	5–47
Number of refereed articles in last 3 years	5	3.7	3.8	0–8
Number of Division of Nursing Research Grants, 1979–1983	6	3	NA	0–12

*M = Mean of program means; range = lowest to highest program mean; SD = standard deviation; NA = not applicable.
†Scales 2 and 15 are described in detail in Holzemer and Chambers (1986).

resent peer review, the number of publications in peer review journals, and the number of research grants received during a fixed period.

FORMAL EVALUATION MECHANISMS

Academic nursing has not yet made a decision about the potential benefits or liabilities of developing formal accreditation procedures for nursing doctoral programs. AACN, through their initiation of the national conference on doctoral criteria, indirectly suggested to the profession that perhaps the AACN would be an appropriate group to accredit nursing doctoral programs. The NLN, which is recognized by the Commission on Post-Secondary Accreditation (COPA) as the accrediting body for academic nursing programs, has recently established a committee to explore NLN's role in such an activity. Because the procedure and criteria developed by NLN for master's degree programs would be similar for doctoral programs—although with significant differences—it would be logical to place this activity with

NLN. An informally organized group, which meets annually and is referred to as the "Doctoral Forum," has also explored issues of accreditation for doctoral programs and reached a consensus that no professional nursing body should adopt a policy of accrediting nursing doctoral programs.

Likewise, it is my recommendation to develop a system that assists nursing doctoral programs to conduct self-evaluation activities similar to those illustrated by the national cooperative studies (Holzemer, 1987), but that no nursing body should adopt any formal accreditation activity. For a relatively low cost, it would be possible to adopt the Graduate Program Self-Assessment questionnaires developed by Educational Testing Service (Clark, 1983), available for both master's and doctoral programs, to provide an important, valid self-evaluation procedure for graduate nursing programs. This activity could be carried out by a national nursing organization.

This type of institutional evaluation is nothing new. There is ample precedent for doctoral programs being evaluated by their own graduate college. At the University of California, San Francisco (UCSF) the Graduate Council, which is a standing committee of the faculty Academic Senate, conducts program reviews of all graduate programs at intervals of approximately 5 years. The purpose of the review is to evaluate the quality and effectiveness of programs leading to graduate degrees. The principal concern of all program reviews is the academic quality of

graduate education at UCSF and the academic welfare of students enrolled in graduate programs (Graduate Council, 1987). Four groups of criteria are examined; these focus on the program, students, faculty, and physical facilities and other resources. The subcommittees selected for these program reviews include persons with expertise in the discipline from outside the University of California, San

---

Suggested guidelines for program review reports from Graduate Council, University of California, San Francisco

I. Program

1. What are the goals of the program? Is it meeting its own goals and the expectations of others? Is it meeting the needs of the discipline, of the university, of society? What is the program's promise for future development and contributions?

2. Are curriculum offerings sufficiently diverse to allow for a broad range of education experiences; for specialization in the major subdivisions of the discipline? How do program requirements (courses, examinations, etc.) compare with those of other graduate programs in the field?

3. Are sufficient resources allocated of the program to allow it to meet its goals? Are the resources allocated used efficiently? Is the program as productive as possible given the resources available to it?

II. Students

1. Are students of high ability attracted to the program? What criteria are used in administrating students to the program? Does the program have an effective plan for recruiting new students?

2. Does the program have established procedures for regularly evaluating student performance? Does the program ensure that adequate information and good advice are provided to students?

3. Are there sufficient opportunities for faculty-student interchange, for the supervision of research projects and teaching activities?

4. Does the program provide sufficient financial support for its students?

5. Do students complete the program within normal time limits? What is the quality and scope of research results or other scholarly work published by graduate students?

6. Are students successful in finding suitable positions upon graduation?

7. What is the morale of the students in the program?

III. Faculty

1. What is the general scholarly quality of the faculty of the program? Does the department recruit and retain faculty members of quality? Is the faculty adequate in numbers and sufficiently diverse in interests for the program offered?

2. Does the department support the teaching and/or counseling activities of the faculty in the graduate program? Is the morale of the staff high?

IV. Physical facilities and other resources

1. Is the physical plan (classrooms, office space, laboratories, study and lounge areas) satisfactory? Is the library adequate to support the instruction and research needs of the program?

2. Is there adequate equipment to support graduate instruction and research? Is there adequate secretarial, technical, and other staff assistance within the department?

Graduate Council. (1987, February). Guidelines concerning program reviews. San Francisco: University of California, San Francisco

Francisco campus who have the obligation to consider making the following recommendations. The subcommittee, after reviewing written materials and conducting site visits, may choose (Graduate Council, 1987):

1. Recommendations to the faculty of the program for modifications and enhancements.
2. Recommendations to UCSF administrators for program modifications, enhancements, and resource allocation.
3. Initiation of the process of disestablishment, in accordance with University of California policy and procedures.
4. Recommendation for commendation of programs operating at high levels of quality and effectiveness.

The suggested guidelines by the UCSF Graduate Council for program review are listed in the box on p. 128. They illustrate the type of indicators a doctoral program must gather for presentation to their graduate college on their quality and effectiveness. If a national organization provided support for this process, but did not create a separate process with additional expenses, it might be favorably reviewed by the leaders of doctoral programs.

In summary, there is a challenge to nursing educators to synthesize the differing sets of criteria being developed, to reach consensus about some common standards while allowing for individuality, and to develop an inexpensive mechanism to provide indicator data to programs on a regular basis. The state of the art of research and graduate education in nursing is healthy, but fragile. Any attempt to control the creativity and scholarship of these developing programs through rigid accreditation procedures will neither support the goals of graduate education nor foster the development of the discipline.

REFERENCES

Chambers, D. B., & Holzemer, W. L. (1988). *Validity and reliability of the Graduate Program Self-Assessment (GPSA) instruments for evaluating nursing doctoral education.* Paper presented at the Annual Meeting of the American Educational Research Association, New Orleans, LA.

Clark, M. (1983). *Graduate program self-assessment service for doctoral programs: Handbook for users.* Princeton, NJ: Educational Testing Service.

Donabedian, A. (1982). *Explorations in quality assessment and monitoring* (Vol. II). Ann Arbor, MI: Health Administration Press.

Downs, F. S. (1988). Doctoral education: Our claim to the future. *Nursing Outlook, 36,* 18–20.

Fox, M. F. (1985). Publications, performance, and reward in science and scholarship. In Smart, J. C. (Ed.), *Higher education: Handbook of theory and research* (Vol 1, pp. 255–282). New York: Agathon Press.

Graduate Council. (1987, February). *Guidelines concerning program reviews.* San Francisco: University of California, San Francisco.

Holzemer, W. L. (1982). Quality in graduate nursing education. *Nursing and Health Care, 3,* 171–189.

Holzemer, W. L. (1986). *Final report. Quality indicators of nursing doctoral programs* (1 RO NU000967.) Bethesda, MD: Division of Nursing, Bureau of Health Manpower, Health Resources Administration, Public Health Service, Department of Health and Human Services.

Holzemer, W. L. (1987). Doctoral education in nursing: An assessment of quality, 1979–1984. *Nursing Research, 36,* 111–116.

Holzemer, W. L., & Chambers, D. B. (1986). Healthy doctoral programs: Relationship of the environment of nursing doctoral programs on faculty and alumni productivity. *Research in Nursing and Health, 9,* 299–307.

Holzemer, W. L., & Chambers, D. B. (1988). A contextual analysis of faculty productivity. *Journal of Nursing Education, 27,* 10–18.

Jamann, J. S. (1985). Proceedings of doctoral programs in nursing: Consensus for quality. *Journal of Professional Nursing, 1,* 90–122.

Joint Committee on Standards for Educational Evaluation. (1981). *Standards for evaluations of educational programs, projects, and materials.* New York: McGraw-Hill.

Leininger, M. (1985). Current doctoral education: A culture of mediocrity or excellence? In J. McClosky & H. Grace (Eds.), *Current issues in nursing* (pp. 219–235). Boston: Blackwell Scientific Publications.

Leininger, M., & Glittenberg, J. (1984, June). *Textual analysis of doctoral nursing dissertation abstracts.* Paper presented at the 1984 Forum on Doctoral Education, Denver, CO.

Mandell, R. D. (1977). *The professor game.* New York: Doubleday.

May, K. M., & Holzemer, W. L. (1985). Master's thesis policies in nursing education. *Journal of Nursing Education, 24,* 10–15.

Murphy, J. F. (1985). Doctoral education of nurses: Historical developments, programs, and graduates. In H. H. Werley & J. J. Fitzpatrick (Eds.), *Annual review of nursing research, 3* (pp. 171–189). New York: Springer-Verlag.

National League for Nursing (NLN) (1983). *Criteria for the evaluation of baccalaureate and higher degree programs in nursing.* New York: Author.

✷ EDITOR'S QUESTIONS FOR DISCUSSION ✷

Discuss possible ethical issues that may be involved regarding students' selecting a topic area for their doctoral dissertation that is specifically related to an ongoing research program of faculty. How might such ethical dilemmas be prevented or resolved? Discuss on what basis or to what extent doctoral dissertations should be a contribution to knowledge development in nursing? Should a thesis be required for all master's students? If so, what should be the basic purpose, limitations, and criteria for a thesis?

How can doctorally prepared faculty be motivated to teach in undergraduate programs while simultaneously developing strong programs of research? How can teaching in both undergraduate and graduate programs enable the best utilization of doctoral preparation, education, and the development of research? What type of criteria might be suggested for doctorally prepared faculty to teach in doctoral programs? What implications are there regarding work load of faculty given Holzemer's suggestions for standards in doctoral programs?

How might doctoral programs be evaluated validly, reliably, and effectively? What are potential problems in the evaluation of doctoral programs? Discuss the legitimacy of the criteria proposed by Holzemer. Discuss the benefits and liabilities of developing formal accreditation procedures for nursing doctoral programs. Should there be a single nursing organization acting as an accrediting body for doctoral education? If yes—which one, why, who should develop the accreditation procedures, and what should be the criteria for persons to qualify as members of an accrediting team or body for the accreditation of doctoral programs? Discuss how a system could be developed to assist nursing doctoral programs to conduct self-evaluation activities. How might external reviewers be selected and utilized for a role in the evaluation of a doctoral program? How can a university use a standing committee's program reviews at intervals as the basis for the evaluation of their doctoral program? What relationships or linkages might be established between faculty, peer, and program evaluation?

18

Common Ground:
International nursing education

Donna B. Jensen, Ph.D., R.N.
Carol A. Lindeman, Ph.D., R.N., F.A.A.N.

Nurses and nursing education exist in every country around the world. The scope of nursing practice and the form of nursing education varies, but it is a truism that wherever there are cities and people, there are institutions for health care and schools for nurses. On the other hand, it is also a truism that the level of nursing education and the resources with which to teach differ significantly around the world. The developed countries of the world have a higher percentage of the gross national product (GNP) designated for health care and have the most resources for nursing education. In the developing countries, however, where the health GNP is lower, nursing education is not a priority item. The disparities are wide between the haves and the have-nots. These disparities need to be acknowledged and studied before any long-term planning can occur to narrow this gap and bring forward what DeSantis describes as "joint international nursing endeavours" (DeSantis, 1987, p. 67). An isolationist view of nursing and nursing education, which at one point in time may have served the countries well, needs to be reexamined and reevaluated with a visionary view on how to bridge cultural lines without becoming intrusive. Cooperative efforts of sharing and collaboration, initiated by those countries who have been more fortunate in gaining resources, will be a key factor in reorienting nursing education and practice in the direction of primary health care for all countries.

LEARNING FROM HISTORY

It was the religious orders that began the training of nurses (Kalisch & Kalisch, 1986), but it was Florence Nightingale who detailed in writing an organized method for the preparation of nurses. Her method has been the major framework used around the world for nursing education. Nightingale began her career in nursing at the deaconess school in Germany where, in 1851, she studied 3 months at the Kaiserswerth training school for nurses. Pastor Fliedner and his wife, Friederike founded the school, and can be credited with opening the door for Nightingale's future accomplishments (Nutting & Dock, 1907-1912). Drawing from her experience in the Crimea, Nightingale's subsequent influence on the British system had far-reaching effects on the neighboring European nursing schools, as well as the colonized regions of countries like Africa, India, and the newly independent United States. Nightingale initiated the legitimization of nursing as a distinct profession that required a special set of mental and physical skills. She began the transition of

131

thinking from nurses as volunteers, hirelings, servants, or dedicated religious nuns and deaconesses to a legitimately earned status in the field of nursing, which could include laypersons. For example, in her *Notes on Nursing* she states that the first rule of nursing is to keep the air within as pure as the air without (Nightingale, 1860). The evolution of this primary statement on nursing to the present can be demonstrated in current activities, such as nursing research on the effects of cotton dust in Thailand's garment factories (Provit, Samporn, & Varatama, 1984) and policymaking conferences on the quality of air by U.S. occupational nurses. These activities reflect action targeted toward health by professionals educated and legitimized to perform these nursing responsibilities while continuing to work within the framework of Nightingale's early thoughts on nursing.

During the colonization periods of the eighteenth and nineteenth centuries, missionaries introduced hospital training schools in all of the colonies (Mule, 1986). In addition, missionaries began schools of nursing in independent countries such as Thailand (Siam) and China. The schools were primarily attached to hospitals as training schools, but in China, before the revolution in 1949, Shanghai University was beginning to educate nurses. Following World War II, the colonization period rapidly began its decline leaving many countries in poverty that was accelerated by the exploitive practices of the colonists (Fischer, 1954). Particularly vulnerable were those nations in Central and South America, Southeast Asia, India, and Africa. These nations began fostering a fierce nationalism, but without the resources to be competitive in the modern world economic scene. Schools of nursing continued, but the health of the people in these poorer countries was far below the standard being set by the then more developed countries. The schools in these poorer countries had limited resources and minimal communication with the outside world.

PATTERNS IN MORE DEVELOPED COUNTRIES

The increased level of economic development in more developed countries has had a major influence on nursing education models. The industrialized countries began actively building both their internal educational structures and their general economic base. In the United States, health care costs were increasing along with expenditures for nursing when, in 1985, total health costs accounted for over 11% of the GNP. At this time funding was available for research in nursing, and schools were being funded with capitation monies to educate nurses. Baccalaureate and master's education for nurses was a part of most major universities, and doctoral programs in nursing began to open (Institute of Medicine, 1983).

This pattern for nursing was not unique to the United States. For example, Japan, Israel, the European continent, and the United Kingdom developed nursing programs that were initially hospital-based, but as the complexity of nursing and health care increased, these programs began moving into a university setting. The United States established the first independent department in nursing at Yale University in 1924 with Annie W. Goodrich as its dean (Kalisch & Kalisch, 1986). The first nursing degree program in the United Kingdom was introduced in 1960 by the Department of Nursing Studies at the University of Edinburgh (Reid, Nellis, & Boore, 1987; Howard & Brooking, 1987). Japan began its first autonomous university programs after the 1967 curriculum revision under the Public Health Nurse, Midwife and Nurse Law (P.M.N. Law). Kojima states that "although the progress of nursing education in Japan is slow in relation to history, tradition, culture, law, etc., it has evolved soundly" (1987, p. 94). The tremendous rate of growth occurring in the United States, its economic system for funding health care, and its relatively unencumbered legacy of tradition and social class restraints, all were factors in the relatively early introduction of an autonomous nursing program within a university setting.

In reality, university-based nursing in most of the more developed countries evolved slowly. In fact New Zealand found that their 1973 attempt at university-based nursing was overturned because a shortage of nurses resulted, that is, "nurses became thin on the ground." For most countries, before an autonomous department of nursing was announced, there were several preceding years in which classes or courses were offered within a university setting or under the auspices of medicine. For example, in the United States a training school for nurses was established at the University of Minnesota in 1909 under the College of Medicine, which began operation 15 years before the Yale University School of Nursing was established. Several universities throughout the country combined academic courses with professional courses in nursing of 4 to 5 years, culminating in an AB or BS degree in nursing. The product of these schools was a generalist in nursing, who would be eligible for the licensing boards' examinations for a registered nurse (RN).

Many other countries began their exploration into university-based nursing by beginning with students who were specializing in administration or education. For example, in 1972, the Catholic Academy for Nursing in Bavaria recognized the need for higher education in nursing. As a specialized school it provided educational programs to prepare RNs, those students who had completed the basic generalist program in nursing at a 3-year diploma school, for courses in education and nursing management (Kellnhouser, 1986). This school was similar to many postbasic nursing schools already in existence in West Germany and throughout the continent. These schools were not university based, but prepared persons for specialization in such areas as critical care nursing, head nurse, nursing service administrator, community health nursing, or as an instructor of nursing. Four years after the Catholic Academy of Nursing's specialized school began, the first bona fide university course of study in West Germany was established as an experimental program at the Free University of Berlin. The program began in the fall of 1976 receiving approval and funding from the Federal-States-Commission for Educational Planning (Hedin, 1987). Virtually all of the more developed countries are educating nurses, who in one form or another, are complying with the International Council of Nurses' (ICN) definition of a nurse, which essentially states that a nurse is one who completes a basic program of study that meets her or his country's qualifications to practice nursing (Styles, 1985). This broad definition is the generic

use of the term *nurse*, in relation to regulating processes for nurses throughout the world, and is further delineated into the variety of categories used to describe the different products of nursing education such as generalist, specialist, basic, and postbasic.

The educational patterns in the different countries are just as diverse as the career pathway, with entry into nursing coming from either less than secondary education or from those persons completing secondary education, depending on the country. These same persons go on to settings of secondary schools, hospitals, independent schools, technical institutes, or universities for their basic nursing education, and may continue on for postbasic education in the same proliferation of settings.

The nursing education patterns of four selected countries are singled out. Our purpose is to demonstrate the versatility and creativity used in developing nursing programs that embody the discrete cultural and socioeconomic constraints imposed on each country.

Canada

Canada has a culture and value system that is reflected in its health care system and role of nursing. The health care system is based on the premise that government has the responsibility to protect citizens from events over which they have no control. Each province is responsible for its own health care system.

Canada has a long tradition of baccalaureate education in nursing having adopted the American model as opposed to the British model. Currently there are 23 baccalaureate programs: 5 are French language programs, 2 are bilingual, and the rest are English. There are 11 master's degree programs, with the first program starting in 1969 at the University of Toronto. There are no doctoral programs in nursing in Canada. The University of Alberta has received approval for a PhD in nursing, but because of the downturn in the economy the program has not been funded. This proposed program reflects the British model of study, emphasizing individual-directed courses of study as opposed to faculty-guided required coursework (Pringle, 1988).

Israel

Jewish higher education is an old phenomenon in Jewish life and its need and worth are an integral part of the culture and social ideology. In the early 1900s the first demand that a university be established in Jerusalem was recorded. The language of instruction was to be Hebrew and there would be three distinct branches of studies: theology, humanity, and natural science.

University education for nurses is a more recent development in Israel and was first identified as a need at the Szold Hadassah School of Nursing, Jerusalem School Committee in 1947. In 1968, following a long process of negotiation and development, the first BA degrees were awarded to nurses completing a postbasic program of study at the Tel Aviv University Department of Nursing. The basic 4-year baccalaureate nursing programs were established later: one in 1975, and one in 1983. During this time, a total of 816 nurses with baccalaureate degrees were prepared in Israel, which is 3.2% of the country's nurses. The first Israeli master's degree program in nursing opened in 1983. Thus far, it has produced six graduates. Although several nurses are currently enrolled in doctoral studies in Israel, they are in programs of behavioral function disciplines such as labor affairs, management, education, and psychology. At this time, the need to establish a doctoral program in nursing has not been pursued (Zwanger, 1988).

Japan

Currently 1% of nurses licensed in Japan have a baccalaureate degree. There are 11 university programs open for student nurse enrollment. Of those, 6 specifically offer a baccalaureate in nursing. The remaining 5 schools are in health-related fields such as health science and public health. After completion of these programs, students may apply for the registered nurse licensure examination. There are 4 master's level programs open for registered nurse enrollment: 2 are in nursing science and 2 in health science. Graduate nurses may enter doctoral programs in medical science, health science, and public health. Two schools are developing doctoral programs that will award the degree in nursing science. One of these schools, St. Luke's College of Nursing, admitted students in 1988.

The proposed curriculum for the doctoral degree in nursing will be structured around a major professor, who has an assistant professor or lecturer and several assistants. Graduate students will learn by doing and working with the faculty. Core courses will be required, but the focus of study will be on the pursuit of specific phenomena culminating in the dissertation (Minami, 1988).

Norway

Norway is a country of approximately four million people. Health care and education, including university education, is paid by the government of Norway. The general social structures are based on the principles of justice, equality, and collectivism. There are approximately 46,000 registered nurses, and their basic education is a 3-year program of study.

Norway has four universities, two of which offer advanced studies in nursing. The four universities are all founded on the traditional European or Germanic university model, in which the students choose courses that support their area of study in the departments of social science, natural science, or humanities. Although there are no doctoral programs in nursing, there is an academic seat or professorship in nursing at the University of Bergen and another similar appointment is being proposed at the Institute for Nursing Science at the University of Oslo. These professors will provide nurses wishing to obtain a doctoral degree the needed professorial mentors (Bunch, 1988).

PATTERNS IN THE DEVELOPING COUNTRIES

The developing countries comply with the same ICN standards and definitions of nursing as the more developed countries. Remarkable strides toward national guidelines for health care and nursing education are evident in these countries, despite the relatively limited resources for both of these items.

The long strides taken by the developing countries have their origin in a landmark conference held in Alma-Ata, U.S.S.R. in 1978 (World Health Organization, 1978). It was there that 23 nations convened under the auspices of the World Health Organization (WHO) and the United Nations Children's Fund (UNICEF) to develop the Alma-Ata doctrine and the subsequent initiative adopted by WHO Member States: "Health for all by the year 2000." Indicators for measuring health status of a community or nation were developed and disseminated along with guidelines for the countries to use in developing national health goals. The focus of these goals was in primary health care (PHC) and in 1985, the Director General of WHO stated:

> WHO has now grasped the significance of nursing potential for PHC. Nurses have already begun to lead the way and have many good successes to show. More and more nurses will become leaders of PHC teams and assume greater responsibility for making decisions. (WHO, 1985)

This leadership responsibility has been most evident in the changes developing countries have made to integrate PHC into nursing education (Bergman, 1986). Since a major objective of PHC is to provide personal and environmental health services to underserved populations, community health nursing has become integrated into the basic and advanced nursing curricula. An example of this effort is the 1-year postbasic community health nursing program in Botswana, which is designed to strengthen preventive and health promotion services in rural areas, where graduates practice in conjunction with regional and district health teams (Anderson, 1987).

Recognizing the increased need for depth and breadth in nursing education, programs are slowly moving into university settings in countries like China, the African States, Thailand, and India. Doctoral education remains associated with related disciplines; many of the graduates from basic programs go abroad to study beyond the baccalaureate level. In this way, graduates return to their country of origin ready to begin nursing programs related to their specific national health goals. Examples of three developing countries with three different approaches to nursing education illustrate the uniqueness of each in contributing to health care.

Thailand

The first nursing school in Thailand was established in 1894 and required 3 years of general schooling before students could enter the 2-year nursing program. Currently there are 44 nursing education institutions under the control of the Ministry of University Affairs, the Ministry of Public Health, the Ministry of Defense, the Ministry of the Interior, and the Red Cross. The faculties of nursing in government universities offer master's degrees in specialties such as medical-surgical and maternity nursing. In 1985, a doctor of public health degree with a major in public health nursing was established at Mahidol University in Bangkok and the first students were enrolled in 1987. Nine credits of core courses are required with the general public health students, the remainder being in the selected area of concentration (Prabha, 1988).

Nepal

Nepal is a small country with a population of 15 million people, 95% of whom live in the rural mountainous areas with little access to the health care system. The major health problems include (a) a relatively high birth and death rate and (b) a high infant mortality rate. It has been determined that the most important group of health workers nearest to the people are nurses working in primary health care (PHC), which has been the basis for a recent curriculum revision. Students prepared to practice in PHC are educated as generalists, to function in a community setting with village groups, families, and individuals. The main objective is to assist these groups to be self-reliant with the available resources in a village development program. The curriculum focuses on learning and understanding community problems, and working with the members of the community.

The curriculum change in all of Nepal was supported by the commitment of His Majesty's Government of Nepal to the concept of health for all by the year 2000. Faculty were encouraged by this commitment to approach a system change in nursing curriculum that was a challenge to both faculty and students (Dass, 1986).

India

India contains one of the world's largest populations. As in other developing countries, the majority of the people reside in rural areas. There is a serious shortage of trained nurses; the institutions charged with training nurses lack both the physical and human resources to do so. In 1981 there were 286 training schools for general nursing and midwifery and 25 postbasic or degree programs. To meet the PHC goals for the year 2000 it is projected that these programs will need to double in size and revise their curricula to educate nurses for primary health care. At this time, the professional and financial incentives necessary to attract and retain qualified persons are inadequate, and the profession, on the whole, suffers from low self-esteem and public respectability (Harnar & Lehman, 1983).

COMMON GROUND

Such a diversity of nursing education, in both the more developed and developing countries, reflects the nature of international nursing. The bonds of tradition, culture, socioeconomics, religion, politics, and geography play a significant role in the development and focus of each educational system. The values and beliefs of each country are communicated in health care provisions for its population and subsequently in its education for nurses.

Each country appears to have its own timetable for the growth and development of nursing programs related to intrinsic factors, as well as the extrinsic forces of pressure, such as that of WHO. With both factors operating in a constant dynamic state, any interference in the process to propose a unified nursing education model would be counterproductive.

On the other hand, finding a common ground may be possible by posing questions, for collaborative discussion between colleagues from different countries, about ways to capture the community involvement emphasized in some programs and the research efforts dominating others. This method of inquiry

uses the principles of intercultural communication to find a series of questions, which may be approached from diverse vantage points. One example in the use of this method occurred in Oregon at a recent international conference of six international nursing colleagues who were invited to discuss international perspectives and implications for doctoral education in nursing (Gaines, 1988). Questions were developed by all of the participants and were clustered into four themes: inquiry, thinking and doing, international responsibility, and the nature of education. The subsequent discussion culminated in the asking of more questions for administrators and faculty of doctoral programs in the United States:

1. Does the United States with 95% of the doctorally prepared nurses and all its resources and wealth have a responsibility to assist other countries to develop nursing leadership? If so, what does this mean in terms of length of program, required content, nature, or research?
2. What are the expectations of nurses with doctoral degrees in respect to the practice of nursing and the discipline of nursing? Are these expectations broad enough to respond to needs in other countries? In this way, both the similarities and differences are exposed to a greater or lesser degree. However, the critical issue is that of providing a larger field of communication that can be pivotal in establishing a common ground for discussions around international nursing education.
3. Is the ideal view that the doctorally prepared nurse be exposed to an alternate conceptualization of practice different from the one that guides our baccalaureate programs?
4. Where do interdisciplinary learning experiences fit in a doctoral program in nursing?
5. Can we justify graduate education for nurses? If so, on what grounds? Should programs be established everywhere? If not, for whom and why? Can we afford higher education for all? Can we afford *not* to have higher education for all?

Through open discussion of questions such as these, both the similarities and differences in cultural perspectives are exposed. The critical issue is establishing a common ground for discussions of international nursing education, from which new perspectives can be gained, and decisions for nursing practice can be made.

REFERENCES

Anderson, S. V. (1987). Response of nursing education to primary health care: The training and practice of post basic community health nurses in Botswana. *International Nursing Review, 34*(1), 17–25.

Bergman, R. (1986). Nursing in a changing world. *International Nursing Review, 33*(4), 110–112.

Bunch, E. H. (1988). Norwegian perspective. In B. Gaines (Ed.), *Proceedings: International implications and perspectives for doctoral education in nursing* (pp. 97–106). Portland, OR: Oregon Health Sciences University.

Dass, U. D. (1986). Basic steps in the review of Nepal's nursing curriculum. *International Nursing Review, 33*(3), 87–89.

DeSantis, L. (1987). Principles of transnational co-operation in nursing. *International Nursing Review, 34*(3), 67–71.

Fischer, L. (1954). *Gandhi: His life and message for the world*. New York: New American Library Incorporated.

Gaines, B. (Ed.). (1988). *Proceedings: International implications and perspectives for doctoral education in nursing*. Portland, OR: Oregon Health Sciences University.

Harner, R. M., & Lehman, B. H. E. (1983). *Nurse education in India: Its relevance in provision of primary health care*. Unpublished report to The USAID, Office of Health and Nutrition, New Delhi.

Hedin, B. A. (1987). Nursing education and social constraints: An in depth analysis. *International Journal of Nursing Studies, 24*(3), 261–270.

Howard, J. M., & Brooking, J. I. (1987). The career paths of nursing graduates from Chelsea College, University of London. *International Journal of Nursing Studies, 24*(3), 181–189.

Institute of Medicine. (1983). *Nursing and nursing education*. Washington, DC: Department of Health and Human Services.

Kalisch, P. A., & Kalisch, B. J. (1986). *The advance of American nursing* (2nd ed.). Boston: Little, Brown.

Kellnhouser, E. (1986). Higher nursing education in Bavaria and in Florida. *International Nursing Review, 33*(2), 56–60.

Kojima, M. (1987). Nursing education in Japan and its future trends. *International Nursing Review, 34*(4), 94–101.

Minami, H. (1988). Reflection of the cultural and social milieu on the development of nursing science in Japan. In B. Gaines (Ed.), *Proceedings: International implications and perspectives for doctoral education in nursing* (pp. 63–74). Portland, OR: Oregon Health Sciences University.

Mule, G. K. (1986). Nursing education in Kenya: Trends and innovations. *International Nursing Review, 33*(3), 83–86.

Nightingale, F. (1860). *Notes on nursing: What it is and what it is not*. London: Harrison.

Nutting, M. A., & Dock, L. L. (1907-1912). *A history of nursing: The evaluation of nursing systems from earliest times to the foundations of the first English and American training schools for nurses* (Vols. 1-4). New York: G. P. Putnam's Sons.

Prabha, L. (1988). Doctoral education in nursing. In B. Gaines (Ed.), *Proceedings: International implications and perspectives for doctoral education in nursing* (pp. 45–62). Portland, OR: Oregon Health Sciences University.

Pringle, D. M. (1988). Multidisciplinary research teams in nursing research and in doctoral education. In B. Gaines (Ed.), *Proceedings: International implications and perspectives for doctoral education in nursing* (pp. 87–96). Portland, OR: Oregon Health Sciences University.

Provit, R., Samporn, T., & Varatama, S. (1984). *The study of health status, health needs, and welfare of female workers in textile mills in traditional and modern factories*. Unpublished manuscript, School of Public Health, Mahidol University, Bangkok, Thailand.

Reid, N. G., Nelis, P. & Boore, J. (1987). Graduate nurses in Northern Ireland: Their career paths, aspirations and problems. *International Journal of Nursing Studies, 24*(3), 215-225.

Styles, M. M. (1985). *Project on the regulation of nursing*. Geneva: International Council of Nurses.

World Health Organization (WHO). (1978). *Primary health care: Impact of the International Conference on Primary Health Care, Alma Ata, USSR*, September 6–12. Geneva: World Health Organization.

World Health Organization (WHO). (1985, April). Press release, 77th WHO Executive Board Meeting, April 1985.

Zwanger, L. (1988). Israeli case. In B. Gaines (Ed.), *Proceedings: International implications and perspectives for doctoral education in nursing* (pp. 17–44). Portland, OR: Oregon Health Sciences University.

✳   **EDITOR'S QUESTIONS FOR DISCUSSION**   ✳

How can the disparities in resources for nursing education nationally and internationally be overcome to become more equitable? What could be the role of leaders and programs of nursing education in the United States for developing countries? What should nursing education leaders in the United States transmit and share with international nursing regarding their experiences, efforts, challenges met and unmet, strategies, processes, and success in promoting and developing professional nursing education? To what extent do consultants have or are provided sufficient information regarding the background, history, and culture of international countries before assisting with the development of nursing programs in other countries?

What are the most critical variables that must be considered in proposing and developing a new nursing education program in another country? What intrinsic and extrinsic forces might be in play in countries that would affect the curriculum for a nursing education program and its possible success? What "common ground" may exist among countries to communicate various issues, raise questions, resolve problems, and plan for more effective nursing education programs in all countries?

Discuss the pros and cons of developing an active, international exchange program for nursing leadership. Suggest what may be the driving forces and restraints in developing such a pro-gram. What resources are essential to initiate an exchange plan? What steps should be included in implementing an international leadership program?

Compare the similarities and differences between the more developed countries and the United States in efforts to promote and develop university-based nursing education programs? How has culture in international countries influenced the development of university-based programs? Discuss the extent to which nursing education and nursing service have been isolated from each other in the United States and internationally, in the underdeveloped and more developed countries. What patterns can you define as fairly consistent in the development of nursing education programs in each of the countries addressed by Jensen and Lindeman?

Discuss the process of developing nursing education programs internationally. How might goals and priorities be established in developing programs internationally? How could the critical areas of nursing practice in each country be defined or identified as a base for developing content for nursing education programs? How might the outcomes of programs be expected to be different in other countries from what is expected of graduates in the United States? Should there be efforts to develop master's and doctoral programs simultaneously with initiating undergraduate education for a given country?

19

Continuing Education:
National and international perspectives

Estelle H. Rosenblum, Ph.D., R.N.

With few exceptions, most adults engage in at least two major learning efforts every year. Some attempt as many as 20. About 70% of all learning projects are planned independently by the adult learner. Learning theorists postulate that there is an inborn desire or motivation in all of us that cries out to be nourished and satisfied above and beyond the need merely to survive (Tough, 1979). That humans do not live by bread alone is far from a cliché. Human beings quest because of an inborn curiosity and desire for novelty, excitement, and growth.

The impetus for continuing education within the discipline of nursing has resulted from nursing's desire for continued growth and development. Nursing has emerged from hundreds of years of a slow and steady development to become a true profession as well as a valued occupation. Every developing profession demands constant educational and information renewal. Before graduation ceremonies are forgotten, each new graduate must make some lifelong learning plans or be relegated as obsolete as an outdated textbook.

Students today leaving schools and colleges differ greatly from their predecessors of hundreds of years ago who learned finite procedures and the exact ways to do things. It is totally different today in a rapidly changing and highly competitive health care environment. We must instill in all adult learners the need for regular updating of obsolete information and the desire for constant renewal, and reassure them that there are many interesting ways to accomplish this goal. Each of us must create our own lifelong learning plans according to our personal needs and styles.

ADULT LEARNING, OR ANDRAGOGY

Many theorists (Bigge, 1982) postulated and Knowles (1984) clarified that the learning needs of adults are far different from the needs of children. Children must be offered the fundamentals of learning in the many guises of natural enfoldment, mental discipline, and apperception. Children are by definition dependent persons, and the teacher becomes the authoritative provider of their beginning explorations in language, reading, writing, and other subject matters.

Adults, by contrast, have already completed the basics and established a large reservoir of experiential learning that makes them independent and in control of their own learning needs. As a continuing education provider, the one complaint that this author has seen occasionally about an education leader that illustrates this thought is the remark, "He (or she) treated us like children." Heaven forbid.

Treating adults like children is a repugnant concept to some but it helps us to understand andragogy, or adult learning. Pedagogy means learning as it applies to children. Andragogy implies that the adult will define his or her own learning needs, be independent, draw on his or her own experiences, and learn material that can be applied *now* or in one's current career. Whereas we educate children for the future, adults require updating that they can use right now. Table 19-1 displays the basic differences between child and adult learners.

Educators have long recognized that learning involves some behavioral change. During the past 20 to 30 years we have seen ideas about learning being tested scientifically, and learning theories postulated and tested. As early as the 1960s, Crow and Crow (1963) defined learning as a process of change that was concerned with the acquisition of habits, knowledge, and attitudes. They postulated that learning enables the individual to make both personal and social adjustments. Since the concept of change is inherent in the concept of learning, any change in behavior implies that learning is taking place or has taken place. Learning that occurs during the process

TABLE 19-1
Differences between child and adult learners

	CHILDREN	ADULTS
Purpose	To prepare for the future	To use now in work or leisure
Orientation	Child is dependent on adult for defining learning content	Adults want to define their own learning needs in a more independent or collaborative style
Approach	Fairly didactic teacher:lectures and guides child	Fairly egalitarian teacher: adults want to participate actively in learning experiences
Experiential	Limited experience to draw on because of age and immaturity	Great experience to draw on because of advanced age and maturity

of change can be referred to as the learning process.

Another definition of learning discusses the interaction of a person with his or her environment. Burton (1963) believed that learning is a change in the individual, owing to the interaction of that individual with the environment, which fills a need and makes him or her more capable of dealing adequately with the environment.

In *Learning Theories for Teachers*, Bigge (1982) synthesizes core concepts offered by many leading learning theorists. Gagne (1972) thought of learning as a change in human disposition or capability that could be retained, which was not simply ascribable to the process of growth. He introduced the concept of information processing and drew a comparison of the mind as being similar to the operations of a computer.

In his seminal work, Skinner (1968) introduced psychological conditioning and advanced the theory that the stimulus-response mechanism was a clear definition of a change in behavior. Stimulus-response conditioning is from the behavioristic model of learning theory and focuses on conditioning with or without reinforcement, defining learning through classic conditioning and instrumental conditioning.

THE HISTORY OF CONTINUING EDUCATION IN PROFESSIONAL NURSING

The term *continuing education* (CE) has been used to synthesize the special learning and renewal that takes place *after* the basic and degree earning education have been completed. The role of universities and other learning institutions in meeting the mandate of continuing education is expected in every modern society.

Nurses who have completed basic degrees (ADN, BSN) look to schools and colleges—and more frequently to hospitals—to provide them with classes and seminars for updating their outdated information, and for offering them the opportunities to upgrade their skills and education. Hospital-based nurses expect their institutions to provide applicable refresher courses. In many clinical settings, there is a system in place for updating and renewing outdated information for quality practice.

Continuing education is the link from basic preparation to advancement in one's career. CE not only upgrades professional information but it can also be a great source of rejuvenation and inspiration. Why shouldn't it be fun—a rhetorical question.

In the 1960s the United States saw a movement toward continuing education that had the nursing world debating whether CE was really necessary, and if it was—should it be mandatory for relicensure. Throughout the country, the standard bearers, as this author likes to think of them, held statewide meetings of nurses and debated how such a movement could be realized. First, since very little had been done in setting up a system for giving credit for these offerings, the challenge across the country became one of providing worthwhile continuing education for nursing practice and at the same time developing a system that was transferable from state to state.

Second, should such a system be incorporated in each state's nurse practice act? Should a nurse be required by law to take CE courses in order to maintain her or his state license for practice? Needless to say, the movement in the 1970s quickly led to many states' adopting standards for CE, setting up systems for continuing education and recognition programs (CEARP). The tedious political and legislative work was begun to raise the standards of practice, so that nurses would be required to update their skills and knowledge.

In the early years, permissive legislation was enacted followed by mandatory laws, for example, the requirement of 20 or 30 hours of CE to renew one's license. Many states adopted a new requirement and continue to do so. If the demand for CE is legislated, the supply of CE offerings in a wide variety of forms will be generated. Thus, the beginning of this major trend has been realized. Universities have offered continuing education and businesses have been formed to market CE offerings.

THE VALUE OF CONTINUING EDUCATION

One of the most frequently debated questions today is whether continuing education actually does change behavior? A correlate question is always,

does it improve patient care? Abruzzese (1987), a national leader in continuing education, lists factors that influence the answer to the question of what is the value of CE? Motivation of the learner, support of supervisory personnel, milieu in which practice occurs, realistic expectation of courses, past experiences of learners, shortage of staff, expertise of teachers, and climate for change are all seen as important factors—if there is to be a change in practice for the better.

Farley (1987) attempted to document a change in nursing practice following a CE offering. Participants were asked to compare their own objectives for the practice setting. Although small in scope and number of subjects, the research is an attempt to transfer learned skills from continuing education into the practice of nursing.

Wake (1987), continuing with the idea of identifying relationships between instructional variables and postteaching change in practice, studied 220 participants. Findings supported the importance of postconference strategies. Suggestions for implementation of new knowledge should be included in CE instruction. Interactive teaching and learning is important in lectures. People must be able to discuss and participate.

The author has found the most cogent result of these studies for adult learners is the finding that the learning must be applicable to current nursing practice. This reiterates the theory of the differences between educating children and adults. Where children are being prepared for the future, adults want to be able to apply the learning in their present work.

Milson and Miaskowski (1987) studied a career nursing CE program and used Knowles's theory of adult learning (1984). Reports from participants in the Adelphi Oncology Certificate Program (Nielsen, Hyman, & Abruzzese, 1979) showed that continuing education influenced professional nursing practice. Participants offered countless reports of activities of leadership and curriculum activities.

Hutton (1987) reviewed research on nurses' attitudes and perceived outcomes and proposed that the fundamental issue posed by mandatory continuing education is the relationship between continuing education and enhanced clinical practice. One consistent theme of this researcher's conclusions is that nurses in states that have mandatory requirements for relicensure favor compulsory participation in continuing education courses, and perceive more benefits than problems with it. The participants did not find the costs prohibitive, and thought that performance was positively affected.

In New Mexico, this author and colleagues conducted a randomized survey using State Board of Nursing membership lists to determine contemporary continuing education needs (Rosenblum, Weiss, & Morris, 1988). The survey was sent to a random sample of 800 registered nurses. In a Sun-belt state like New Mexico with a rapidly growing population and much new migration, there is a population mix of native born with many recently arrived nurses. A response rate of close to 37% (294 respondents) revealed the following demographics: *Educational background of respondents*—over two-thirds (70.52%) of the respondents were either ADN or diploma graduates. One-fourth were BSN graduates, while only 6% held master's degrees or above. *Employment status*—approximately two-thirds (63.95%) of the respondents worked full-time. The median salary level of those respondents who worked full-time was between $21,000 and $25,999 per year. The part-time nurses who responded earned less than $15,000.

The purpose of this study was to compare statewide demographics with other published studies and to gain a baseline for assessing continuing education needs as described by those surveyed. More than 99% of the respondents in the study indicated that they would attend and pay for relevant continuing education in their work community. The most important reasons for selecting a CE program were topic of the program (80.14%), cost (42.55%), and number of credit hours or CEARP units (36.27%). Only a small percentage listed a speaker as being important to their choice. From this study the author and colleagues learned that the most popular topics are legal and ethical issues followed closely by physical assessment and health promotion.

THE ACCREDITATION PROCESS IN CONTINUING EDUCATION

The Council on Continuing Education of the American Nurses' Association (ANA) offered leadership in the quest for quality in both CE offerings and providers. ANA attempted to set up a system that was fair and equitable and finally to develop a national accreditation mechanism that could be uniform across states and territories.

At the June 1988, ANA Convention, the Board of Directors took action that culminates more than a decade of dedicated work toward this goal. There is now one national accreditation body in the ANA that is responsible for policymaking and implementation. The historical review of the major continuing education achievements of the American Nurses' Association is presented in Table 19-2.

Approximately 38 states and the District of Columbia currently meet the stringent standards for accredited approvers and 13 specialty nursing associations are approved for offerings. Note that not all states have received this accreditation. Perhaps the best way to explain this phenomenon is to pause and think about the leadership and determination of those individual nurses who dedicated themselves to the task of initiating a continuing education system in their individual states.

Accreditation in states is almost always in the hands of volunteers. There may be paid executive directors but this author suspects that they will admit readily that such movements as these are the achievements of their dedicated member volunteers. CE does not just happen. It has to be made to happen.

INTERNATIONAL CONTINUING EDUCATION ACROSS THE GLOBE

In 1980, this author first submitted an application to the continuing education unit of the American Nurses' Association (ANA) to approve an international program in continuing education for nurses. Professional Seminar Consultants (PSC) developed program offerings and was given approval to offer these programs for 2 years. PSC is accredited by the ANA Board on Accreditation as a provider of inter-

TABLE 19-2
Historical Perspective

1981	ANA Accreditation Board (now called Board of Accreditation) began evaluating the nursing continuing education accreditation and approval system to ensure a comprehensive, consistent and easily understood national system.
1981–1984	[Board of Accreditation] developed several models which were reviewed in the field by all accredited organizations and internal ANA units including the Constituent Forum.
Dec 1984	Board of Directors approved revised accreditation system.
Jan 1985– Mar 1986	Board on [sic] Accreditation and Regional Accreditation Committees developed policies, procedures and criteria for the revised system.
Nov 1985	Orientation meeting by the Board of Accreditation for accredited providers. Some significant changes to the system were requested by the approvers.
Dec 1985	Board on [sic] Accreditation met to incorporate changes.
Mar 1986	Board on [sic] Accreditation met to finalize system.
Oct 1986	New accreditation manuals [were] distributed to users of [the] system. New accreditation fee schedule [was] announced.
Dec 1986	Board of Directors agreed that the governance structure needed to be examined from a cost-effective standpoint. Board of Directors directed the Cabinet on Nursing Education to prepare [a] report for [the] June 1987 meeting.
Mar 1987	"Proposed Plan" for a modified governance structure for Accreditation of Continuing Education in Nursing was reviewed by the Cabinet on Nursing Education. The Cabinet on Nursing Education met, considered the "Proposed Plan," and developed additional areas of concern regarding modifications to the structure. The Cabinet also deemed it appropriate that those most involved with the accreditation system have an opportunity to review and comment. The Cabinet also sought guidance from the Board of Directors.
Apr 1987	The Cabinet on Nursing Education reported to the Board [of Accreditation] and recommended that implementation of the new system be delayed until February 1988. The Cabinet also asked the [Board of Accreditation] to "clearly delineate the goals of the accreditation program. Specifically, should the program be a profit generating (money-making) activity or a subsidized membership service?" The Board of Accreditation accepted the Cabinet's report and the first recommendation. No action was taken on the second recommendation.
Jun 1987– Sep 1987	Review of the "Proposed Plan" and the Cabinet on Nursing Education's additional areas of concern by the Board of Accreditation, regional accreditation committees, and Executive Committee of the Council on Continuing Education. Responses were sent to the Cabinet on Nursing Education.
Aug 1987	Began implementation of newly revised accreditation system.
Sep 1987	New accreditation fee schedule [was] announced.
Oct 1987	The Cabinet on Nursing Education met and considered consensus reports. The Cabinet on Nursing Education decided on recommendations to the Board [of Accreditation] that would make the system self-supporting in 4 years while maintaining the quality of accreditation.
Dec 1987	The Cabinet on Nursing Education report with recommendations are considered by the Board [of Accreditation.]
Apr 1988	ANA Board of Directors reviews results of a study on accreditation that involved many organizations and groups. The Board [of Directors] approved the recommended modifications in the accreditation governance structure, including the following items: (1) There will be one national body consisting of 14 members that will be responsible for both policy and implementation. Five of the 14 members will serve as the policymaking committee. (2) The accreditation period will be changed from 4 years to 6 years.

Craddock A. (1988, July 8). Data are from personal communication with A. Craddock, Program Manager, Credentialing Center for Credentialing Services, American Nurses' Association.   *Continued.*

TABLE 19-2
Historical Perspective—cont'd

	(3) Site visits will remain a part of the accreditation process. (4) There will continue to be two application review cycles each year.
Jun 1988	The ANA Board of Directors took action in April 1988 and June 1988 that provides for the additional modifications to the accreditation program and governance structure as follows: *Structure:* There will be one national accreditation body, called the American Nurses' Association, Board of Accreditation, responsible for both policymaking and implementation. *Size:* The new Board of Accreditation will consist of 14 members who are responsible for implementation; 5 of these members will also serve as the executive committee, which will be the policymaking body. *Period of accreditation:* The accreditation period for both providers and approvers will be increased from 4 to 6 years. The change will be implemented beginning with organizations applying for accreditation on August 1, 1988. The fee for accreditation will change proportionally to reflect the additional 2 years. *Site visits:* Site visitors will continue as part of the accreditation process. Members of the current regional accrediting committee and the Board of Accreditation continued their present terms through August, 1988. The new 14-member Board of Accreditation became operational on September 1.

national continuing education programs. The office for International Operations is located in Kansas City, Missouri and the office for Professional Continuing Education is based in Albuquerque, New Mexico. In 1980, five study tours were planned. One year later, the number of tours increased to 30. Nursing leaders such as Belinda Puetz, Eileen Jacobi, and Lucie Kelly, joined this author and a small group of medical leaders to visit the Soviet Union in 1981 (Rosenblum, 1982). During this meeting of key professionals, additional seminars were planned through the auspices of PSC.

In the years that followed (1983, 1985, 1987), there were three 2-year accreditation cycles. In 1988 PSC was awarded full provider status of continuing education by the ANA for 4 years. These efforts have resulted in more than 600 study tours drawn from a pool of more than 1000 nurse educators who have visited nursing groups and toured in more than 20 countries on every continent. More than 13,000 American nurses have participated as registrants.

Opportunity

International continuing education has been a major turning point for the author, for the national advisory committee that serves PSC, for the hundreds of educational leaders who direct the learning, and for the thousands of registrants who participate, as well as for the host groups that receive these distinguished lecturers. When the author keynoted the Hong Kong Nurses' Association's first conference in 1985, she was surrounded by Chinese colleagues whose friendship will always be cherished. Had it not been for this opportunity in international CE, they would never have met. They would never have had a steady stream of visiting scholars to lecture, share information, and challenge them to lead their nursing groups in the quest for professionalism (Rosenblum, 1986a, 1986b). Many education leaders and registrants, who have participated in the tours, would never have had the opportunity to learn directly from them about health care in their countries.

Across the world in Kenya, the Kenya Nurses' Association meets each PSC group of nurses and together they share new knowledge and common nursing interests. For them there is an opportunity to have excellent visiting educators and to build their nursing fellowship fund. For the American nurse registrants, program evaluations consistently show a deepened appreciation for what dedicated African nurses can do in situations that constantly challenge one's initiative and resources. The values that are developed through this unique programming may be difficult to measure in actual clinical behavioral change, but professional enrichment is enhanced nevertheless. And so it goes, the constant learning and relearning, the cultural awakenings and the fears that are abated, the networks that are formed, the friendships that are made.

The need to encourage international collaboration in research efforts is imperative, as we see our profession emerging with a true scientific basis for practice. Sigma Theta Tau, Inc. is leading internationally in this continuing education endeavor by conducting international meetings and helping to set up chapters abroad.

Many educators have said that the teacher is the architect and the builder of behaviors. We need to expand on our narrow school-learning to see the broad relations of our life experiences. We need constant renewal in learning in order to understand anything at all. We must build our experiential base, challenge our intellect, and expand our horizons. Continuing education on the local, national, or international level is a marvelous vehicle for such a learning adventure.

REFERENCES

Abruzzese, R. S. (1987). Effects of continuing education: Where's the proof? [Editorial]. *Journal of Continuing Education in Nursing, 18*(6), 183.

Bigge, M. L. (1982). *Learning theories for teachers* (4th ed.). Harper & Row: New York.

Burton, W. H. (1963). Basic principles in a good teaching-learning situation. In L. D. Crow & A. Crow (Eds.), *Readings in human learning* (pp. 7–19). New York: McKay.

Crow, L. D., & Crow, A. (Eds.). (1963). *Readings in human learning*. New York: McKay.

Farley, J. (1987). Does continuing nursing education make a difference? *Journal of Continuing Education in Nursing, 18*(6), 184–187.

Gagne, N. L. (1972). *Teacher effectiveness and teacher education*. Palo Alto, CA: Pacific Books.

Hutton, C. A. (1987). Impact of mandatory continuing education: A review of research on nurses' attitudes and perceived outcomes. *Journal of Continuing Education in Nursing, 18*(6), 209–213.

Knowles, M. S. (1984). *The adult learner: A neglected species* (3rd ed.). Houston: Gulf Publishing.

Milson, B., & Miaskowski, C. (1987). The influence of an oncology nursing education program on nursing practice. *Journal of Continuing Education in Nursing, 18*(6), 193–199.

Nielsen, B., Hyman, R. B., & Abruzzese, R. (1979). Designing cancer nursing courses for community hospitals. *Cancer Nursing, 2*, 109–116.

Rosenblum, E. H. (1982). *Nursing in the Soviet Union*. Oceanside, NY: Professional Seminar Consultants.

Rosenblum, E. H. (1986a). East meets West: Sino-American curriculum visit collaboration for baccalaureate education in China now and in the future. *Hong Kong Nursing Journal [Hsiang-kang Hu Li Tsa Chih]*, November issue (41), 8–14.

Rosenblum, E. (1986b). Trends in nursing: In view of Halley's comet. *Hong Kong Nursing Journal [Hsiankang Hu Li Tsa Chih]*, November issue (41), 29–34.

Rosenblum, E. H., Weiss, J., & Morris, L. (1988). *Statewide continuing education needs assessment:* New Mexico. Unpublished manuscript, University of New Mexico, College of Nursing, Albuquerque, New Mexico.

Skinner, B. F. (1968). *The technology of teaching*. New York: Appleton-Century-Crofts.

Tough, A. (1979). *The adult's learning projects: A fresh approach to theory and practice in adult learning* (2nd ed.). Austin, TX: Learning Concepts.

Wake, M. (1987). Effective instruction in continuing nursing education. *Journal of Continuing Education in Nursing, 18*(6), 188–192.

✳   **EDITOR'S QUESTIONS FOR DISCUSSION**   ✳

What strategies might be offered to encourage professional socialization as lifelong learning? What should be the role of continuing education in the life of the professional nurse in contrast to formal academic programs? Discuss the pros and cons of mandatory continuing education for relicensure. Discuss strategies by which international continuing education programs that are most relevant for the practice of nursing might be developed, offered, monitored, and evaluated. What criteria should be enforced for a continuing education program and offering? What application from Jensen and Lindeman (Chapter 18) may be made to and for international continuing education programs?

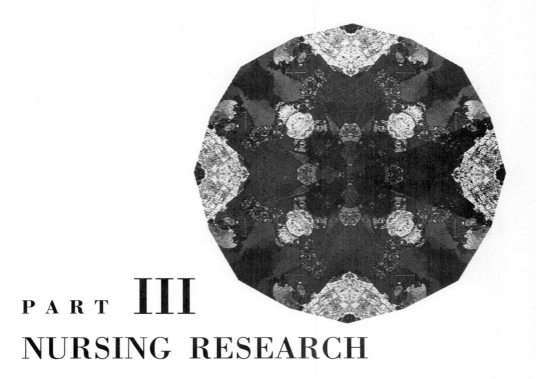

PART III
NURSING RESEARCH

Symmetrical patterns of geodetic design are woven in the nursing kaleidoscope to mirror a broad spectrum of research questions that need to be addressed. Preconceived ideas regarding the appropriate utilization of research methods are being challenged. Research horizons are being expanded through a spectrum of various methodological hues. The nursing curiosity is being stimulated. Nursing questions are unfolding. Blindness becomes sight and darkness becomes light through the stained glass of discovery and surprise. Nursing is projecting its own world of vision through advancing nursing research.

The magic of pattern is unveiled through kaleidoscopes. A look at what can be perceived as abstract within the confines of the mind is glimpsed. Likewise the chapters in this section reflect only a glimmer of the concerns in the emerging realm of nursing research.

Carol Deets in Chapter 20 focuses on the four concepts of the nursing metaparadigm. Evidence of research to test one or more of the concepts and to develop the metaparadigm is extremely minimal. Alternative foci are suggested for scientific research in nursing.

Eleanor Donnelly and Carol Deets demonstrate in Chapter 21 that there exists a comparable relation of consequence between theory and observation in the conduct of scientific inquiry irrespective of the research methods employed. The authors illustrate their point by two methodological examples drawn from their separate research agenda.

The debate as to the research methods or strategies to acquire the fullest understanding of nursing phenomena is further addressed by Marilyn Stember and Nancy Hester in Chapter 22. They reaffirm that inquiry must integrate approaches. The authors offer an unifying paradigm to extend beyond existing methods. Their desire is to articulate an approach for integrating and synthesizing knowledge derived through multiple ways of knowing.

Nursing as a science of human care has led researchers to the phenomenological method of inquiry. Marilyn Ray in Chapter 23 presents an exposition of phenomenology and its implications for nursing. The meaning of lived experience, health, and health care can be more completely understood through phenomenological research.

Meta-analysis as a quantitative method in reviewing and conducting research is described by Elizabeth Devine in Chapter 24. Some of the advantages and disadvantages of the method are presented in a general overview of the method.

In Chapter 25 Jacqueline Clinton explores the thorny issues engulfing the development of scientists and nursing research in the academic setting. Significant strategies are offered to address the numerous challenges. A community of nursing scholars is essential for advancing nursing as a science.

The relevance of research for nursing practice and the role of the clinical nurse researcher are highlighted in Chapter 26, by Karen Haller. She identifies the various models used to generate nursing research. Haller outlines research programs that are housed in practice settings. The role of the nurse researcher is thoroughly examined in terms of structure, process, and outcomes.

It is clear that research—and kaleidoscopes—encourage people to look at their environment in a different way. There are systematic steps to follow to reach the world of inquiry. For nursing, research is an integration of knowledge and understanding just as color and the various hues of the kaleidoscope show the beauty of pattern unfolding.

20

Nursing's Paradigm and a Search for Its Methodology

Carol A. Deets, Ed.D., R.N.

About 10 years ago, several prominent nurse authors suggested that the most expeditious approach to ensure that nursing was recognized as a science (or at least an applied science) would be to determine the concepts that would be the cornerstones of the nursing paradigm (Bush, 1979; Fawcett, 1978, 1983; Flaskerud & Halloran, 1980; Newman, 1983). Apparently their reasoning was based on (a) Kuhn's (1962) contention that a mature science was characterized by agreement among its scientists on one paradigm and the "more esoteric type of research it permits" (p. 11); (b) the belief that members of the profession would focus their research in terms of these concepts; and (c) the expectation that a true paradigm would develop faster as a result of this concentrated effort. The hope of the prominent nurse authors was that Kuhn's idea of a paradigm could be useful in allowing nursing to become a science in much less time than if nature was allowed to take its normal, slow, torturous path of theory development.

With little effort, these authors were able to generate considerable interest in four concepts—environment, nursing, man or person, and health. Books on the nursing process were revised to include these four concepts if they were not already there, or to make the concepts more prominent if they had been previously considered. The authors who purported to deal with nursing theory also revised their work to illustrate how it addressed the four concepts if they had not previously done so. Did these changes produce the desired result? Are nurse researchers developing a paradigm in nursing based on the cornerstone concepts? The purposes of this chapter are to assess the current research (a) to determine if the four concepts are being studied specifically in terms of a paradigm, and (b) to see if indeed there is an identifiable paradigm emerging.

The criterion for making a judgment about the first purpose—determining whether the concepts were being studied as part of a paradigm—was that the author made such a statement. Kuhn's (1962) criteria were used for making a judgment concerning the second purpose. Kuhn contended that a paradigm functioned much like a map, assisting research practitioners in deciding what should and should not be addressed. From his perspective, a paradigm includes agreement among the practitioners as to the theory, methods to use in conducting the research, and standards for those who conduct research under its rubric. The paradigm also becomes the content taught those aspiring to become members of that scientific community. There is no question that content related to the four paradigm concepts is being taught. The problem in deciding about the emergence of a paradigm is whether or not there is (a) an identified theory being produced through research, (b) consensus on the use of methodology, and (c) standards for the conduct of research. The first two criteria are the ones used in assessing the second purpose of this chapter. Since an emerging paradigm is expected, it would be unrealistic to find agreed-on standards for the conduct of research.

OVERVIEW OF KUHN'S IDEA OF A PARADIGM

Kuhn (1962) developed the idea of paradigms as a result of his attempt to theorize about the development of science. He studied mature sciences by tracing the development of their paradigms. Why did one paradigm gain sufficient status in a science to preclude the viewing of reality from a competing point of view in that science? Kuhn described the circumstances that led to the changing of scientific ideas within a community of scholars during the period of change. He also described the changes in scientific ideas after a competing paradigm emerged. In essence, he felt that when a paradigm became the accepted one, its acceptance by that science's scholars was the result of the fact that the paradigm's theory was best able to explain the phenomena of interest. He found that the paradigm's research methods were often developed as the theory developed, and that they reflected technical as well as theoretical advances. Specific concepts become the hallmark of the science because of their centrality to their theory. The paradigm grew as the research findings produced information that was employed to refine the theory and its explanatory power. The accumulation of this research-based information often took considerable time—50, 100, or even more years—and these were mature sciences, not aspiring ones.

In its rush to mature, nursing has attempted to short-circuit the process of developing a tradition, by the massing of research information to decide the paradigm's concepts and then conducting the research. Positions can be taken to support and refute the wisdom of this position, but in truth, only time will reveal the result of the gamble. That is why an assessment of progress to date has value.

REVIEW OF THE LITERATURE

The only work that attempts to review previous research and its influence on theory development in nursing is Silva's article (1986), in which she sought to determine the status of efforts to test nursing theory. She considered Johnson, Roy, Orem, Rogers, and Newman to be nurse theorists.

Basically Silva (1986) found that nurses reported using a nursing model (a) as a framework, but did little with it—24 of 62 studies fell in this category; (b) as a means for organizing their study—29 of 62 studies; and (c) to test a proposition—9 of 62 studies. Both this author and Silva consider the third use of a model to represent a testing of a theory. Unfortunately only 3 of these 9 studies were identified by Silva (1986). Of these 3 studies, only 1 addressed a paradigm concept and that concept was health. In fact, health was operationally identified through the variables of time and motion; thus, even this study really did not meet the criterion for testing a paradigm concept. One of Silva's conclusions was that more theory testing has not occurred because of a lack of commitment to such activities in the discipline. The author of this chapter proposes that nursing theories do not provide nurse researchers with the direction they need to conceptualize their studies.

The fact is that only 1 of the 62 articles reviewed by Silva (1986) addressed one of the cornerstone concepts and that one—only indirectly since it could be attributed to a time factor. Silva's work was published in 1986 and thus means that the majority of the research surveyed was conducted before 1985. Sufficient time may not have transpired for nurse researchers to have heeded the recommendations to conceptualize research using the four cornerstone concepts, actually implemented the research, and published the results of such research.

METHODOLOGY

The population of published articles for the study that is the subject of this paper were those articles published in *Advances in Nursing Science*, *Nursing Research*, *Western Journal of Nursing Research*, and

Research in Nursing and Health during 2 years, 1986 and 1987. The studies included in the sample were those in which the four paradigm concepts were addressed. There was one exception to the 1986, 1987 dates: the April 1988 issue of *Advances in Nursing Science* that was dedicated to theory and practice. The 1988 inclusion increased the probability that the articles might address at least one of the four concepts.

For inclusion of a study, the authors had to indicate that in some way the study addressed one or more of the paradigm concepts. This criterion soon proved too limiting, and thus an article was included in this study if its purpose or if the data collected addressed one of the four concepts.

If the concept "health" was described in terms of health behaviors (or health beliefs, or similar applied terms), the article was not included as a health concept article. There seems to be a very different concept of health as a goal, as separate from behaviors taken to gain or maintain a healthy status. The concept "nursing" was considered to represent the process and not the profession. The concepts of "environment" and of "man" or "person" were expected to function as wholes, not parts of the total, for example, the concept "self-esteem" was not considered the same as man or person.

The review of published articles was limited to 2 years because there was no need to replicate Silva's (1986) work. Perhaps her results will have influenced current nurse researchers to conduct more rigorous testing of theory studies.

When so few articles that met the criteria were found, the *Annual Review of Nursing Research* (Vols. 4, 5, and 6) for 1986, 1987, and 1988 were also reviewed. Since the reviews were designed to address some aspect of nursing research, the inclusion of a paradigm concept seemed probable.

When a study was identified as an appropriate data source, the following information was noted:

1. The specific paradigm concept that was addressed and the expected relationship with other concepts—especially paradigm concepts;
2. The methodology employed in the study that

was identified, with no judgment on its appropriateness or rigor of the method; and

3. The presence or absence of theory testing in the study that was determined employing the same criteria as Silva (1986).

There were no attempts to judge the adequacy of the methods employed in the review of each of the studies, but rather the emphasis was to identify what type of method was associated with each concept and its theory (framework). Since the presence of a theory is expected in a paradigm, the framework offered by the researcher in each of the studies was also noted—again, the concern was to identify those theories that were consistently employed when a specific concept or set of concepts was considered.

FINDINGS

Of over 300 published articles reviewed, only 6 met the criteria for inclusion. The concepts health and nursing were each addressed in 2 articles. The concepts environment and person were each cited in 1 article. In only 2 of the reviewed articles did the authors indicate that their work was in any way related to efforts to develop a paradigm, to test 1 or more of its concepts, or to provide any cues that might suggest this was their purpose.

The only work this author found that addressed the concept of environment was Williams's review chapter (1988), which restricted the environment to the physical factors linked to patient care. About half of the articles reviewed in the study were not published in the nursing literature. Of those published in the nursing literature, sensory deprivation, excessive noise, and the effects of different stimuli on the elderly tended to be the foci rather than a testing of the concept environment. Williams concluded that "the physical environment for patient care has commanded limited attention from nurse researchers" (1988, p. 77).

There were 2 articles on an aspect of the health concept. One article (Laffrey, 1986a) was concerned with the development of a tool to measure the meaning of health, whereas the second article was the report of a study. In developing the tool, Laffrey

(1986a) considered perception of health in four dimensions: clinical (absence of illness), functional or role performance, adaptive (flexible adjustment), and eudaimonistic (exuberant well-being). She then discussed the importance of health as a concept to nursing because it was a paradigm concept—but not in terms of developing or testing the paradigm. In the second article (Laffrey, 1986b), differences between two groups were tested, but none were significant. In this study, Laffrey found the correlation coefficients of health concept with health behaviors scores significant for both groups, indicating that beliefs covary with behavior. Interestingly, the health concept scores were not separated into the four dimensions.

There were 2 articles that addressed the concept nursing; however, neither were reports of research. One was by Schlotfeldt (1987), and the other by Kasch (1986). My conclusion is that the major contribution of Schlotfeldt's article is its clearly stated message that nursing diagnoses will not and cannot lead to theory development in nursing. Although this reality is evident by observing the results of developing an extensive taxonomy of diagnoses in medicine, there is still considerable effort being expended by nurses to develop theory from the taxonomy of nursing diagnoses.

Kasch's article (1986) was designed to address clearly the concept nursing as part of the paradigm. The purpose of this article was to suggest that the best way to conceptualize nursing action was to consider it in terms of a social interaction process. The thesis of the article is based on a symbolic interactionist perspective, which some shortsighted nurses might reject because it comes from another discipline. The philosophical orientation outlined in the article is an argument for supporting the type of research studies that are being published in the nursing journals, that is, perceptions and beliefs of clients about their ability to manage their condition. Kasch did not place the other paradigm concepts into a relationship with health, and in fact, her arguments could result in reducing the role of environment.

Schultz's article (1987) was the only one that addressed the concept man or person. Kasch (1986) and Schultz (1987) were the only authors who contended that they were addressing a cornerstone concept of the nursing paradigm. Schultz presented the argument that person(s) was (were) usually conceptualized inappropriately. In order to include terms such as *family* and *communities* that have an interactional connotation, Schultz asserted that the concept person must be conceptualized as more than just aggregates (the summing of units).

The second purpose of this author's study was the attempt to identify common measurement and research techniques that should be there if a paradigm was indeed emerging. Most methodologies employed in the 6 studies were simplistic in nature, reflecting tool development, comparison of groups, or presenting a logical, philosophical argument. No attempt at theory testing was found in any of the 6 articles.

Serendipitous Findings

There were some interesting findings across the 300-plus reviewed studies. First—and in this author's view, a very positive one—the topics that have been studied and reported during the last 2 years seem to cluster into categories that may have theoretical importance. On the other hand, there were a few studies that dealt with specific physiological phenomena, for example, blood pressure, skin, and oxygenation, with even fewer studies dealing with specific procedures, for example, intramuscular (IM) sites and temperatures. These procedural studies tend to reflect problem solving rather than research-oriented studies, in that the issue inherent in the studies was which one of several sites (or techniques) is best.

The bulk of studies addressed some aspect of the personal experience of the clients, for example, personal adjustment, beliefs, perceptions, and the influence of this personal experience on the ability of clients to manage their condition. Most of these studies relied on theoretical efforts that came from other paradigms such as stress and coping, attitude theory, and role attainment rather than any of the nursing models.

The second interesting and important finding is that several of the studies addressed an interaction of some aspect of the physical with some aspect of the experiential. This category included studies on pain management, sleep-wake patterns, and why clients make the decisions they do with respect to the management of their health problems. The number of studies investigating interactional questions will probably increase as more is learned about the personal experience of clients. This is an area in which nurses may make unique contributions to science.

Another observation that probably reflects the limited nature of the investigation and the youth of theory development in nursing is the fact that few articles are by the same researcher addressing the same research interest. In the reviewed journals, there was only one author who had two articles that included the same concept in both studies. Unfortunately this observation is typical. Instead of authors belonging to a tradition and working within that tradition over several years and many studies, a review of the literature indicates that nurse researchers seem to change orientations and interests, seldom pursuing any one in depth. This is unfortunate because continued work in one area is the only way one can obtain sufficient knowledge to have the potential of adding new knowledge.

An anticipated problem by this author was that the different ways of measuring a concept would result in data that represented different concepts, for example, Spielberger's state anxiety as measured by the State-Trait Inventory does not measure the same concept as Taylor's Manifest Anxiety test (Spielberger, Gorsuch, Luschene, Vagg, & Jacobs, 1983). Measurement techniques that reflect different theoretical orientations, even though the concept's label is the same, do not produce measurement of comparable concepts. Until more research is executed employing the same concept, this will not be a problem. Perhaps by then nurse researchers will have matured sufficiently to anticipate and not commit this error.

DISCUSSION

The authors of opinion-based literature repeatedly assert that there is agreement on the four cornerstone concepts of health, nursing, environment, and man or person. Perhaps it is this very agreement that stands in the way of research being conducted on the four concepts or their interrelationships. These concepts may be considered by many nurses to exist as realities. If they are a reality, why bother testing them any further? Of course, that is just the point. These concepts cannot be realities if they are part of a theoretical paradigm that must be composed of theoretical abstractions. They must be abstractions that reflect the reality that nurses have attempted to explain and to understand through the theories. And these theoretical propositions must be tested!

The absence of articles addressing the cornerstone concepts may reflect the strict interpretation of the concepts employed in the assessment. If the research did not address man as a whole rather than a part, the article was not included in the sample. In other words, all articles that addressed aspects of the self (self-esteem, role, values, perceptions, and the like) or the individual in the context of a larger unit (social support, psychosocial adjustment, and so on) were omitted. As stated previously, health behaviors and health beliefs were not considered as instances of the health concept. This author's definitions of the four concepts might have been too restrictive.

Another explanation for the findings is that it is not possible to build paradigms from the top down (identify concepts leading to theory) rather than from the bottom up (develop theory that guides in the identification of concepts) as conceptualized by Kuhn (1962). To support this explanation, one must first assume that Kuhn's approach to the development of science is appropriate. There are no data to support this assumption and there are many rival hypotheses on how sciences develop; thus, the viability of this argument is questionable.

Another way to address this problem would be to consider the expansive nature of the concepts and the phenomena they are attempting to explain. If the phenomenon is nursing care, how can concepts that are so inclusive possibly explain the specific aspects of care?

In summary, the four concepts of environment, nursing, man or person, and health do not seem to offer much in terms of theory development. Whatever the explanation for not finding research results that support the development of a paradigm, the fact remains that there is little support for the viability of the concepts, much less the paradigm. After almost 10 years, there are two obvious questions. If there have not been data to support the development of the four cornerstone concepts and thus *the paradigm*, what is the rationale employed by the nurse educators who continue to develop curricula and teach nursing as if the four cornerstone concepts are realities? The second question may have even more impact on the future: If young nursing scholars have been socialized into a nonexisting paradigm and attempt to conduct their research within that paradigm, how greatly will they be distracted and deflected from producing the much-needed scientific research in nursing?

REFERENCES

Bush, H. A. (1979). Models for nursing. *Advances in Nursing Science, 1*, 13–21.

Fawcett, J. (1978). The 'what' of theory development. In J. Fawcett (Ed.), *Theory development: What, why, how?* New York: National League for Nursing.

Fawcett, J. (1983). Hallmarks of success in theory development. In P. L. Chinn (Ed.), *Advances in nursing theory development* (pp. 3–15). Rockville, MD: Aspen Publications.

Flaskerud, J. H., & Halloran, E. J. (1980). Areas of agreement in nursing theory development. *Advances in Nursing Science, 3*, 1–7.

Fitzpatrick, J. J., & Taunton, R. L. (Eds.). (1987). *Annual Review of Nursing Research, Vol. 5*. New York: Springer.

Fitzpatrick, J. J., Taunton, R. L., & Benoliel, J. Q. (Eds.). (1988). *Annual Review of Nursing Research, Vol. 6*. New York: Springer Publishing.

Kasch, C. R. (1986). Toward a theory of nursing action: Skills and competency in nurse-patient interaction. *Nursing Research, 35*, 226–230.

Kuhn, T. S. (1962). *The structure of scientific revolutions*. Chicago: University of Chicago Press.

Laffrey, S. C. (1986a). Development of a health conception scale. *Research in Nursing and Health, 9*, 107–113.

Laffrey, S. C. (1986b). Normal and overweight adults: Perceived weight and health behavior characteristics. *Nursing Research, 35*, 3–86.

Newman, M. A. (1983). The continuing revolution: A history of nursing science. In N. L. Chaska (Ed.), *The nursing profession: A time to speak* (pp. 385–393). New York: McGraw-Hill.

Schlotfeldt, R. M. (1987). Defining nursing: A historic controversy. *Nursing Research, 36*, 64–67.

Schultz, P. R. (1987). When client means more than one: Extending the foundational concept of person. *Advances in Nursing Science, 10*, 71–86.

Silva, M. C. (1986). Research testing nursing theory: State of the art. *Advances in Nursing Science, 9*, 1–11.

Spielberger, C., Gorsuch, R., Luschene, R., Vagg, P., & Jacobs, G. (1983). *Manual for the State-Trait Anxiety Inventory* (form Y). Palo Alto, CA: Consulting Psychologists Press.

Werley, H. H., Fitzpatrick, J. J., & Taunton, R. L. (Eds.). (1986). *Annual Review of Nursing Research, Vol. 4*. New York: Springer Publishing.

Williams, M. A. (1988). The physical environment and patient care. In J. J. Fitzpatrick, R. L. Taunton, & J. Q. Benoliel (Eds.), *Annual review of nursing research* (Vol. 6, pp. 61–84). New York: Springer Publishing.

✳   **EDITOR'S QUESTIONS FOR DISCUSSION**   ✳

Discuss Deets's criteria for including a research article in her study. Were the criteria that she employed too restrictive? Would you agree with her definitions of the concepts? What other types of studies might have been considered in the review and why? Discuss the extent that agreement exists regarding the specific meaning of the nursing metaparadigm concepts among nurse theorists and researchers. What relationships may exist between the lack of commonly accepted concept definitions and the apparent lack of theory testing in nursing? Provide examples of measurement techniques that reflect different theoretical orientations of a single concept. Provide examples of different ways of measuring a concept that might result in data that represent different concepts. Can those data and findings then be compared? Is the issue that there is disagreement on the operational definitions of the cornerstone concepts but not on the concepts themselves? What kinds of problems are posed for comparing measurement of concepts and results of measuring concepts when more than one operational definition of a concept is involved?

Why may or may not nursing diagnoses lead to theory development in nursing? What might be the relationship and significance between developing an extensive taxonomy of diagnoses in medicine and the results of those efforts, and the efforts to develop theory in nursing from nursing diagnoses? How can concepts that are broadly defined explain specific aspects of care? As long as the so-called parts of the man or person concept are linked in a study in some fashion is not the whole being studied? To what extent do you agree or disagree with the author's conclusion regarding the usefulness of the four concepts for theory development in nursing? Provide evidence whereby curricula have been developed as if the four concepts are realities. What alternatives to the so-called accepted paradigm would you suggest for focus and development of scientific research in nursing?

21

Theory-Laden Observation:
Two examples

Eleanor Donnelly, Ph.D., R.N.
Carol A. Deets, Ed.D., R.N.

After an early infatuation with quantitative methods, nursing has begun to question the appropriateness of these methods for some of the questions it seeks to address. In this regard, nursing's intellectual odyssey seems to parallel that of education's, in which the adoption of an alternative in the form of qualitative methods has had a somewhat longer history. Having initially associated the use of quantitative methods with the practice of science, both groups are struggling to justify the incorporation of qualitative methods in their respective research endeavors. This struggle is reflected in a burgeoning literature. Shulman (1981), Smith (1983), Lincoln and Guba (1985), Smith and Heshusius (1986), Miller (1986), Firestone (1987), and Jacob (1988) in education; and Tinkle and Beaton (1983), Goodwin and Goodwin (1984), Leininger (1985), Sandelowski (1986), Powers (1987), Duffy (1987), and Phillips (1988) in nursing, are illustrative of but by no means exhaustive of the ongoing discussion.

Justifications for qualitative methods tend to highlight differences between these and quantitative methods, often characterizing the two as being on opposite ends of a continuum, for example, theory developing versus theory testing, nonexperimental versus experimental, "soft" science versus "hard"

science. Most unsettling in this arena of discourse has been the tendency to describe the use of *kinds of methods*, whether qualitative or quantitative, as *kinds of research* and to propose alternative sets of criteria for evaluating their adequacy.

In the authors' view, a pseudoproblem has been created. A mistaken belief about what constitutes science has been coupled with a failure to recognize that methods are simply ways of making observations. The problem dissolves when the essence of science is understood to be theory construction, and methods are seen to be what they are in the context of their use. Whether the methods of observation are qualitative or quantitative, the authors' maintain that an equivalent relation between theory and observation must hold. The purpose of this chapter is to demonstrate that there does indeed exist a similar relation of consequence between theory and observation in the conduct of scientific inquiry, irrespective of the research methods employed. How this relation is manifested is illustrated with two examples drawn from the authors' individual research agenda.

Both authors are interested in human cognition: the first (ED) in cognitive models of face-to-face interaction; the second (CD) in the role of attitudes or beliefs as predictors of behavior. Both want to know what some sector of the stream of experience looks like in order to understand better how the mind works. The authors are willing to entertain seriously the notion that these phenomena—cognitive models and attitudes or beliefs—exist not just as inventions of their minds but as real things subject to empirical investigation. To access the sectors of interest, subjects are asked questions about those sectors. With regard to the first author's interest, they are asked about occasions of face-to-face interaction. With respect to the second author's interest, they are asked about their attitudes or beliefs related to the enactment of specific behaviors. The authors believe the subjects' replies will be reflective of the content and structure of their experiences in these domains. The authors have elected, however, to explore and describe different aspects of the stream of experience, and they have chosen different ways to conduct that exploration. The first author (ED) has adopted a theory-generating approach and employs qualitative methods; the second author (CD) employs a theory-testing approach and quantitative methods. The authors regard these combinations of approach and method as outcomes of personal preferences and socialization experiences in their respective graduate programs. There is for them no necessary connection between phenomenon of interest and method of observation, between approach and method, or between design and method. Both regard themselves as conducting scientific inquiry and believe that the same criteria of adequacy should be applied to their respective endeavors.

SCIENTIFIC INQUIRY AND OBSERVATION

Research is either theory oriented or not. For the authors, theory-oriented research by definition is scientific inquiry. This means that an investigator is interested in patterns, regularities, or recurrences that the investigator attempts to describe and explain. There is an active search for a fit between description and explanation. The phenomena of focus are examined in order to infer the principles that underlie their organization or structure. The examination of these phenomena is conducted according to the method common to all scientific inquiry: an in-

vestigator obtains data by means of the senses and attempts to account for the data by means of explanations that, in turn, are themselves subjected to corroboration by the investigator's return to sense data. Particulars are of interest only insofar as they may illuminate the general.

It is a truism within the philosophy of science that all observations are selective in terms of some point of view, some theoretical stance, some bias (Brown, 1977; Hanson, 1958; Kaplan & Manners, 1972; Kuhn, 1962; Popper, 1963). An investigator cannot help but see the phenomena of interest in terms of some theoretical or conceptual orientation. Any description varies with the theoretical framework within which it is generated—even if that framework remains largely implicit for the person who generates the description. In other words, all observation by an investigator in the course of scientific inquiry is theory-laden. The more explicit the theoretical orientation is, the better guide it will be to the examination of relevant properties and events.

A theory directs an investigator's examination as to what to observe, but a given orientation does not contain within it any directives as to what method or methods to use for making observations. An investigator is free to choose whatever means of observation suggest themselves as enabling of the research objectives. A method qualifies as scientific depending on the kind of project within which it is embedded. Observations in and of themselves, however they are made, are neither scientific nor nonscientific. They may be made for a variety of ends—some scientific, some not, as in news reports. Nor is systematicity of observation in an effort to find out something sufficient to confer scientific status, as in the compilation of the United States census. When a method of observation is used to collect data within a context of scientific inquiry as previously described, it is then that the authors would regard such a method as scientific.

TWO EXAMPLES

In what follows, the authors each discuss some of the more conspicuous ways in which their respective theoretical orientations inform their decisions of what to observe and how to go about conducting those observations given the methods they have chosen. The first example is based on the first author's (ED) experience in conducting inquiry into subjects' cognitive models of face-to-face interaction. To make observations pertinent to her interests, she employs qualitative methods. The second example is based on the second author's (CD) experience in conducting inquiry into subjects' attitudes or beliefs in terms of Rosenstock's health belief model (HBM) (1966). She employs quantitative methods to make observations pertinent to her interests.

Cognitive Models of Face-to-Face Interaction

Cognitive models is the first author's (ED) answer to the question: What are interactants interacting in terms of? It is her belief that all experience is mediated by interpretation. In other words, people behave in terms of their interpretations of what is going on. She refers to subjects' interpretations of occasions of face-to-face interaction as cognitive models. And, because different people take different courses of action when confronted with the same objective conditions, She assumes that there are related differences in their cognitive models. The author wants to know what these models look like, how they are constructed, and how they relate to subsequent actions on the part of subjects.

To make observations of these models, the author must entertain some notion of what they look like (Donnelly, 1985, 1986, 1987; Donnelly & Moneyham, 1988 Dougherty, 1978, 1984a, 1984b; Dougherty & Morrissey, 1987). At present these cognitive models are conceived as configurations of temporally and hierarchically related sets of interpretations of interactional events. The interpretations are selective, differentially foregrounded, and multimodal in nature. They are conceived as consisting of two kinds of meaning designated as grounded meanings and valuative meanings in the author's framework. These occur ontologically as a unity, but are sometimes separable in discourse and are separable for purposes of analyses in making comparisons across subjects. Grounded meanings are interpretations of events at the level of recognition and identification.

Valuative meanings are interpretations of events at the level of their significance for a subject.

There are two kinds of cognitive models: schemata and signs. Schemata are models of an occasion as a class of experience. Signs are models of an occasion as an instance of experience. Schemata, formed by earlier experiences, influence the apprehension of current experience. They function as sets of expectations providing subjects with a framework of interpretation for successive occasions of face-to-face interaction. Both kinds of models bear the impress of a subject's epistemic orientation to a given kind of occasion. This orientation is a perspective based on what subjects view as desirable to have happen and from which they assess what does happen. It is inferable on the basis of the selection of grounded meanings and associated valuative meanings making up a given model.

To access subjects' cognitive models of face-to-face interaction, the author asks them to participate in two open-ended interviews, which are subject-structured, and to tell her about occasions of face-to-face interaction with which they are familiar. In a given study she asks them in the first interview to describe and to give their opinions about what typically occurs in an occasion selected for investigation. Then in the second interview she asks them to view a videotape recording of an actual instance of the occasion and to describe and to give their opinions about what is occurring in that particular occasion. These interviews are audiotape-recorded with verbatim transcripts serving as the data for analysis. The author also employs ethnographic observation as a means of identifying occasions that are psychologically relevant for subjects and as a means of gaining firsthand exposure to the kinds of events subjects refer to in their interviews.

This conception of cognitive models is an evolving one. It has emerged as a consequence of an interest in seeing things from the subject's point of view and a desire to segment the flow of behavior in a theoretically motivated, rather than ad hoc, fashion. The notion of cognitive models has been developed by imagining what such phenomena might look like, given what is known about the mind and given what is reflected and thus revealed about their content and structure in subjects' interviews about occasions of face-to-face interaction.

The Interplay of Theory and Observation

In what follows, the author demonstrates how her theoretical orientation influences the way in which the phenomena of interest are circumscribed, what questions subjects are asked, and how these questions are posed in the course of employing qualitative methods. A subject is asked about an occasion of face-to-face interaction because of the way in which the author imagines the stream of experience to be organized. There are no obvious discontinuities in the stream of experience, just the seamless flow of interpretations of ongoing happenings. It is the author's belief that some interpretations stand on their own as discrete phenomena. Other interpretations derive their significance from the parts they play within more encompassing ones. The task is to circumscribe the phenomena so that they are rendered undistorted and empirically relevant for inspection. Those interpretations that cohere as wholes, being functionally complete in their psychological relevance, are ones that are stored in memory as such and that serve as foci for the organization of behavior in the course of natural, purposeful activity. Interpretations of occasions of face-to-face interaction have been chosen for study because they appear to cohere as psychologically relevant wholes. Subjects readily label occasions and share their memories of them. This ease of labeling and recounting seems to be a pancultural phenomenon strongly supportive of the proposal that occasions of face-to-face interaction punctuate the stream of experience. Thus is the theoretical orientation seen to provide direction for delimiting the very object of study.

Interviews are conducted with a subject in which verbal reports of the focal occasion are elicited on the basis of the assumption that cognitive representation and linguistic representation of the occasion are both efforts to model the same experience. It is further assumed that there is a homology of content and structure between the two, with the former being reflected in the latter. These assumptions function within the theoretical orientation to provide the investigator with a warrant for examining what subjects say in order to observe what is going on in their minds.

The interviews are open-ended and subject-structured, that is, the investigator confines herself to pursuing matters that are first identified by a subject, to ensure that what emerges on interview is a faithful representation of a subject's interpretation. For the investigator to ask specific questions in terms of her own ideas of what the experience might be like would be to run the risk of selecting and differentially foregrounding her own event interpretations rather than a subject's. The interviews are audiotape-recorded and transcribed verbatim for similar reasons. These fixed records of a subject's report minimize the possibility of the investigator's imposing her own interpretation of the occasion and help ensure an undistorted observation of a subject's interpretations in terms of what he or she attended to and what kinds of sense he or she made of what goes on. The stage of development of the theoretical orientation is here seen to influence how the data are collected. At a later stage, as more is understood about the content and organization of subjects' cognitive models, more specific questions can be directed to subjects as is shown in the next two illustrations.

In both interviews a subject is asked to describe and to give opinions about the occasion in order to access the two kinds of meanings, postulated as comprising any given event interpretation. By asking a subject to describe what happens, the investigator attempts to tap into a subject's array of grounded meanings. By asking a subject to give opinions about what happens, the investigator attempts to tap into the associated valuative meanings. Once in possession of a subject's array of grounded meanings and valuative meanings, the investigator is able to infer a subject's epistemic orientation, that is, the perspective from which the occasion is monitored and appraised.

A subject is asked to describe and give opinions about an occasion as it typically occurs and as it occurs as an actual instance because present experience is held to be interpreted in terms of past experience. By asking about an occasion as it typically occurs, the investigator attempts to tap into a subject's framework of expectations or schema model of the occasion. By asking about an occasion as a particular instance, the investigator attempts to tap into a subject's specific representation, or sign model, of the occasion. A subject's schema model and sign model can then be compared to examine the nature of the relationship between the two.

As can be seen from the preceding discussion, what the investigator takes to be data about cognitive models and what she looks for in those data derive directly from her theoretical orientation. This orientation directs her to the examination of subject-structured verbal accounts of occasions of face-to-face interaction as reflections of subjects' cognitive models. Asking subjects to describe and to give their opinions about an occasion as it typically occurs and as it actually occurs grows out of the investigator's conception of the nature and characteristics of the cognitive models she is attempting to observe. And what she subsequently looks for in the data she collects are properties or characteristics that are corroborative or elaborative of her basic conception of those cognitive models. In other words, the investigator looks for what she expects to see, and what she sees tells me about what she is looking for.

Health Belief Model

The second author (CD) believes that individuals organize their attitudes or beliefs with regard to specific behaviors in terms of past experiences. In essence, she wants to know why people do the things they do and she believes that if enough is known about their attitudes or beliefs it will be possible to predict what people will do in certain situations.

The health belief model (HBM) addresses the author's interests and is compatible with her presuppositions about attitudes or beliefs. In the HBM the relevant attitudes or beliefs are conceptualized as perceived susceptibility to, and seriousness of a condition, along with perceived benefits of and barriers to enacting the designated behavior; and these are the summed cognitive valuations of past experiences

related to the behavior of interest (Rosenstock, 1966, 1974).

If subjects believe that they have been susceptible to events, over time they begin to perceive themselves more likely to be susceptible when in a new setting or situation. The same line of reasoning applies to seriousness, in that previous perceptions of seriousness influence current ones. On the other hand, benefits and barriers reflect the view people have of the positive and negative results of previously performing that behavior or one similar to it. Those persons who perceive themselves able to cope with most situations will see fewer barriers to the enactment of a behavior, whereas individuals who see many barriers are less likely to perceive many benefits to performing a specific behavior.

These attitudes or beliefs, individually or in concert, should predict the occurrence of the specific behavior. For instance, persons most likely to get a flu shot will be those who perceive themselves as more likely to get the flu than others (high susceptibility), as more likely to have a bad case of the flu if they get it (high seriousness), as willing to take the time to get a flu shot (high benefits), and as seeing no problem in getting to the clinic (low barriers).

To access subjects' attitudes or beliefs regarding the HBM, the author asks them to complete a specially designed paper and pencil instrument. Not only are the attitudes or beliefs assessed, but often information about the enactment of the behavior of interest is also obtained.

The HBM is evolving, but considerable development is needed. While there is some confidence in this set of attitudes or beliefs as the empirically significant ones for predicting behavior, there are still questions about the relationships among the members of the set. What is the role of each? Do they function in some specific combined relationship? These are the kinds of questions to which the author and her doctoral students have devoted their attention.

Interaction of Theory and Observation

Observations are made through the use of instruments. These tools must reflect the theoretical constructs if the results of the study are employed for theory testing. What follows is a description of the process to ensure this match (content validation).

The specifically developed instrument is the mechanism by which subjects are asked questions about their attitudes or beliefs. The questions are designed to assess the subjects' attitudes or beliefs regarding susceptibility, seriousness, benefits, and barriers. The subjects answer the questions by selecting a response from those provided, typically "strongly agree" to "strongly disagree." The author views the responses as representing the content and structure of the subjects' stream of experience as it relates to the behavior of interest. The instrument is composed of summated rating scales. The starting point in the development of four scales to measure susceptibility, seriousness, benefits, and barriers is to create statements that reflect the theoretical definition of each. The goal in developing each scale is to identify a range of statements that adequately reflect the domain represented by the attitude or belief. To do this, the developer must know the theory's nuances so that interpretation of the theoretical definitions is appropriate. The process of generating statements is a complex, time-consuming one, which begins by translating the theoretical definitions into the specific research situation. Statements must be assessed to make sure they reflect the subjects' perspective with respect to the attitudes or beliefs. "Benefits" is defined as all the positive aspects of performing a behavior (taking an action). For the most part it is easy to identify the benefits persons consider when trying to decide if they should enact the behavior of interest. People perform the same behavior for many different reasons, all of which could be subsumed under the construct of benefits. The same can be said for why people elect not to enact a behavior, that is, barriers to taking the action. "Barriers" is defined as the perceived cost to the individual in performing the behavior. If formulating benefit or barrier statements is a problem, information can be gathered from the research literature on why patients do or do not do the behavior of interest or change their behavior and adopt a new one (the one of interest). Based on experience and the literature, about 10 to 15 statements are constructed to

reflect the possible range inherent in the benefits and barriers to enacting the behavior.

Identifying the range of statements that reflect the ideas of susceptibility to and the seriousness of the condition is more complex than for benefits and barriers. To do this, the theoretical definitions must be carefully translated. "Susceptibility" is defined as the degree to which persons perceive themselves subject to the risks inherent in a condition. "Seriousness" is the degree a condition is perceived to negatively affect individuals (Rosenstock, 1966, 1974). In each, the word *condition* is the critical aspect of the theoretical definition. The term *condition* is not restricted to a disease condition; thus, the model addresses behaviors in addition to those that are disease related. Identifying the specific condition is essential to ensure good measurement. First the behavior of interest is identified. Then working backward, it is possible to identify the specific condition that is most closely related to that behavior. For instance, when the behavior was "use of seat belts," the condition was injury caused by auto accidents (S. S. Gerhart, personal communication, 1988; Lishner, McDonald, Sheehan, & Wassem, 1985). When Sheehan (1987) studied the behavior—participating in therapy—the condition was considered the possibility of a relapse requiring rehospitalization. Once the condition was determined, the development of susceptibility and seriousness items was possible.

After sufficient statements are generated, they are compared with Champion's items (1981, 1984). Champion developed the first instrument with good internal-consistency reliability and construct validity to measure systematically susceptibility, seriousness, benefits, and barriers. Although the behavior in Champion's instrument was the doing of a self breast examination, the stems of many statements she developed are usable with other behaviors. For example, the statement "I believe I have a good chance of getting breast cancer" is a susceptibility statement. Substituting the condition of interest for Champion's condition "breast cancer" creates a statement known to measure the construct of susceptibility. Across studies by Champion (1981), Baugh (1983), Emerson (1984), Blatchley (1984), Hadley

(1986), McKee (1986), Sawin, (1987), Sheehan (1987), Wilder (1987), and S. S. Gerhart (personal communication, 1988), statements have been identified that consistently measure a construct, thus ensuring that scores of these scales are addressing the same phenomena.

Since the task is to represent the persons' meaning of each statement from their perspectives, additional analyses are conducted once the data are collected. The instrument was developed from the researcher's perspective, no matter how great the effort to represent the subjects' views. By conducting confirmatory factor analysis, evidence for how well the items functioned within their scales can be obtained (construct validity). If the subjects interpreted all of the items developed to measure susceptibility in a similar fashion, these items will load on one factor independent of the other items. The loading of items for a scale independent of the other items should also occur for each of the other scales. The use of Cronbach's alpha technique can also provide information on the contribution of each item to its scale. Revision of the scales based on the information provided by these analyses increases the researcher's confidence that she has indeed represented the intent of the subjects.

In summary, the valuation of past experiences with regard to specific behaviors are represented by the attitudes or beliefs inherent in the HBM. The theory directly influences interpretations of observations of these attitudes or beliefs. All items of the instrument are designed to measure the theoretical definitions; thus, the observations are of susceptibility to and seriousness of a condition and perceived benefits and barriers to enactment of the behavior. The author believes that the responses to these scales reflect the content and structure of the subjects' experiences with respect to the behavior of interest. From information about the content and structure of their experiences, the investigator expects to predict occurrence of future behavior.

CONCLUSION

In this chapter, the authors have presented a brief summary of their respective theoretical orientations and the kinds of methods they employ in addressing their research interests. Although the methods for making observations of their phenomena differ, they have shown how theory and observation manifest a comparable relationship in their respective endeavors. That this should be the case, although one of them employs qualitative methods and the other quantitative methods, underscores what is both fundamental and common to their work: subscription to the canons of scientific inquiry. When methods of observation, of whatever ilk, are pressed into the service of scientific inquiry ipso facto they become scientific. It then becomes a question of preference and training as to whether one uses qualitative methods or quantitative methods, or some combination of the two. With this understanding, it follows that nurse scientists are free to choose the means of observation most enabling of their pursuits.

REFERENCES

Baugh, C.L. (1983). *Prediction of smoking behavior using the HBM, HLOC and self-esteem*. Unpublished doctoral dissertation, Indiana University, Indianapolis, IN.

Blatchley, E. (1984). *An extension of the health belief model with the construct learned helplessness*. Unpublished doctoral dissertation, Indiana University, Indianapolis, IN.

Brown, H. I. (1977). *Perception, theory and commitment: The new philosophy of science*. Chicago: University of Chicago Press.

Champion, V. L. (1981). *Tool construction for measurement of health belief model constructs*. Unpublished doctoral dissertation, Indiana University, Indianapolis, IN.

Champion, V. L. (1984). Instrument development for health belief model constructs. *Advances in Nursing Science, 6*(3), 73–85.

Donnelly, E. (1985). Signs of a problematic person. In J. Deely (Ed.), *Semiotics 1984* (pp. 435–450). Lanham: University Press of America.

Donnelly, E. (1986, November). *Collecting and analyzing interpretations of clinical encounters*. Paper presented at the Thirteenth Annual Patient Care Research Colloquium, Indianapolis, IN.

Donnelly, E. (1987). Descriptions as reflections of cognitive representations of face-to-face interactions. In J. Evans & J. Deely (Eds.), *Semiotics 1983* (pp. 591–602). Lanham: University Press of America.

Donnelly, E., & Moneyham, L. L. (1988). Interpreting premenstrual syndrome: A clinical encounter. In J. N. Deely (Ed.), *Semiotics 1987*. Lanham: University Press of America. (pp. 95-104).

Dougherty E. (1978). Segmenting the behavior stream: Verbal reports as data. *Semiotica, 24*, 221–243.

Dougherty E. (1984a). *Cognitive models of face-to-face interaction: A semiotic approach*. Unpublished doctoral dissertation, State University of New York at Buffalo, NY.

Dougherty E. (1984b). A semiology of interaction: Posing the problem. *Semiotica, 50*, 213–220.

Dougherty E., & Morrissey, S. (1987). Everyday activities as signs: A case study. In J. Deely & J. Evans (Eds.), *Semiotics 1982* (pp. 69–80). Lanham: University Press of America.

Duffy, M. E. (1987). Methodological triangulation: A vehicle for merging quantitative and qualitative research methods. *Image, 19*, 130–134.

Emerson, L. A. (1984). *Variables affecting postoperative activity levels*. Unpublished doctoral dissertation, Indiana University, Indianapolis, IN.

Firestone, W. A. (1987). Meaning in method: The rhetoric of quantitative and qualitative research. *Educational Researcher, 16*, 16–24.

Goodwin, L. D., & Goodwin, W. L. (1984). Qualitative vs. quantitative research or qualitative and quantitative research? *Nursing Research, 36*, 378–380.

Hadley, S. A. (1986). *Prediction of work status following coronary artery bypass surgery: A test of the health belief model*. Unpublished doctoral dissertation, Indiana University, Indianapolis, IN.

Hanson, N. R. (1958). *Patterns of discovery*. Cambridge: Cambridge University Press.

Jacob, E. (1988). Clarifying qualitative research: A focus on traditions. *Educational Researcher, 17*, 16–24.

Kaplan, D., & Manners, R. A. (1972). *Culture theory*. Englewood Cliffs, NJ: Prentice-Hall.

Kuhn, T. S. 1962. *The structure of scientific revolutions*. Chicago: University of Chicago Press.

Leininger, M. M. (1985). *Qualitative research methods in nursing*. Orlando, FL: Grune & Stratton.

Lincoln, Y., & Guba, E. (1985). *Naturalistic inquiry*. Beverly Hills, CA: Sage Publications.

Lishner, K., McDonald, M., Sheehan, M., & Wassem, R. (1985). *The HBM as a predictor of seat belt use*. Unpub-

lished manuscript, Indiana University, School of Nursing, Indianapolis, IN.

McKee, N. J. (1986). *The health belief model, state locus of control and state-anxiety and participation in screening for cervical cancer*. Unpublished doctoral dissertation, Indiana University, Indianapolis, IN.

Miller, S. (1986). Some comments on keeping the quantitative-qualitative debate open. *Educational Researcher, 15*, 24–25.

Phillips, J. R. (1988). Research blenders. *Nursing Science Quarterly, 1*, 4–5.

Popper, K. (1963). *The logic of scientific discovery*. New York: Harper & Row.

Powers, B. A. (1987). Taking sides: A response to Goodwin and Goodwin. *Nursing Research, 36*, 122–126.

Rosenstock, I. M. (1966). Why people use health services. *Memorial Fund Quarterly, 44*, 94–121.

Rosenstock, I. M. (1974). Historical origins of the health belief model. *Health Education Monographs, 2*, 1–8.

Sandelowski, M. (1986). The problem of rigor in qualitative research. *Advances in Nursing Science, 8*, 27–37.

Sawin, K. (1987). *The impact of the HBM, desire for control, perceived control and modifying variables on young women's contraceptive use*. Unpublished doctoral dissertation, Indiana University, Indianapolis, IN.

Sheehan, M. (1987). *The HBM as a predictor of involvement in treatment in hospitalized clients*. Unpublished doctoral dissertation, Indiana University, Indianapolis, IN.

Shulman, L. S. (1981). Disciplines of inquiry in education: An overview. *Educational Researcher, 10*(6), 5–12.

Smith, J. K. (1983). Quantitative versus qualitative research: An attempt to clarify the issue. *Educational Researcher, 12*(3), 6–13.

Smith, J. K., & Heshusius, L. (1986). Closing down the conversation: The end of the quantitative-qualitative debate among educational inquirers. *Educational Researcher, 15*(1), 4–12.

Tinkle, M. B., & Beaton, J. L. (1983). Toward a new view of science: Implications for nursing research. *Advances in Nursing Science, 5*(2), 27–36.

Wilder, M. G. (1987). *Utilizing the health belief model to predict the delivery of patient education by registered nurses*. Unpublished doctoral dissertation, Indiana University, Indianapolis, IN.

✳   **EDITOR'S QUESTIONS FOR DISCUSSION**   ✳

What is the essence of science and nursing science? Must there be a relationship between the methods that are chosen to make observations and the theory base one is using? Provide examples to illustrate your points from various research studies. Is there a relation of consequence between theory and observation in the conduct of scientific inquiry irrespective of the research methods used? Provide examples for your beliefs. Provide examples of phenomena that may be studied within the realm of nursing in which observations can be or have been made through both qualitative and quantitative approaches and where either one or the other approach was used to address the same research question. Is the method utilized by Donnelly in describing the development of cognitive models an inductive or deductive approach to theory development? How might the investigator prevent bias in data analysis and interpretation of the data in using qualitative and quantitative methods? How can the investigator control for his or her own bias in perceptions or observations of certain phenomena? What are the two kinds of meanings postulated as making up any given event interpretation? Provide examples in which these two types of meanings are evident or can be evident. How might investigator bias occur and be controlled in using quantitative methods?

How is it possible to predict what people may or may not do in certain situations if you know enough about their attitudes and beliefs? How can response set bias be controlled? What type of statistical techniques can be used to determine whether or not there is some specific combined relationship between the variables inherent in the HBM or whether one variable must exist before another? Discuss the advantages and disadvantages of using both qualitative and quantitative approaches in a study. Discuss how reliability and validity might be established in the two approaches for studies as exemplified by the authors. Discuss the development of Likert-type scales. To what extent is the scale a continuum in a response? How is the midpoint on the scale interpreted? How is reliability and validity best established in the development of scales?

22

Research Strategies for Developing Nursing as the Science of Human Care

Marilyn L. Stember, Ph.D., R.N.
Nancy K. Hester, Ph.D., R.N.

Not long ago, the noted anthropologist Dr. Norrie Flightengale came to the United States to study nursing research and describe the people who were calling themselves nurse researchers. In Dr. Flightengale's recent report, she identified two distinct nations of nurse researchers: "Quantifica" and "Qualifica." Interestingly the two nations were not geographically distinct; identifiable cultural groups were scattered throughout the land. The size of the groups varied, but the larger concentrations of both nations were located in institutions of higher learning. Their strength and cultural identity were often associated with the persuasion of the tribal leader, most often called a Dean. As members of the culture moved from place to place, they became active missionaries for the culture, thus contributing to the proliferation of the

"Quantifica" or "Qualifica" nations. Dr. Flightengale noted that both cultural groups were actively engaged in intensive nation-building activities. A variety of mechanisms were used such as local brainwashing rituals (e.g., doctoral research courses) and national congregational meetings (e.g., research conferences). Flightengale's analyses of her field notes provide descriptions of the salient features of the two nations.

Quantifica as a nation is distinguished by the members' affinity to numbers. They enjoy counting, scaling, calculating, and performing complex mathematical procedures such as matrix algebra, statistics, and structural equations. Religion is not an important theme, for faith alone is not acceptable. Real things can be observed and measured.

Flightengale noted with interest that the Quantifica nation has a particular historical link with ancient Greek culture. Alpha, beta, chi, gamma, lambda, and other Greek letters are frequently used in their vocabulary. She noted that not all of these patterns were understood (e.g., chi was often associated with a square [chi-square] but not with other geometric structures).

At the heart of the work-tasks of the Quantificas is theory building, and the most common ritual practiced by every member is verification of theory.

Primary sources of funding for the authors' research studies cited include D.H.H.S., Division of Nursing, (RO1 NU00993), "A Study of School Nurses' Use of Project HealthPACT," Marilyn L. Stember, P.I.; N.I.H., National Center for Nursing Research (R23 NR01382), "Procedures Assessing Pain in Children," Nancy O. Hester, P.I.; and N.I.H., National Center for Nursing Research (RO1 NR01964) "Nurse Clinical Decision-Making: Pain in Children," Nancy O. Hester, P.I.

The ritual begins when a new theory is born or an old theory is found. The theory becomes the center of attention as the members scurry about busily with activities to design and implement the critical test of the theory. The theory must be very clear with concepts both conceptually and operationally defined. Designs are developed to control threats to internal and external validity. Samples are carefully selected in advance to be representative and to control for unwanted variation. And the ritual would be incomplete without statistical analyses and generalizations to appropriate populations.

Quantificas work objectively, standing apart from the work they study, trying to understand the phenomenon in an unbiased way. And Dr. Flightengale noted that although Quantifica researchers use double-blind experiments, the researchers are rarely seen with white canes or blindfolds.

In the Quantifica nation, members play with building blocks of knowledge. They often take one block and see how it fits with other blocks. Using scientific techniques throughout their careers, they build the blocks to see larger and larger patterns. They like the idea of models because models help to represent and communicate the reality of nursing. In a recent survey of 1256 randomly selected students, Operationalization 101, Generalizability 202, Verification 307, and Error Terms 406 were among the most favorite subjects in this culture.

Nursing research is quite different in the "Qualifica" nation. In this nation, several subcultures exist: phenomenological, ethnographic, ethnonursing, hermeneutic, humanistic, and philosophical inquiry. Persons who belong to the different subcultures prefer to be known by these names in the same way that persons who profess to be Christians may nevertheless prefer to be known as Catholic, Lutheran, Episcopalian, Presbyterian, Adventist, Fundamentalist, or Baptist. They hold to these more specific labels in an attempt to differentiate their particular doctrines from those of others (who, needless to say, have turned from the True way).

The members of Qualifica are self-oriented, believing that they themselves are very important instruments in the research process. They participate and interact in the experience, reconstruction, interpretation, and understanding. They begin their task-accomplishing ritual by claiming to never know for what they are looking. They select a general topic, a natural setting, at least one informant, and plan their research as they are doing it. Discovery of meanings is the objective. To do this, they participate fully in the situation using personal understanding, common sense, introspection, and imagination as they interact with informants. Pursuing the whole of the experience is highly valued. They use intuition, reflection, theme analysis, and metaphors to describe the wholeness of the experience.

In socializing new researchers, the mentors in this culture teach the young that subjectivity prevails. In attempts to search for the meaning of experience, researchers try to capture the work as it is immediately experienced. Happenings in the world are not viewed as ordered; rather they occur in simultaneous and changing patterns. In the curriculum, Complexity 102, Diversity 205, Indeterminacy 310, and Experiencing 403 are among the most popular classes.

In noting how these two cultures of nurse researchers related, Dr. Flightengale noted that the two nations frequently have clashes, often guerilla style, followed by periods of "cold war." The nations hold formal debates to argue the advantages and disadvantages of qualitative and quantitative methods. These findings disturbed Dr. Flightengale, who wondered: Why is it that these nations cannot be at peace and work together? Wouldn't the development and advancement of nursing knowledge benefit from the work of both nations?

This fictitious story obviously exaggerates the prevailing polarity in nursing research. However, considerable disagreement exists over the appropriateness of various methods and paradigmatic stances for conducting research in nursing. The heart of the debate is the distinction between quantitative and qualitative methods. Quantitative methods include the techniques of randomized experiments, quasi-experiments, multivariate statistical analyses, and time series analyses. In contrast, qualitative methods include ethnography, phenomenology, hermeneutics, and philosophical inquiry. Each group has acquired a constituency of advocates who think that their preferred methods are best suited for developing and advancing nursing science.

A full appreciation of how the debate between method-types is being waged may facilitate an understanding of the fallacies in current thinking. The debate is not merely a disagreement over the relative advantages and disadvantages of qualitative and quantitative methods; it is a fundamental clash between paradigms. Each method-type is associated with a separate and unique paradigmatic perspective, and these two perspectives are in conflict. As Rist (1977) stated the case, "Ultimately, the issue is not research strategies, per se. Rather, the adherence to one paradigm as opposed to another predisposes one to view the world and the events within it in profoundly different ways" (p. 43).

In this chapter we present the argument that viewing nursing as the science of human care requires the "transcendent paradigm." Within the framework of nursing as human science, we consider the conflicts between prevailing paradigmatic viewpoints and redefine the issues raised by the debate. Because the transcendent paradigm goes beyond the limits of philosophical stances and research methods, it empowers investigators to examine the fullest context of human phenomena. Two examples from studies contributing to the science of human care are presented to illustrate the use of the transcendent paradigm, to highlight research strategies for nursing, and to describe the potential benefits of the transcendent paradigm.

NURSING AS THE SCIENCE OF HUMAN CARE

Nursing as the science of human care is based on the assumptions that nursing is a human science and that human care is a dominant domain and unifying goal of nursing. As a human science, nursing seeks to integrate empirical knowledge with esthetics, humanities, and art (Watson, 1985a). As a human care science, the focus is on developing the knowledge that is central to nursing. As Watson (1985b) stated, "human care is the heart of nursing" (p. 346). Likewise, Leininger (1981, 1984) has emphasized that "caring is the central and unifying domain for the body of knowledge and practices in nursing" (1981, p. 3). This human care perspective encompasses the nursing-client-health-environment approach (Bilitski, 1981; Kim, 1983; Newman, 1983) and other descriptions of nursing (e.g., Donaldson & Crowley, 1978).

Our view of nursing as the science of human care is comprehensive and encompassing. It includes development of knowledge requisite for the science of human care in areas including (a) assessment of human conditions; (b) explication of human experiences with and responses to various health and illness conditions; (c) examination of the management of human conditions; (d) description of attributes of caring relationships; and (e) the study of systems for the delivery of human care. Inquiry in the science of human care can focus on various units of analyses including cells, systems, individuals, families, groups, communities, and organizations in a variety of contexts. While critics may decry the lack of specificity within our perspective, Visintainer (1986) has identified similar breadth as a strength for clinical applications.

In explicating the science of human care, nursing inquiry must include a multiplicity of methods to acquire the fullest understanding of human phenomena (DeGroot, 1988; Fitzpatrick & Abraham, 1987; Gortner, 1983; Gortner & Schultz, 1988; Schultz, 1987; Tripp-Reimer, 1985). Inquiry must facilitate the integration of knowledge from the biomedical, behavioral, and sociocultural sciences with the arts and humanities to create new nursing knowledge. Through strategies of integration and synthesis, the world of objectivity can be linked with the subjective world of human experience. To accomplish this linkage, the prevailing paradigms must be transcended.

PARADIGMATIC CONSIDERATIONS

The concept of paradigm as discussed by Kuhn (1970) refers to a world view or general perspective for viewing some complexity of the real world that becomes embedded in the orientation of those who subscribe to the paradigm. Two predominant world views have emerged—qualitative and quantitative. Those who contrast these paradigms usually provide a list of attributes that distinguish these world views. For example, Rist (1977) offers 3 attributes, Reichardt and Cook (1979) provide 11, and Guba (1978) lists 14. Essentially, the quantitative paradigm is characterized as analytical empiricism, particularistic, hypothetico-deductive, objective, and outcome-oriented. In contrast, the qualitative paradigm is phenomenological, holistic, inductive, subjective, and process-oriented.

Such paradigmatic characterizations are based on an assumption that is of direct consequence to the debate over methods: methods are directly linked to a paradigm. With many scholars (e.g., Donaldson & Crowley, 1978; Kuhn, 1970) having argued for a singular paradigm to guide progress in science, nursing as a discipline has been forced to choose between these mutually exclusive and antagonistic world views and subsequently must also choose between the method-types. Thus an allegiance to a philosophical paradigm has provided the means for choosing between method-types. In other words, the worldview has dictated the methods of inquiry that researchers use to examine human phenomena. Intentionally or not, this assumption ultimately has led to the conclusion that qualitative and quantitative methods themselves can never be used together.

Reichardt and Cook (1979) and Goodwin and Goodwin (1984) have argued that an inconsistency does not inherently exist in subscribing to one paradigm and employing the methods of the other method-type; philosophical paradigms do not logically determine the choice of research method. A researcher who uses quantitative procedures is not necessarily a logical empiricist, and conversely, a researcher who uses qualitative procedures is not necessarily a phenomenologist. Reichardt and Cook (1979) provided examples demonstrating that qualitative procedures are not necessarily naturalistic, unobtrusive, and subjective, and quantitative procedures are not necessarily controlled, obtrusive, and objective. They also emphasized that qualitative procedures are not always grounded, exploratory, and inductive, and quantitative procedures are not always ungrounded, confirmatory, and deductive.

A similar view was proposed by Glaser and Strauss (1967), the fathers of grounded theory, who stated, "There is no fundamental clash between the purposes and capacities of qualitative and quantitative methods. . . . We believe that each . . . is useful for both verification and generation of theory, whatever the primacy of emphasis" (pp. 17–18). They noted that qualitative methods need not only be used to discover interesting questions to ask and that quantitative procedures need not be the only methods for answering them. Rather, each general approach can serve both functions. Contrary to the

positions of Phillips (1988) and Powers (1987), we believe that a strict adherence between philosophical paradigms and the use of qualitative and quantitative strategies does not optimally facilitate the development of nursing knowledge. As Judson (1980) stated, "Science is enormously disparate . . . Nobody has succeeded in catching all this in one net; . . . behind the diversity lies a unity" (p. 112).

RESOLUTION

Scholars must address an important question: To what end does the continuation of the debate serve in regard to the development and advancement of nursing as the science of human care? Can either paradigm by itself adequately generate solutions to the crucial problems in nursing? The debate continues to perpetuate a host of false dichotomies and adds to those previously identified by Watson (1981). Differences in the quantitative and qualitative methods do not necessarily mean that one method is superior to the other (Chinn & Jacobs, 1978; Duffy, 1987; Norbeck, 1987), nor does it mean that there should be a hierarchy of research designs (Brink & Wood, 1983; Ryan, 1983) with the descriptive work preceding the experimental designs. Neither does a shift from analytical empiricism to phenomenology and existentialism (Watson, 1985a, 1985b) seem to be the best solution for nursing.

Coexistence Model

Parallel coexistence (like parallel play during early childhood) of these paradigms is one way to solve the problem. For example, Allen, Benner, and Diekelmann (1986) proposed that the coexistence of three philosophical paradigms (analytical empiricism, Heideggerian phenomenology, and critical social theory) could do more for nursing than adoption of any single model. While the coexistence perspective is more palatable than choosing one paradigm, coexistence does not necessarily foster interplay across the paradigms nor does it ensure the end to current debate. Thus the separatists will continue their advocacy of uncontaminated methods, while combinationists will continue to select, sometimes indefensibly, methods from any or all coexisting paradigms. In the meantime, the development and advancement of nursing knowledge may continue to suffer.

Transcendent Paradigm

The preferred solution is the creation of a new paradigm that transcends the aforementioned issues. Focusing nursing as the comprehensive science of human care, redefining the paradigms as complementary rather than contradictory, and viewing methods as logically independent of the prevailing paradigms permit the evolution of a new paradigm for nursing science: the transcendent paradigm. The transcendent paradigm not only permits but empowers investigators to examine the fullest context of human phenomena by using multiple philosophies and methods.

The transcendent paradigm was named because its intent is to go beyond the limits or the boundaries of the prevailing paradigms. Not simply the combinationist perspective described by Leininger (1985), it seeks to transcend the limits of philosophical stances, research methods, data collection, and analytical procedures. For example, the nature of reality is singular and multiple, objective and subjective, as well as particularistic and holistic. Similarly, the paradigmatic assumption regarding the nature of truth is that the world is stable and dynamic. Individual uniqueness and generalizations across individuals are both highly valued.

While investigators will have the freedom to choose a mix of methodological attributes from currently prevailing paradigms that best fit the demands of the human phenomena under study, the hope is that new or revised modes of inquiry that advance nursing as the science of human care will evolve. Two exemplars of research conducted by the authors are presented for the purpose of illustrating the potential benefits of the transcendent paradigm,

Exemplar 1

Hester and colleagues (Foster & Hester, 1989; Hester, 1979, 1987, 1989; Hester & Barcus, 1986; Hester & Ray, 1987; Hester, Foster, & Kristensen, in press) have conducted research on the human phenomenon of pain as experienced by children, ages 4 through 13 years. In examining this human condition Hester used different research strategies within and across the studies. Each strategy was deliberately chosen to address the specific research question. Examples of the methods used include:

1. Psychometric studies for the development of an instrument to assess pain.
2. Descriptive studies for: (a) observing children's responses to pain; (b) eliciting cues nurses and parents use in assessing pain in children; (c) understanding the experience of pain from the child's perspective; and (d) describing children's perceptions of what others could do to help during the pain experience (i.e., caring behaviors).
3. Correlational studies for determining relationships: (a) among various behavioral responses to painful situations and self-reported measures of pain; (b) between parents' and nurses' classification of pain cues and levels of pain reported by children, nurses, and parents; and (c) between nurses' rating of children's pain and use of pharmacological agents by the nurse.
4. Hermeneutic approach for qualitatively assessing Watson's carative factors with caring behaviors described by children.
5. Case study methodology for exploring the decision making of nurses in regard to children in pain.

Through the use of multiple research strategies, Hester and her colleagues expanded the clinical knowledge base concerning caring for the child in pain. Knowledge has advanced in the following areas: the child's experience of the human condition of pain, the child's responses to pain, nurses' and parents' assessment of pain, and therapeutic management including the use of pharmacological agents and caring behaviors.

Exemplar 2

Stember and her colleagues (Stember, 1986, 1987a, 1987b, 1988; Stember & Malkewicz, 1988; Stember, Rogers, & Stiles, 1986a, 1986b; Stember, Stiles, & Rogers, 1987) conducted a major study on children, 6 through 13 years of age, and their participation in health care. Stember replicated the following research strategies in each of seven sites:

1. Experimental design for testing the effectiveness of an intervention for increasing children's level of participation in health care.
2. Psychometric studies for developing and testing instruments.
3. Artistic assessment of children's drawings as another vehicle into the child's world.
4. Ethnographic sociolinguistic approach (using videotaping and participant observation) for understanding how the nurse and child interact during health visits.
5. Community assessment for understanding the contexts of the settings for the studies.

Within and across sites, data and findings from the research designs were triangulated. Through integration and synthesis, an understanding of the children's health consumerism perspectives and the influence of the contextual variables on children's perceptions and participation in health care evolved.

These two exemplars are different in that Hester's work involved different methods of inquiry within and across studies, while Stember's work involved different methods within one study. Use of the transcendent paradigm facilitated knowledge development. Adherence to one of the prevailing paradigms would have greatly limited these contributions to nursing.

CONCLUSION

Advancing nursing as the science of human care necessitates a serious consideration of the transcendent paradigm. This paradigm allows for viewing existing paradigms as complementary rather than antagonistic; it allows for the use of multiplicity of methods within and across studies; and it encourages new strategies for inquiry.

One challenge of the transcendent paradigm is to generate new methods of inquiry (e.g., holographic methods, photographic documentaries, literary analyses [Watson, 1985[b]]) that better examine nursing phenomena. Another challenge is to expand approaches that assist in integrating and synthesizing the knowledge generated through various research strategies. Various forms of triangulation have been suggested (Duffy, 1987; Hinds & Young, 1987; Jick, 1979; Mitchell, 1986). Bockmon and Riemen (1987) suggested the metaphor of the Chinese symbol for Tao to symbolize the intermingling of two opposites to form a harmonious whole. Schultz (1987, 1988) and Tinkle and Beaton (1983) advocated the dialectic approach in which the paradigms are given equal status and "dialectical reasoning assists in reconciling two seemingly contradictory responses" (Schultz, 1988, p. 9). These and other modes of integration need further articulation so that knowledge derived through multiple ways of knowing can be synthesized for nursing science.

The transcendent paradigm can overcome the limitations imposed by the prevailing debate between quantitative and qualitative methodologies. By unifying and going beyond the discordant paradigms, it can inspire researchers to develop fully and creatively nursing as the science of human care.

REFERENCES

Allen, D., Benner, P., & Diekelmann, N. L. (1986). Three paradigms for nursing research: Methodological implications. In P. L. Chinn (Ed.), *Nursing research methodology: Issues and implementation* (pp. 23–38). Rockville, MD: Aspen Publications.

Bilitski, J. S. (1981). Nursing science and the laws of health: The test of substance as a step in the process of theory development. *Advances in Nursing Science, 4*(1), 15–29.

Bockmon, D. F., & Riemen, D. J. (1987). Qualitative versus quantitative nursing research. *Holistic Nursing Practice, 2*(1), 71–75.

Brink, P. J., & Wood, M. J. (1983). *Basic steps in planning nursing research, from question to proposal* (2nd ed.). Monterey, CA: Wadsworth Health Sciences Division.

Chinn, P. L., & Jacobs, M. K. (1978). A model for theory development in nursing. *Advances in Nursing Science, 1*(1), 1–11.

DeGroot, H. A. (1988). Scientific inquiry in nursing: A model for a new age. *Advances in Nursing Science, 10*(3), 1–21.

Donaldson, S. K., & Crowley, D. M. (1978). The discipline of nursing. *Nursing Outlook, 26*(2), 113–120.

Duffy, M. E. (1987). Methodological triangulation: A vehicle for merging quantitative and qualitative research methods. *Image, 19*(3), 130–133.

Fitzpatrick, J. J., & Abraham, I. L. (1987). Toward the socialization of scholars and scientists. *Nurse Educator, 12*(3), 23–25.

Foster, R. L. & Hester, N. O. (1989). The relationship between assessment and pharmacologic interventions for pain in children. In S. K. Funk, E. M. Tornquist, M. T. Champagne, L. A. Copp, & R. A. Wiese (Eds.), *Key aspects of comfort: Management of pain, fatigue, and nausea* (pp. 72–79). New York: Springer Publishing.

Glaser, B. G., & Strauss, A. L. (1967). *The discovery of grounded theory: Strategies for qualitative research*. New York: Aldine Publishing Company.

Goodwin, L. D. & Goodwin, W. L. (1984). Qualitative vs. quantitative research or qualitative and quantitative research? *Nursing Research, 33*(6), 378–380.

Gortner, S. R. (1983). The history and philosophy of nursing science and research. *Advances in Nursing Science, 5*(2), 1–8.

Gortner, S. R., & Schultz, P. R. (1988). Approaches to nursing science methods. *Image, 20*(1), 22–24.

Guba, E. G. (1978). *Toward a methodology of naturalistic inquiry in educational evaluation*. Los Angeles: University of California, Los Angeles, Center for the Study of Evaluation.

Hester, N. O. (1979). The preoperational child's reaction to immunizations. *Nursing Research, 28*(4), 250–255.

Hester, N. O. (1987). *Child participation in the pain experience*. Unpublished manuscript.

Hester, N. O. (1989). Comforting the child in pain. In S. K. Funk, E. M. Tornquist, M. T. Champagne, L. A. Copp, & R. A. Wiese (Eds.), *Key aspects of comfort: Management of pain, fatigue, and nausea* (pp. 290–298). New York: Springer Publishing.

Hester, N. O., & Barcus, C. (1986). *The human experience of pain for hospitalized children*. Unpublished manuscript.

Hester, N. O., Foster, R. L., & Kristensen, K. (in press). Measurement of children's pain: Generalizability and validity of the Pain Ladder and the Poker Chip Tool. *Advances in pain research and therapy: Proceedings of the First International Symposium on Pediatric Pain*. New York: Raven Press.

Hester, N. O., & Ray, M. D. (1987). *Assessment of Watson's carative factors: A qualitative research study*. Unpublished manuscript.

Hinds, P. S., & Young, K. J. (1987). A triangulation of methods and paradigms to study nurse-given wellness care. *Nursing Research, 36*(3), 195–198.

Jick, T. D. (1979). Mixing qualitative and quantitative methods: Triangulation in action. *Administrative Science Quarterly, 24*, 602–611.

Judson, H. F. (1980). The rage to know. *The Atlantic Monthly, 245*, 112–117.

Kim, H. K. (1983). *The nature of theoretical thinking in nursing*. Norwalk, CT: Appleton-Century-Crofts.

Kuhn, T. S. (1970). *The structure of scientific revolutions* (2nd ed.). Chicago: University of Chicago Press.

Leininger, M. (1981). The phenomena of caring: Importance, research questions, and theoretical considerations. In M. Leininger (Ed.), *Caring: An Essential Human Need. Proceedings of the Three National Caring Conferences* (pp. 3–15). Thorofare, NJ: Charles B. Slack, Inc.

Leininger, M. (1984). Care: The essence of nursing and health. In M. Leininger (Ed.), *Care: The essence of nursing and health* (pp. 3–15). Thorofare, NJ: Charles B. Slack, Inc.

Leininger, M. (1985). Nature, rationale, and importance of qualitative research methods in nursing. In M. Leininger (Ed.), *Qualitative research methods in nursing* (pp. 1–25). Orlando, FL: Grune & Stratton.

Mitchell, E. S. (1986). Multiple triangulation: A methodology for nursing science. *Advances in Nursing Science, 8*(3), 18–26.

Newman, M. A. (1983). The continuing revolution: A history of nursing science. In N. L. Chaska (Ed.), *The Nursing profession: A time to speak* (pp. 385–393). New York: McGraw-Hill.

Norbeck, J. S. (1987). In defense of empiricism. *Image, 19*(1), 28–30.

Phillips, J. R. (1988). Research blenders. *Nursing Science Quarterly, 1*(1), 4–5.

Powers, B. A. (1987). Taking sides: A response to Goodwin and Goodwin. *Nursing Research, 36*(2), 122–126.

Reichardt, C. S., & Cook, T. D. (1979). Beyond qualitative versus quantitative methods. In T. D. Cook & C. S. Reichardt (Eds.), *Qualitative and quantitative methods in evaluation research* (pp. 7–32). Beverly Hills, CA: Sage Publications.

Rist, R. (1977). On the relations among educational research paradigms: From disdain to detente. *Anthropology and Education Quarterly, 8*, 42–49.

Ryan, N. M. (1983). The epidemiological method of building causal inference. *Advances in Nursing Science, 5*(2), 73–81.

Schultz, P. R. (1987). Toward holistic inquiry in nursing:

A proposal for synthesis of patterns and methods. *Scholarly Inquiry for Nursing Practice: An International Journal*, *1*(2), 135–145.

Schultz, P. R. (1988). A dialectical model of nursing. Unpublished manuscript.

Stember, M. L. (1986). *Assessing children's view of health visits through use of drawings*. Unpublished manuscript.

Stember, M. L. (1987a). *Children's consumer behavior concerning health*. Unpublished manuscript.

Stember, M. L. (1987b). *Children's participation in their health*. Unpublished manuscript.

Stember, M. L. (1988). *Kids as consumers: Effectiveness of HealthPACT*. Final Grant Report, Submitted to DHHS/NCNR, Washington, DC.

Stember, M. L., & Malkewicz, J. (1988). *Accessing views of health through children's drawings*. Unpublished manuscript.

Stember, M. L., Rogers, S. J., & Stiles, M. (1986a). *Measuring children's health habit behavior*. Unpublished manuscript.

Stember, M. L., Rogers, S. J., & Stiles, M. (1986b). *Parental influence on children's health attitudes and behaviors*. Unpublished manuscript.

Stember, M. L., Stiles, M. K., & Rogers, S. (1987). Severity and vulnerability in school age children. *Issues in Comprehensive Pediatric Nursing*, *10*(4–5), 263–272.

Tinkle, M. B., & Beaton, J. L. (1983). Toward a new view of science: Implications for nursing research. *Advances in Nursing Science*, *5*(2), 27–36.

Tripp-Reimer, T. (1985). Combining qualitative and quantitative methodologies. In M. Leininger (Ed.), *Qualitative research methods in nursing* (pp. 179–194). Orlando, FL: Grune & Stratton.

Visintainer, M. A. (1986). The nature of knowledge and theory in nursing. *Image*, *18*(2), 32–38.

Watson, J. (1981). Nursing's scientific quest. *Nursing Outlook*, *29* (7), 413–416.

Watson, J. (1985a). *Nursing: Human science and human care. A theory of nursing*. Norwalk, CT: Appleton-Century-Crofts.

Watson, J. (1985b). Reflections on different methodologies for the future of nursing. In M. Leininger (Ed.), *Qualitative research methods in nursing* (pp. 343–349). Orlando, FL: Grune & Stratton.

✳ EDITOR'S QUESTIONS FOR DISCUSSION ✳

How does the transcendent paradigm encompass other descriptions of nursing's domain? What are the three concerns identified by Donaldson and Crowley regarding the domain of nursing? Provide examples of the quantitative and qualitative paradigms as characterized by the authors. Discuss whether or not you agree that the world view dictates the methods of inquiry researchers might use to examine phenomena. How do the statements of these authors compare with those made by Donnelly and Deets (Chapter 21)? What are the two so-called mutually exclusive and antagonistic world views referred to by the authors? Respond to the authors' questions regarding the resolution of the debate concerning world views. How is the transcendent paradigm more than a combinationist perspective paradigm as described by Leininger? What is meant by triangulation? What are the various forms of triangulation that have been suggested to integrate and synthesize knowledge?

23

Phenomenological Method for Nursing Research

Marilyn A. Ray, Ph.D., R.N.

A new awareness has occurred within the scientific community of nursing. In the last decade researchers and theorists began to recognize that an incongruity existed between nursing philosophy and nursing research. As new or resynthesized philosophical ideas in nursing emerged, such as nursing as a human science, nursing as the science and art of human caring, clients as experiencing persons, and the importance of the context in human interaction, scholars began questioning the typically used medical atomistic causal model as the avenue of investigation. The beliefs about the holistic person whose language and behavior is experiential and the beliefs about the contextual grounding of experience led nurse researchers to a method of inquiry that is more adequate for the study of human beings wherein the situated meanings of human experience can be understood. Thus the phenomenological method—expressed as a philosophy, approach, and method was introduced into nursing research (Benner, 1985; Cohen, 1987; Davis, 1978;

Munhall & Oiler, 1986; Oiler, 1982; Omery, 1983; Parse, Coyne, & Smith, 1985; Paterson & Zderad, 1976; Ray, 1985, 1987; Reeder, 1984, 1985, 1987; Watson, 1985).

Phenomenological research is the study of lived experience. Phenomenology's purpose is to seek a fuller understanding through description, reflection, and direct awareness of a phenomenon to reveal the multiplicity of coherent and integral meanings of the phenomenon (Ray, 1985). By the practice of reflection in phenomenological research, the phenomenologist develops a mindful wonder, a caring attunement about living and about what it means to live a life. Phenomenology is the study of essence—what makes something what it is. "Phenomenology is the ministering of thoughtfulness" (Van Manen, 1984a, p. 1).

The focus of phenomenology is to describe experience as it is lived (Oiler, 1982). Thus human experience is the beginning point of phenomenology.

The purpose of this chapter is to present an exposition of phenomenology. It aims at discussing the origins and evolution of phenomenology and its implications for nursing. The final portion of the chapter focuses briefly on a process for conducting phenomenological research.

The author wishes to acknowledge the mentorship of Dr. Max Van Manen, Professor, University of Alberta, Edmonton, Canada for his help with the phenomenological method.

ORIGINS AND EVOLUTION OF PHENOMENOLOGY

The phenomenological movement in philosophy arose in Germany before the turn of the century and now occupies a distinguished place in 20th century philosophy, especially as it relates to the human sciences. For the purposes of clarity, human science is a name used to group a variety of qualitative approaches and orientations to research, such as ethnography, phenomenology, hermeneutics, ethnomethodology and critical social theory. The term *human science* was coined by Dilthey in the 19th century who argued that human phenomena (mental, social, historical) differed from natural phenomena (physical, chemical, behavioral, and animal) and therefore required interpretation and understanding (hermeneutics) rather than external observation and explanation as used in the natural sciences. Human science is involved with all the disciplines of the humanities, social sciences, and nursing, where interpretation and meaningful expressions of the active inner, cognitive, and spiritual aspects of human beings in social, historical, or political contexts is sought (Human Science in Education Project, 1985).

The phenomenological movement was divided into three phases: preparatory, German, and French (Cohen, 1987). In the preparatory phase, phenomenology as a method of inquiry first appeared in the writings of the philosopher Brentano in the last half of the 19th century. It was further developed in the early 20th century, in the German phase, by Edmund Husserl who is referred to as the primary philosopher of phenomenology. In the French phase of the phenomenological movement other philosophers, such as Heidegger, Merleau-Ponty, Marcel, and others expanded both the philosophy and the method of phenomenology.

Husserl (1936/1970), the father of the phenomenological movement, related phenomenology to the question of knowing. How do human beings know? How is knowledge manifested to us? As such, Husserl's phenomenology is an epistemology—a theory of knowledge (Natanson, 1973; Reeder, 1985). Husserl was disenchanted with the scientific position of positivist-empiricism, that is, the final truth lay in facts alone. He believed that the study of philosophy should not only have rigor but a new humanism. The fundamental principle of Husserl's phenomenology is the following: "No opinion is to be accepted as philosophical knowledge unless it is seen to be adequately established by observation of what is seen as itself given 'in person' [phenomenon in itself]" (Wagner, 1983, p. 46). In short, Husserl believed that ideas that order and give form to experience create our lived experience (Polkinghorne, 1983).

Husserl specified how the philosopher can recover by the process of phenomenological reduction (structured reflection) or the practice of thoughtfulness, the ability to describe with scientific exactness the life of consciousness in its original encounter with the world (Ray, 1985). Hence phenomenology and, more precisely, phenomenological reduction is concerned with the demonstration and explanation of the activities of consciousness—a true science of the mind (Schutz, 1967). In his last major work, *The Crisis of European Sciences*, Husserl formulated the notion of the "Lebenswelt," the lifeworld—the everyday world in which we live in, the natural, taken-for-granted attitude (Natanson, 1973). This notion of the lifeworld became instrumental in the development of the more existentially oriented phenomenology in the French phase of the phenomenological movement.

Existential phenomenology aims to describe how phenomena present themselves in lived experience, in human existence. For example, for Heidegger, phenomenology was an ontology, a study of the modes of being in the world (Gadamer, 1976). For Merleau-Ponty (1962), phenomenology related to experienced space, time, body, and human relations as we live them.

In many ways the expansiveness of this movement can be witnessed in all disciplines. In the science of physics there is a search for the holographic unfolding of life (Chivington, 1983). In the arts, the phenomenology of aesthetic experience has gained momentum (Dufrenne, 1973). Psychology has progressed in some circles to the position of psychology as a human science advanced by Giorgi (1985), and sociology is evolving to a sociological phenomenology (Schutz, 1967). Although anthropologists have been advocates of description, understanding, and the explication of the meaning of behavior within social and cultural contexts, serious questions have been raised in relation to the definition of meaning in anthropology, the role of reflection in ethnographic understanding, and the extent to which Western thought and methods have shaped the interpretation of other cultures (Parkin, 1982). Phenomenology offers anthropologists access to the nature of the experience itself. In nursing, phenomenology has gained respect in research as the most valid approach to the study of nursing as a human science, and to the art and science of human caring (Leininger, 1985; Munhall & Oiler, 1986; Parse et al., 1985; Paterson & Zderad, 1976; Ray, 1985, 1987; Watson, 1985).

IMPLICATIONS OF PHENOMENOLOGY FOR NURSING AND NURSING RESEARCH

Nursing as a human science, and the philosophy, science, and art of human caring is the new view of nursing (Watson, 1985; Munhall & Oiler, 1986). Phenomenology offers a means by which human phenomena (mental, social, and historical), or the lived experiences of the "lifeworld" of nurses and the persons to whom they are responsible, can be studied and understood. Phenomenology as a philosophy and a method is a fundamental way through which the nurse clinician or researcher at the beginning of an enterprise secures an absolute foundation for herself or himself. This absolute foundation is the cumulative consciousness of her or his lifeworld, made explicit by the rigorous process of structured reflection, which informs how she or he structures the way she or he views and experiences the ever-changing world of immediate experience. In this sense, the nurse-phenomenologist's task through self-reflection is to bring to clarity what is implicit in the experience in question—what is the meaning of the world for me? Phenomenology offers a means by which a nurse can constantly discover and rediscover her or his awareness of the world (Ray, 1985). One must know and understand the self first before entering into the lifeworld of another.

In nursing, the logical positivist or causal model

for scientific inquiry has dominated. However, to permit the discovery of universal meaning in nursing, to interpret the meanings of holistic persons, and to understand comprehensive approaches to nursing as a human science, not only traditional empirical observations are necessary, but also the discovery and interpretation of what it means to be human through phenomenology is essential.

The prevailing view (logical positivism) and the phenomenological view of science were compared and contrasted by Reeder (1984). The author pointed out that when attempting to make inquiry objective, or developing evidence gleaned from concentrating on only five sense (seeing, hearing, touching, tasting, smelling) perceptible things, certain aspects of life such as feeling, imagining, anticipating, willing, loving, and intuiting were screened out. In contrast Reeder pointed out that the phenomenological view incorporates all phenomena of experience—phenomena in present consciousness, from the past through recollection, and from the future through anticipation. Therefore, in the phenomenological view, experience is not limited to sensory experience, but includes multiple modes of awareness known as integral evidence, which is referred to by Husserl as the "principle of intentionality" or "consciousing the world." The evidence of the knower and the known are not separate but integral (Reeder, 1984). As Reeder emphasized, "the known is recognized as crucial in the critique of knowledge" (1984, p. 21). This becomes a central factor in why phenomenology is so important to nursing's philosophy of science, research, and clinical practice. By understanding that the knower and the known are integral and not separate as the ground of philosophy and science, the principle of intentionality demonstrates that strictly objective evidence as put forth in traditional science is impossible in a discipline that refers to its philosophy as holistic and precisely, its epistemology as knowledge generated from experiencing human persons, and its practice as contextual and interhuman. The principle of intentionality offers a new way for the philosopher, researcher, and clinician to interpret the nature of consciousness, and of a person's involvement in the world, which is taken for granted or which is dominated by the results of the objective sciences (Natanson, 1973). For nursing, phenomenology as the rigorous science of meaning offers nursing a way to ground its claims as a human science. Phenomenology, as Natanson (1973) elucidated "honors the integrity of the aspect [particular] and the whole, the unit, and the horizon in which it is viewed, the concrete and the universe in which it comes into clarity" (p. 205).

The implications of the phenomenological method for nursing, thus, are far-reaching. Because nursing claims to be holistic and interactive, there is an integral relationship between the nurse and the client, between the nurse and the community. Nursing must pursue the humanistic and spiritual elements, or what it means to be human and to be spiritual, by discovering the meaning of human caring for persons and communities of persons. If certain human attributes, such as empathy, sympathy, compassion, comfort, respect, hope, and trust have been identified as caring (Leininger, 1981), what depth of meaning do they have in the "lived-world" of nurses and their clients? What depth of meaning is there in caring for community—the community of persons, the global community? To the nurse the beauty of her or his own existence, and of each person's unique existence, and of what that existence means can enhance nursing as a human science, and provide a deeper understanding of the nature of nursing itself.

THE PHENOMENOLOGICAL METHOD

Through the enrichment of existential (being-in-the-world) and hermeneutic (interpretive) thought, phenomenology as methodology concerns itself with gaining access to the outer world (lifeworld) from the inside of human experience (consciousness), through structured reflection leading to transcendental subjectivity (unmediated intuition) and thematic understanding of the meaning of experience (Van Manen, 1984a, 1984b Wagner, 1983;). To understand the essence or what makes something what it is, language is the means—both spoken language from face-to-face communication and its conversion into written language or text. Phenomenologists reduce

observations, impressions, and experiences of the reality of concern to descriptions and thematic interpretations, or linguistic constructions of the meaning of a phenomenon. What is ultimately offered is phenomenological theory—a unity of meaning of the whole of an experience (Van Manen, 1984a; Wagner, 1983). Phenomenological inquiry is "a creative attempt to somehow capture a certain phenomenon of life in a linguistic description that is both holistic and analytical, evocative and precise, unique and universal, and powerful and eloquent" (Van Manen, 1984a, p. 6).

METHODOLOGICAL OUTLINE FOR PHENOMENOLOGICAL RESEARCH

Central aspects of the phenomenological method follow, which are adapted from the ideas of the contemporary phenomenologist, Van Manen (1984a, 1984b). The method appears as a linear process however, when doing phenomenology, for the work is interwoven and a part of the researcher's creativity. The reader also should turn to the literature for a variation of phenomenological approaches (e.g., see Ray, 1987).

Turning to the nature of lived experience (orienting to the phenomenon).   Centering is a way of putting oneself in the frame of mind for "doing" phenomenology. It is a contemplative act wherein the phenomenologist experiences herself or himself in full depth so as to experience the other (Reeder, 1985). Then one can develop a commitment of turning to an abiding concern. Heidegger remarked, "To think is to confine yourself to a single thought till it stands still like a star in the world's sky" (Van Manen, 1984a, p. 3).

Formulating the phenomenological question. Phenomenology does not ask the "how" of something from the perspective of cause and effect. It asks, what is the nature of the experience or meaning of something so that a phenomenon can be better understood. The "whatness" of experience is the key to phenomenological questioning. The essence of the question, said Gadamer, is the opening up and keeping open the possibilities. "We live and become the question" (Van Manen, 1984a, p. 8). As Van

Manen (1984a, 1984b) pointed out, in the researcher's abiding concern of questioning, he or she finds himself or herself interested to be or to stand in the midst of something—in that which makes the question possible in the first place. It teaches us to wonder, to question deeply, the very thing that is being questioned by the question (Van Manen, 1984a, p. 8).

Bracketing and explicating assumptions and preunderstandings. In phenomenology, the researcher brackets out presuppositions. Bracketing (suspension, discounting) refers to holding in abeyance those elements that are irrelevant to the experience (Ray, 1985). Bracketing is a setting aside or detaching the meaning that a phenomenon has for the researcher (Parse, et al., 1985). All information, such as a review of the literature, should be bracketed or accomplished after the research is completed. In addition, the researcher should explicate his or her own assumptions about a phenomenon first, so not to interpret or apply objective evidence to the nature of the phenomenon, before coming to grips with the significance of the phenomenological question and phenomenological data (Van Manen, 1984a).

INVESTIGATION OF THE PHENOMENON

Generating data. Phenomenological research is called generating data. It is the part of the research process where the researcher is educated, that is, finding ways to develop deeper understandings of the phenomenon under investigation. "All understanding is ultimately self understanding," stated Van Manen (1984a, p. 12). Epoché is also practiced and refers to the avoidance of prejudging the data. As one receives the data of experience, one should just "sit with it, and let it speak" (Reeder, 1985). The point of phenomenological research is "to borrow" other people's experiences in order to come better to an understanding of the deeper meaning or significance of an aspect of human experience in the context of the whole of human experience (Van Manen, 1984a). The ethics of informed consent to participate in a nursing research study must apply.

In generating data, the techniques used are interviewing or conversing with participants, personal experience, case studies, literature, music, art, etymological tracings, and so forth. In nursing, the dominant technique is the process of interviewing participants. In phenomenological research, the number of participants can vary but a small sample (5 to 10 people) yields significant data.

The interview process relies upon the life experiences of the participant through genuine dialogue, which can be spoken or silent. The essential element of genuine dialogue is seeing the other or experiencing the other side. For the researcher, prior knowledge of the phenomenon under study is "put into brackets" during interviews. Later, during thematic interpretation, the knowledge bracketed can be unbracketed and considered as it relates to the study as a whole. The interview generally is audiotaped and transcribed; however, descriptive field notes may be written. Any descriptive statement about any kind of phenomenon is a phenomenological datum (Wagner, 1983).

Phenomenological analysis. After the generation of data, the audiotapes are transcribed into textual accounts, and the researcher first gives a direct linguistic description of experience as it is written without causal explanations or interpretive generalizations. The researcher follows the clues as the world of experience is opened up or disclosed, and records whatever comes into awareness as reflective analysis or thoughtfulness is practiced. Disclosures will be synthesized as insights or unmediated intuition. The researcher lets the capacity of knowing surface. The researcher explores the phenomena in all possible ways to see how phenomena present themselves. All that occurs to the researcher should be written down (Van Manen, 1984a, 1984b).

Conducting thematic analysis, and uncovering thematic aspects in the lifeworld descriptions provide the foundation from which the structures of experience can be identified. Themes relate to what the segment of data is all about, or to a partial descriptor of the phenomenon (Tesch, 1987). Although phenomenological themes usually are more than singular statements (concepts or categories), such as thematic descriptions or phrases, often a singular concept may be present or sustained in the course of becoming aware of the phenomenon. To identify themes is to find the threads that weave the experience together (Van Manen, 1984a, 1984b).

Reflecting on the data leads by the process of intuition to the apprehension of the gestalt, the universal essence, or the unity of meaning that can often occur prior to the completion of the thematic analysis. Intuition relates to the mode of awareness in which the object intended by it, does not only have meaning but is originally given in consciousness. To possess the character of intuition, one arrives at knowledge that grasps the ideal (essential image), or the unity of meaning (Ray, 1985), and subsequently can be represented as an aspect of phenomenological theory. Intuition enables the researcher to grasp the essence of the universal validity of the phenomenon in contrast to accidental, individual features (Wagner, 1983).

The work of other scholars can become a source of knowledge for the researcher, that is, "bracketed" experiences or knowledge become "unbracketed" to advance phenomenological description and interpretation to phenomenological theory. Select literature enables the researcher to reflect more deeply on the experience and can add to the development of phenomenological theory. Thus phenomenological theory is an integration of the participants' description of their experience, the researcher's description and interpretation of the data, the researcher's intuitive grasp of the whole of the experience (the unity of meaning), the researcher's use of cumulative knowledge (literature) of the phenomenon under investigation, and the researcher's creativity in organization and explication of the phenomenon as theory.

To evaluate the credibility of the process, the researcher may appeal to the participants to enter into a dialogic reflection on the question and the researcher's interpretive and intuitive data. In this interaction, participants self-reflectively orient themselves to the experience that brings the significance of the phenomenon into view (Van Manen, 1984a).

PHENOMENOLOGICAL WRITING

Phenomenological writing is attending to the speaking and varying of language (Van Manen,

1984a, 1984b). The researcher's writing can be organized around the themes, which can be explained as follows: descriptions of the phenomenon, thematic developments, varying the examples, unity of meaning, engaging with the thinking of other scholars, and theory development.

SUMMARY

In this chapter the philosophy of phenomenology and the phenomenological method were presented. Phenomenology is a way to recover and maintain the humanistic and scientific claims nursing posits by locating insights into the meaning of human existence. This ideal of science is an approach to nursing research and practice that can offer continued growth and revelation, attentiveness and awareness to the meaning of nursing, and the meaning of nursing for nurses and clients as that meaning continually comes into existence (Ray, 1985, p. 91). As Schutz remarked, "phenomenology allows us to bring back 'the full humanity of the thinker into the theoretical field'" (Quoted in Wagner, 1983, p. 206).

REFERENCES

Benner, P. (1985). Quality of life: A phenomenological perspective on explanation, prediction, and understanding in nursing science. *Advances in Nursing Science,* *8*(1), 1–14.

Chivington, P. (1983). *Seeing through your illusions.* Denver: G-L Publications.

Cohen, M. Z. (1987). A historical overview of the phenomenological movement. *Image, 19*(1), 31–34.

Davis, A. J. (1978). The phenomenological approach in nursing research. In N. Chaska (Ed.), *The nursing profession: Views through the mist* (pp. 186–197). New York: McGraw-Hill.

Dufrenne, M. (1973). *The phenomenology of aesthetic experience.* (E. Casey, A. Anderson, W. Domingo, & L. Jacobson, Trans.). Evanston, IL: Northwestern University Press.

Gadamer, Hans-Georg. (1976). *Philosophical hermeneutics.* (D. Linge, Ed. and Trans.). Berkeley: University of California Press.

Giorgi, A. (Ed.) (1985). *Phenomenology and psychological research.* Pittsburgh,: Duquesne University Press.

Human Science in Education Project. (1985). University of Alberta, Faculty of Education. Edmonton, Alberta, Canada: University of Alberta Press.

Husserl, E. (1970). (Trans.) *The crisis of European sciences and transcendental phenomenology*. Evanston, IL: Northwestern University Press. (Original work published 1936)

Leininger, M. (Ed.) (1981). *Caring: An essential human need*. Thorofare, NJ: Charles B. Slack, Inc.

Leininger, M. (Ed.) (1985). *Qualitative research methods in nursing*. New York: Grune & Stratton.

Merleau-Ponty, M. (1962). *Phenomenology of perception*. London: Routledge & Kegan Paul.

Munhall, P., & Oiler, C. (1986). *Nursing research: A qualitative perspective*. Norwalk, CT: Appleton-Century-Crofts.

Natanson, M. (1973). *Edmund Husserl: Philosopher of infinite tasks*. Evanston, IL: Northwestern University Press.

Oiler, C. (1982). The phenomenological approach in nursing research. *Nursing Research, 31*(3), 178–181.

Omery, A. (1983). Phenomenology: A method for nursing research. *Advances in Nursing Science, 5*(2), 49–63.

Parkin, D. (Ed.) (1982). *Semantic anthropology*. New York: Academic Press.

Parse, R., Coyne, A., & Smith, M. (1985). *Nursing research: Qualitative methods*. Bowie, MD: Brady Communications.

Paterson, J., & Zderad, L. (1976). *Humanistic nursing*. New York: John Wiley & Sons.

Ray, M. (1985). A philosophical method to study nursing phenomena. In M. Leininger (Ed.), *Qualitative research methods in nursing* (pp. 81–92). New York: Grune & Stratton.

Ray, M. (1987). Technological caring: A new model in critical care. *Dimensions of Critical Care Nursing, 6*(3), 166–173.

Reeder, F. (1984). Philosophical issues in the rogerian science of unitary human beings. *Advances in Nursing Science, 8*(1), 14–23.

Reeder, F. (1985). Guest Lecturer. *Qualitative research course*, University of Colorado, School of Nursing, Denver, Colorado.

Reeder, F. (1987). The phenomenological movement. *Image, 19*(3), 150–152.

Schutz, A. (1967). *The phenomenology of the social world*. Evanston, IL: Northwestern University Press.

Tesch, R. (1987). Emerging themes: The researcher's experience. *Phenomenology and Pedagogy: A Human Science Journal, 5*(3), 230–241.

Van Manen, M. (1984a). *"Doing" phenomenological research and writing* (Monograph 7). Edmonton, Alberta, Canada: Faculty of Education Publication Services, University of Alberta.

Van Manen, M. (1984b). Practicing phenomenological writing. *Phenomenology and Pedagogy: A Human Science Journal, 2*(1), 36–69.

Wagner, H. (1983). *Phenomenology of consciousness and sociology of the life-world*. Edmonton, Alberta, Canada: University of Alberta Press.

Watson, J. (1985). *Nursing: Human science and human care*. Norwalk, CT: Appleton-Century-Crofts.

✳ EDITOR'S QUESTIONS FOR DISCUSSION ✳

How is the knower and the known integral as the base for science? How can the depth of meaning of one's own experience and existence provide a deeper understanding of the nature of nursing? What is the connection between intentionality and a science of meaning for nursing as a human science? Provide some examples by which phenomenology as a method is applicable to nursing. Discuss to what extent the complex linguistic constructions of the meaning of a phenomenon can hinder, rather than help, the evolution of nursing as a science of caring. What is the essence of nursing practice as an experience? Formulate some phenomenological questions from nursing practice. What does the author mean by "all information . . . should be bracketed" after the research is completed? Provide some examples of bracketing and unbracketing information.

24

Meta-analysis:
A new approach for reviewing research

Elizabeth C. Devine, Ph.D., R.N.

WHAT IS META-ANALYSIS?

Just as no heap of stones is a house, no amount of research is a sufficient knowledge base for a science or discipline until it is assembled, organized and interpreted. With the accumulation of research in the social, behavioral, and health care sciences, researchers have developed increasing interest in deriving knowledge from and resolving contradictions among studies of the same phenomenon (Beecher, 1955; Feldman, 1971; Feldman & Newcomb, 1969; Light & Smith, 1971; Rosenthal, 1969; Taveggia, 1974). This has led to the development of several different methods whose common purpose is to improve both the quality and the outcome of research reviews.

The most widely used term to describe these new methods of research reviewing is meta-analysis. However, there are almost as many different terms as there are major proponents of the process. Some of the other popular terms include quantitative research synthesis, research integration, quantitative reviewing, and quantitative assessment of research. For simplicity, throughout this chapter the term *meta-analysis* is used to describe these new approaches to reviewing research, and meta-research will be used to describe the mode of inquiry that relies on the analysis of the results of prior research to answer research questions. Examples are limited to reviews of studies on the effects of a treatment. However, it should be noted that meta-analysis can be done with correlational studies as well. Readers should refer to the work of Hunter, Schmidt, and Jackson (1982), Glass, McGaw, and Smith (1981), and Hedges and Olkin (1985) for a more detailed discussion of the use of meta-analysis with correlational research.

The term meta-analysis was created in 1976 by Gene Glass. In his seminal paper on forms of analysis, Glass described primary analysis, secondary analysis, and a new form of analysis that he labeled the meta-analysis of research. These three forms of analysis are defined as follows: *primary analysis* is the original analysis of data in a study; *secondary analysis* is the re-analysis of data to answer the original research question with better statistical techniques, or to answer new questions with previously collected data; and *meta-analysis* is the statistical analysis of a large collection of results from individual studies for the purpose of integrating findings (Glass, 1976).

The common thread behind the various procedures called meta-analysis is that survey and statistical methods are applied to the review of existing research with overlapping substantive content. As such, meta-analysis is a study of studies. The processes involved in conducting meta-research are very much like those used in primary research. Research questions are formed. Populations of interest are identified. Selection criteria are created. Data collection instruments are created and tested. Data are collected, evaluated, analyzed, and interpreted. Finally, results are disseminated. The big distinction between meta-research and primary research is that instead of collecting data from individuals, groups, institutions, or archives as one might do in primary research, in meta-research data are collected mainly from research reports. Each individual study is, in essence, a subject in the sample. The characteristics and outcomes of studies are coded to provide data for the meta-analysis. (Occasionally meta-analysts obtain additional data from the researchers who conducted the primary studies being reviewed in the meta-analysis.)

The basic statistics used by meta-analysts to aggregate results across studies are not new. Many of them date from the 1930s or before (Hedges & Olkin, 1985). However, these statistics were not used widely until the idea of meta-analysis began to gain momentum in the latter 1970s.

There are two completely different approaches to combining evidence from different studies. One of these relies on estimating treatment effects (effect sizes) across studies, and the second relies on testing for the statistical significance of combined study results. In this chapter, the former is called the effect size approach to meta-analysis, and the latter is called the combining probabilities approach.

The effect size approach involves calculating an equivalent metric for the outcomes of all studies so that the results of different studies can be combined. Effect size *(ES)*, based on Cohen's statistic δ (Cohen, 1969), is the most frequently used equivalent metric in meta-analysis of research on the effects of a treatment. With a two-group experimental study, *ES* is calculated by dividing the difference between the posttreatment groups means on the dependent variable by a measure of standard deviation. (Some meta-analysts advocate using the standard deviation of the control group, while others suggest using the pooled-within-group standard deviation. The advantages and disadvantages of both approaches are discussed in detail elsewhere [Hedges & Olkin, 1985].) Regardless of the original scale of the dependent variable, *ES* is in standard deviation units. When the desired outcome of a treatment (e.g., decreased anxiety) has a high score on some outcome measures and a low score on others, a convention must be adopted to ensure that all outcomes in the desired direction have the same sign. For example, one might take the absolute value of the calculated *ES* statistic and give it a positive sign if the experimental group had less anxiety than the control group, and a negative sign if the reverse were true.

Because *ES* contains information about both the direction and magnitude of between-group differences after the treatment, and because all outcomes are converted to a common scale (standard deviation units), it is easy to aggregate results across studies using either descriptive or inferential statistics. (See Hedges & Olkin [1985] for a complete discussion of statistical methods for meta-analysis including a discussion of multivariate models for effect size.) For those studies in which means and standard deviations are not available, often it is possible to estimate *ES* from certain statistical values (e.g., *t*-values or proportions). Tables and formulas for those calculations are presented by Glass et al. (1981).

The effect size approach to meta-analysis also can be used with correlational research. With these types of studies various measures of correlation usually are converted to Pearson's *r* or to *ES*. In either case, the equivalent metric conveys information about the direction and magnitude of association, and can be aggregated across studies.

The second major statistical approach to meta-analysis involves combining probabilities or exact *p*-values from a series of studies. The *p*-values are analyzed to determine the overall level of significance of the results obtained from the studies. The procedures involved in conducting a combining probabilities type of meta-analysis are described in detail elsewhere (Rosenthal, 1978, 1979, 1984). The procedures involved in an effect size meta-analysis are described by Glass et al. (1981), Hunter et al.

(1982), Cooper (1982, 1984), and Light and Pillemer (1984).

One advantage of the combining probabilities approach is that procedures exist (Rosenthal, 1979) to calculate what has come to be called the fail-safe N, that is, the number of additional studies yielding nonsignificant results that would be needed to reverse the overall test of significance. This is useful because no matter how diligently one looks for studies, it is likely that some relevant studies will not be found. The problem with this is twofold. First, all studies are not equally easy to find. For example, studies published in journals are easier to find than are unpublished studies (including unpublished theses and dissertations). Second, published and unpublished studies do not necessarily have the same results. Addressing this issue, Rosenthal identified what he has called a file drawer problem. At the extreme, one can imagine an ineffective treatment that has been tested in 100 studies. In this hypothetical example, even though the treatment *really* has no effect, the null hypothesis probably will be rejected in 5 of the 100 studies simply because of chance differences. Given the admitted inclination of researchers, reviewers, and editors to publish more readily those studies reaching traditional levels of statistical significance (Greenwald, 1975), the 5 studies in which the null hypothesis was rejected erroneously are probably more likely to be published than the 95 studies in which the null hypothesis was correctly upheld. Rosenthal proposed, rather colorfully, that many of these 95 studies may be tucked away in the file drawers of the researchers who conducted them.

The extent to which a file drawer problem or a publication bias (as Glass et al. [1981] refer to this problem) might affect the veracity of reviews based on published research, should be a major concern to all consumers of research. With the combining probabilities approach, one can calculate the fail-safe N. With the effect size approach, one can make special efforts to obtain unpublished studies and then determine empirically whether the direction and magnitude of effects are similar to the published studies.

Despite allowing the reviewer to calculate the fail-safe N, the combining probabilities approach to meta-analysis currently is used primarily in conjunction with the effect size approach, rather than as the sole form of analysis. Its major weakness is that it provides no information about the magnitude of effect or association. This is problematic because with a large enough sample, trivial effects or correlations can be statistically significant.

Both approaches to meta-analysis help the reviewer overcome the most common problem in reviewing research. This problem is: How can one summarize past research succinctly when (a) many different versions of the independent variable were implemented, (b) many different target populations were studied, and (c) many different measures of the same outcome construct were used? For example, one might be interested in the effects of providing information about usual sensations experienced in the perioperative period on the postoperative pain experienced by adult surgical patients. Let us suppose that in one study pain was measured by a questionnaire, in a second study it was measured by counting the amount of analgesics used, and in a third study it was measured by having nurses observe patients and assign ratings. Assuming that one is willing to accept all the outcomes being aggregated as measures of the construct pain, with meta-analysis it is simple to aggregate the results across studies. Using the effect size approach, one aggregates the calculated *ES* values rather than the same outcomes in the original scales. With the combining probabilities approach, the scale of the outcome measures in individual studies is not considered at all because one aggregates the exact p-values obtained in the primary studies in an overall test of significance.

The issue of aggregating studies with different versions of the treatment and with different populations of interest is more conceptual. With meta-analysis there are no inherent limits to what can be aggregated using either *ES* values or exact p-values. One must be limited by good sense and theory, taking care not to do violence to the data. As Presby (1978) noted, overly broad categories of interventions can obscure important differences between treatments. Similar problems can occur if one lumps all recipients of a fairly global type of treatment into a single analysis. As with any aggregation it is essential to examine relevant subgroups to ensure that important interactions are not aggregated away.

WHY DO WE NEED META-ANALYSIS?

Any single study cannot be definitive. Even in a study with flawless research design and high quality measurement, chance between-group differences in outcome could lead a researcher or clinician to conclude erroneously that a certain treatment is beneficial. To rise above this inherent weakness of single studies, replications of research are advocated and reviews of research used to summarize what is known and what critical studies are yet to be done. To a large extent meta-analysis was developed because traditional methods for reviewing existing research were found to be inadequate. While most traditional reviews of research are qualitative in nature, meta-analysis is quantitative; however, this is not a qualitative versus quantitative issue. The main problem with traditional reviews is that current standards for generating credible research results usually are not applied; hence the product is often questionable. Comparisons of traditional and meta-analytical approaches to research reviewing are presented in detail elsewhere (Cook & Leviton, 1980; Cooper & Rosenthal, 1980).

To document the state of the art of traditional research reviews, Jackson (1978) examined a random sample of 36 major review papers from leading journals in education, psychology, and sociology. He drew the following conclusions about the status of research synthesis:

1. Reviewers frequently fail to examine critically the evidence, methods, and conclusions of previous reviews on the same topic.
2. Reviewers often focus on only a subset of the relevant studies in an area, the subset is rarely a representative sample, and the methods for selecting the specific studies are seldom specified.
3. Reviewers frequently rely on crude representations of study findings, such as statistical significance.
4. Reviewers sometimes fail to recognize that random sampling error can play a role in creating variability among study results.
5. Reviewers usually report so little about their methods of reviewing that the reader cannot judge the validity of the conclusions.

Three things are important to note here. First, while these problems are specific to research reviews, there are direct analogies to primary research. These deficiencies would not be accepted in primary research, and they should not be accepted in meta-research. Clearly, research reviewing should be held to the same standards of scientific rigor as primary research. Second, *none* of these problems is inherent in a narrative review of research. The case can be made that the decision to use quantitative or qualitative methods to summarize past results is separate from issues of methodological quality of the review. Finally, because a review is quantitative does not ensure that these problems will not be present. Several excellent critiques of existing meta-analyses have been published (Ganong, 1987; Sacks, Berrier, Reitman, Ancona-Berk, & Chalmers, 1987).

However, there are two reasons why meta-analysts may be more likely to avoid the pitfalls of traditional research reviewers identified by Jackson (1978). First, anyone reading the meta-analysis literature should be cognizant of the aspects of traditional research reviews that have been criticized. Based on this knowledge the reviewers should be able to take steps to avoid these weaknesses. These steps include critically reviewing past reviews on the same topic; conducting a comprehensive search for relevant research, and including unpublished studies (e.g., theses and dissertations) in the review when appropriate; examining the consistency of outcomes using homogeneity tests (Hedges & Olkin, 1985; Hunter et al., 1982) to avoid misinterpreting between-study differences in the magnitude of effect or association; and reporting the specific methods and procedures used in conducting the review.

Second, when meta-analysts use the effect size approach they can avoid overdependence on statistical significance tests. Instead of relying on significance tests, conclusions can be based on the magnitude of treatment effect or, with correlational research, the size of the association.

WHAT ARE THE ADVANTAGES OF META-ANALYSIS FOR NURSING?

Meta-analysis represents a revolution in research reviewing. In time, the haphazard and subjective old-style literary reviews no longer will be acceptable contributions to the scientific literature. The methodological standards developed under the rubric of meta-analysis will serve to improve the quality of research reviews, and this should help to improve the accumulation of past research into a knowledge base for nursing.

Another revolutionary aspect of meta-analysis is that analyses often are based on an equivalent metric (e.g., effect size). Focusing on the size of effect or relationship is advantageous in three ways. First, while interpreting the results of an effect size type of meta-analysis requires that readers understand the concept of effect size, the conclusions of meta-analyses are usually more direct than those of traditional literary reviews. In addition, the implications of these conclusions are usually clearer for clinicians and policymakers.

Second, the conclusions of a meta-analysis are usually more definitive about the effect of a treatment than those of a traditional review of the same research. With meta-analysis one has the power to detect a consistent effect, even if most of the individual studies do not reach traditional levels of statistical significance. This aspect of meta-analysis is especially important for clinical nursing research, in which it is often difficult to obtain large samples and sufficient statistical power to detect clinically relevant effects. In the past, dependence on statistical significance as the sole measure of treatment effectiveness decreased the ability of nurse clinicians, researchers, and theorists to take full advantage of past nursing research. Sensitivity to the direction and magnitude of study outcomes should help us discover what can be known from prior research.

In addition to identifying what is known from past research, comprehensive meta-analytical reviews are useful in identifying questions that need to be addressed in future research. The third advantage of an effect size type of meta-analysis is that it can provide estimates of the magnitude of a treatment's effect and information on sample variability. These data are useful for ad hoc statistical power calculations for new studies of the same phenomenon.

SUMMARY

In summary, meta-analysis is not a panacea that always yields unambiguous and scientifically accurate results. As any other methodology, it can be used inappropriately or uncritically. Further, it is limited by the methodological and theoretical strengths of the original studies being analyzed. Despite these problems, meta-analysis can be a vast improvement over traditional reviews of research. Consumers of research and research reviewers need to know about meta-analysis and its potential contribution to nursing research.

In a single chapter a complete introduction to such a complex topic is impossible. Readers are encouraged to consult the many methodological and issue-oriented papers and books cited in this chapter. In addition, meta-analyses with relevance to public health have been summarized by Louis, Fineberg, and Mosteller (1985), and a complete volume of the *Evaluation Studies Review Annual* has been devoted to meta-analysis (Light, 1983). There are also several published meta-analyses on topics of interest to nurses. These include patient education (Devine & Cook 1983, 1986; Hathaway 1986; Mazzuca 1982; Mumford, Schlesinger, & Glass 1982); stereotyping by nurses (Ganong, Bzdek, & Manderino, 1987); nonnutritive sucking in preterm infants (Schwartz, Moody, Yarandi, & Anderson 1987); tardive dyskinesia (Morgenstern, Glazer, Niedzwiecki, & Nourjah, 1987); psychotherapy (Smith, Glass, & Miller, 1980); and deinstitutionalization of the mentally ill (Straw, 1983).

REFERENCES

Beecher, H. K. (1955). The powerful placebo. *Journal of the American Medical Association, 159*(2), 1602–1606.

Cohen, J. (1969). *Statistical power analysis for the behavioral sciences*. New York: Academic Press.

Cook, T. D., & Leviton, L. C. (1980). Reviewing the literature: A comparison of traditional methods with meta-analysis. *Journal of Personality, 48*(4), 449–472.

Cooper, H. M. (1982). Scientific guidelines for conducting integrative research reviews. *Review of Educational Research, 52*(2), 291–302.

Cooper, H. M. (1984). *The integrative research review*. Beverly Hills, CA: Sage Publications.

Cooper, H. M., & Rosenthal, R. (1980). Statistical versus traditional procedures for summarizing research findings. *Psychological Bulletin, 87*(3), 442–449.

Devine, E. C., & Cook T. D. (1983). A meta-analytic analysis of effects of psychoeducational interventions on length of post-surgical hospital stay. *Nursing Research, 32*(5), 267–274.

Devine, E. C., & Cook, T. D. (1986). Clinical and cost relevant effects of psychoeducational interventions with surgical patients: A meta-analysis. *Research in Nursing and Health, 9*(2), 89–105.

Feldman, K. A. (1971). Some observations on reviewing and integrating. *Sociology of Education, 44,* 86–102.

Feldman, K. A., & Newcomb, T. M. (1969). *The impact of college on students.* San Francisco: Jossey-Bass.

Ganong, L. H. (1987). Integrative reviews of nursing research. *Research in Nursing and Health, 10*(1), 1–11.

Ganong, L. H., Bzdek, V., & Manderino, M. A. (1987). Stereotyping by nurses and nursing students: A critical review of research. *Research in Nursing and Health, 10*(1), 49–70.

Glass, G. (1976). Primary, secondary, and meta-analysis of research. *Educational Research, 5,* 3–8.

Glass, G., McGaw, B., & Smith, M. L. (1981). *Meta-analysis in social research.* Beverly Hills, CA: Sage Publications.

Greenwald, A. G. (1975). Consequences of prejudice against the null hypothesis. *Psychological Bulletin, 82*(1), 1–20.

Hathaway, D. (1986). Effects of preoperative instruction on postoperative outcomes: A meta-analysis. *Nursing Research, 35*(5), 269–275.

Hedges, L. V., & Olkin, I. (1985). *Statistical methods for meta-analysis.* New York: Academic Press.

Hunter, J. E., Schmidt, F. L., & Jackson, G. B. (1982). *Meta-analysis cumulating research findings across studies.* Beverly Hills, CA: Sage Publications.

Jackson, G. B. (1978). *Methods for reviewing and integrating research in the social sciences.* (Final report to the National Science Foundation for Grant No. DIS 76-20309). Washington, DC: Social Research Group, George Washington University.

Light, R. J. (Ed.) (1983). *Evaluation studies review annual, Vol. 8.* Beverly Hills, CA: Sage Publications.

Light, R. J., & Pillemer, D. B. (1984). *Reviewing research: The science of summing up.* Cambridge: Harvard University Press.

Light, R. J., & Smith, P. V. (1971). Accumulating evidence: Procedures for resolving contradictions from among different research studies. *Harvard Educational Review, 41*(4), 429–471.

Louis, T. A., Fineberg, H. V., & Mosteller, F. (1985). Findings for public health from meta-analyses. *Annual Review of Public Health, 6,* 1–20.

Mazzuca, S. (1982). Does patient education in chronic disease have therapeutic value? *Journal of Chronic Disease, 5*(7), 521–529.

Morgenstern, H., Glazer, W. M., Niedzwiecki, D, & Nourjah, P. (1987). The impact of neuroleptic medication on tardive dyskinesia: A meta-analysis of published studies. *American Journal of Public Health, 77*(6), 717–724.

Mumford, E., Schlesinger, H. J., & Glass, G. (1982). The effect of psychological interventions on recovery from surgery and heart attacks: An analysis of the literature. *American Journal of Public Health, 72*(2), 141–151.

Presby, S. (1978). Overly broad categories obscure important differences between therapies. *American Psychologist, 33*(5), 514–515.

Rosenthal, R. (1969). Interpersonal expectation. In R. Rosenthal & R. L. Rosnow (Eds.), *Artifacts in behavioral research* (pp. 182–277). New York: Academic Press.

Rosenthal, R. (1978). The "file drawer problem" and tolerance for null results. *Psychological Bulletin, 86*(3), 638–641.

Rosenthal, R. (1979). Combining results of independent studies. *Psychological Bulletin, 85*(1), 185–193.

Rosenthal, R. (1984). *Meta-analytic procedures for social research.* Beverly Hills, CA: Sage Publications.

Sacks, H. S., Berrier, J. A., Reitman, D., Ancona-Berk, V. A., & Chalmers, T. C. (1987). Meta-analyses of randomized controlled trials. *New England Journal of Medicine, 316*(8), 450–455.

Schwartz, R., Moody, L., Yarandi, H., & Anderson, G. (1987). A meta-analysis of critical outcome variables in nonnutritive sucking in preterm infants. *Nursing Research, 36,* 292–295.

Smith, M. L., Glass, G., & Miller, T. I. (1980). *The benefits of psychotherapy.* Baltimore: Johns Hopkins University Press.

Straw, R. (1983). Deinstitutionalization in mental health: A meta-analysis. In R. J. Light (Ed.), *Evaluation studies review annual, Vol. 8* (pp. 253–278). Beverly Hills, CA: Sage Publications.

Taveggia, T. C. (1974). Resolving research controversy through empirical cumulation: Toward reliable social knowledge. *Sociological Methods and Research, 2*(4), 395–407.

✳   EDITOR'S QUESTIONS FOR DISCUSSION   ✳

What are the advantages and disadvantages of meta-analytical research? How valid and reliable can meta-research data obtained from research reports be? What is meant by treatment effects? What is meant by the concept of effect size? What kind of suggestions could be made to address the problem of publication bias? How are the conclusions of meta-analysis more definitive regarding the effect of a treatment than those of a traditional review? How can one be reasonably assured that the data are not being distorted when examining relevant subgroups of the aggregates that were studied? Provide examples of research questions that could be addressed by using meta-analysis. Why is it important to be able to detect a consistent effect in a number of studies relating to clinical nursing research?

25

Methods for Facilitating Faculty Research

Jacqueline F. Clinton, Ph.D., R.N., F.A.A.N.

Factors affecting the evolution of nursing research in the United States have been well documented by numerous scholars (Abdellah, 1977; Abdellah & Levine, 1986; Batey, 1978; Bunge, 1958; Cross, 1977; Gortner & Nahm, 1977; Hyde, 1977; Kalisch, 1977; Werley, 1962; Wilson, 1984). One major factor in the twentieth century has been nursing education's movement into institutions of higher learning. This includes the establishment of baccalaureate programs in the nursing major, growth of graduate programs in nursing, and increased access to doctoral level education for nurses in numerous fields of study including nursing.

NURSING'S PRESENCE IN INSTITUTIONS OF HIGHER LEARNING: THE RESEARCH IMPERATIVE

The movement of nursing into the university environment has served to upgrade nursing education, bring recognition and prestige to nursing as a legitimate and autonomous discipline, and provide nursing faculty and students with access to a wide array of resources necessary for scholarly work. Nursing faculty and educational administrators also are cognizant that the privilege of being in a community of scholars involves specific responsibilities. In the majority of institutions of higher learning, faculty in the sciences are expected to be productive in three general areas: teaching excellence (the dissemination and debate of existing knowledge in the field), community service (the application of knowledge), and research or other scholarly activity (the generation and testing of new knowledge).

Historically, nursing's achievements in these three areas have been uneven. Teaching excellence was the major emphasis in the first half of the century and reflects that nurses' early entry to graduate preparation was predominantly in the field of curriculum and instruction. Community service has also been an area wherein nursing faculty excel because of the fact that nursing is an applied discipline; that is, nurses are action-oriented with a deep sense of social commitment. Research productivity of nursing faculty has had a more irregular track record that can be linked to several key factors: (a) opportunities for research training in doctoral and postdoctoral programs; (b) heavy teaching loads and other job expectations within schools of nursing; (c) the reward structure within the university as a whole including merit raises, promotion, and tenure; (d) the extent to which a school of nursing's reward structure mirrors that of the larger institution; (e) the degree to which faculty colleagues create and maintain an interpersonal milieu of encouragement for, and expectations about, research-related activities; and (f) the availability and integration of graduate students within faculty research activities.

THE RESEARCH IMPERATIVE WITHIN THE LARGER SOCIAL CONTEXT

The development and testing of a scientific body of knowledge is currently the most critical factor to the advancement of professionalism in nursing. It is the public who ultimately authorizes what constitutes the scope of practice for any human service discipline. The public expects such disciplines to base their practice on systematic knowledge that has been tested and retested. Nurses have learned that organized nursing's political strategies for advancing professional status or changing public policy are remarkably ineffective in the absence of carefully documented evidence that nursing makes significant contributions to the welfare of the public. Nursing faculty in institutions of higher learning carry a special responsibility in this regard because of their advanced preparation and expertise in research and their charge to create and disseminate new knowledge in the field.

In addition to nursing's move into institutions of higher education in the United States during this century, another gain for nursing research occurred in 1986 with the establishment of the National Center for Nursing Research (NCNR) within the National Institutes of Health (NIH) (Merritt, 1986). For the first time, nursing research entered the mainstream of health research in the United States. Nursing has now taken its place in and has full access to a larger community of health scientists. Jacox (1986) refers to it as the "coming of age" of nursing research. The creation of the NCNR represents public confidence and commitment that nurses are accountable for generating the knowledge base of their practice. In essence, society's expectation that nurses conduct research in their field is greater than ever before.

PROMOTING FACULTY RESEARCH PRODUCTIVITY

Since 1953 one of the most salient developments promoting nursing research has been the growth of centers or offices of nursing research, the majority of which are located in academic settings in the United States (International Council of Nurses, 1984). The overall mission of such units is generally to facilitate research conducted by nursing faculty and students as well as by nurses in the community. The organizational characteristics of these centers that are conducive to research productivity have been well described by others (Batey, 1978; Gortner, 1985; Pranulis & Gortner, 1985). Published evidence that the existence of nursing research centers positively influences scholarship and overall excellence in schools of nursing has been summarized by Clinton, Wahl, and Kelber (1987).

While the published literature on centers for nursing research contains considerable information on the organizational structure, mission, goals, and services of such entities, there remains insufficient published information on the specific details of how to support faculty research productivity. This includes the day-to-day considerations and strategies that can be employed by schools of nursing to facilitate research, regardless of the existence of a structural unit devoted to research. Further, very little is published on faculty's learning needs related to research. The purpose of this chapter is to explore such strategies in light of the needs of the developing scientist and the role of senior faculty.

NEEDS OF NEW DOCTORATES

Similar to other academic departments within the university environment, nursing schools are rapidly moving toward the minimum requirement of the doctorate for appointment to tenure track positions. Unlike in the past when nurses with earned doctorates were regarded by their colleagues as "senior experts" in the field, it is now being recognized that nurses with recent doctorates are neophytes whose development as scientists has just begun. Their growth as scientists is inextricably linked to the extent to which their immediate environment provides resources and support for research, particularly during the first 3 years postdoctorally.

A primary need of the new investigator is access to a wide variety of resources necessary to develop a research program. The first resource needed is

of productive research environments in nursing. *Western Journal of Nursing Research, 7*, 127.

Tripp-Reimer, T. (1986). Health heritage project: A proposal submitted to the Division of Nursing. *Western Journal of Nursing Research, 8*, 207–224.

Werley, H. (1962). Promoting the research dimension in the practice of nursing through the establishment and development of nursing in an institute of research. *Military Medicine, 127*, 219–231.

Wilson, H. S. (1984). Research in nursing has a history. *Journal of Nursing Administration, 12*, 4–5.

✳ EDITOR'S QUESTIONS FOR DISCUSSION ✳

Suggest specific strategies as to how faculty may meet the demands for superior teaching and simultaneously develop strong research programs. How might faculty role demands be effectively balanced? Should criteria be established by which faculty are allocated more time than others for developing their research programs? If so, what criteria might you suggest? What strategies would you suggest for negotiating time to develop and conduct research?

How can information regarding resources, support services, and funding sources be more appropriately shared, organized, and distributed for faculty? What should be the components of a faculty research program? How might the components be supported by administration on an ongoing basis? How might teaching assistants and graduate student assistants be used for the purposes of developing and strengthening the research programs of faculty? What mechanisms and criteria might be established for the use of research assistants in a school of nursing? How might a one-to-one consultation service be provided for nursing faculty to conduct research? What accountability mechanisms might be established in relation to research development programs?

26

The Clinical Nurse Researcher Role in a Practice Setting

Karen B. Haller, Ph.D., R.N.

The need for research-based practice and data-based management has prompted some clinical agencies to initiate nursing research and development programs. It is hoped that these programs will promote the integration of nursing research in service settings and generate practice-relevant studies.

A growing number of hospitals, for example, are establishing and maintaining practice-based nursing research programs. This trend received formal recognition and support from the American Hospital Association in their publication, *Strategies: Integration of Nursing Research into the Practice Setting* (1985). In this statement, a commitment to the values of practice-based nursing research in an economically constrained environment was made: "Nurse executives are urged to view the environment's economic constraints as an incentive to the integration of research into the practice setting, instead of as a prohibiting factor" (p. 1).

The clinical research programs developed to date vary in design, functions, resources, and project applications. Structurally, however, they tend to be patterned after one of three basic models identified by Engstrom (1984): (a) a university-based program, (b) an agency-based program, or (c) a collaborative model. University-based research is usually conducted by academicians and their graduate students,

using clinical facilities as their laboratories. Agency-based research is conducted primarily within the walls of a sponsoring clinical organization and, as Engstrom notes, "the researcher is an instrument through which the hiring agency can seek answers to specific questions" (p. 77). The Veterans Administration has successfully implemented agency-based research programs in many of their hospitals. Collaborative models employ structural arrangements that pool the resources of academe and health care centers in order to conduct research. One approach to facilitating collaborative research is to have researchers hold joint appointments in both the university and clinical sectors. The University of Arizona (Chance & Hinshaw, 1980) pioneered such an approach, and other institutions have successfully emulated this type of collaborative model.

Nursing research has traditionally been housed in universities. Universities provide the resources and the environment in which scholarly work can progress. With researchers using the university-based model, the nursing profession has steadily increased the quality and the quantity of its research over the past 30 years.

The isolation of research in academic institutions, however, results in several problems for practice professions like nursing. First, expert practicing nurses and nursing administrators are often excluded from the process by which research problems are identified and priorities are set for study. This exclusion has contributed to the lack of research on issues that are important for clinical practice. Second, the results of research are often made available to other researchers at scientific meetings and in research journals, but not directly disseminated to practitioners in a meaningful form.

Agency-based and collaborative models enhance clinicians' and administrators' participation in research from the initial problem identification through dissemination of study results. In both agency-based and collaborative models, a key person in the success of the research program is the nurse scientist assigned to facilitate research. This person should have a doctorate, relevant clinical and research experience, and personal qualities that are assets in working with clinicians.

ROLE OF THE CLINICAL NURSE RESEARCHER

The role of the clinical nurse researcher who works primarily in a practice setting includes management responsibilities as well as responsibilities for facilitating research (Hagle, Kirchhoff, Knafl, & Bevis, 1986). As manager of a research program, the nurse must assure that the goals of the program are consonant with the mission of the agency. As research facilitator, the scientist must ensure that the research work of staff is sound and can be implemented.

Management Responsibilities

The aims and objectives of a research program in a service setting should complement the nursing department's philosophy and goals (Smeltzer & Hinshaw, 1988). It is the clinical nurse researcher's role to implement the organization's research mission. It would be inappropriate, for example, to embark on an ambitious program of fundamental research if the mission of the agency is directed toward research utilization.

Other management responsibilities of clinically based researchers may include monitoring research activities in the institution by reviewing proposals from investigators seeking access to clinical populations or support from nursing staff. It is important to keep line managers aware of current research activity in an institution. The research scientist in a nursing department often participates in the administrative work of the agency by serving on committees that use research methods, such as the quality assurance committee or the product evaluation committee. If the nursing research program is to be fully integrated into the mainstream of research in an agency, then it is essential that the nurse researcher sit on the Institutional Review Board for the Protection of Human Subjects.

Research Responsibilities

Research responsibilities of the nurse scientist in an agency program involve (a) promoting a positive climate for research and scholarly activities, (b) assisting members of the nursing staff to carry out activities that support the research functions of the department, and (c) conducting one's own research.

Efforts to promote and maintain an effective research environment in a service setting are directed toward removing the obstacles to nursing research, as well as installing an awareness of the value of research to the discipline. Obstacles to nursing research are widely known to be lack of expertise and time. Most practicing nurses lack academic preparation sufficient for conducting research; concomitantly, they lack socialization to appropriate research roles (Fawcett, 1984). In nursing, and particularly in service settings, there has been little opportunity to work under a research mentor and be socialized as a researcher. May, Meleis, and Winstead-Fry (1982) have discussed the importance of mentorship in developing the nursing scholar. Another obstacle is widespread misunderstanding of research and, as a result, nurses tend to avoid research activities. The obstacle of limited time is real and must be effectively circumvented by a research program in order for it to be productive.

Strategies for removing the obstacles to research activity in service settings center on increasing the visibility of nursing research, demonstrating the utility of research findings, and providing access to research expertise. Visibility of nursing research can be increased in an institution by including research and researchers in agency programs; for example, research findings can be incorporated regularly into staff development or continuing education offerings. A series of research presentations has been successfully implemented by nursing departments in some academic health care centers; for example, the Department of Nursing at Foster G. McGaw Hospital, Loyola University of Chicago, sponsors an annual series of research lectures for hospital staff. When well-known researchers are brought in to discuss their work with clinicians and administrators, it is possible to arrange consultations for staff who are interested in the methodology or the content area under study. Occasionally, such consultations lead to opportunities for collaboration; the researcher provides methodological expertise and academic resources, while the clinician contributes clinical expertise and access to study populations.

Other strategies for increasing the visibility of nursing research may be implemented by the clinical nurse researcher. A "contents service," in which the tables of contents from nursing research journals are circulated to all clinical units, can be effective in keeping busy staff aware of current research. Newsletters or annual reports that feature the scholarly and research work of staff promote nursing research both inside and outside the nursing department, as well as recognize the contributions of the institution's researchers. For example, The Johns Hopkins Hospital publishes *Hopkins Nurse*, a newsletter with a center tearout section that abstracts publications and presentations by nursing staff.

The axiom that "nothing succeeds like success" holds true in research endeavors. When a project has findings of clinical import, it is important to make them available and visible. Releasing an announcement of the findings to nursing units, key people in other departments, and the press are effective means of garnering interest and support. Currently, projects that measure cost-effectiveness are highly valued. Building cost measures into clinical tests is a useful strategy for broadening a project's potential audience.

The main thrust of an active research program in a clinical setting is to facilitate research by making expertise available to clinicians who lack the formal preparation to conduct studies independently. Expertise is often made available to clinicians by "team building." A clinician who has identified a researchable problem is put in touch with a researcher who is willing to consult or collaborate on the project; in addition, most projects require statistical consultation, a part-time research assistant, and secretarial services to develop the proposal. By building a team around the clinician who is a research novice, access to research expertise and mentorship is afforded. In addition, the provision of personnel resources lessens the time that will be necessary for the clinician to be away from her or his patients.

Structure, Process, and Outcomes of Research Programs

Like all roles, the role of clinical nurse researcher can be considered in terms of its structure, its processes, and its outcomes. Each of these aspects are discussed.

Structure. The structure in which the nurse researcher functions consists of the design for the research program, the program functions, and the resources available to the program. In service settings, the three most commonly used designs to carry out research work are research committees with rotating chairpersons, a single research specialist hired to direct the program, and research departments. Program functions are the objectives determined by the nursing department. Some departments may limit their function to evaluation and approval of proposals from outside investigators, while more aggressive departments may design and carry out multiple projects of their own. Program resources vary by the type of research program established; however, the American Hospital Association (1985) recommends "hard monies" to fund whatever is undertaken. An aggressive program, one whose primary goals are the conduct of significant studies and the application of research findings to practice, needs sufficient resources. Secretarial support, the services of an automated library, computer facilities with statistical and programming services, as well as research and development funds, are essential.

Process.   The work of the nurse researcher requires many processes. As program manager, the scientist advises the management team on research-related matters. As research facilitator, the scientist actively consults with investigators and collaborates with research teams. Ideally the clinical nurse researcher also conducts a personal program of research.

Outcomes.   There are multiple consumers for the products of nursing research and, therefore, multiple outcomes desired from research programs in clinical settings. For patients, the ultimate goal of nursing science is research-based practice with predictable outcomes. For expert practitioners, the involvement in research may be expected to add breadth or depth to their professional lives. Administrators in organizations where patients and practitioners interact may desire greater cost-effectiveness from the client and clinician encounter as a result of their financial investment in research and development. The extent to which research programs in clinical agencies have been able to achieve these outcomes has not been well documented, and there is a need for systematic evaluation.

RESEARCH ACTIVITIES APPROPRIATE IN CLINICAL SETTINGS

It is helpful to define research broadly in service settings. Stetler (1983) codified and clarified the continuum of research work that is possible in hospitals. This continuum begins with routine projects in which research methods can be useful. Common projects include product evaluation, quality monitoring, patient classification, nursing productivity measurement and monitoring, development of research-based patient care standards, documentation for policy and procedure development, research utilization aimed at improved cost-effectiveness and quality of care, and evaluating infection control initiatives. The continuum of possible research work ranges beyond these routine applications to include other research utilization and evaluation activities, as well

as fine replication studies and original pieces of research.

While the range of research work appropriate for clinical agencies is not restricted, pressures in the service setting tend to focus research efforts on generating solutions to immediate problems. Hinshaw and Smeltzer (1987) note that although pressure for tangible outcomes to solve agency problems often supercedes the nursing discipline's need to generate new knowledge and test theory, both goals can be achieved in clinical research programs. They suggest two strategies for ensuring that agency research contributes both to the development of knowledge and the provision of data for directing institutional policy. The first strategy is to use "frameworks that organize research questions in terms of the empirical data needs, but also places (sic) the variables and the data in perspective to the abstract concepts that are represented" (p. 21). Thus, knowledge can be developed with the same data that were generated for internal policy decisions. Second, Hinshaw and Smeltzer suggest that replication of small, local studies in multiple sites is an effective means of meeting specific agencies' needs for data while building knowledge.

Traditional, university-based researchers have advantages in conducting independent, original research. Not the least of these advantages are the presence of colleagues trained in research methods during doctoral and postdoctoral study, the time afforded to research as a legitimate activity in academia, and the recognition given successful researchers. Nevertheless, there are some research activities that are best carried out in clinical agencies, under the direction of skilled nurse researchers. Agency-based research programs have the advantages of access to expert clinicians and study populations. Therefore, the following research activities are most appropriately carried out in clinical agencies. It is in these areas that service settings are likely to make their largest contributions to nursing science:

1. Identification of problems for future nursing research.
2. Collection of data for nursing studies.
3. Facilitation of nursing research conducted in clinical settings.

4. Use of research methods to enhance the quality of nursing department activities such as audits, patient classification, and quality monitoring.
5. Consultation or collaboration with researchers to enhance the clinical relevance of nursing research by identifying significant variables to include in studies.
6. Application of research-based knowledge in practice.

RESEARCH ACTIVITIES ACCORDING TO EDUCATIONAL PREPARATION

Those who have run clinical research programs (e.g., Stetler, 1984) have found it helpful to define research involvement broadly so that it encompasses facilitating research conducted by others, using research methods in routine problem solving, and utilizing as well as conducting, research. This broad definition begs the question of who is responsible for carrying out the various research-related activities, since all nurses cannot be expected to carry out all functions. The American Nurses' Association (ANA) (1981) has taken the position that there are research activities appropriate for nurses at each level of academic preparation and, collectively, these activities account for the broad range of research responsibilities that exist. The ANA classification of research activities by educational preparation is presented in the accompanying box, Guidelines for the Investigative Function of Nurses, p. 199.

The associate degree graduate, for example, is expected at least to assist in problem identification and data collection. The baccalaureate graduate can be held accountable for applying established research-based knowledge to clinical practice. The master's degree graduate should assist others in applying research findings to practice, conducting quality monitoring activities, and collaborating on investigations. Those prepared at the doctoral level are charged with providing leadership for conducting research that contributes to theory, developing methods, and integrating new knowledge into practice. All nurses are expected to support and facilitate the

scientific work of their colleagues (Haller, 1986).

The ANA's typology of research responsibilities by educational preparation has been the target of some criticism in the nursing community. Criticisms center on whether educational programs adequately prepare nurses to assume the research responsibilities delineated for the various degree programs, and whether the distinction between role responsibilities for graduates from the two types of doctoral degrees (professional, meaning DNSc, EdD, and others, versus the research-oriented PhD) is valid. Fawcett (1985) has addressed some of the criticisms of the ANA document and has emphasized that the guidelines serve as a "suggestion for maximizing nurses' participation in research, while at the same time not establishing expectations that are inappropriate for the individual nurse, based on his or her educational preparation" (p. 77). Fawcett recognizes that the guidelines may be helpful to clinicians who wish to participate in research activities by defining appropriate objectives for them. The guidelines help educators by suggesting what research content needs to be emphasized in the various programs, and how this content builds sequentially with advancing degrees. The guidelines may also help nurse administrators to develop appropriate research criteria for clinical ladders and performance appraisal systems. If followed, the guidelines allow consistency in expectations for research among those who work in practice, education, and administration.

INTEGRATING RESEARCH INTO NURSING DEPARTMENTS

The clinical nurse researcher is often explicitly or implicitly charged with integrating research functions and responsibility for them into the nursing system. This is particularly true if the researcher is the first person to hold such a position in the agency. There are standard means by which to integrate functions and responsibilities in all systems, and the researcher can use these mechanisms to advance nursing research. For example, a nursing research committee is a useful organizational entity for broadening participation in research and advising

Guidelines for the investigative function of nurses

Associate degree in nursing

1. Demonstrates awareness of the value or relevance of research in nursing.
2. Assists in identifying problem areas in nursing practice.
3. Assists in collection of data within an established structured format.

Baccalaureate in nursing

1. Reads, interprets, and evaluates research for applicability to nursing practice.
2. Identifies nursing problems that need to be investigated and participates in the implementation of scientific studies.
3. Uses nursing practice as a means of gathering data for refining and extending practice.
4. Applies established findings of nursing and other health related research to nursing practice.
5. Shares research findings with colleagues.

Master's degree in nursing

1. Analyzes and reformulates nursing practice problems so that scientific knowledge and scientific methods can be used to find solutions.
2. Enhances the quality and clinical relevance of nursing research by providing expertise in clinical problems and by providing knowledge about the way in which these clinical services are delivered.
3. Facilitates investigations of problems in clinical settings through such activities as contributing to a climate supportive of investigative activities, collaborating with others in investigations and enhancing nursing's access to clients and data.
4. Conducts investigations for the purpose of monitoring the quality of the practice of nursing in a clinical setting.
5. Assists others to apply scientific knowledge in nursing practice.

Doctoral degree in nursing or a related discipline

A. Graduate of a practice-oriented doctoral program
1. Provides leadership for the integration of scientific knowledge with other sources of knowledge for the advancement of practice.
2. Conducts investigations to evaluate the contribution of nursing activities to the well-being of clients.
3. Develops methods to monitor the quality of the practice of nursing in a clinical setting and to evaluate contributions of nursing activities to the well-being of clients.

B. Graduate of a research-oriented doctoral program
1. Develops theoretical explanations of phenomena relevant to nursing by empirical research and analytical processes.
2. Uses analytical and empirical methods to discover ways to modify or extend existing scientific knowledge so that it is relevant to nursing.
3. Develops methods for scientific inquiry of phenomena relevant to nursing.

From the American Nurses' Association, Commission on Nursing Research (1981). *Guidelines for the investigative function of nurses* (Publication No. D-69). Kansas City, MO: Author. Reprinted with permission.

research nurses. Written policies can be used to institutionalize and legitimize research activities. A policy about who may conduct research and how proposals are reviewed is essential. This policy should also clarify the relationship between the objectives and functions of the nursing research review, and those of the institution's human subjects' review. In general, nursing research committees consider administrative issues such as the time required of staff to support a study, whether a sufficient sample can be found, and similar issues. Human subjects' review focuses on ethical issues, including the cost-benefit ratio of the proposed study. A policy for supporting travel to professional meetings that gives priority to staff who are presenting research papers is another means to foster and reward research initiatives. Perhaps the most effective way to set expectations for research and reward participation is by integrating criteria that address research into the nursing performance appraisal system.

CHALLENGES FACING PRACTICE-BASED RESEARCHERS

As research programs in clinical settings proliferate and mature, and as increasing numbers of nurse researchers work in nonacademic settings, there will be an opportunity to resolve a number of challenges currently facing the profession. First among these challenges is the integration of nursing research into the overall research effort of health care institutions. Medical centers, which were developed for and are now known for their medical research, need to be developed also as "nursing centers" that are known for their nursing research. As Oberst (1980) has noted, nurses who work in these large and powerful medical systems function daily in the midst of "a ready-made, well-controlled research situation with access to large subject populations" (p. 459). Infrequently have nurses taken advantage of the medical research environment to promote their own scholarship and advance their own research interests. Nursing has not fully placed its people into the mainstream of a system for conducting and implementing research that already exists in university-affiliated health care centers.

A second challenge facing practice-based researchers is the need to garner an increased proportion of the internal and external funds available for research work. These funds will help support individual work and lend the credibility of peer review to research conducted in agency programs with practitioners. Third, the outcomes of agency-based research programs and clinical nurse researchers' work must be measured. The long-term success of research programs in service settings will be determined by their ability to contribute to knowledge and to quality patient care. Finally, there needs to be some attention given to the professional development, mentorship, and peer support of the clinical nurse researcher who works as the only scientist in a nursing department. Networks and consortium arrangements, as well as other mechanisms, are useful in assisting those who are new to the position and providing input to seasoned clinical researchers. These, then, are the challenges facing clinical nurse researchers in the 1990s.

REFERENCES

American Hospital Association. (1985). *Strategies: Integration of nursing research into the practice setting*. Chicago: Author.

American Nurses' Association, Commission on Nursing Research. (1981). *Guidelines for the investigative function of nurses*. (Publication No. D-69). Kansas City, MO: Author.

Chance, H.C., & Hinshaw, A.S. (1980). Strategies for initiating a research program. *Journal of Nursing Administration, 10*(3), 32–39.

Engstrom, J. (1984). University, agency, and collaborative models for nursing research: An overview. *Image, 16,* 76–80.

Fawcett, J. (1984). Hallmarks of success in nursing research. *Advances in Nursing Science, 7,* 1–11.

Fawcett, J. (1985). A typology of nursing research activities according to educational preparation. *Journal of Professional Nursing, 1,* 75–78.

Hagle, M.E., Kirchhoff, K.T., Knafl, K.A., & Bevis, M.E. (1986). The clinical nurse researcher: New perspectives. *Journal of Professional Nursing, 2,* 282–288.

Haller, K.B. (1986). Research in clinical settings. *MCN, 11,* 290.

Hinshaw, A.S., & Smeltzer, C.H. (1987). Research challenges and programs for practice settings. *Journal of Nursing Administration, 17*(7/8), 20–26.

May, K.L., Meleis, A.I., & Winstead-Fry, P. (1982). Mentorship for scholarliness: Opportunities and dilemmas. *Nursing Outlook, 30,* 22–28.

Oberst, M.T. (1980). Nursing research: New definitions, collegial approaches. *Cancer Nursing, 3,* 459.

Smeltzer, C.H., & Hinshaw, A.S. (1988). Research: Clinical integration for excellent patient care. *Nursing Management, 19,* 38–40, 44.

Stetler, C.B. (1983). Nurses and research: Responsibility and involvement. *NITA: The Official Journal of the National Intravenous Therapy Association, 6,* 207–212.

Stetler, C.B. (1984). *Nursing research in a service setting*. Reston, VA: Reston Publishing.

✳ **EDITOR'S QUESTIONS FOR DISCUSSION** ✳

Discuss the various issues involved in providing joint appointments between universities and clinical settings for conducting research. How may roles, authority, responsibility, and accountability of the senior clinical nurse researcher be defined in both settings? Indicate strategies for negotiating shared research resources between the two types of institutions, such as financial, personnel, technological, and other support services. How can clinical nurse research joint appointments be accounted as facilitating revenue for clinical agencies as well as academic settings.?

Indicate some specific concerns that need to be addressed in developing a research-based practice, and program of research. How might research programs be evaluated? What type of research questions should be addressed that may generate solutions to concerns of nursing practice? Indicate some specific frameworks that might be used to organize research questions in terms of the needs for empirical data?

How can knowledge be developed and theory be tested from the same data that were generated for internal policy decisions of an institution? Provide specific examples of research studies that might be conducted in clinical agencies that address each of the six areas suggested by Haller. Provide specific examples of research activities that are appropriate for nurses at each level of academic preparation. How can nursing staff be involved in the implementation and evaluation of scientific studies and findings? Discuss the types of negotiations and agreements that need to take place among colleagues in conducting research as a group. Provide examples of using the ANA guidelines concerning research responsibilities of graduates from various nursing education programs as the basis for the design of curriculum. Provide specific examples on how nurses can maximize being in a medical research environment to promote their own scholarship and advance nursing research.

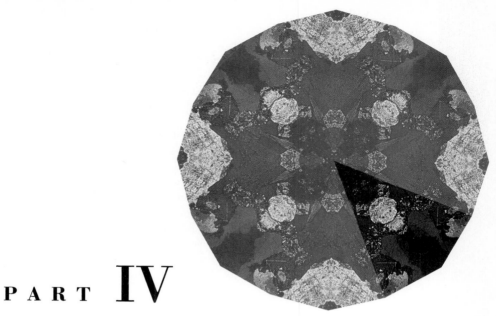

PART IV
NURSING THEORY

The numerous pieces of glass and color forming the many images in a kaleidoscope are like the many concepts propounded for specific nursing conceptual frameworks, models, and the development of nursing theory. Particles of various elements form a complete picture within the kaleidoscope much like portions of abstract thoughts and ideas spin into place for a whole view of nursing and nursing theory.

Numerous turns of the kaleidoscope cylinder show significant similarities and differences within the chapters pertaining to nursing theory. The chapters highlight the form and substance of knowledge development for nursing and professional practice.

Edna Menke in Chapter 27 critiques the development of nursing knowledge. She suggests that nurse scholars make a commitment to advance knowledge in a substantive area.

In Chapter 28 Sara Fry identifies the stages that have marked the various formulations of theory in nursing. Fry urges the maturation of a philosophy of nursing science as the base for further knowledge building within nursing.

Barbara Sarter in Chapter 29 explores a number of viewpoints regarding nursing's philosophy of science. She analyzes the emerging philosophical commitment of nursing and goes beyond the limits of previous theory.

Differentiating the light or paradigm that directs research is essential to understanding and applying research findings. In Chapter 30 Margaret Newman illumines the confusion that occurs when investigations set in one paradigm are used to test theories derived from another, or when different levels of reality are used to connote each other. She directs attention to the need for nursing to clarify its paradigm.

Violet Malinski in Chapter 31 explicates the meaning of the Rogerian perspective as a knowledge base for nursing. She explores the progressive worldview in nursing through the discussion of selected research.

The premise of Maeona Kramer in Chapter 32 is that holistic care in nursing can be facilitated by knowledge development and utilization that is more compatible with the tenets of holism. Consequently she traces the tenets and the history of holistic health. Kramer further suggests approaches for empirical knowledge development and application consistent with holism.

Jacqueline Fawcett in Chapter 33 illustrates concrete application of knowledge development for nursing. Specifically she focuses on the nursing practice implications of selected conceptual models of nursing.

The patterning of concepts and principles in this section introduces various views of people and environment for nursing science. Experiences in life as a human being and professional whisper secrets to a person for their kaleidoscope and that of the profession. The kaleidoscope of experience infuses the mind with color. Thus many unique and distinct color patterns of knowledge are formed, organized, tested, and made ready for application in nursing practice.

27

Rhetoric and Reality in the Development of Nursing Knowledge

Edna M. Menke, Ph.D., R.N.

Knowledge development is essential for the evolution of nursing science. Nursing knowledge comprises theories and facts that explore, describe, predict, and prescribe nursing practice in relationship to human responses to actual or potential health problems (American Nurses' Association, 1980; Hinshaw, 1985). Nursing knowledge should improve the care of individuals, families, and communities. Nursing is a science of the twenty-first century (Peplau, 1987; Watson, 1987). Compared with other sciences, nursing science is still in its early stages of development and will evolve only if nurse scholars continue to be knowledge seekers and develop a highly organized, cumulative, specialized field.

Nursing knowledge refers to knowledge developed for the discipline through any of the ways of knowing. Ways of knowing or pursuing truth in any discipline can be traced to early philosophers, such as Plato and Socrates. Carper (1978) identified the patterns of knowing from nursing literature as empirics, in the science of nursing; esthetics, in the art of nursing; personal knowledge; and ethics, the component of moral knowledge in nursing. All of these ways are important in developing knowledge. Ellis

(1983) argued for the importance of philosophical inquiry for the development of nursing knowledge. Belenky and her colleagues (1986) derived five epistemological perspectives of women's ways of knowing from interview data of a diverse group of female respondents. The perspectives are silence, received knowledge, subjective knowledge, procedural knowledge, and constructed knowledge. Constructed knowledge is defined as that in which women view all knowledge as contextual, experience themselves as creators of knowledge, and value both subjective and objective strategies. According to Jean Watson (1987), nurse scientists have primarily used procedural knowledge and have "bootlegged" other knowledge from different disciplines. Nurse scholars need to be involved primarily with the development and testing of constructed knowledge; however, subjective and procedural knowledge are important in advancing the development of nursing knowledge. Constructed knowledge can be developed through theory development strategies that are derived from nursing models or theories from other disciplines.

The development of nursing knowledge has supposedly come a long way in the past decade. Evidence of this growth can be seen in the quality and quantity of journal articles, chapters, and books that pertain to nursing knowledge. Other evidence is the number of theory- or knowledge-based conferences, for example, knowledge-based research conferences and state of the art conferences related to a particular area of knowledge, such as the family, care of the elderly, and health promotion.

There has been a great deal of rhetoric about the development of nursing knowledge; in reality, though, what has actually occurred? Rhetoric refers to what nurse scholars from a metatheorist perspective are saying what should be done versus what is actually occurring in knowledge development. Rhetoric refers to conveying one's knowledge through language on any given subject, in this case knowledge development in nursing. The purpose of this chapter is to address the rhetoric and reality issues in the development of nursing knowledge.

HISTORICAL DEVELOPMENT

The development of nursing knowledge can be traced to Florence Nightingale in 1859 when she theorized about nursing in her book, *Notes on Nursing* (Nightingale, 1859/1969; Johnson, 1968, 1978). Nightingale advocated the use of systematic observation to discover the laws of life and death. She provided definitions of health, disease, and nursing, as well as emphasizing the importance of environmental aspects of nursing care. Almost a hundred years elapsed before other nurse scholars developed substantive knowledge for nursing. In 1952 the journal *Nursing Research* was published. During its first few years, the majority of manuscripts pertained to nurse research activities, characteristics about nurse activities, or personality variables related to specific specialization in nursing. According to Gortner (1983), there were 10 times as many studies of nurses compared with patient care studies. Many of the manuscripts were coauthored by nurses and persons from other disciplines or written exclusively by persons from other disciplines. Nursing knowledge or nursing science was rarely mentioned in the literature until the late 1950s (Carper, 1978). The era before 1960 in nursing theory was prescientific.

The launching of the scientific era in nursing can be traced to the 1960s. Several theory conferences were held at Case Western Reserve University, the University of Kansas, and the University of Colorado (Meleis, 1985; Nicholl, 1986). At one of these conferences Dickhoff and James (1968) presented a theory-of-theories paper on the status of nurse theory. This paper was revolutionary in advocating the development of prescriptive theory for practice. Nurse scholars were quite critical of the paper, for knowledge development was essentially just beginning and some nurse scholars were attempting to develop a grand theory to guide practice and knowledge development. Obviously this was not a realistic endeavor, since none of the more established sciences have a grand theory that guides their discipline in knowledge development. The paper by Dickhoff and James (1968) resulted in heuristic discussions among the community of nurse scholars. Ellis (1968) delineated characteristics to evaluate theories. Abdellah (1968) identified a group of nurse scholars whom she considered the pioneer knowledge developers. This group included Florence Blake, Rita Chow, Lydia Hall, Virginia Henderson, Madeline Leininger, Ida Orlando, Hildegard Peplau, Reva Rubin, and Ernestine Wiedenbach. Other pioneers that should be mentioned are Dorothy Johnson, Myra Levine, Catherine Norris, and Dorothea Orem. In retrospect, the early nurse scholars laid the foundation for delineating the phenomena that should be the focus of inquiry within the discipline.

The state of knowledge evolved in the 1970s to the point at which it could be labeled scientific (Andreoli & Thompson, 1977; Menke, 1983). Emphasis was placed on how to develop theory and on the nature of knowledge that was necessary to advance the discipline. Jacox (1974) and Hardy (1973) wrote classic papers on how to develop theory and Newman (1979) wrote a book on how theory should be developed. The influence of positivism and the social sciences were evident in the approaches to theory development advocated by these authors. Practice theory was advocated for the advancement of nursing knowledge (Dickhoff & James, 1968; Jacox, 1974). Beckstrand (1978a, 1978b, 1980) took issue with the tenet that practice theory is a viable means for developing knowledge. Beckstrand argued for nurse scholars to develop scientific and philosophical knowledge (Menke, 1983). Several new nursing models were developed by King (1971), Neuman (1974), Newman (1979), Rogers (1970), Roy (1970), and Watson (1979). Some of the publications in *Nursing Research* focused on the testing and development of substantive knowledge about specific phenomena in nursing. The theory or framework used was derived from knowledge primarily in other disciplines. Two new journals, *Advances in Nursing Science* and *Research in Nursing and Health*, were established. Nurse scholars were beginning to critique what was being said about knowledge development and the substantive works written by nurses (Fawcett, 1978; Hardy, 1978; Stevens, 1979). In essence, a cadre of metatheorists emerged who were primarily faculty in graduate programs, doctoral students in nursing, and graduates of doctoral programs in nursing. A metatheorist is a person who evaluates the knowledge development in a discipline or a specific area of a discipline.

Knowledge development has continued to grow in the 1980s. Some nurse scholars and students of these scholars have refined and/or tested parts of their models or have derived theories from their models (King, 1981; Malinski, 1986; Newman, 1986; Orem, 1985; Roy, 1981, 1987; Roy & Roberts, 1981; Rogers, 1987; Watson, 1985). Some new nursing models or theories have emerged (Fitzpatrick, 1983; Parse, 1981, 1987; Parse, Coyne, & Smith, 1985). Books as well as collections of papers have been published about knowledge development in nursing, and nursing models (Fawcett, 1984a; Fitzpatrick & Whall, 1983; George, 1985; Marriner, 1986; Meleis, 1985; Nicholl, 1986; Walker & Avant, 1983; Winstead-Fry, 1986). Some new journals, *Nursing Science Quarterly* and *Scholarly Inquiry for Nursing Practice: An International Journal*, and the book, *Annual Review of Nursing* were initiated. Nurse scholars have debated the appropriateness of the philosophical perspectives underlying knowledge development, the structure of knowledge, and male dominance in approaches to knowledge development (Chinn, 1985; MacPherson, 1983; Thompson, 1985). Meleis (1987) has encouraged nurse scholars to stop focusing on the snytax and get on with the actual development of substantive knowledge for the discipline.

Nursing knowledge is being developed from the nursing models and knowledge from other disciplines. The emphasis is on knowledge for practice; however, some nurses are developing philosophical, historical, and ethical knowledge. The majority of the knowledge is being developed by doctorally prepared nurses and doctoral students who are committed to advancing the discipline. Few nurse scholars have developed knowledge in a substantive area over a period greater than 10 years. Exemplar models of this kind of knowledge development are the works of Kathryn Barnard (1980) in mother-child interaction, Jean Johnson and her colleagues (1978) on the effects of information for coping with stressful situations, Regina Lederman (1985) on psychosocial adaptation in pregnancy, and Ramona Mercer (1986) on maternal role attainment. Other nurse scholars are in the process of developing substantive knowledge, for example, in the areas of health promotion, family functioning, parenting, social support, stress and coping, family stress, health restoration, transitioning, and community competence. The majority of these scholars are using knowledge from other disciplines to develop new knowledge for nursing.

This brief historical overview of knowledge development indicates that there has been progress. The progress can be attributed to the growth in the community of nurse scholars, as well as more nurses earning doctoral degrees in nursing instead of other disciplines. These nurses have been socialized into the importance of being productive scholars. Doctoral programs in nursing have come of age in the 1980s. Faculty and students involved with doctoral programs are focusing their inquiry on phenomena that are important for the discipline. The critical issue is whether the outcome of such inquiry will be the growth of substantive knowledge that will make a difference ultimately in caring for individuals, families, and communities in promoting or restoring their health.

PARADIGMATIC INFLUENCES

The paradigmatic influences must be considered in critiquing the development of nursing knowledge. In the last decade nurse scholars have advanced the development of paradigms or world views for structuring the discipline's reality. Indicators of this progress have been the development of a metaparadigm, the conceptualization of two major paradigms, and the delineation of domains for structuring nursing knowledge (Fawcett, 1984b; Kim, 1983, 1987; Meleis, 1985, 1986; Parse, 1987; Parse, Coyne, & Smith, 1985). Person, environment, health, and nursing are the concepts that make up the metaparadigm (Fawcett, 1984b). The totality paradigm and the simultaneity paradigm are the two major paradigms (Parse, 1987). Kim (1983, 1987) has delineated the domain concepts for structuring knowledge as client, environment, client-nurse, and practice. Nurse scholars have questioned the philosophical underpinnings of nursing knowledge, and the appropriateness of the paradigms, and have made a plea to stop debating the structure and focus on the development of knowledge (Fry, 1987; Meleis, 1985, 1986, 1987; Watson, 1985).

Fawcett (1984a) proposed a metaparadigm that has been used to analyze and structure knowledge development derived from nursing models and theories. Metaparadigm refers to a statement or group of statements identifying a discipline's relevant phenomena. The metaparadigm comprises four concepts: person, environment, health, and nursing, and the three themes from the work of Donaldson and Crowley (1978). There is evidence of some support for the metaparadigm (Chinn, 1983; Fitzpatrick & Whall, 1983; Flaskerud & Halloran, 1980; Menke, 1983; Wagner, 1986). Implicit in the metaparadigm is the notion that there are existing paradigms or disciplinary matrixes that are the nursing models in the discipline. Conway (1985) has questioned the use of "nursing" as being an appropriate concept in the metaparadigm and has recommended the clarification of nursing's preparadigm in the development of the metaparadigm. Hardy (1978, 1983) has taken issue with the metaparadigm, contending that nursing is at a preparadigm stage in its development. Brodie (1984) has contended that nursing knowledge has not advanced to where a metaparadigm can exist. Ramos (1987) has used Toulmin's work (1972) to advocate not having a metaparadigm, which will bring premature closure to the discipline.

The nursing models developed by nurse scholars are examples of some of the disciplinary matrixes that need to be considered in evaluating the progress that has been made in the development of nursing knowledge. The purpose of the nursing models was to guide practice and develop knowledge for the discipline. Nightingale (1859/1969) developed the first nursing model. Some other early nursing models were those developed by Henderson (1964, 1966), Levine (1969), Orlando (1961), Peplau (1952), and Wiedenbach (1964). Contemporary nursing models include the works of King (1971, 1981), Leininger (1976), Neuman (1974), Newman (1979, 1986), Orem (1971, 1985), Parse (1981), Rogers (1970, 1987), Roy (1970, 1981, 1987), and Watson (1979). Some of these nursing models have been used to derive nursing theories (King, 1981, 1987; Malinski, 1986; Parse, Coyne, & Smith, 1985; Parse, 1987; Roy & Roberts, 1981); however, there are skeptics who view these models as ideologies that are untestable (Avant, 1988; Stevenson & Woods, 1986). Others contend that the nursing models need to be used to derive nursing knowledge for the advancement of nursing science (Menke, 1983; Parse, 1987). In Loomis's study (1985) of dissertations, she found that the majority of nurse scholars focused on phenomena related to clinical practice, but few used one of the nursing models. Silva (1987) found that little inquiry had been done that tested aspects of the nursing models and the inquiry that had been done had major methodological problems.

Parse, Coyne, and Smith (1985) delineated the man-environment totality paradigm and the man-environment simultaneity paradigm as being the two major paradigms for the discipline. According to Parse (1987) the totality paradigm predominates in nursing. Historically, the totality paradigm is rooted in Nightingale's conceptualization of nursing. The paradigm can be characterized as being behavioristic or mechanistic and being related to medical science. In the totality paradigm, man is

> a total, summative organism whose nature is a combination of bio-psycho-social-spiritual features. This worldview specifies the environment as the internal and external stimuli surrounding man. Man adapts and interacts with the environment to maintain balance and achieve goals (Parse, 1987, p. 4).

Health is a dynamic state and the process of physical, psychological, social, and spiritual well-being. The models or theories of King (1981), Orem (1985), and Roy (1987) are examples of the totality paradigm. Quantitative research methods are generally used in studying phenomena from the totality paradigm.

The simultaneity paradigm can be traced to Rogers's unitary human being model (Parse, 1987). In this paradigm, man is viewed as a unitary being who is more than and different from the sum of his parts and is in continuous mutual interrelationship with the environment. Health is a process of becoming, a set of value priorities, and how an individual is experience personal living. In addition to Rogers's model, Parse's "man-living-health theory" (1981) is an example of the simultaneity paradigm. Qualitative methods are generally used to study phenomena from the simultaneity paradigm.

Few nurse scholars have expressed support or rejection of the two paradigms. Peplau (1987) has contended that for the first time in nursing there are two paradigms, which should influence knowledge development. It is too early to ascertain the impact of the two paradigms on the advancement of nursing knowledge.

Kim (1983, 1987) and Meleis (1985, 1986, 1987) have emphasized the importance of delineating domains for knowledge development. A *domain* is a broad concept that can be used to categorize subconcepts and allows for revisions and discovery of the domain. Kim (1987) has advocated four domains that can be used to categorize the essential concepts in nursing. The domains are client, environment, client-nurse, and practice. According to Kim, all knowledge developed in the domains must ultimately relate to client care if nurses are truly developing nursing knowledge. Meleis (1986) has identified the domain concepts as client, environment, interaction, nursing process, transitions, and nursing therapeutics. Meleis has advocated the use of multiple theories and methods to develop knowledge about these domain concepts. In addition, nurse scholars should assume accountability for focusing their inquiry on the domain concepts.

Positivism has been the dominant philosophy-of-science influence on the development of nursing knowledge. Positivism, which is based on formal logic, operationalism, and mathematics, was the dominant philosophy of science from 1920 to 1960 (Suppe & Jacox, 1985). Most nurse scholars who earned their doctorates in nurse scientist programs or other disciplines were socialized into positivism as being the way to develop science. The appropriateness of positivism as a philosophical orientation has been questioned as more nurse scholars have studied philosophy and are cognizant of this perspective's being considered obsolete by philosophers. Likewise, some nurse scholars have rejected positivism and advocate historicist or humanist philosophical perspectives as being appropriate to develop knowledge about the humanistic phenomena of nursing (Munhall & Oiler, 1986; Parse, 1987; Thompson, 1985; Watson, 1985). Evidence of positivism is strong in the nursing theory and research literature (Fawcett & Downs, 1986; Walker & Avant, 1983).

Kuhn's work (1970, 1977) with paradigms and the progress of science through revolution has had a major influence on the development of nursing knowledge. Kuhn's work is based on a natural science model. Even though Kuhn is a historist, his work has been attacked by other philosophers (Laudan, 1977, 1984; Toulmin, 1972) and some nurse scholars (DeGrout, 1988; Ramos, 1987). Laudan (1984) has made a case for knowledge not being developed through revolution but by evolution. Fry (1987) has thought that Laudan's work offers a view of scientific rationality that can be used in developing the philosophy of nursing science. Laudan has provided a method by which scientific change within nursing can be assessed. Ramos (1987) has taken issue with Kuhn as being inappropriate for nursing science on the basis that his conceptualizations of paradigms have no explanatory power. Striving for consensus on which philosophical perspective should be used in nursing is unrealistic. Each philosophical perspective has a place in the discipline. Nurse scholars need to be cognizant of which philosophical perspective they are using in their inquiry. Some nurse scholars should be involved in developing the philosophy of nursing science.

FACILITATION OF KNOWLEDGE DEVELOPMENT

The development of systematic knowledge should be a priority in planning the discipline's future (Schlotfeldt, 1988). A tapestry must be woven that provides patterns for knowledge that will ultimately influence the practice of nursing. This tapestry could be developed by using the metaparadigm or the domains delineated by Kim (1987) or Meleis (1987). Whichever approach is used, the knowledge could be developed from the nursing models or substantive knowledge that has been developed by nurse scholars or scholars in other disciplines.

Young faculty members and doctoral students need to be enculturated early to the importance of having a systematic program for the development of and contribution to nursing knowledge in a substantive area. These students should work collaboratively with other scholars, ideally mentors, in building knowledge. Deans and other seasoned nurse scholars need to develop methods to work with doctorally prepared nurses who are not committed to knowledge development for the discipline. These efforts may help these nurses to become productive scholars. Faculty should develop focused inquiry programs that involve collaborative work with students and faculty. In addition, collaboration with faculty and students from other disciplines can facilitate knowledge development. Collaboration might be done with nurse scholars at other academic or health care settings.

Nurse scholars must use a variety of approaches in developing knowledge. This means that qualitative or qualitative methods might be used. No longer can nurse scholars afford to debate which method results in "good" science. Rather, the emphasis should be on the method that is appropriate for the type of inquiry. All kinds of inquiry are necessary to form a knowledge base for the discipline of nursing. Nurse scholars have the opportunity to advance knowledge development so that nursing is truly the science of the twenty-first century.

REFERENCES

Abdellah, F. G. (1968). The nature of nursing science. *Nursing Research, 18,* 390–393.

American Nurses' Association (ANA). (1980). *Nursing: A social policy statement.* Kansas City, MO: Author.

Andreoli, K. G., & Thompson, C. E. (1977). The nature of science in nursing. *Image, 9,* 32–37.

Avant, K. C. (1988). [Review of *"Case Studies in Nursing Theory" by P. Winstead-Fry]. Image, 20,* 55.

Barnard, K. E. (1980). *Nursing child assessment satellite training instructor's manual.* Seattle: University of Washington.

Beckstrand, J. (1978a). The notion of practice theory and the relationship of science and ethical knowledge to practice. *Research in Nursing and Health, 1,* 131–136.

Beckstrand, J. (1978b). The need for a practice theory as indicated by the knowledge used in the conduct of practice. *Research in Nursing and Health, 1,* 175–179.

Beckstrand, J. (1980). A critique of several conceptions of practice theory in nursing. *Research in Nursing and Health, 3,* 69–80.

Belenky, M. F., Clinchy, B. M., & Tarule, J. M. (1986). *Women's ways of knowing.* New York: Basic Books.

Brodie, J. N. (1984). [A response to Dr. J. Fawcett's paper—"The metaparadigm of nursing: Present status and future refinements."] *Image, 16,* 87–89.

Carper, B. A. (1978). Practice oriented theory. Part I: Fundamental patterns of knowing in nursing. *Advances in Nursing Science, 1,* 13–23.

Chinn, P. L. (1983). Nursing theory development: Where we have been and where we are going. In N. L. Chaska (Ed.), *The nursing profession: A time to speak* (pp. 394–405). New York: McGraw-Hill.

Chinn, P. L. (1985). Debunking myths in nursing theory and research. *Image, 17,* 45–49.

Conway, M. E. (1985). Toward greater specificity in defining nursing's metaparadigm. *Advances in Nursing Science, 7,* 73–82.

DeGrout, H. A. (1988). Scientific inquiry in nursing: A model for a new age. *Advances in Nursing Science, 10,* 1–21.

Dickhoff, J., & James, P. (1968). Theories of theories. *Nursing Research, 17,* 197–206.

Donaldson, S. K., & Crowley, D. M. (1978). The discipline of nursing. *Nursing Outlook, 26,* 113–120.

Ellis, R. (1968). Characteristics of significant theories. *Nursing Research, 17,* 217–333.

Ellis, R. (1983). Philosophic inquiry. In H. H. Werley & J. J. Fitzpatrick (Eds.), *Annual Review of Nursing Research, Vol. 1* (pp. 211–228). New York: Springer Publishing.

Fawcett, J. (1978). The relationship between theory and research: A double helix. *Advances in Nursing Science, 1,* 49–62.

Fawcett, J. (1984a). *Analysis and evaluation of conceptual models of nursing*. Philadelphia: F. A. Davis.

Fawcett, J. (1984b). The metaparadigm of nursing: Present status and future refinements. *Image, 16*, 84–87.

Fawcett, J., & Downs, F. (1986). *The relationship between theory and research*. Norwalk, CT: Appleton-Century-Crofts.

Fitzpatrick, J. J. (1983). The life's perspective model. In J. J. Fitzpatrick & A. L. Whall (Eds.), *Conceptual models of nursing: Analysis and application* (pp. 303–322). Bowie, MD: R. J. Brady.

Fitzpatrick, J. J., & Whall, A. L. (1983). *Conceptual models of nursing: Analysis and application*. Bowie, MD: R. J. Brady.

Flaskerud, J. H., & Halloran, E. I. (1980). Areas of agreement in nursing theory development. *Advances in Nursing Science, 3*, 1–7.

Fry, S. A. (1987, March). *Pragmatism, the aims of science, and nursing science*. Paper presented at the Fourth Annual Nursing Science Colloquium, Boston University, Boston, MA.

George, J. B. (Ed.) (1985). *Nursing theories: The base for professional nursing practice* (2nd ed.). Englewood Cliffs, NJ: Prentice-Hall.

Gortner, S. R. (1983). The history and philosophy of nursing science and research. *Advances in Nursing Science, 6*, 1–8.

Hardy, M. E. (1973). Theories: Components, development, evaluation. *Nursing Research, 23*, 100–107.

Hardy, M. E. (1978). Perspectives on nursing theory. *Advances in Nursing Science, 1*, 37–48.

Hardy, M. E. (1983). Metaparadigms and theory development. In N. L. Chaska (Ed.), *The nursing profession: A time to speak* (pp. 427–437). New York: McGraw-Hill.

Henderson, V. (1964). The nature of nursing. *American Journal of Nursing, 64*, 62–68.

Henderson, V. (1966). *The nature of nursing: A definition and its implications for practice, research and education*. New York: Macmillan.

Hinshaw, A. S. (1985, March). *Nursing science: Perspectives on theory*. Paper presented at the Second Annual Nursing Science Colloquium, Boston University, Boston, MA.

Jacox, A. (1974). Theory construction in nursing. *Nursing Research, 23*, 4–13.

Johnson, D. E. (1968, April). *One conceptual model of nursing*. Paper presented at Vanderbilt University, Nashville, TN.

Johnson, D. E. (1978). State of the art of theory development. In *Theory Development: What, why, how*. New York: National League for Nursing.

Johnson, J. E., Rice, V. H., Fuller, S. S., & Endress, M. P. (1978). Sensory information, instruction in a coping strategy, and recovery from surgery. *Research in Nursing and Health, 1*, 4–17.

Kim, H. S. (1983). *The nature of theoretical thinking in nursing*. Norwalk, CT: Appleton-Century-Crofts.

Kim, H. S. (1987). Structuring the nursing knowledge system: A typology of four domains. *Scholarly Inquiry for Nursing Practice: An International Journal, 1*, 99–110.

King, I. M. (1971). *Toward a theory of nursing*. New York: John Wiley & Sons.

King, I. M. (1981). *A theory for nursing: Systems, concepts, process*. New York: John Wiley & Sons.

King, I. M. (1987). King's theory of goal attainment. In R. R. Parse (Ed.), *Nursing science: Major paradigms, theories, and critiques* (pp. 107–114). Philadelphia: W. B. Saunders.

Kuhn, T. S. (1970). *The structure of scientific revolutions* (2nd ed.). Chicago: University of Chicago Press.

Kuhn, T. S. (1977). *The essential tension*. Chicago: University of Chicago Press.

Laudan, L. (1977). *Progress and its problems*. Berkeley: University of California Press.

Laudan, L. (1984). *Science and values*. Berkeley: University of California Press.

Lederman, R. P. (1985). *Psychosocial adaptation in pregnancy: Assessment of seven dimensions of maternal development*. Englewood Cliffs, NJ: Prentice-Hall.

Leininger, M. (1976). *Transcultural nursing: Concepts, theories, and practices*. New York: John Wiley & Sons.

Levine, M. E. (1969). *Introduction to clinical nursing*. Philadelphia: F. A. Davis.

Loomis, M. E. (1985). Emerging nursing knowledge. In J. C. McClosky & H. K. Grace (Eds.), *Current issues in nursing* (2nd ed.) (pp. 171–181). Boston: Blackwell Scientific Publications.

MacPherson, K. I. (1983). Feminist methods: A new paradigm for nursing research. *Advances in Nursing Science, 6*, 17–25.

Malinski, V. M. (Ed.). (1986). *Explorations on Martha Rogers' science of unitary human beings*. Norwalk, CT: Appleton-Century-Crofts.

Marriner, A. (1986). *Nursing theorists and their work*. St. Louis: C. V. Mosby.

Meleis, A. I. (1985). *Theoretical nursing: Development and progress*. Philadelphia: J. B. Lippincott.

Meleis, A. I. (1986). Theory development and domain concepts. In P. Moccia (Ed.), *New approaches to theory development* (pp. 3–22). New York: National League for Nursing.

Meleis, A. I. (1987). Revisions in knowledge development: A passion for substance. *Scholarly Inquiry for Nursing Practice: An International Journal, 1,* 5–19.

Menke, E. M. (1983). Critical analysis of theory development in nursing. In N. L. Chaska (Ed.), *The nursing profession: A time to speak* (pp. 416–426). New York: McGraw-Hill.

Mercer, R. T. (1986). *First-time motherhood.* New York: Springer-Verlag.

Munhall, P. L., & Oiler, C. J. (1986). *Nursing research: A qualitative perspective.* Norwalk, CT: Appleton-Century-Crofts.

Neuman, B. (1974). The Betty Neuman health care systems model: A total person approach to patient problems. In J. P. Riehl & C. Roy (Eds.), *Conceptual models for nursing practice* (2nd ed., pp. 119–134). New York: Appleton-Century-Crofts.

Newman, M. A. (1979). *Theory development in nursing.* Philadelphia: F. A. Davis.

Newman, M. A. (1986). *Health as expanding consciousness.* St. Louis: C. V. Mosby.

Nicholl, L. H. (Ed.) (1986). *Perspectives on nursing theory.* Boston: Little, Brown.

Nightingale, F. (1969). *Notes on nursing.* New York: Dover. (Original work published 1859)

Orem, D. E. (1971). *Nursing: Concepts of practice.* New York: McGraw-Hill.

Orem, D. E. (1985). *Nursing: Concepts of practice* (3rd ed.). New York: McGraw-Hill.

Orlando, I. J. (1961). *The dynamic nurse-patient relationship.* New York: G. P. Putnam.

Parse, R. R. (1981). *Man-living-health: A theory for nursing.* New York: John Wiley & Sons.

Parse R. R. (1987). *Nursing science: Major paradigms, theories, and critiques.* Philadelphia: W. B. Saunders.

Parse, R. R., Coyne, A. B., & Smith, M. J. (1985). *Nursing research: Qualitative methods.* Bowie, MD: J. Brady.

Peplau, H. E. (1952). *Interpersonal relations in nursing.* New York: G. P. Putnam.

Peplau, H. E. (1987). Nursing science: A historical perspective. In R. R. Parse (Ed.), *Nursing science: Major paradigms, theories, and critiques* (pp. 13–34). Philadelphia: W. B. Saunders.

Ramos, M. C. (1987). Adopting an evolutionary lens: An optimistic approach to discovering strength in nursing. *Advances in Nursing Science, 10,* 19–26.

Rogers, M. E. (1970). *An introduction to the theoretical basis of nursing.* Philadelphia: F. A. Davis.

Rogers, M. E. (1987). Rogers' science of unitary human beings. In R. R. Parse (Ed.), *Nursing science: Major paradigms, theories, and critiques* (pp. 139–146). Philadelphia: W. B. Saunders.

Roy, C. (1970). Adaptation: A conceptual framework in nursing. *Nursing Outlook, 18,* 42–45.

Roy, C. (1981). *Introduction to nursing: An adaptation model.* Englewood Cliffs, NJ: Prentice-Hall.

Roy, C. (1987). Roy's adpatation model. In R. R. Parse (Ed.), *Nursing science: Major paradigms, theories, and critiques* (pp. 35–46). Philadelphia: W. B. Saunders.

Roy, C., & Roberts, S. (1981). *Theory construction in nursing: An adaptation model.* Englewood Cliffs, NJ: Prentice-Hall.

Schlotfeldt, R. M. (1988). Structuring nursing knowledge: A priority for creating nursing's future. *Nursing Science Quarterly, 1,* 35–38.

Silva, M. C. (1987). Conceptual models of nursing. In J. J. Fitzpatrick & R. L. Taunton (Eds.), *Annual review of nursing research, Vol. 5* (pp. 229–246). New York: Springer Publishing.

Stevens, B. J. (1979). *Nursing theory: Analysis, application, evaluation.* Boston: Little, Brown.

Stevenson, J. S., & Woods, N. F. (1986). Nursing science and contemporary science: Emerging paradigms. In G. Sorenson (Ed.), *Setting the agenda for the year 2000: Knowledge development in nursing* (pp. 6–20). Kansas City: American Academy of Nursing.

Suppe, F., & Jacox, A. K. (1985). Philosophy of science and the development of nursing theory. In H. H. Werley & J. J. Fitzpatrick (Eds.), *Annual review of nursing research, Vol. 3* (pp. 241–267). New York: Springer Publishing.

Thompson, J. L. (1985). Practical discourse in nursing: Going beyond empiricism and historicism. *Advances in Nursing Science, 7,* 59–71.

Toulmin, S. (1972). *Human understanding (Vol. 1).* Princeton, NJ: Princeton University Press.

Wagner, J. D. (1986). *Nurse scholars' perceptions of the nursing metaparadigm.* Unpublished doctoral dissertation, Ohio State University, Columbus, OH.

Walker, L. O., & Avant, K. C. (1983). *Strategies for theory construction in nursing.* Norwalk, CT: Appleton-Century-Crofts.

Watson, J. (1979). *Nursing: The philosophy and science of caring.* Boston: Little, Brown.

Watson, J. (1985). *Nursing: Human science and human care.* Norwalk, CT: Appleton-Century-Crofts.

Watson, J. (1987, May). *The science of caring*. Paper presented at the Nurse Theorist Conference Discovery International, Pittsburgh, PA.

Wiedenbach, E. (1964). *Clinical nursing: A helping art*. New York: Springer Publishing.

Winstead-Fry, P. (Ed.). (1986). *Case studies in nursing theory*. New York: National League for Nursing.

✳ EDITOR'S QUESTIONS FOR DISCUSSION ✳

What is the purpose of a philosophy of science in relation to developing knowledge for nursing? What philosophy of science perspectives are influencing the development of nursing knowledge? What do you believe is the most appropriate philosophical perspective to develop knowledge about the humanistic phenomena of nursing? What is the difference between developing a philosophy of nursing science and developing systematic knowledge of nursing or for nursing? Discuss the extent that there are kinds of metaphysical commitments held on the part of nurse scholars, rather than actual paradigms. Are concepts things in and of themselves rather than things that derive their meaning from the theoretical framework in which they are imbedded? How appropriate is it to try to impose consensus definitions concerning concepts? Does not a consensus definition of concepts limit the development of nursing knowledge?

How appropriate is holistic practice and applying the principles of holism for developing theory and science? How can a scientist study nursing phenomena that are empirically relevant without distorting the phenomena? What nursing phenomena are relevant for the development of nursing knowledge and science? To what extent is positivism more concerned with methodology than the phenomena being studied? Indicate examples of areas for substantive knowledge development in nursing. How might substantive knowledge development make a difference in caring for individuals, families, and communities in promoting or restoring their health? Why have nurse scholars not as yet sufficiently used the two paradigms of totality and simultaneity to influence knowledge development?

28

The Development of Nursing Science:
Theoretical and philosophical issues

Sara T. Fry, Ph.D., R.N.

OVERVIEW OF ISSUES

The development of nursing science has been identified as having many stages (Meleis, 1985). Crucial to this development has been the drive to develop nursing theory and the attempt to do metatheory or theorizing about the logical and methodological foundations of nursing knowledge.

The drive to develop nursing theory has been marked by nursing theory conferences (Dickoff & James, 1968; Dickoff, James, & Wiedenbach, 1968a, 1968b; Norris, 1969, 1970), the proliferation of theoretical and conceptual frameworks for nursing (Johnson, 1980; King, 1981; Neuman, 1982; Newman, 1979; Orem, 1980; Parse, 1981; Rogers, 1970, 1980; Roy, 1981), and the formal teaching of theory development in graduate education in nursing (Murphy, 1985). The attempt to do metatheory in nursing has been marked by the development of many schemata for the analysis and evaluation of theory (Chinn & Jacobs, 1987; Ellis, 1968; Fawcett, 1984; Fitzpatrick & Whall, 1983; Stevens, 1984); a fascination with the philosophy of science (Fawcett, 1978, 1984; Meleis, 1985; Suppe & Jacox, 1985); and confusion among theory development strategies, metatheory, and choice of quanti-

tative versus qualitative research methodologies (Silva & Rothbart, 1984; Thompson, 1985).

Throughout these developments, a number of theoretical and philosophical issues have arisen. This article analyzes the prominent issues in a dialectical fashion (Hegel, 1929). By positing the thesis and the antithesis of each issue, it is hoped that a synthesis of issues will mark the next stage of nursing's theoretical development into the 21st century.

THEORETICAL ISSUES

Discussions about nursing theorizing have a tendency to be hampered by covert, unresolved issues about the nature of theory. Theorists and metatheorists in nursing often have different ideas about the nature of theory but these ideas are not usually subjected to critical analyses. The result is a number of issues about nursing theorizing that can best be called "theoretical issues" because they all seem to hinge on how we view nursing theory. These issues are analyzed under the following headings: (a) borrowed versus unique nursing theory, (b) closed versus open-ended nursing theory, (c) structured versus unstructured nursing theory, (d) monistic versus pluralistic nursing theory, and (e) revolutionary versus evolutionary theory development.

Borrowed Versus Unique Nursing Theory

A primary issue in discussions of nursing theorizing is the issue of whether theory should be unique to nursing or borrowed from other disciplines. Early attempts to argue for unique nursing theory took the form of supporting practice theory as a conceptual framework for ultimately creating change in a nursing client or nursing situations (Dickoff, James, & Wiedenbach, 1968a; Jacox, 1974; Wald & Leonard, 1964). Levels of theory were proposed that inevitably led to situation-producing or prescriptive theories in order to produce change, in which change was viewed as the desirable outcome of nursing theorizing and nursing actions. Situation-producing theory, according to Dickoff and James (1968), is the highest level of theory. It is prescriptive in that it supplies directives for carrying out activities that will, in fact, produce desired situations. Theorizing is not simply an academic or even a scientific enterprise; the purpose of theorizing in nursing is to produce change in the patient or nursing situations as effected by the nurse.

A basic premise of this type of theory is the notion that nurses should develop theories that are grounded in the discipline of nursing and that guide the actions of the discipline. The ultimate goal is prescriptive theory that stresses justification rather than discovery. A second premise is that any theory that evolves out of the practice arena of nursing is substantially nursing. Although one might borrow theory and apply it to the realm of nursing actions, it is transformed to nursing theory because it addresses phenomena within the arena of nursing practice. Thus practice theory is ultimately unique to nursing. The goal of nursing theorizing should be the development of practice theories since these will, of necessity, reflect the values and standards of nursing and be the types of theories ultimately capable of producing change in the patient.

The notion of a unique theory *of* nursing is usually juxtaposed to the notion of a borrowed theory *in* nursing. Advocates of borrowed theory argue that nursing is an applied science and, as such, depends on the theories of other disciplines for its theoretical foundations. Beckstrand (1978a, 1978b, 1980), for example, persuasively argued that the practical knowledge used in nursing is not different from the knowledge of science or ethics. By examining selected aspects of practical knowledge in nursing (the knowledge of how to control, how to make change, and what is good), she established a case for debunking practice theory as unique to nursing. The result was the replacement of practice theory with scientific theory and moral theory; in other words, borrowed theory.

Other theorists in nursing have supported the borrowed theory notion by advocating systems theories of nursing (King, 1981; Neuman, 1982), humanistic theories of nursing (Parse, 1981; Paterson & Zderad, 1976; Watson, 1985), and adaptation theories of nursing (Roy, 1981). According to Johnson (1968), borrowed theory is "that knowledge which is developed in the main by other disciplines and is drawn upon by nursing" (p. 206). However, it gains a new perspective when it is applied to the realm of nursing practice or the phenomena of nursing concern. Does this mean that it is truly "borrowed"? According to some scholars, the notion of "borrowed theory" is a fallacy since no one ever owns knowledge. If knowledge is never the exclusive ownership of any one discipline, then the use of knowledge generated by any discipline is not truly "borrowed." It is simply used and applied to describe, explain, and predict phenomena significant to the scope of inquiry or the practice of the discipline.

This seems to be the view that is currently favored by many nurse theorists and scholars in nursing. It is the nursing perspective that guides the conceptualization of theories. It is also the synthesis of extant theories with the nursing perspective that allows theorizing to be truly unique to nursing problems. While theory itself is not unique, the phenomena of nursing concern tend to support the unique use of theory within the realm of nursing concern. They may even give rise to the generation of knowledge that has application beyond the realm of nursing practice and that can be used by theorists in other disciplines. Knowledge so generated might be useful to other disciplines in which the application of theory to human events is concerned, although the theories themselves might describe, explain, and predict phenomena specific to the domain of nursing.

Closed Versus Open-Ended Theorizing

Some nurse scholars writing about nursing theorizing have tended to view the nature of theory in terms of closed theory; that is, theory in which theoretical meanings are defined in terms of observational language and no theoretical meanings are relevant apart from observational language (Ellis, 1968; Hardy, 1974; Jacox, 1974; McKay, 1969). As noted by leading philosophers of science, the language of science before the 1960s was typically viewed as having its own descriptive vocabulary (Suppe, 1982). Theory contained (a) an observation vocabulary that described what could be directly observed, and (b) a theoretical vocabulary that related to the observation vocabulary. In other words, the nature of theory was such that the only theoretical terms permitted in a theory were those terms whose meanings were explicitly defined in terms of the observation vocabulary.

Philosophers of science who held this view of theorizing were logical positivists and supported a philosophical school of thought based on empiricism and the German antimetaphysical movement after Hegel (Suppe, 1977). Later on, this trend within the philosophy of science was dubbed "The Received View on Theories (RV)" (Putnam, 1962; Suppe, 1977). RV thinking was the basis of most of the analysis and evaluation of theory within sociology, psychology, and education before the 1960s and had a very strong influence on nursing theorizing through the 1970s (Ellis, 1968; Hardy, 1974; Jacox, 1974; McKay, 1969). The most unfortunate aspect of this influence is that it continued in nursing long after the highly restrictive methodology of RV concerning the nature of theory fell out of favor within the philosophy of science and long after it was abandoned by other disciplines. The result is that nursing metatheory suffers from an impoverished methodology and has led to scientific studies that are likewise theoretically impoverished (Suppe, 1982; Webster, Jacox, & Baldwin, 1981).

Other efforts in nursing theorizing, however, have contained views that have not been "the dogmatic regurgitation of out-dated, discredited, or even currently fashionable positions with philosophy of science" (Suppe, 1982, p. 11). This is open-ended theorizing that is sensitive to the advantages of nonclosure on methodological issues in theorizing. It allows for a coexistence of different views toward nursing knowledge development and a pluralism among nursing theories and conceptual frameworks (Cull-Wilby & Pepin, 1987; Walker, 1983). It also allows for growth of information as derived from practice and from new perspectives on the phenomena of nursing concern (Visintainer, 1986).

Structured Versus Unstructured Theory

The issue of structure versus nonstructure in nursing's theorizing is not widely discussed. Nursing has assumed that theory must have structure and that this structure should resemble the structure of scientific theories. Again, this means that theoretical terms and their relationships should be explicitly linked to the observation terms of a theory, which refer, in turn, to empirically observable entities. It also means that there can be no theoretical terms without observation language, and vice versa. Unstructured theorizing, on the other hand, allows for both theoretical and observation terminology with no identifiable links to other terms or to empirically verifiable entities. It also does not presume predetermined categories of disciplinary knowledge reflected in theory.

Nursing assumptions about the structure of theory are readily evident in most of the early writings about nursing theorizing in the literature (Donaldson & Crowley, 1977, 1978; McKay, 1977) and persist in contemporary views of nursing knowledge development (Levine, 1988; Schlotfeldt, 1988). Building on the ideas of Schwab (1964a, 1964b) and others (Phenix, 1964; Robey, 1973) McKay (1977) urged nursing to develop conceptual and syntactical structures by which nursing truth would be ascertained and verified. Both structures would presumably identify the discipline of nursing *as nursing* and set the stage for articulation of the nursing perspective. In a similar vein, Schlotfeldt recently argued that "one of the highest priorities for creating an appropriate future for nursing is that of identifying, *structuring* [italics added for emphasis], and continuously advancing the knowledge that underlies the practices of professionals in the field" (1988, p. 35). Both of these examples assume an unexplicated store of knowledge about nursing that awaits discovery, identification, and structuring before it can be used in nursing theorizing.

The structuring of the subject matter of nursing has been consistently emphasized throughout nursing's history. It persists in the nursing diagnosis movement, whereby nursing knowledge of the patient is structured into categories and forms of language that seemingly tell us something about the patient. A fundamental goal of this movement is to construct nursing theory that incorporates the categories of knowledge created and that uses the forms of language so described (Kritek, 1978). Such knowledge is nursing knowledge when it is articulated in the particular language framework called "nursing diagnoses." The nursing diagnosis form of language is believed to be an accurate reflection (or image) of the actual status of the patient and becomes foundational to theorizing about the patient's health status.

The most interesting aspect of the structure-of-the-discipline approach in nursing is the mistaken belief that the "real" structure of nursing has been preordained and is simply waiting for nurse scholars to discover it and present it to the members of the discipline (Donaldson & Crowley, 1977). It is presumed to be already "out there" and waiting to be explicated. Once it is explicated, unique nursing theorizing will result because such theorizing will then be done within the explicated structure. Explicating the substantive structure (conceptualizations) of nursing will tell us the scope and subject of nursing inquiry; explicating the syntactical structure (research methodologies and truth criteria) will tell us how to proceed in our research efforts.

It is interesting that many other disciplines have already abandoned this need to structure the knowl-

edge of their disciplines. Indeed, contemporary scholars in other disciplines are moving toward the "deconstruction" of inquiry and are dismantling the structures of knowledge that, according to them, have constrained and confined the limits of human inquiry within their respective disciplines (Culler, 1982; Norris, 1985). They are moving toward recognition of the social construction and justification of knowledge and are, in some cases, adopting a "historicist" approach to inquiry (Bernstein, 1983). Nursing might consider whether or not these latter approaches have implications for the development of nursing knowledge. Nurse scholars might also want to assess critically the advantages (and disadvantages) of theorizing according to the presumed need to structure nursing knowledge in identifiable forms and categories.

Monistic Versus Pluralistic Theorizing

One of the central issues in discussions of nursing theorizing has been the issue of whether nursing needs a single theory or whether the discipline can support several theories of nursing. While some theorists have advocated a single, grand theory for nursing (Rogers, 1970), others have urged the proliferation of many theories as appropriate to nursing's present stage of theory and knowledge development (Meleis, 1985, 1987a, 1987b). This seems to be the consensus of most scholars in nursing, at the present time; pluralism is desired and encouraged.

However, there is some indication that grand theories are enjoying a revival in other disciplines (Skinner, 1985). Across the human sciences, for example, an interest in large-scale, normative systems of thought is beginning to appear in legal, political, moral, and social theorizing (Dworkin, 1977; Gadamer, 1975; Habermas, 1971; Parfit, 1984; Rawls, 1971). The goal seems to be that of constructing a systematic theory of the nature of man and society. Central to all of these attempts is the idea of a framework that gives meaning and significance to individual phenomena and that guides understanding and action. Nursing might want to remain open to the emergence of a grand theory of nursing. Indeed, some contemporary nurse theorists (Kritek, 1978) are already wondering whether the nursing diagnosis movement might produce nursing's "grand theory" in the not-too-distant future.

Revolutionary Versus Evolutionary Theory Change for Nursing

In debating how to consider and conceptualize change in nursing theorizing, nurse scholars have often appealed to the work of Kuhn (1970) and his notion of scientific revolutions. Scientific change, he claimed, follows a period of crisis involving the appearance of many anomalies that cannot be explained by presently accepted theories. As theories compete to explain the anomalies, the crisis is resolved when one theory triumphs over all other theories. A new period of science is then initiated when a paradigm or disciplinary matrix is accepted and recognized by the members of the science. A period of normal science follows within this research paradigm. The entire transition from the time of crisis to the period of normal science marks the scientific revolution. Knowledge develops within the discipline by the recognition of one paradigm over others (Kuhn, 1970).

This idea has been very popular in writings about nursing theorizing. Nursing themes are described in Kuhnian terms such as "paradigms" or "metaparadigms" (Fawcett, 1984); nursing science is described as "preparadigmatic" (Hardy, 1978); and at least one contemporary nursing scholar has written about the shared "exemplars" of expert nurse practitioners (Benner, 1984). Yet the views of Kuhn have been sharply criticized by philosophers of science and others during the last 15 years. Why does this notion of revolutionary change continue to remain so attractive to nursing?

There is strong reason to believe that a revolutionary view of scientific change is not consistent with the experience of scientific theorizing during the past decade. For these reasons, a few nurse scholars (Meleis, 1985; Ramos, 1987) have looked toward an evolutionary model of scientific change as an explanatory model for nursing theorizing. Evolutionary theory views change as something that occurs over time. Building on the evolution theory of Dar-

win, Toulmin (1972) formulated an impressive account of knowledge development in the sciences, which assumed a cumulative pattern rather than a convergent one, as claimed by Kuhn (1970).

Unfortunately, it is not clear that nursing's scientific development is any more evolutionary than it is revolutionary. There simply does not seem to be evidence that nursing theorizing is following the pattern of the cumulative model described by Toulmin (Meleis, 1985). Furthermore, it is not certain that a cumulative model of scientific change is even desirable for a science such as nursing. If this is the case, what other means are there to describe and explain the nature of scientific change within the discipline of nursing?

NEW DIRECTIONS FOR NURSING SCIENCE: BEYOND THEORY AND METATHEORY

In a critique of Kuhn and his account of scientific revolutions, Laudan (1984) has attempted to expose the major flaws of the Kuhnian model of scientific change and provide a plausible account of theorizing. He states unequivocally that it is time to acknowledge that Kuhn's *Structure of Scientific Revolutions* ought no longer be regarded as a credible account of scientific change. Kuhn's account is simply not the best or even the latest word on scientific rationality. This is the assumption behind Laudan's seminal work, *Progress and its Problems* (1977). Laudan's account of scientific progress and his formulation of research traditions is thus an alternative to the Kuhnian model of scientific revolutions.

The Aims of Science

For Laudan (1984), scientific change occurs in an evolutionary manner. However, the aim of science is not to establish truth about the world as we know it but simply to solve problems (Laudan, 1977). Implicitly adopting the pragmatic notion of practical outcomes (problem-solving effectiveness), Laudan proposes a view of scientific rationality that is both refreshing and exciting in terms of contemporary discussions on nursing theorizing and the philosophy of nursing science.

Laudan's point is that if scientific progress consists in a series of theories that represent an ever closer approximation to the truth, then science cannot be shown to be progressive. However, if one adopts the pragmatic maxim that (a) science is a system of inquiry for the solution of problems, (b) scientific progress consists in the solution of an increasing number of important problems, and (c) rationality consists in making choices that will maximize the progress of science, then we might be able to show to what extent science (and specific sciences, in particular) constitutes a rational and progressive system (1977).

Laudan (1977) recognizes that this type of formulation runs the risk of entailing that we find ourselves adopting theories that are progressive and rational but false. However, we should not despair over this situation. Many scientific theories in the past have been demonstrated to be false; this will continue to happen in the future. Acknowledging this state of affairs is not a judgment that science has not progressed. Any theory of science will be worthy to the extent that it solves problems and contributes to scientific progress. As Laudan (1977) states, "the workability of the problem-solving model is its greatest virtue. In principle we can determine whether a given theory does or does not solve a particular problem" (p. 127).

The Philosophy of Nursing Science

What Laudan (1977, 1984) offers nursing is a view of scientific rationality that can be properly called the philosophy of nursing science. However, his approach does *not* tell us how we should develop theory or how to test theory, as some nurse researchers have apparently claimed (Silva & Rothbart, 1984). Laudan's model of scientific rationality (1977) only applies to how we might evaluate a particular nursing theory against the types of problems in nursing practice that one commonly brings theory to bear upon. And that is *all* any account in the philosophy of science can do: it simply gives the nurse philosopher or the metatheorist a selection of criteria

by which we might begin to assess scientific change and progress within nursing.

Therefore, the development of the philososophy of nursing science has to do with the assessment of theories that have been brought to bear on problems that require nursing interventions. According to Laudan (1977), one way to do this is to assess the problem-solving effectiveness of the nursing theory in terms of its empirical problems solved, conceptual problems generated, and anomalous problems continued or left hanging. It involves a pragmatic calculus of problem-solving effectiveness.

Given the state of discussion in nursing on the need for a relevant set of criteria for the evaluation of theories, Laudan's work is very timely. He offers the philosopher of science and those who function in nursing as philosophers of science a way to explain consensus as well as dissent in our accounts of scientific change. To the extent that such a model of scientific rationality is adopted and used within nursing, the discipline's future efforts at metatheory will be beneficial to the development of the philosophy of nursing science, and vice versa.

REFERENCES

Beckstrand, J. (1978a). The notion of a practice theory and the relationship of scientific and ethical knowledge to practice. *Research in Nursing and Health, 1,* 131–136.

Beckstrand, J. (1978b). The need for a practice theory as indicated by the knowledge used in conduct of practice. *Research in Nursing and Health Care, 1,* 175–179.

Beckstrand, J. (1980). A critique of several conceptions of practice theory in nursing. *Research in Nursing and Health Care, 3,* 69–80.

Benner, P. (1984). *From novice to expert: Excellence and power in clinical nursing practice.* Menlo Park, CA: Addison-Wesley.

Bernstein, R. J. (1983). *Beyond objectivism and relativism: Science, hermeneutics, and praxis.* Philadelphia: University of Pennsylvania Press.

Chinn, P. L., & Jacobs, M. (1987). *Theory and nursing: A systematic approach* (2nd ed.). St. Louis: C. V. Mosby.

Culler, J. (1982). *On deconstruction: Theory and criticism after structuralism.* Ithaca, NY: Cornell University Press.

Cull-Wilby, B. L., & Pepin, J. T. (1987). Towards a coexistence of paradigms in nursing knowledge development. *Journal of Advanced Nursing*, *12*, 515–521.

Dickoff, J., & James P. (1968). A theory of theories: A position paper. *Nursing Research*, *17*, 197–203.

Dickoff, J., James, P., & Wiedenbach, E. (1968a). Theory in a practice discipline: Part I. Practice oriented theory. *Nursing Research*, *17*, 415–435.

Dickoff, J., James, P., & Wiedenbach, E. (1968b). Theory in a practice discipline: Part II. Practice oriented research. *Nursing Research*, *17*, 545–554.

Donaldson, S. K., & Crowley, D. M. (1977). Discipline of nursing: Structure and relationship to practice. In M. V. Batey (Ed.), *Communicating nursing research*, *Vol. 10* (pp. 1–22). Boulder, CO: WICHE.

Donaldson, S. K., & Crowley, D. M. (1978). The discipline of nursing. *Nursing Outlook*, *26*, 113–120.

Dworkin, R. (1977). *Taking rights seriously*. Cambridge, MA: Harvard University Press.

Ellis, R. (1968). Characteristics of significant theories. *Nursing Research*, *17*, 217–222.

Fawcett, J. (1978). The relationship between theory and research: A double helix. *Advances in Nursing Science*, *1*, 49–62.

Fawcett, J. (1984). *Analysis and evaluation of conceptual models of nursing*. Philadelphia: F. A. Davis.

Fitzpatrick, J., & Whall, A. (1983). *Conceptual models of nursing: Analysis and application*. Bowie, MD: R. J. Brady.

Gadamer, H. G. (1975). *Truth and method*. New York: Crossroads Publishing.

Habermas, J. (1971). *Knowledge and human interests*. Boston: Beacon Press.

Hardy, M. E. (1974). Theories: Components, development, evaluation. *Nursing Research*, *23*, 100–107.

Hardy, M. E. (1978). Perspectives on nursing theory. *Advances in Nursing Science*, *1*, 27–48.

Jacox, A. (1974). Theory construction in nursing: An overview. *Nursing Research*, *23*, 4–13.

Johnson, D. E. (1968). Theory in nursing: Borrowed and unique. *Nursing Research*, *17*, 206–209.

Johnson, D. E. (1980). The behavioral system model for nursing. In J. P. Riehl & C. Roy (Eds.), *Conceptual models for nursing practice* (pp. 207–254). New York: Appleton-Century-Crofts.

Hegel, G. W. F. (1929). *The science of logic*, Vols. 1 and 2. (W. H. Johnston & L. G. Struthers, Trans.) London: Oxford University Press. (Original work published 1812–1816)

King, I. M. (1981). *A theory for nursing: Systems, concepts, process*. New York: John Wiley & Sons.

Kritek, P. B. (1978). The generation and classification of nursing diagnoses: Toward a theory of nursing. *Image*, *10*, 33–40.

Kuhn, T. S. (1970). *The structure of scientific revolutions* (2nd ed.). Chicago: University of Chicago Press.

Laudan, L. (1977). *Progress and its problems*. Berkeley, CA: University of California Press.

Laudan, L. (1984). *Science and values: The aims of science and their role in scientific debate*. Berkeley, CA: University of California Press.

Levine, M. E. (1988). Antecedents from adjunctive disciplines: Creation of nursing theory. *Nursing Science Quarterly*, *1*, 16–21.

McKay, R. (1969). Theories, models, and systems for nursing. *Nursing Research*, *18*, 393–399.

McKay, R. P. (1977). Discussion: Discipline of nursing—syntactical structure and relation with other disciplines and the profession of nursing. In M. V. Batey (Ed.), *Communicating nursing research*, *Vol. 10* (pp. 23–30). Boulder, CO: WICHE.

Meleis, A. I. (1985). *Theoretical nursing: Development & progress*. Philadelphia: J. B. Lippincott.

Meleis, A. I. (1987a). Revisions in knowledge development: A passion for substance. *Scholarly Inquiry for Nursing Practice: An International Journal*, *1*, 5–19.

Meleis, A. I. (1987b). Theoretical nursing: Today's challenges, tomorrow's bridges. *Nursing Papers*, *19*, 45–56.

Murphy, J. F. (1985). Doctoral education of nurses: Historical developments, programs, and graduates. In H. H. Werley & J. J. Fitzpatrick, (Eds.), *Annual Review of Nursing Research*, *Vol. 3*. New York: Springer Publishing.

Neuman, B. (1982). *The Neuman systems model: Application to nursing education and practice*. Norwalk, CT: Appleton-Century-Crofts.

Newman, M. A. (1979). *Theory development in nursing*. Philadelphia: F. A. Davis.

Norris, C. (1985). *Contest of faculties: Philosophy and theory after deconstruction*. New York: Methuen.

Norris, C. M. (Ed.). (1969, 1970). *Proceedings, first, second, and third nursing theory conferences*. Lawrence, KS: University of Kansas.

Orem, D. E. (1980). *Nursing: Concepts of practice* (2nd ed.). New York: McGraw-Hill.

Parfit, D. (1984). *Reasons and persons*. New York: Oxford University Press.

Parse, R. R. (1981). *Man-living-health: A theory of nursing*. New York: John Wiley & Sons.

Paterson, J. G., & Zderad, L. T. (1976). *Humanistic nursing*. New York: John Wiley & Sons.

Putnam, H. (1962). What theories are not. In E. Nagel, P. Suppes, & A. Tarski (Eds.). *Logic, methodology, and the philosophy of science: Proceedings of the 1960 International Congress* (pp. 240–251). Stanford, CA: Stanford University Press.

Phenix, P. (1964). *Realms of meaning*. New York: McGraw-Hill.

Ramos, M. S. (1987). Adopting an evolutionary lens: An optimistic approach to discovering strength in nursing. *Advances in Nursing Science, 10*, 19–26.

Rawls, J. (1971). *A theory of justice*. Cambridge: Harvard University Press.

Robey, D. (Ed.) (1973). *Structuralism: An introduction*. Oxford, England: Clarendon Press.

Rogers, M. (1970). *An introduction to the theoretical basis of nursing*. Philadelphia: F. A. Davis.

Rogers, M. (1980). Nursing: A science of unitary man. In J. P. Riehl & D. Roy (Eds.). *Conceptual models for nursing practice* (2nd ed.). (pp. 329–337) New York: Appleton-Century-Crofts.

Roy, C. (1981). *Introduction to nursing: An adaptation model*. Englewood Cliffs, NJ: Prentice-Hall.

Schlotfeldt, R. M. (1988). Structuring nursing knowledge: A priority for creating nursing's future. *Nursing Science Quarterly, 1*, 35–38.

Schwab, J. F. (1964a). Problems, topics, and issues. In S. Edam (Ed.), *Education and the structure of knowledge*. Chicago: Rand McNally.

Schwab, J. F. (1964b). Structure of the disciplines: Meanings and significance. In G. W. Ford & L. Pugno, (Eds.), *The structure of knowledge and the curriculum* (pp. 1–30). Chicago: Rand McNally.

Silva, M. C., & Rothbart, D. (1984). An analysis of changing trends in philosophies of science on nursing theory development and testing. *Advances in Nursing Science, 6*, 1–13.

Skinner, Q. (Ed.) (1985). *The return of grand theory in the human sciences*. Cambridge: Cambridge University Press.

Stevens, B. (1984). *Nursing theory: Analysis, application and evaluation* (2nd ed.). Boston: Little, Brown.

Suppe, F. (1982). Implications of recent developments in philosophy of science for nursing theory. In *Proceedings of the Fifth Biennial Eastern Conference on Nursing Research* (pp. 10–16). Baltimore: University of Maryland School of Nursing.

Suppe, F. (Ed.). (1977). *The structure of scientific theories*. Urbana: University of Illinois Press.

Suppe, F., & Jacox, A. (1985). Philosophy of science and the development of nursing theory. In H. H. Werley & J. J. Fitzpatrick (Eds.), *Annual review of nursing research* (pp. 241–267). New York: Springer.

Thompson, J. (1985). Practical discourse in nursing: Going beyond empiricism and historicism. *Advances in Nursing Science, 7*, 59–71.

Toulmin, S. (1972). *Human understanding, (Vol. 1)*. Princeton, NJ: Princeton University Press.

Visintainer, M. A. (1986). The nature of knowledge and theory in nursing. *Image, 18*, 32–38.

Wald, F. S., & Leonard, R. C. (1964). Toward development of nursing practice theory. *Nursing Research, 13*, 309–313.

Walker, L. O. (1983). Theory and research in the development of nursing as a discipline: Retrospect and prospect. In N. L. Chaska (Ed.), *The nursing profession: A time to speak* (pp. 406–415). New York: McGraw-Hill.

Watson, J. (1985). *Nursing: Human science and care*. Norwalk, CT: Appleton-Century-Crofts.

Webster, G., Jacox, A., & Baldwin, B. (1981). Nursing theory and the ghost of the received view. In J. C. McCoskey & H. K. Grace (Eds.), *Current issues in nursing* (pp. 26–35). Boston, MA: Blackwell Scientific Publications.

✳ EDITOR'S QUESTIONS FOR DISCUSSION ✳

How can developing nursing theory from the science perspective of particulars result in practice theory that emphasizes a holistic perspective? Is the goal of prescriptive theory to indicate how to alter a situation rather than stress change per se or discovery? What is the difference between borrowed theory and knowledge that is unique for a discipline? How does Fry differ from other theorists regarding the goal of nursing theorizing?

Is there a preordained structure for the development of nursing knowledge? Explain the various transitions in the development of nursing knowledge. Can the transition or transitions be defined in terms of revolution or evolution? If they are neither, how can the nature of changes in theory development in nursing be explained? Discuss what Laudan means by "problem solving." Is he addressing how to fix particulars, or discussing theoretical or conceptual problems in describing and explaining how the world works? How does Laudan's view of scientific rationality address or relate to some of the issues raised concerning Beckstrand's alleged beliefs about practice theory? How can one evaluate whether or not a theory of science contributes to scientific progress?

Philosophical Foundations of Nursing Theory:
A discipline emerges

Barbara J. Sarter, Ph.D., R.N.

The history of philosophy in nursing, until recently, has been primarily a history of philosophy of science in nursing. Philosophy of science is a branch of philosophy that analyzes and evaluates the nature of scientific knowledge. It has become clear, however, that a philosophy of science cannot be developed independently of other philosophical dimensions of a discipline. The other major branches of philosophy—metaphysics, logic, epistemology, and ethics—are all interrelated with philosophy of science. Metaphysics investigates the essential nature of reality; logic, the rules of rational thought; epistemology, the nature of knowledge; and ethics, the nature of the good. The efforts by nursing theorists in the 1960s and 1970s to describe the character of scientific knowledge without establishing nursing's other philosophical commitments led to the espousal of an unnecessarily limited view of science, commonly referred to as the "received view." Nursing suffered a virtual "identity crisis" as it compared itself to the received view and found that its theory and research efforts did not meet the standards set forth in the physical sciences.

The 1980s have been characterized by nursing scholars' expansion of philosophical inquiry into metaphysics, ethics, and epistemology, with a concerted focus on the development of a coherent and complete philosophical foundation for the discipline of nursing. With the emergence of a disciplinary metaparadigm of holism, caring, and multiple modes of knowing, the revision of nursing's philosophy of science has become an essential and active arena for scholarship. As the 1990s approach, nursing scholars are acutely aware that the domain of human responses in health and illness requires a view of science quite different from that which has served the physical and natural sciences so well. We explore in this chapter the emerging philosophical commitments of nursing theory and their implications for a philosophy of nursing science. As a background for this analysis, our attention turns first to an overview of some of the common issues that have been explored by philosophers of science and the positions taken in the received view. Next, the emerging metaphysical and ethical commitments of our discipline are identified, and finally a philosophy of science appropriate for the emerging discipline of nursing is proposed.

MAJOR ISSUES IN PHILOSOPHY OF SCIENCE

Perhaps the most enduring and controversial issue in the history of the philosophy of science is that of induction versus deduction. This controversy, in turn, is based on a wide divergence of viewpoints on the nature of the "real world" and how it can be known. Concerning these latter questions, a continuum of opinion exists, with materialism and idealism at opposite ends. Materialism is the philosophy wherein only that which is perceivable through the five senses, that is, matter, is real. All phenomena are explainable in terms of interactions among material, observable events. Idealism is the view that reality is of the nature of mind (objective idealism), or that only mental events are real (subjective idealism). Strict materialists reject the reality of mind independent of matter, whereas strict idealists reject the reality of matter independent of mind. The nature of "true" knowledge, then, will vary accordingly. For the materialist, the only reliable source of knowledge is perception. This view is known as empiricism. Idealism turns to the mind, or thought, as its source of knowing. Rationalism and intuitionism uphold reason and intuition, respectively, as the mental processes that can reveal the true nature of the world.

Carrying this contrast one step further, we arrive at our initial distinction between the inductive and deductive paths of science. The inductive path begins with the objects of perception, that is, with single observable events, and makes generalizations or theories on the basis of these observations. The deductive approach begins with theories formulated or selected by the researcher and then tests them in the empirical world. Both approaches rely, whether initially or finally, on empirical observation. This is the *essence* of science, as opposed to other ways of knowing. If the reality of the empirical world is denied altogether, as it is by some philosophers, we can no longer talk of science at all. The differences between induction and deduction lie (a) in the relative weight given to observation and theory, and (b) in the order of their appearance in the process of scientific investigation. There is also a fundamental difference in the logic of these two approaches.

The process of inductive reasoning is based on a basic philosophical assumption—that of the uniformity or regularity of nature. David Hume (1711–1776), whose thought remains a focus of intense discussion, challenged this assumption by maintaining that we can never be certain that events which we have not yet experienced will resemble those that we have witnessed (Oldroyd, 1986). This has come to be known as the "problem of induction" and it indeed poses a serious problem to proponents of the inductive method. Is it justifiable to make generalizations on the basis of a specific set of empirical observations? Science has attempted to deal with this problem by setting forth strict rules regarding sampling and the logical steps involved in inductive reasoning.

Those scientists and philosophers who have supported the deductive approach to science have found the "problem of induction" to be insoluble. Their effort, then, is to begin with the formulation of a theory or hypothesis (derived from reason, intuition, and/or experience) and to proceed to "test" this theory in one of several ways. In general, a theory is tested by deducing (logically deriving) what observable events should or should not occur if it were true. The theory is corroborated if these deductions prove to be consistently accurate. Verification of a theory is the purpose of an individual research effort. This means that the scientist hypothesizes events that will occur if the theory is true; and if they are actually found, the theory has been verified.

Karl Popper (1968), one of the most influential contemporary philosophers of science, maintains that *falsification* is the only legitimate method for deductive theory testing. He asserts that verification is induction in reverse, and that both have the same logical fault of assuming that future cases will be the same as past cases. Popper (1968) concludes, therefore, that searching for refutations, rather than verifications, of a theory is the best way to test it. Popper adds that the falsifiability of a theory is what makes it scientific, as opposed to philosophical. If it is *logically* capable of being refuted by experience, it is a scientific theory. This does not mean that it must *actually* be refuted; it simply must be formulated in such a way that (a) some statements about a particular observable event can be derived from it and (b) at least one of these statements, if true, will contradict the theory.

The issue of causality is another critical and fundamental area of exploration for philosophy of science. Perhaps the first Western philosopher to deal with causality was Aristotle. Aristotle (1929) identified four possible types of causation: the material cause, the efficient cause, the formal cause, and the final cause. The first two are retained in modern concepts of causality, whereas the last two have been rejected since the "scientific revolution" of the 17th century. The material cause is simply the matter or substance out of which an object or organism is made. The efficient cause is the agent involved in shaping the matter, or it is the immediately preceding event. To describe the idea of formal cause, terms such as blueprint, essence, and pattern have been used. Aristotle believed that there is an inner, innate "form" which causes an organism to develop as it does. Lastly, final causation is that in which the end, final result, or goal exerts a causal influence on the development of the entity.

Hume (1888/1968), in addition to rejecting the uniformity of nature, also rejected the concept of causality, since it is not directly observable. All that is observed is that two events repeatedly occur close together in time and space. On this basis, an inference is made that one event "causes" the other. This inference is a kind of induction that, in the future, "B" will always occur if "A" has occurred; and since to Hume induction is not valid, neither is the inference of causality. Hume recognized the pragmatic value of the concept of causality, however, and even developed a set of rules for the inference of causality.

Despite Hume's challenge, philosophers did not entirely abandon the concept of causality. Immanuel Kant (1724–1804) maintained that causation is an innate category or perceptual mold of the human mind (Kant, 1933). Causal relationships may not really "exist," but the mind automatically interprets its perceptions in terms of causation. Kant made the same claim concerning the concepts of space and time.

Modern philosophers have also kept alive the discussion of causality. Nagel (1961) identified four patterns of scientific explanation and placed causality as a subset of the first:

1. *Deductive:* The explicandum (that which is being explained) is a logically necessary consequence of the explanatory premises.
2. *Probabilistic:* The explanation contains a statistical assumption about some class of elements, whereas the explicandum is a statement about a specific member of that class.
3. *Teleological:* The explanation describes the function that an event performs in maintaining or creating certain traits of a system to which the event belongs, or it states the role an event plays in accomplishing some goal.
4. *Genetic:* The explanation sets out the sequence of major events through which an earlier system has been transformed into a later one.

A third critical issue in the philosophy of science is the problem of error. Error here refers to a situation in which an observed event is different from that which would be expected according to the theory under investigation. The classic empiricist point of view, expressed centuries ago by Sir Francis Bacon (1561–1626), is that lack of objectivity, or observer bias, is the source of all error (Bacon, 1905). This is based on an inductivist view of theory, in which the source of all knowledge lies in perception. If the observer's mind is "pure," that is, free of all preconceived ideas, the observations will be accurate and hence the theory will be correct. The modern school of logical positivism believes that the problem of error is one of language when observations become symbolized. The emphasis of the positivists, then, is on accurate definitions that state the observable conditions under which a sentence containing the term is true or false.

Among those who favor the deductivist approach, several different interpretations of error are possible. Popper (1968), as implied above, believes that errors serve as refutations of a theory and are extremely valuable in theory development. The scientist must try his best to refute the theory being tested. A strong theory will survive this test. Thomas Kuhn (1970) maintains that errors indicate the need for further development of a theory, but unless the errors (or "anomalies") become so numerous that the community of scientists makes a decision to reject the theory entirely, errors do not refute the theory.

In summary, the major issues that are dealt with in philosophy of science include those of induction versus deduction, causality, and the problem of error. This is by no means a complete list of the complex problems that are dealt with in this discipline, nor have all the positions taken been explored in the preceding paragraphs. For example, there are those who maintain that science has no *single* method (Feyerabend, 1975) and still others who emphasize the role of intuition, or personal knowledge, in scientific discovery (Polanyi, 1958). Next, we more specifically address the "received view" of science, which in the early 20th century became the dominant and very effective standard for the physical sciences and whose influence permeated the natural and human sciences as well.

THE RECEIVED VIEW

The school of logical positivism (or logical empiricism) provides the philosophical foundation of the received view. In its name lies the key to its beliefs and method. Positivism is the philosophy that the natural sciences are the only reliable form of knowledge. Combining positivism with logic, this school has held as its major goal the development of a set of logical rules for the use of language that will render a given theoretical proposition either empirically verifiable or meaningless. Stated as the "verifiability principle," the belief is that the meaning of a proposition consists of its method of verification. If no empirical verification of a statement is possible, it is meaningless. Thus linguistic analysis becomes the philosophical method of logical positivism. The statements of philosophers and scientists are logically analyzed for their verifiability through empirical observation (Hutchison, 1977; Oldroyd, 1986; Russell, 1945).

The emphasis of the received view of science, then, is on the "reduction" of theoretical propositions and concepts into observable discrete phenomena that can be objectively measured. Ideally a direct correspondence must be made between a concept and a "fact." In this view, however, lies another central problem in the philosophy of science—the relation between theory and fact. The early logical positivists believed that a one-to-one correspondence between concepts and facts could be established—that somehow, the two exist in a pure form without any mutual influence. Currently most philosophers agree that this sets up a false dichotomy, that nearly all facts are "theory-laden" and all concepts are influenced by perceptions. The empirical world is perceived through the filter of the mind, and theory is based on some kind of experience.

The received view, for this and other reasons, has come under increasing skepticism, particularly among members of the social and human sciences. There may possibly be pure facts in the physical world, but in the realm of human life and society this distinction crumbles. It is questioned whether it is possible to identify "facts" in this arena with complete objectivity, and even if so, whether this will provide us with the kind of knowledge of human life that we are seeking. This is a question currently under intense discussion among nursing scholars, who realize that nursing's implicit philosophical commitments may require more than the received view of science.

NURSING'S PHILOSOPHICAL COMMITMENTS

Let us explore some of these philosophical commitments, or metaparadigmatic beliefs, of the discipline of nursing. Some nursing scholars (Uys, 1987) have argued that many of nursing's so-called theories are actually philosophies. Whether one agrees with this statement or not, it is true that nursing theories are laden with philosophical assumptions, either implicit or explicit. In a recent analysis (Sarter, 1988a) of the nursing theories of Rogers (1970, 1980, 1983, 1986), Parse (1981), Watson (1985), and Newman (1986), a pattern of recurrent philosophical themes was identified. The themes are:

1. *Process:* There is a view of constant change, evolutionary in nature, predictable to a degree, but always innovative and creative.

2. *Consciousness:* The evolutionary process is one of the evolution of human consciousness, proceeding toward a state of self-transcendence in which one's separateness from the environment dissolves. Health is maximal in this state of self-transcendence or spiritual awareness.

3. *Openness:* The interaction between person and the world is dynamic, continuous, and necessary for personal development.

4. *Harmony:* Harmony within the various dimensions of the individual and harmony between person and environment are important aspects of health.

5. *Noncausality:* In general, the theorists analyzed reject the validity of searching for simple causal relationships in human health and illness.

6. *Space-time:* Space-time forms a nonlinear, fluid, relative matrix in which past and future merge into present, and distance is not an insurmountable barrier to interactions among persons and events.

7. *Pattern:* Pattern is a unique, holistic, non-physical, organizing force of the individual which is always changing in the process of human evolution.

In addition to these themes, which are common to the previously mentioned theories, there is general consensus that the discipline of nursing embraces a holistic and humanistic viewpoint with a fundamental ethic of caring. There is the pragmatic goal of promoting optimum health in the recipients of nursing care. Is the received view of science compatible with this complex of philosophical commitments? Even if so, is it adequate in itself to guide the entire range of nursing research? The consensus is that it is not (Leininger, 1985; Meleis, 1985; Watson, 1985). The reduction of the object of nursing research—human responses in health and illness—to a single observable variable cannot be upheld as the *only* valid way of developing nursing knowledge. The utility and power of the received view need not be denied, but nursing must expand its view of science and of valid knowledge in order to nurture its unique philosophical stance.

A PHILOSOPHY OF SCIENCE FOR NURSING

Let us return to the three issues described earlier and attempt to outline some possible positions that are consistent with nursing's philosophy of holism, humanism, and caring. Concerning the issue of induction versus deduction, it appears desirable to embrace both of these approaches to scientific method. The problem of induction will be particularly acute when one is attempting to make generalizations on the basis of observations of unique individuals. But, it would be dangerous to formulate our theories, concepts, and propositions without drawing on nursing experience. It will also be unacceptable to develop theories deductively without requiring that they be validated in the pragmatic sphere of nursing practice.

Induction and deduction can be seen as complementary and equally important phases of nursing science. Whether one begins with experience or with theory, the circle must be completed. If a theory is inductively developed, it must be made generalizable to a larger population and then tested again empirically. If a theory is deductively formulated, it must be tested in the empirical world and then altered according to the results of this testing. Our definition of "empirical" requires some expansion beyond the positivist meaning of "observable through the five senses." For example, if we insist on a traditionally empirical criterion for the presence of pain, we will not admit the existence of pain in a patient unless it is observable. Clearly, this is not how nursing approaches its phenomena of concern. Pain exists whenever a person says that it does. Subjective as well as objective experience must be incorporated into the empirical realm.

Scientific explanation in nursing may be profitably modeled after the Aristotelian system of causality. In addition to material and efficient causation, which we have noted to be largely rejected by modern philosophers, the modes of formal and teleological causation may provide fruitful avenues for explanations of human responses in health and illness. The "pattern" of the human being in Rogerian theory is analogous to the "form" of an organism in Aristotelian philosophy (Sarter, 1988b). Both concepts refer to a holistic inner organizing principle that molds a unique individual. The evolutionary nature of nursing theory is highly compatible with teleological explanation, in which a process or event is interpreted in terms of its contribution to a certain developmental trend or goal. For example, Newman (1986) describes both health and illness as aspects of an overall process of expanding consciousness.

Nagel's framework (1961) also provides a useful model of scientific explanation for nursing. Nagel describes deductive, probabilistic, teleological, and genetic patterns of scientific explanation (see the definitions presented earlier). Nursing phenomena may be explored using any of these patterns. The latter two have been rarely utilized in nursing but appear to present fruitful areas for exploration.

Concerning the problem of error, all the approaches examined above may be utilized in nursing science. Researcher or observer bias must be recognized as a potential problem. Operational definitions pose problems for the validity and reliability of measurement tools. The value of errors as refutations of a theory should be acknowledged, as well as their role in indicating areas in need of theoretical refinement. And certainly Kuhn (1970) is correct in stating that when the number of anomalies unexplainable by a current theory increases to a critical point, a radical change in the discipline's theoretical matrix may be necessary. Polanyi's assertion (1958) that errors are ultimately judged by the personal intuition of the scientist is also an appropriate view for nursing science.

The discussion of scientific method in the nursing literature has often taken the form of a debate about quantitative versus qualitative research methods. The above analysis has deliberately avoided posing this dichotomy. It is believed that the framework of a philosophy of science for nursing presented earlier will accommodate both of these methods, making them equally valid in the development of nursing's knowledge base. Quantitative methods emphasize reductionistic objective measurement and statistical analysis, whereas qualitative methods focus on holistic verbal description and analysis. Both are concerned with empirical experience, and both deserve credit as rigorous scientific methodologies. It may be

helpful to view qualitative research as being inductive in nature, and quantitative as being deductive in the positivist tradition.

The goals of science are the description, explanation, prediction, and control of phenomena. Each of these goals should draw on a variety of methods, and their interrelationships should be acknowledged. The hallmark of science is rigorous and systematic investigation. Nursing science requires a broad interpretation of its mission and its methods. The vast range and nature of human experience requires openness to multiple ways of knowing and of scientific investigation.

REFERENCES

Aristotle. (1929). *The physics* (P. H. Wicksteed & F. M. Cornford, Trans.). Cambridge: Harvard University Press.

Bacon, F. (1905). New organon. In J. M. Robertson (Ed.), *The philosophical works of Francis Bacon* (pp. 256–387). New York: Dutton.

Feyerabend, P. (1975). *Against method: Outlines of an anarchistic theory of knowledge*. Atlantic Highlands, NJ: Humanities Press.

Hume, D. (1968). *A treatise of human nature*. London: Oxford University Press. (Originally published 1888)

Hutchison, J. (1977). *Living options in world philosophy*. Honolulu: University Press of Hawaii.

Kant, I. (1933). *Critique of pure reason* (2nd ed.). (N. K. Smith, Trans.) London: Macmillan.

Kuhn, T. (1970). *The structure of scientific revolutions*. Chicago: University of Chicago Press.

Leininger, M. (Ed.). (1985). *Qualitative research methods in nursing*. New York: Grune & Stratton.

Meleis, A. I. (1985). *Theoretical nursing: Development and progress*. Philadelphia: J. B. Lippincott.

Nagel, E. (1961). *The structure of science*. New York: Harcourt.

Newman, M. (1986). *Health as expanding consciousness*. St. Louis: C. V. Mosby.

Oldroyd, D. (1986). *The arch of knowledge: An introductory study of the history of the philosophy and methodology of science*. New York: Methuen.

Parse, R. (1981). *Man-living-health: A theory of nursing*. New York: John Wiley & Sons.

Polanyi, M. (1958). *Personal Knowledge: Towards a post-critical philosophy*. London: Routledge & Kegan Paul.

Popper, K. E. (1968). *The logic of scientific discovery*. New York: Harper.

Rogers, M. E. (1970). *An introduction to the theoretical basis of nursing*. Philadelphia: F. A. Davis.

Rogers, M. E. (1980). Nursing: A science of unitary man. In J. Riehl & C. Roy (Eds.), *Conceptual models for nursing practice* (2nd ed., pp. 329–337). Norwalk, CT: Appleton-Century-Crofts.

Rogers, M. E. (1983). Science of unitary human beings: A paradigm for nursing. In I. Clements & F. Roberts (Eds.), *Family health: A theoretical approach to nursing care*. New York: John Wiley & Sons.

Rogers, M. E. (1986). Science of unitary human beings. In V. Malinski (Ed.), *Explorations on Martha Rogers'*

science of unitary human beings (pp. 3–14). Norwalk, CT: Appleton-Century-Crofts.

Russell, B. E. (1945). *A history of Western philosophy*. New York: Simon & Schuster.

Sarter, B. (1988a). Philosophical sources of nursing theory. *Nursing Science Quarterly, 1*(2).

Sarter, B. (1988b). *The stream of becoming: A study of Martha Roger's theory*. New York: National League for Nursing.

Uys, L. (1987). Foundational studies in nursing. *Journal of Advanced Nursing, 12*, 275–280.

Watson, J. (1985). *Nursing: Human science and human care: A theory of nursing*. Norwalk, CT: Appleton-Century-Crofts.

✳ EDITOR'S QUESTIONS FOR DISCUSSION ✳

What are the differences between induction and deduction in approaching the development and testing of theory? Discuss what is known as the "problem of induction." How justifiable is it to make generalizations on the basis of specific empirical observations? Why does Popper suggest that searching for refutations rather than verification is the best way to test a proposed theory? To what extent is Popper a transitional figure between logical positivism and historicism? How are the criticisms of the received view and positivism addressed in the philosophical perspectives of historicism?

Can the inductive approach be equated with the perceived view of science and the deductive approach be associated with the received view of science? What is the relationship between inductive and deductive approaches with qualitative and quantitative methods? Provide examples in which both the received and perceived views are necessary for the development of nursing knowledge. How does Sarter's discussion concerning research approaches support the content offered by Donnelly and Deets (Chapter 21)? What implications exist in Sarter's chapter for the issues addressed by Stember and Hester (Chapter 22)? Does not Sarter's statements concerning the use of "error" contradict Bacon's idea of error? Provide examples on how subjective experience can be rendered objective or empirical.

30

Nursing Paradigms and Realities

Margaret A. Newman, Ph.D., R.N., F.A.A.N.

Knowing what paradigm guides one's research is the *key* to findings and, ultimately, to discerning the nature of nursing practice. I would like to share my experience of what happens when one mixes paradigms and different levels of reality.

MAJOR PARADIGMS OF HEALTH

Clarifying one's paradigm is particularly important in regard to the phenomenon of health. There are basically two paradigms of health (Capra, 1982; Ferguson, 1980; Parse, 1981; Watson, 1985). The major and prevailing paradigm is health as the absence of disease. Health as absence of disease varies along a continuum that ranges from high-level wellness at the positive end to the disease state at the negative end. In-between are various stages of adaptation to disease and absence of disease without the extra dimensions implied by the high-level wellness concept. Smith's philosophical study (1981) of the concept of health describes these varying perspectives of health within the absence of disease paradigm. She categorizes the literature about health as clinical, adaptive, role performance, and eudaimonistic. Clinical refers primarily to the medical clinical model and relates to the absence or presence of symptoms of disease. In terms of the above continuum, it would relate to both disease and absence of disease in terms of

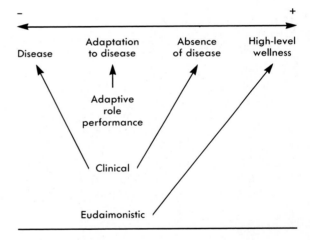

FIGURE 30-1

Paradigm of health as the absence of disease.

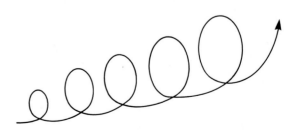

FIGURE 30-2

Paradigm of health as a unitary evolving pattern of person-environment interaction.

prevention (Fig. 30-1). The adaptive and role-performance categories are consistent with the stage of adaptation to disease. The eudaimonistic category would be consistent with high-level wellness. The work of a large number of nursing theorists and researchers emanates from this paradigm of health.

The other major paradigm of health is person-centered and encompasses disease as a meaningful aspect of the dynamic pattern of the whole of an evolving person-environment. This paradigm refers to a rhythmic process of increasing complexity. It is a spiraling progression of the unitary person-environment pattern to higher levels of development (Fig. 30-2). Martha Rogers (1970) was the first nursing theorist to explicate this paradigm, and a number of other theorists have adopted it as the basis for their work.

So we in nursing find ourselves operating in at least these two major paradigms, and we sometimes get them mixed up. It is possible to do research using the *same* constructs to reflect *different* paradigms—a predicament that leads to misunderstanding and confusion. To maintain communication within our ranks, we need to be clear on our respective paradigms.

INFLUENCE OF A PARADIGM ON THE MEANING OF RESEARCH FINDINGS

A paradigm is an overall perspective on things, a worldview. In this case we are talking about a perspective of health. The following accounts illustrate how two different paradigms of health influence the conceptualization and interpretation of similar pieces of research, resulting in findings that are difficult to interpret unless the guiding paradigm is clarified.

My perspective of health fits within the general paradigm of evolving pattern of the whole person-environment. Health is the process of expanding consciousness; all manifestations of life evolving, including disease and disability, reflect this pattern of expanding consciousness (Newman, 1979; 1983; 1986). Consciousness is defined as the capacity of the system (person) to interact with the environment.

Movement, time, and space are identified as manifestations of consciousness, that is, the changing pattern of the person's interaction with the environment. Movement and time were operationalized for the purposes of my early research (Newman, 1972, 1976).

Engle (1981) decided to follow up this research with a study of movement and time in elderly women. Her intent, as mine, was to gain a better understanding of how these concepts describe health. She consulted with me regarding operationalization of the concepts and methodological questions and designed her research to test and extend the work I had started. I was eager to participate in a reciprocal exchange of findings and extension of the theory, but after a while I became aware of an uneasy feeling that Engle and I were not talking about the same thing. I was unable to identify the incongruity until she published her research results (Engle, 1984, 1986). Then *her* perspective of health, her paradigm, became clear. Engle's concept of health, as operationalized in her research, is one of functional ability. This measure of health was found to correlate positively with rate of movement, and Engle concluded that speed of movement was an indicator of health. The relevance of this correlation stems from its interpretation in terms of the paradigm of health as the absence of disease: Functional ability would be a measure of role performance within this continuum.

In a paradigm of pattern, which is the foundation for my theory, the viewpoint of more or less healthy is antithetical to the perspective of the paradigm. Health *is* the pattern. Rate of movement is a reflection of the pattern, but it is not a quantification of health. It is not possible within the theory of health as expanding consciousness to conclude that the faster one moves, the healthier one is. The linear, polar notion of more or less ability is replaced by a notion of pattern.

The communication barrier between Engle and me stemmed from the fact that we were operating from different paradigms of health. The operationalization of major concepts in these two research endeavors was the same, but they were being played in two different ballparks, unbeknown, at least for a while, even to the players. Engle was viewing health as more or less functional ability; in that context, faster movement meant healthier. My view of health was an evolving pattern of person-environment interaction (emphasizing the concepts of movement-time-space-consciousness); in that context, faster (or slower) movement helped to describe the total pattern of health.

In another study designed within the context of my general theory of expanding consciousness, the investigators (Nojima et al., 1987) hypothesized that higher consciousness would be related to greater functional ability. Here again the latter variable places the research within an absence of disease paradigm. They found, however, that more disabled persons had higher indices of consciousness than less disabled persons. Rather than representing a rejection of the theory of health as expanding consciousness, as the authors thought, this finding provides data that support a pattern of expanded consciousness in persons whose movement is restricted. It has a completely different interpretation within a paradigm of pattern of the whole person-environment.

These examples are shared to illustrate the difficulties encountered when it is not clear which paradigm guides the conceptualization and interpretation of the research. We have been reared in a society dominated by the absence of disease paradigm. Nurses have sensed intuitively that there is more in the experience of health and illness than the linear, quantitative approach can offer. Sometimes we glimpse the pattern of the whole person-environment for an instant, but then lose that insight, temporarily. There is delight in suddenly seeing the whole pattern and yet confusion because it is not yet grasped entirely. And so we flip back and forth between the two paradigms, perhaps unknowingly. It is like having two jigsaw puzzles cut by the same form but portraying different pictures. The pieces of the two may be interchangeable but meaningless unless they are fit into the picture from which they originated.

LEVELS OF REALITY

Another way in which one's paradigm influences research findings is by specifying what data are acceptable. The paradigm of health as absence of disease is grounded in the scientific method and requires data that are observable and measurable. Such data would be classified in a level of reality referred to as the "see-touch" realm, and perhaps the "behavioral" realm (LeShan & Margenau, 1982). In addition to these realms, LeShan and Margenau (1982) suggest that there are at least three other different constructions of reality: the microcosmic realm, the macrocosmic realm, and the realm of inner experience. Nurses clearly function in the realities of the see-touch realm, the behavioral realm, and the realm of inner experience. The see-touch realm is the most familiar and is quantifiable; pallor, temperature, and pulse are familiar measurements within this realm. The behavioral level is another realm with which nurses are very familiar; this realm includes observations of the way a person talks, what a person chooses to do, who a person relates to, and how a person relates. That too is somewhat quantifiable although the quantities lose some of the meaning in the act. The last realm of reality, that of inner experience, is an important aspect of the health experience; however, phenomena such as joy and sorrow are not quantifiable and cannot be comprehended with see-touch methods. A paradigm that requires observable, "objective" data precludes direct study of the realm of inner experience.

Data from different realms are not contradictory, but each reality has its limits. Different rules apply and therefore observations at one level may not be transferable to another level. Table 30-1 illustrates differences in physical and social reality in terms of the concepts of time and space as suggested by LeShan and Margenau (1982, pp. 157–159).

An example of an attempt to capture one level of reality by measuring another level is seen in studies of time perception. The meaning of subjective time (an inner experience) is limited by measuring it in terms of clock time (a combination of the behavioral and see-touch realms). The different levels are not contradictory; however, the connection between

TABLE 30-1
Different levels of reality of time and space

	PHYSICAL REALITY	SOCIAL REALITY
Time	Flows evenly	Flows unevenly
	Past and present causality	Future causality
	Experience as present	Experience of present contains past and future
	Everywhere the same	Differs according to culture and social class
	Clock time	Personal time
Space	Geographical	Behavioral
	Two feet apart	Too close/too far
	Geometric	Personal
	House	Relation to other family members — shared space/private space

TABLE 30-2
Correspondence of NANDA dimensions of person-environment interaction with levels of reality

LEVELS OF REALITY	DIMENSIONS OF INTERACTION
See-touch	Exchanging Moving Perceiving
Behavioral	Choosing Communicating Relating
Inner experience	Feeling Knowing Valuing

them is not always apparent. The physical measurement is the "tip of the iceberg" or one arc of a circle. One cannot expect direct correspondence between the part and the whole, *but* the partial information afforded by the physical measurement *is* part of the pattern of the whole person-environment and therefore can be a clue to the pattern.

The intuitive leap that a nurse makes on the basis of very vague, unarticulated information is an example of seeing the pattern of the whole person-environment from partial information. It is the reading of the hologram.* It is allowing that tiny bit of information to project the whole.

The different levels of reality are not mutually exclusive, but we sometimes have difficulty communi-

---

*The hologram has been widely used as a model that illustrates the phenomenon of information of the whole being imbedded in the part. A fuller discussion of this phenomenon as a model for practice is included in Newman, M. A. (1986). *Health as expanding consciousness (pp. 70–72)*. St. Louis: C. V. Mosby.

cating across realms. What we comprehend probably depends on our own levels of reality. When I first began to work with the nine dimensions of person-environment interaction that constitutes the framework for nursing diagnosis adopted by the North American Nursing Diagnosis Association (NANDA) (Newman, 1984; Roy et al., 1982), I was aware that my analyses of case study material usually clustered in the categories of exchanging, communicating, and relating. If I could get sufficient data to describe these dimensions of interaction, I could begin to identify their patterns. In retrospect, I see that the levels of reality of these dimensions were more readily observable. At any rate, the pattern of the whole person-environment emerged from partial information. As additional data pertaining to these and other dimensions came forth, of course, the pattern was elaborated and refined.

The nine dimensions of person-environment interaction reflect the three levels of reality described above (Table 30-2). Just to take three nursing practice observations that went into developing the dimensions as examples, one can see how they reflect these different realities. Urinary incontinence, for example, would go into the category of exchanging and is a phenomenon that can be observed and quantified. Abusive behavior would fit into the relating category and is consistent with the definition of behavior as being observable behavior above the reflex level. Low self-concept would fit in the knowing/feeling/valuing categories and is a phenomenon of inner experience. Data from each of these levels of reality are partial reflections of the pattern of the whole person-environment. If these data pertained to one person, the pattern of that whole person-environment would begin to reveal itself.

Since nurses must take into consideration these different levels of reality, either we must be able to switch back and forth between paradigms, or perhaps the paradigm guiding our practice and our investigations must be broad enough to incorporate differing perspectives and methods.

WHAT ARE THE ESSENTIAL QUESTIONS?

A paradigm of research specifies the kinds of questions that will be asked. We need to ask ourselves, as Rosemary Ellis (Nursing Theory Think Tank Conferences, 1978–1984) asked many times: *What are the essential questions in nursing?*

As I ponder research in other areas, I am struck with some major overriding question that researchers in the field are trying to answer? In biological rhythms, first there was the question of rhythmicity itself—is it a characteristic of all living systems? And all processes within living systems? Then if this is so, where does it come from? Is there an exogenous force or an endogenous clock that maintains the rhythmicity? Volumes of research are devoted to this latter question.

In the area of hemispheric dominance, the question is what are the respective functions of the two cerebral hemispheres? Again, volume after volume of research addresses this basic question and describes the relationship of the two hemispheres in different conceptual terms, as well as the specifics of the various observable functions. The questions engendered by this basic question will keep scientists in the field occupied for many years to come.

The major question in the life sciences is how do new forms of life come into being. This is the question addressed by Sheldrake's hypothesis of morphic

resonance* and by Prigogine's theory of dissipative structures†. Investigators in laboratories all over the world are pursuing this question.

What then is the guiding, essential question in nursing? The process of theory building is not just an accumulation of facts. It is one powerful, unifying idea evolving. As we become clear on the worldview of nursing, what major question must we answer? I submit it has something to do with how nurses facilitate the health of human beings. The way that the question is asked and the answers that we get, however, depends on which paradigm of health is in place. The question asked by the absence of disease paradigm is: What is the etiology, treatment, and prevention of disease? In the paradigm of health as pattern of the evolving whole person-environment, a question, still focusing on the disease situation, could be: What is the pattern of the whole person-environment depicted by the disease? A further question within a paradigm that depicts nursing as a partnership in the patterning of person-environment development might be: What is the quality of relationship that makes it possible for the nurse and patient to connect in a transforming way?

SUMMARY

We have reached a stage in the development of nursing science when we must be clear about the paradigm that guides our research and must distinguish research relating to one paradigm from that

---

*Sheldrake's hypothesis of morphic resonance states that the characteristic forms and behavior of physical, chemical, and biological systems are determined by invisible organizing fields, referred to as morphogenetic fields, the effect of which is not diminished by space or time and is cumulative. This theory lends an explanation to the observed phenomenon that the difficulty of synthesizing new compounds becomes increasingly easier once the compound has been formed the first time, and this facility is apparent in laboratories great distances from each other (Sheldrake, 1981).

†Prigogine's theory of dissipative structures posits that all dynamic systems fluctuate, but rather than averaging out, the process becomes supraordinate to the random perturbations and shifts to a new, higher order, more complex structural form. (Prigogine, I., Allen, P.M., & Herman, R. [1977]).

which relates to another. The major prevailing paradigms in nursing today are derived from the prevailing paradigms of health: health as absence of disease, and health as the evolving pattern of person-environment. Research findings will have vastly different meaning depending on which paradigm guides the conceptualization and interpretation. Paradigms determine the research questions to be asked and the data to be sought. A paradigm that integrates different levels of reality would be consistent with the content of nursing practice.

REFERENCES

Capra, F. (1982). *The turning point*. New York: Simon & Schuster.

Engle, V. (1981). A study of the relationship between self-assessment of health, function, personal tempo and time perception in elderly women (Doctoral dissertation, Wayne State University, 1981). *Dissertation Abstracts International*, 42/03B, DEN81-17056.

Engle, V. (1984). Newman's conceptual framework and the measurement of older adults' health. *Advances in Nursing Science*, 7, 24–36.

Engle, V. (1986). The relationship of movement and time to older adults' functional health. *Research in Nursing and Health*, 9, 123–129.

Ferguson, M. (1980). *The aquarian conspiracy: Personal and social transformation in the 1980's*. Los Angeles: J. P. Tarcher.

LeShan, L., & Margenau, H. (1982). *Einstein's space and van Gogh's sky*. New York: Macmillan.

Newman, M. A. (1972). Time estimation in relation to gait tempo. *Perceptual and Motor Skills, 34*, 359–366.

Newman, M. A. (1976). Movement tempo and the experience of time. *Nursing Research, 25*, 273–279.

Newman, M. A. (1979). *Theory development in nursing*. Philadelphia: F. A. Davis.

Newman, M. A. (1983). Newman's health theory. In I. Clements & F. Roberts (Eds.), *Family health: A theoretical approach to nursing care* (pp. 161–175). New York: John Wiley & Sons.

Newman, M. A. (1984). Nursing diagnosis: Looking at the whole. *American Journal of Nursing, 84*, 1496–1499.

Newman, M. A. (1986). *Health as expanding consciousness*. St. Louis: C. V. Mosby.

Nojima, Y., Oda, A., Nishii, H., Fukui, M., Seo, K., & Akiyoshi, H. (1987). Perception of time among Japanese inpatients. *Western Journal of Nursing Research, 9*, 288–300.

Parse, R. R. (1981). *Man-living-health*. New York: John Wiley & Sons.

Prigogine, I., Allen, P. M., & Herman, R. (1977). *Long-term trends and the evolution of complexity*. In E. Laszlo & J. Berman (Eds.), *Goals in a global community: The original background papers for Goals for Mankind* (Vol. 1, pp. 1–63). New York: Pergamon Press.

Rogers, M. E. (1970). *An introduction to the theoretical basis of nursing*. Philadelphia: F. A. Davis.

Roy, C., Rogers, M. E., Fitzpatrick, J. J., Newman, M. A., Orem, D., Feild, L., Stafford, J. J., Weber, S., Rossi, L., & Krekeler, K. (1982). Nursing diagnosis and nursing theory. In M. J. Kim & D. A. Moritz (Eds.), *Classification of nursing diagnoses* (pp. 26–40). St. Louis: C. V. Mosby.

Sheldrake, R. (1981). *A new science of life: The hypothesis of formative causation*. Los Angeles: Tarcher.

Smith, J. (1981). The idea of health: A philosophic inquiry. *Advances in Nursing Science, 3*, 43–50.

Watson, J. (1985). *Nursing: The philosophy and science of caring*. Boulder, CO: Colorado Associated University Press.

✳   EDITOR'S QUESTIONS FOR DISCUSSION   ✳

Provide examples from research in which the same constructs are used reflecting different paradigms. Indicate examples of using different levels of reality from paradigms. Propose alternative ways of defining concepts and paradigms. According to Newman, is expanding consciousness the paradigm or is it a major concept? How does Newman define the concept of health?

How might high-level wellness be a construct that is defined in two different ways for two different paradigms? Provide examples of different paradigms of health and different constructs of the same health paradigm evident in the works of nurse theorists. What applications are there in Newman's presentation about paradigms for Lyon's definitions of wellness, illness, and disease (Chapter 34)? Provide examples of nursing research in which the linear, polar notion of more or less ability is replaced by a notion of pattern. What are the essential questions in nursing that should be addressed? Propose research designs and methodology that could be utilized to address the research questions raised by Newman.

31

The Meaning of a Progressive World View in Nursing:

Rogers's science of unitary human beings

Violet M. Malinski, Ph.D., R.N.

Rogers's (1970, 1986, 1987) Science of Unitary Human Beings offers a new world view from which to derive theories about how people evolve. Using this framework, nurses can develop modalities to enhance clients' knowing participation in the continuous process of change. The world view underlying this framework is a progressive one, in the sense of moving and evolving, and is different from much of contemporary nursing. However, it is a view that shows parallels with other progressive world views currently emerging across a variety of disciplines.

THE SCIENCE OF UNITARY HUMAN BEINGS

Rogers defines nursing as a basic science having a philosophy of wholeness; the science provides the basis for knowledgeable nursing actions. The unitary human being interacting with the environment is the phenomenon of concern to the discipline of nursing (Rogers, 1970, 1986, 1987). "Unitary" means whole, and Rogers (1986) uses "field" to convey "a means of perceiving people and their respective environments as irreducible wholes" (p. 4). The person-environment field process is characterized by energy patterning of low or high frequency. The nature of the patterning is continuously changing and always creative. Rogers (1986) defines patterning "as the distinguishing characteristic of an energy field perceived as a single wave" (p. 5).

Patterning is a major concept in Rogers's (1986) principles of homeodynamics (resonancy, helicy, and integrality). According to *resonancy*, human and environmental field patterning change continuously, flowing in higher frequencies. *Helicy* identifies the innovative and probabilistic (noncausal), increasing diversity of this field patterning. *Integrality* specifies the continuous mutual process of human and environmental fields; person and environment are unitary (whole) rather than separate entities.

Manifestations of field patterning emerge within this continuous mutual process. Rogers has identified motion, time, and sleep as examples of such manifestations (Malinski, 1986, p. 9). For example, since change is probabilistic and diverse, these manifestations are postulated to flow for motion as slower motion, faster motion, seems continuous; for time experienced as slower, as faster, as timelessness; and for sleep, as longer sleeping, longer waking, beyond waking.

Rogers (1987) identified two theories derived

237

from this conceptual system, the theories of accelerating change and emergence of paranormal phenomena. According to the theory of accelerating change, change is continuous, innovative, and probabilistic, characterized by higher-frequency field patterning. This means that "norms" are not valid yardsticks. For example, this theory suggests that hyperactive children manifest accelerated field rhythms rather than symptoms necessitating medical intervention. The theory also suggests that the process of aging is rich in potentials for freedom, learning, and creative participation rather than decay and decline.

The theory of the emergence of paranormal phenomena suggests that experiences ordinarily labeled "paranormal," such as precognition, clairvoyance, or healing at a distance, are quite "normal" within a four-dimensional view of reality. Each human-environmental field process experiences a relative present that is four-dimensional, meaning that it is nonlinear and without space and time constraints. Four-dimensionality suggests nonordinary experiencing.

Unitary human beings, integral with the environment, can participate knowingly in change, actualizing some potentials over others (Rogers, 1970, 1986, 1987). Following this assumption Barrett (1986) derived a theory of power from the science of unitary human beings, defining power as "the capacity to participate knowingly in the nature of change characterizing the continuous (re)patterning of human and environmental fields" (p. 174). As manifestations of power, Barrett identified awareness, choices, freedom to act intentionally, and involvement in creating changes. Unitary humans *participate* in the mutual human-environment field patterning process rather than adapting to or altering the environment.

PROGRESSIVE WORLD VIEWS IN CONTEMPORARY THOUGHT

While Rogers's science has seldom been included in overviews of new paradigms, the Rogerian perspective is compatible with other systems of thought that share a progressive world view. This section explores the progressive world view as manifested in the works of two scientists, physicist David Bohm and chemist Ilya Prigogine, and the relationships to Rogers's science of unitary human beings. Emphasis is on the meaning of this view of "reality" to nursing. Bohm and Prigogine are only two of many authors whose works could be included here. I chose them because their ideas seem to parallel those advanced by Rogers and have appeared in print for over 10 years, stimulating lively scholarly debate.

David Bohm's World View

Wholeness and interconnectedness resonate through Bohm's view of the world (1980, 1985). He describes a "universe of unbroken wholeness" (Bohm, 1980, p. xv), supported by relativity and quantum theories. There is no dichotomy between consciousness and external reality, animate and inanimate matter; all are aspects of one, of the whole (Bohm, 1980; Bohm & Peat, 1987).

For the individual there is no distinction between mind and body. Bohm (1985) coined the terms *soma-significance* and *signa-somatic* to describe the flow of energy within soma (physical) and significance (mental, the meaning attributed to an experience), which he sees as two aspects of one process. Whereas "psycho-somatic" conveys the idea of two separate entities (mind and body) in mutual interaction with each other, Bohm suggests that they are manifestations of one reality. That reality is the flow of energy within the soma-significant and signa-somatic process. Rather than mind affecting matter and vice versa, "any change of meaning is a change of soma, and any change of soma is a change of meaning" (Bohm, 1985, p. 76).

Order and movement and flow, a process of enfolding and unfolding, are primary concepts for Bohm, whereas time and space are not. In keeping with the absence of dichotomies, Bohm does not distinguish order from disorder but talks of orders of varying degrees of complexity. This continuum flows from simple orders, which can be associated with prediction, to random orders of infinite degrees, which can only be associated with intuitive understanding to which a grasp of context (again, perception of the whole) is key (Bohm, 1980; Bohm & Peat, 1987). Bohm has described four kinds of orders—generative, implicate, explicate, and super-implicate—as a continuum which shades off into each other leaving no clear boundaries.

Bohm's work in quantum mechanics led him to formulate an interpretation of quantum theory. His interpretation suggests that there is a hidden order at work, rather than the picture of chaotic, disconnected particles presented in other formulations of quantum mechanics. Other physicists have been reluctant to consider his theory because it implies nonlocal interconnectedness that transcends traditional views of space and time (Bohm & Peat, 1987), a universe in which everything is fundamentally interconnected. This hidden order or source of wholeness is the implicate order in which all is enfolded (or nonmanifest) until unfolded and manifested in the explicate order, the three-dimensional world of experience that people accept as "reality." Because of the perceived dominance of the explicate order, the world is seen as composed of elementary particles or building blocks that are independent of each other and can be assembled to form a whole entity. The implicate order, however, suggests a very different reality, one of undivided wholeness in which parts are derived only as abstractions of the whole (Bohm, 1980).

The generative order, fundamental to nature and consciousness, is a more inward order that facilitates the expression of creativity. The generative and implicate orders form the actual ground of all experiencing (Bohm & Peat, 1987). The super-implicate order implies a higher ordering field which enfolds the implicate itself, "a super-information field of the whole universe" (Weber & Bohm, 1986a, p. 33). The super-implicate field is continuous, nonlinear, and nonlocal, meaning everything is connected at once (Bohm & Peat, 1987).

Seeing the whole versus seeing the part is integral to whether humans live their lives as separate or connected beings, alienated or empathic. Bohm suggests that it shapes one's attitude about world hunger, as well as the ability to live in a creative rather than destructive way (Bohm, 1985; Bohm & Peat, 1987).

Relationship to the science of unitary human beings

Both Rogers and Bohm start with a field view of the world that suggests openness, nonlinearity, and revised views of time and space. Wholeness and simultaneity of connections throughout the field imply integrality, what Rogers describes as a continuous, mutual process of human and environmental fields. Bohm describes this in his soma-significant and signa-somatic relationship process, which is actualized by meaning and intention. Energy is movement. It is given form by meaning, and meaning can only be grasped in the total context. This suggests that person and environment participate in a mutual process; changing the meaning can change the experience.

For example, imagery as a nursing modality for clients with cancer is congruent with Rogers's and, it would appear, with Bohm's view. Bohm (Weber, Bohm, & Sheldrake, 1986) stated, "the aim to be whole inspires the search for a coherent meaning" (p. 123), noting that an incoherent meaning implies people are unhealthy in some way. Because of his underlying view of wholeness, Bohm went further, stating that any part that is unhealthy implies that the whole is unhealthy "because we are all in each others' contexts" (Weber, Bohm, & Sheldrake, 1986, p. 123). In the Rogerian view we are integral with another's environmental field, and that person is integral with ours.

Rogers (personal communication, 1987) maintains that only motion and pattern are inherent in the field. Bohm (1980) discussed the primacy of motion of the field as the flowing process of enfolding and unfolding, "Undivided Wholeness in Flowing Movement" (sic) (p. 11). Pattern parallels order. Both see change as essential, continuous, innovative, and nondeterministic. Bohm does not use the term *negentropic* but discusses the process of change in a way similar to Rogers, that is, the universe is intrinsically creative and innovative, which he describes as a process of learning and experimenting, a participatory creating of reality (Weber & Bohm, 1986b).

Rogers's conceptualization of four-dimensionality resonates with the implicate order. Both are timeless

(Rogers, 1986, 1987; Bohm, 1980; Weber & Bohm, 1986a). Rather than a linear progression, time is flowing movement, as is space (Weber & Bohm, 1986a). The three-dimensional or explicate view of time and space are only abstractions; people abstract events and boundaries from the flow and think of them as the reality. The implicate or four-dimensional view is nowhere yet everywhere; "elsewhen" rather than now, earlier, or later.

Unity in diversity, or the idea of the universal and the particular, is another theme in common. The individual's patterning is unique, probabilistic, and innovative, yet relative diversity in unitary human patterning can be summarized through Rogers's description of the manifestations of field patterning, noted earlier. The principles of homeodynamics form the "ground" of emergence for human-environmental field patterning. Bohm sees true individuality emerging only when the person is grounded in the whole; a fragmented self/whole perception means a fragmented self. This is a different view from that offered by Rogers, who sees the unitary human as always whole.

Ilya Prigogine's World View

Wholeness, order, irreversibility, diversity, innovative change, and a reconceptualization of time characterize Prigogine's work (Prigogine, 1980; Prigogine & Stengers, 1984; Weber & Prigogine, 1986). Like Rogers and Bohm, Prigogine (Prigogine & Stengers, 1984) identifies the emergence of a new world view in which a central thesis is the unity of person and nature. It signals a move away from the mechanistic conceptualization of person and universe. Reality is conceived as a participatory process, that is, there is no "objective observer."

Prigogine's work focuses on the second law of thermodynamics, which postulates an increase in entropy (increase in disorder, depletion of energy) and gradual breakdown of systems. He demonstrates that this works in the mechanical world of at-equilibrium conditions but not in the living world. Living systems are open and dynamic, thus far-from-equilibrium. He calls such systems "dissipative struc-

tures" which, by their very interaction with the environment, dissipate the entropy and increase in complexity rather than decay into simpler structures. The processes described are not mechanistic or predetermined but stochastic or random processes that are inherently creative.

Prigogine (1980) and Prigogine and Stengers (1984) offer a new view of the second law of thermodynamics based on the concepts of probability and irreversibility, which implies randomness, as the basis for an evolutionary paradigm in physics, the physics of becoming. Irreversibility and nonequilibrium are the sources of order, bringing "order out of chaos" (Prigogine & Stengers, 1984, pp. 287, 292). This means that matter at equilibrium conditions behaves like separate particles that only know their own neighbors and are acted on by short-range forces, but matter at far-from-equilibrium conditions is interconnected by a pattern of long-range correlations. "Local" events reverberate throughout the whole system.

At nonequilibrium conditions sudden shifts occur, giving rise to bifurcations (branching). Symmetry does not exist. For example, billiard balls are molded into a triangle by the rack. The balls are at equilibrium until struck with the cuestick. Sudden shifts then occur, with the balls rushing off in different directions, creating a complex, asymmetrical, dynamic pattern with multiple options for play.

Nonequilibrium also breaks the symmetry of the classical view of time as a straight line containing past, present, and future. Prigogine describes time as an irreversible arrow containing the past and the present; the future is not yet there, for "time is creation" (Weber & Prigogine, 1986, p. 190).

Relationship to the science of unitary human beings

According to Rogers (1986, 1987), openness and pattern are building blocks of the science of unitary human beings. To be open means to be infinite; person and environment are postulated to be coextensive with the universe. Prigogine acknowledges this link of person and nature. In emphasizing this interdependence he believes it may be possible to show that there is no dichotomy between life and nonlife, between the biological and the mechanical, with these separated in some way from the human domain; "we are embedded in the world as a whole (Weber & Prigogine, 1986, p. 186). Prigogine's dissipative structures are open systems whose very interaction with the environment means that they grow in complexity and diversity. Nothing is predetermined. Indeed, predeterminism, with the implication of absolute knowledge, fosters intolerance and violence (Weber & Prigogine, 1986). The phrase, "the reenchantment of nature," appears in Prigogine and Stengers' book (1984) and the title of Weber's dialogue with Prigogine (1986). It is intended to convey the sense of wonder and awe, the ability to see entirely new options, that accompanies the introduction of diversity and innovation in the new world view offered in his work.

Prigogine's reconceptualization of the second law of thermodynamics supports Rogers's view of change in the principle of helicy as innovative, probabilistic, and characterized by increasing diversity and of the continuous mutual human-environmental field process in the principle of integrality. His concept of irreversibility parallels Rogers' nonrepeating rhythmicities. In Rogers's view, for example, there is no such thing as regression. Movement is unidirectional, never flowing backward. Change is probabilistic, not predetermined.

THE MEANING OF A PROGRESSIVE WORLD VIEW FOR NURSING

The views described represent a radical shift in how people experience their reality. They entail a move away from a mechanistic, reductionistic view in which (a) the whole is seen as an assemblage of parts that are interchangeable (donor organs, the artificial heart); (b) the cell is a basic building block; (c) prediction and control are both possible and desirable; and (d) the scientific ideal is the objective observer, separate from that which is observed, whose methods yield some ultimate truth. Homeostasis, equilibrium, and adaptation are concepts appropriate to this view.

The progressive world view, with its emphasis on wholeness, context, totally open systems, and continuous, creative change suggests that (a) the observer is not separate from the observed; (b) there is no ultimate truth, but multiple realities and options; and (c) prediction and control are neither possible nor desirable. The human being cannot be defined only by the physical body; well-being is to be examined in the broader context of the whole.

Rogers has suggested that conditions like cancer may be evolutionary emergents. Prigogine suggests that shifts at nonequilibrium conditions change the order of a system, moving it into a more complex pattern, a process characterized by turbulence while it is occurring. Because these shifts are random processes, prediction of "outcomes" is not possible. Perhaps cancer and acquired immunodeficiency syndrome (AIDS) are examples of such fluctuations for humankind. People with AIDS have begun to say, "Do not call me a victim; that tells me I am powerless. Do not assume I will die, for then I cannot hope to learn a way to live with AIDS." Perhaps what they are asking for are ways to participate in the patterning process, as for example a person with AIDS who spoke of his hope to learn to live with AIDS through the transforming medium of his art.

The life process is experienced differently in a progressive world view than in the traditional, mechanistic, reductionistic view. In nursing this is particularly evident in the science of unitary human beings, as can be seen in the phenomena identified for research within this world view. As examples, in 1979 Ference (1986) explored relationships among time experience, creativity, differentiation, and human field motion, developing a tool to measure the latter. Macrae (1982) examined time experience and human field motion in meditators and nonmeditators. Ludomirski-Kalmanson (1984) explored the experience of human field motion of blind and sighted individuals in the presence of red and blue environmental lighting (described briefly below). Cowling (1986) explored the relationships of mystical experience, differentiation, and creativity. Barrett (1986) derived a theory of power and a tool to measure power as knowing-participation-in-change. Sanchez

(1986) looked at empathy, diversity, and telepathy in mother-daughter dyads. McEvoy (1987) explored relationships among the dying experience, paranormal events, and creativity in adults. Paletta (1987) explored the manifestation of temporal patterning and developed the Temporal Experience scales.

Ludomirski-Kalmanson's Light Study

Color is one manifestation of environmental field patterning, and human field motion is one manifestation of the human field. Open fields are integral or continuous with each other. In a four-dimensional framework, sight is not a necessary prerequisite to the experience of color. Thus Ludomirski-Kalmanson (1984) hypothesized that the experience of human field motion is faster with blue light (short wavelength, high frequency) compared with red light (long wavelength, low frequency) in *both* sighted and blind adults. Human field motion is the "experiential, multidimensional position of the human energy field pattern" (Ference, 1979, p. 11).

The investigator covered the walls and floor of the experimental room with white cloth to provide 80% reflection of room light. Subjects wore black robes to provide maximum absorption of light. Ludomirski-Kalmanson randomly assigned subjects to the red and blue lighting conditions. She selected an exposure of 30 minutes to the first experimental light, 30 minutes to white light, and 30 minutes to the second experimental light. Following each exposure to the experimental lighting, the subject completed the Ference human field motion test (copies in braille for the blind subjects) and verbally responded to a short Post-Experimental Questionnaire. The data were analyzed by two-factor analysis of variance with repeated measures. Her hypothesis was supported ($p < .001$).

The ability to experience light is not dependent on the ability to visually perceive light. As the science of unitary human beings suggests, the unitary human is a field, not a physical body that processes stimuli by means of sense perception. The field is whole, regardless of whether visual perception is present or absent. As stated in the principle of integrality, human and environment are in continuous mutual process. This study supports the idea that the experience of human field motion is faster in an environment characterized by higher frequency light, regardless of whether or not subjects can see the light.

Nursing Practice

Rogers (1986, 1987) describes the continuous mutual process of human and environmental fields as one that changes continuously and creatively. People are integral with this continuous process; they flow with it. Thus they can participate knowingly in the flow or process of change.

Knowing participation means that individuals can "share in the creation of their human and environmental reality" (Barrett, 1984, p. 119). The concept of sharing in creating human and environmental reality, in participating knowingly in the process of change, suggests that people can participate knowingly in their own process of well-being. "Reality" is dynamic and continuously changing rather than static; it is a participatory experience rather than an objective one.

For example, a person knows that he or she is liable to become depressed during the winter months. Knowledgeable participation in the nature of the change process for this person might include full-spectrum lighting (approximates natural sunlight) in the home and work environments, energizing music, and ice skating or roller skating as a means of experiencing faster motion. The specific choices would vary for each person, but they reflect the idea of knowing participation in the human-environmental field process.

As previously mentioned, Barrett (1986) developed the Power as Knowing-Participation-in-Change tool using the indicators of "awareness," "choices," "freedom to act intentionally," and "involvement in creating changes." She uses this tool with clients in her private practice of health patterning. "Assisting clients with their knowing participation in change is called health patterning" (Barrett, 1988, p. 50). Client scores assist the nurse and client in "deliberative mutual patterning" of the environmental field "to promote harmony related to health events" (Barrett, 1988, p. 50), similar to the example of the person with depression.

The Nursing Service at the San Diego Veterans Administration Medical Center adopted the science of unitary human beings as the framework for nursing practice in 1983 (Link, 1988). This includes the introduction of nursing modalities such as therapeutic touch, relaxation, and imagery.

SUMMARY

The science of unitary human beings describes people as open systems in continuous process with their environment, forming a unitary whole that cannot be taken apart. People and environment are postulated to change in creative, probabilistic ways that cannot be predicted from knowledge of the "status quo." Knowing participation entails respect for autonomy and choice. The system is active, not reactive. The Rogerian science provides a knowledge base specific to nursing that assists in the provision of creative, knowledgeable nursing care to humankind.

REFERENCES

Barrett, E. A. M. (1984). *An empirical investigation of Martha E. Rogers' principle of helicy: The relationship of human field motion and power*. Unpublished doctoral dissertation, New York University, New York City.

Barrett, E. A. M. (1986). Investigation of the principle of helicy: The relationship of human field motion and power. In V. Malinski (Ed.), *Explorations on Martha Rogers' science of unitary human beings* (pp. 173–188). Norwalk, CT: Appleton-Century-Crofts.

Barrett, E. A. M. (1988). Using Rogers' science of unitary human beings in nursing practice. *Nursing Science Quarterly, 1*, 50–51.

Bohm, D. (1980). *Wholeness and the implicate order*. Boston: Routledge & Kegan Paul.

Bohm, D. (1985). *Unfolding meaning: A weekend of dialogue with David Bohm*. London: Ark Paperbacks.

Bohm, D., & Peat, F. D. (1987). *Science, order, and creativity*. New York: Bantam Books.

Cowling, W. R. (1986). The relationship of mystical expe-

rience, differentiation, and creativity in college students. In V. Malinski (Ed.), *Explorations on Martha Rogers' science of unitary human beings* (pp. 131–143). Norwalk, CT: Appleton-Century-Crofts.

Ference, H. M. (1979). *The relationship of time experience, creativity traits, differentiation, and human field motion: An empirical investigation of Rogers' correlates of synergistic human development*. Unpublished doctoral dissertation, New York University, New York City.

Ference, H. M. (1986). The relationship of time experience, creativity traits, differentiation, and human field motion. In V. Malinski (Ed.), *Explorations on Martha Rogers' science of unitary human beings* (pp. 95–106). Norwalk, CT: Appleton-Century-Crofts.

Link, V. (1988, June). San Diego VA nursing service adopts science of unitary human beings as the framework for nursing practice. *Rogerian Nursing Science News, Newsletter of the Society of Rogerian Scholars*. (Available from the Society of Rogerian Scholars, P.O. Box 362, Prince Street Station, New York, NY 10012).

Ludomirski-Kalmanson, B. G. (1984). *The relationship between the environmental energy wave frequency pattern manifest in red light and blue light and human field motion in adult individuals with visual sensory perception and those with total blindness*. Unpublished doctoral dissertation, New York University, New York City.

McEvoy, M. D. (1987). *The relationships among the experience of dying, the experience of paranormal events, and creativity in adults*. Unpublished doctoral dissertation, New York University, New York City.

Macrae, J. A. (1982). *A comparison between meditating subjects and non-meditating subjects on time experience and human field motion*. Unpublished doctoral dissertation, New York University, New York City.

Malinski, V. (1986). Further ideas from Martha Rogers. In V. Malinski (Ed.), *Explorations on Martha Rogers' science of unitary human beings* (pp. 9–14). Norwalk, CT: Appleton-Century-Crofts.

Paletta, J. L. (1987). *The relationship of temporal experience to human time*. Unpublished doctoral dissertation, New York University, New York City.

Prigogine, I. (1980). *From being to becoming: Time and complexity in the physical sciences*. San Francisco: W. H. Freeman & Co.

Prigogine, I., & Stengers, I. (1984). *Order out of chaos: Man's new dialogue with nature*. Boulder, CO: New Science Library.

Rogers, M. E. (1970). *An introduction to the theoretical basis of nursing*. Philadelphia: F. A. Davis.

Rogers, M. E. (1986). Science of unitary human beings. In V. Malinski (Ed.), *Explorations on Martha Rogers' science of unitary human beings* (pp. 3–8). Norwalk, CT: Appleton-Century-Crofts.

Rogers, M. E. (1987). Rogers's science of unitary human beings. In R. R. Parse (Ed.), *Nursing science: Major paradigms, theories, and critiques* (pp. 139–146). Philadelphia: W. B. Saunders.

Sanchez, R. (1986). *The relationship of empathy, diversity, and telepathy in mother-daughter dyads*. Unpublished doctoral dissertation, New York University, New York City.

Weber, R., & Bohm, D. (1986a). The implicate order and the super-implicate order. In R. Weber (Ed.), *Dialogues with scientists and sages: The search for unity* (pp. 23–49). New York: Routledge & Kegan Paul.

Weber, R., & Bohm, D. (1986b). Creativity: The signature of nature. In R. Weber (Ed.), *Dialogues with scientists and sages: The search for unity* (pp. 91–101). New York: Routledge & Kegan Paul.

Weber, R., Bohm, D., & Sheldrake, R. (1986). Matter as a meaning field. In R. Weber (Ed.), *Dialogues with scientists and sages: The search for unity* (pp. 105–123). New York: Routledge & Kegan Paul.

Weber, R., & Prigogine, I. (1986). The reenchantment of nature. In R. Weber (Ed.), *Dialogues with scientists and Sages: The search for unity* (pp. 181–197). New York: Routledge & Kegan Paul.

✳ EDITOR'S QUESTIONS FOR DISCUSSION ✳

What is the essential phenomenon of concern to the discipline of nursing according to Rogers? Discuss how unitary humans participate in a mutual human-environment field patterning process rather than adapting to or altering the environment. Discuss how the Rogerian perspective is compatible with other systems of thought that share a world view. What other persons advance a progressive world view? What kind of stature do D. Bohm, I. Prigogine, and R. Weber enjoy in their own discipline? What is the significance for nursing and the development of nursing knowledge to explore the works of these persons?

How widely accepted is the "world view"? How can or does the progressive world view examine well being in the broader context of the whole? What is the relevance for nursing of the progressive world view as compared with the traditional mechanistic reductionistic view? What is the relevance for the Science of Unitary Human Beings and the development of nursing knowledge of the studies by Macrae, Ludomiski, Kalmanson, and McEvoy? How can the Science of Unitary Human Beings be a framework for nursing practice? How does science of unitary human beings inform the art of nursing?

32

Holistic Nursing:

Implications for knowledge development and utilization

Maeona K. Kramer, Ph.D., R.N.

Without question, nurses claim to approach their practice from a holistic perspective. In its popular meaning, holistic nursing moves beyond disease management and requires that nurse and patient collaborate toward health. Collaboration with the intent of achieving holistic health mandates a focus on the whole person, including the environment within which individuals are located. Few clinicians would admit to focusing only on curing disease while ignoring social, psychological, and spiritual factors affecting recovery.

Nurses who practice holistically are acutely aware of impediments to maintaining a whole person perspective. Our "health care" system is, in reality, an "illness cure" system that reflects a nonholistic view of health as the absence of disease. Care fragmentation and institutionalized power relations within medical care facilities render patients and nurses powerless in working collaboratively toward a positive health state. Careful thought about the context of care delivery confirms the difficulty of providing holistic care (Freund, 1984).

If nursing is to embrace seriously the tenets of holism, impediments to holistic practice need scrutiny. Such an examination must take many directions, for multiple factors affect how nurses function. These include nurses' socialization within their educational system; the sociopolitical context within which health care is marketed and delivered; institutionalized power relations in the larger society, which are reflected in nurses-as-female and physicians-as-male roles; and knowledge development strategies within the profession.

What nurses individually and collectively "know" certainly affects practice. It follows that holistic practice will be more effectively realized if our professional efforts in relation to knowledge development and utilization are consistent with the tenets of holism. Knowledge that is consistent with holistic tenets will not remove all, or even most, barriers to holistic nursing. Nor can it be presumed that knowledge supporting holistic tenets will be easily transferred into practice (Freund, 1984). However, a basic examination of what holism implies in relation to processes and goals for knowledge development in nursing provides one means for realistically approaching the ideal of holistic care.

The collaboration of Peggy L. Chinn in formulating the ideas related to creation, expression, and evaluation of knowledge is gratefully acknowledged.

THE TENETS OF HOLISM

To state that holism connotes a "whole person view" is not wrong, but it does not discriminate the holistic perspective from whole person views that are not holistic. In order to comprehend the implications of holism for the development of nursing knowledge and its utilization in practice, the concept needs elucidation. Understanding holism's range of meanings clarifies its present and potential use within nursing. It should be recognized that regardless of careful efforts to clarify meaning, the term is destined to remain somewhat obscure. Like the concept of "quality," it can be understood and recognized but is described poorly in words. Despite a range of meanings and difficulty of capturing in language what holism implies, there is a central core of meaning that elucidates the basic qualities of the universe and living entities when they are labeled "holistic."

The words "holism" or "wholism"—for they are here synonymous—derive from "holos," which has a root meaning of "complete, entire, total." A central tenet of holism is that living organisms are unified and indivisible units. The words "unified" and "indivisible" are highly significant, implying that if "parts" or "elements" of a whole *are* designated, those parts are both interrelated and interdependent and form a unique totality. In the holistic perspective, the designation of "parts" and "whole" is relative (Lemko, 1981). "Parts" may refer to elements of a whole living organism, or "parts" may refer to individual living organisms within a larger environment. In nursing practice, discrete individuals are commonly viewed as the "whole" that comprises interrelated parts or elements. The elements of holism have often been expressed in adaptations of open systems theory. The holistic unit—an individual—is viewed as interrelated to larger system structures such as a family, community, social system, or universal consciousness. Thus a common theme within various versions of holism is a *connectedness* of wholes and parts, however designated, and the recognition that *any unit is simultaneously both whole and part*.

The elements of holism further imply that the interdependent "parts" of an organism critically determine the nature of the entire unit. When the parts of any whole are in interrelationship, they exhibit characteristics or behave in ways that are not evident when the unity is broken. Thus in a holistic view, the whole cannot be understood by the isolated examination of parts. If parts are isolated in an attempt to understand them, the interrelationships—and therefore the whole—no longer exist and the characteristics of the whole are no longer evident. This feature of holism is the basis for the common phrase, "the whole is greater than the sum of its parts." The unique behavior characteristic of unified wholes, termed "synergy," may be thought of as the "something greater" or perhaps the more neutral "something different" about the whole that is not expressed by a study of parts (Cmich, 1984). Thus holism is not an ideology captured by viewing wholes as the additive sum of separate parts. That is, in holism interrelatedness coexists with interdependence and the organism is not just a living machine.

The synergistic behavior exhibited by holistic organisms tends toward increasing complexity or negentropy (Rogers, 1970). When holism is embraced, a view of matter, life, and mind is also assumed. In this view life is not fixed, constant, and unalterable, but rather it is changing and active, creating new patterns that are expressed by the unified whole.

HOLISTIC HEALTH

Not surprisingly, the tenets of holism and the assumptions about the nature of reality that it makes are reflected in the holistic view of health. Nursing's long-standing emphasis on health and caring and de-emphasis on curing reflects its claims of holism. Three central themes related to health emerge from the tenets of holism: (a) health is a reflection of the whole individual; (b) health is active, changing, and creative; and (c) health is characterized by progressive harmony and integration within a naturally healing organism (Cmich, 1984; Edlin & Golanty, 1982; Gross, 1980). These themes lay the foundation for understanding the role and focus of knowledge development for holistic nursing practice.

A holistic health focus requires viewing the living

organism as a unit with both health and ill-health reflecting throughout its entirety. Thus attention to an ill "part" must be tempered by a view to the whole. Not only will the properties of the parts continue to integrate to create a new and unique whole, but the whole will also determine the interaction of the parts, including the features of an "ill" part. Although easy to say, it remains difficult to maintain this whole person view, for it requires attending to elements and whole "all at once." A holistic view of health, nonetheless, requires a perspective on multiple interactions among and between parts as making up a unique indivisible unit.

In a holistic perspective, the unique indivisible unit is active and creative. That is, it continually changes in novel ways. Health, therefore, is not a static state but a dynamic process reflecting continual change in the person's life. Wellness, despite shared commonalities across individuals, remains unique to the person and is an expression of integrated wholeness. In the holistic view, the negentropic change of increasing patterning and complexity is characterized by a progressive harmony and integration within the person and between the person and the environment (Cmich, 1984). Thus the tenets of holism, when applied to holistic health, become translated into assertions or implications that the continual change of a holistic organism is a naturally healing change that is in a good and valued, that is, "healthy" direction. The reader should be aware that there are challenges to the point of view that the creative change of holistic organisms is in a valued direction (Woodhouse, 1981). Nonetheless, in the holistic view of health the goal is not to return the person to a previous state of "health," for that is not possible anyway, but rather to assist the individual toward a new "level" of health. The holistic view holds the individual ultimately responsible for health, and individuals are deemed both capable and responsible for choosing experiences that will enhance health. In the holistic view, the health care provider is not in a detached power position in relation to clients. Rather, both are active and committed participants in enhancing growth toward health. The provider may have information of benefit to the client for making health-related choices, and provid-

ers are viewed as responsible for collaboratively sharing such information.

In summary, the holistic organism—for our purposes a human individual—is an indivisible whole. Parts, if designated, are interconnected interdependently to produce unique whole behavior that is not evidenced by separate parts. Moreover, this organism is both part and whole simultaneously, that is, part of a larger whole and whole in and of itself. The unique behavior exhibited by the human individual is negentropic in nature, meaning it changes in the direction of increasing patterning and complexity. Health for the holistic organism is an alterable process. Through client-provider collaboration, the individual is not only cared for in a traditional sense but moved toward options that enhance freedom and responsibility in choosing health. Curing disease does not assure health nor equate with it. Rather, a progressive harmony and integration within a unified, naturally healing whole reflects health.

NURSING'S KNOWLEDGE DEVELOPMENT TRADITION

The tenets of holism and subsequent implications for holistic health provide a healthy challenge to standards for knowledge development in nursing. Empirical science represents nursing's predominant inquiry mode, and although necessary, it is an insufficient guide for holistic practice. Development of knowledge for holistic practice will require not only a departure from the predominant value for empirical knowledge, but it will demand developing processes for creating, representing, and evaluating other knowledge patterns.

Traditional scientific empiricism was based in a worldview that spawned knowledge development approaches consistent with it. The worldview underlying scientific empiricism was not holistic, but atomistic. Atomists held that discrete units of sensory data were the ultimate source of knowledge. These sense data were directly observable units with behavior that was separate from and unaffected by the observer. The atomistic parts making up the whole unit were governed by linear time, and the separateness of the parts allowed for dichotomization. With dichotomization, counting of units was possible and number counts expressed in statistics became the basis for making decisions about the truth or falsity of supposed causal relationships formulated as hypotheses. The features of atomism perpetuated a science that regarded the parts as appropriate objects for study, and knowledge of the parts translated into probability predictions about the whole.

The demise of traditional empirics as the *supreme* form of knowledge occurred, in part, when the observation of finer and finer discrete units revealed errors in the epistemic base. To reiterate, traditional empirics refers to science embodying assumptions and processes necessary to establish causal relationships. Increasing sophistication in investigating the empirical, largely caused by technology, in combination with discoveries in modern physics eroded the supremacy of the concept of linear time and, subsequently, of causality. The singular existence of discrete atomistic units and finity was shown to be empirically unsound. Simply put, at one level of observation, there were no basic units of sense data that could be observed independently of the observer. Instead a world of interchanging mass and energy, in which observer altered observed and in which time was relative, was revealed. In summary, empirical science perpetuated a vision of reality that assumed objective observables, physical dichotomies, assumptions of linear time, and the supremacy of parts in the quest for empirical generalizations about the whole of physical reality.

Nursing adopted the methods of traditional science for generating knowledge, despite their inadequacy to answer important practice questions. During the late 1960s, nursing literature began to reflect a strong bias toward empirical science. The scientific model of knowledge development had produced dramatic technological and humanitarian advances in society. Nursing embraced it as a way to develop nursing's scientific base and achieve rank and status with other academic disciplines.

Despite recognition of the value of other knowledge patterns in nursing and their continued use in practice, remnants of a primary value for traditional science are quite evident in nursing today. Priority is given to experimental research approaches and the search for causal relationships in controlled contexts by hypothesis testing. Rather than valuing descriptions of phenomena, there are strivings to go "beyond" descriptions and quantify variables using valid and reliable instruments. Although the foregoing represents an extreme view within nursing, both our values and preoccupations provide evidence of leanings toward a primary value for empirical science.

It merits mention that the methods and goals of traditional empiricism changed considerably as its limitations were uncovered and it was applied to human sciences such as nursing. For example, empirical knowledge came to include descriptive research findings, "descriptions" resulting from application of phenomenological methods, grounded theory, as well as products of experimental research. Despite a liberalization of what constituted empirical approaches, empirics as the only approach to knowledge development remained insufficient, and nursing was never very successful in bringing "scientific" knowledge to bear on practice. Although multiple reasons for this phenomena may be cited, a plausible explanation is that the holistic concerns of nursing could not be fully answered by embracing an empiricist approach to knowledge development. Regardless of how liberal the view of empiricism, the underlying view of reality it assumed was partial. The products of empirical science were meaningful and useful within a reality in which discrete units were observable, linear time could be assumed, and language could express that reality. However, nursing realities without these features existed, and different approaches to knowledge development needed to be named and recognized as valuable.

Carper (1978) has suggested that nursing utilizes and requires knowledge patterns in addition to empirics. A major significance of Carper's work is that it named knowledge patterns other than empirics at a time when examining and legitimating knowledge forms different from the products of traditional science was of interest. It is noteworthy that Carper's original patterns included empirics—and thus a version of traditional science. Since scientific empiricism is a useful approach to knowledge development for holistic health promotion, the suggestion is not to abandon it. The notion of retaining empirics may seem paradoxical when the tenets of holism and the requirements of empirics are scrutinized. Nonetheless, nursing will benefit from considering how empirical knowledge that is more consistent with the tenets of holism might be created. In considering "holistic empirics," holism suggests two things: empirical knowledge must be as consistent with holistic tenets as possible, and it must be integrated with other patterns of knowledge to yield goals consistent with holistic health.

HOLISM: IMPLICATIONS FOR EMPIRICS

Summarizing from Carper's (1978) work, empirics—in this instance, the science of nursing—is knowledge representing abstracted generalities. It is mediate, that is, it consists of knowledge acquired and transmitted through the understanding of meaning associated with commonly held language symbols. Empirical knowledge is public, verifiable, and common.

Empirical knowledge is created through attempts to understand reality through its description, explanation, and prediction (Chinn & Jacobs, 1987). Thus, empirics accrues by systematically accounting for an empirical—or sensory perceivable—reality. This "accounting for" process is often traditional experimental or descriptive research. However, it also may be an "accounting for" using methods that fall outside accepted meanings of research. The research products and descriptions constituting empirics are often thought of as evolving into theory, or from theory, but not all empirical knowledge is generated out of or moving toward theory. Although empirical knowledge is commonly expressed in nursing as theories and conceptual frameworks, facts and nonfactual interpretations of reality also constitute empirical knowledge. What makes empirics "empirics" is its accrual from direct or indirect sensory experience, its expression in language that is structured and linear in form, and an appeal to common sensory experience to render it "good." The public and common features of empirics rely on the assumption that meaning of language symbols used to express empirical knowledge is shared across knowers. The

assumption that empirical sensory experience is similarly experienced and described across persons forms the basis for the valued characteristic of reliability. Validity, also important to judging empirical knowledge, implies that such knowledge describes, explains, and predicts the reality to be understood.

Clearly some nursing realities conform to the requirements of empirics. Empirics is useful in accounting for phenomena that have some stability across persons and time and that can be captured and expressed in language. There are patterns in our practice that recur, and knowledge of past occurrences recovered through application of empirical knowledge development processes is useful in shaping the present and future.

Empirical knowledge created that is consistent with holistic care goals would require some alteration in expectations held for empirical knowledge. First, the notion that empirical knowledge is useful for "control" of empirical reality needs to be abandoned. Retaining description, explanation, and prediction as uses for empirics remains appropriate, for these descriptors characterize how empirical knowledge enhances understanding of empirical realities. Although "control" may seem a suitable role for knowledge, it implies a completeness of structured knowledge that is practically unachievable in a holistic universe. Moreover, expecting to control some reality named "health" implies health is a static end state, rather than an ongoing process.

Secondly, empirics as a tool for holistic health care is inconsistent with structuring the purposes for empirical knowledge hierarchically. This hierarchy is classically expressed as descriptions leading to explanations that, in turn, form a foundation for predictions. For empirics to be consistent with holism, descriptions need to be valued for the knowledge they impart, and not seen as the first step to explanatory and predictive knowledge. When the purposes of empirical knowledge are viewed as evolving only hierarchically, the implicit assumption is that for observed phenomena there is only one description, explanation, and prediction possible that is connected to a stable reality base. Holism supports the view that there are multiple descriptions of the same phenomena, as well as multiple explanations and predictions not connected to a stable reality base. Although some descriptions may be incorporated into explanations that then constitute the basis for predictions, such hierarchically developed knowledge does not constitute the sum total of empirics. It is quite possible to evolve clinically useful and valuable predictive knowledge without first describing and explaining the underlying phenomena. A focus on the hierarchical steps of first describing, then explaining, and finally predicting phenomena detracts from the development of useful predictive knowledge. Moreover, a shift toward viewing empirics as enhancing understanding is facilitated if requirements for its hierarchical evolution are abandoned.

Thirdly, a holistic view of empirics will require recognition of the limitations of language in establishing meaning for underlying ideas within empirical knowledge forms. Language is said to be limited because our words and symbols are insufficient to capture the complexity of nursing's practice reality. For example, imagine encountering a hospitalized client who is acutely ill with overwhelming sepsis. Imagine further, attempting to describe and explain in words the person's coping behavior. Although some aspects of coping can be captured in language, the coping experience is so complex and dependent on interacting and changing situational variables that it cannot be fully conveyed in words. Also the meaning associated with language expressions contained in empirical knowledge forms are not givens, but are deliberate choices. Health within theories used in nursing, for example, can mean a condition that is the opposite of illness or a condition that can coexist with illness. In many ways, the broad abstract concepts of importance in nursing, such as health and coping, provide particular difficulty in making choices that communicate meaning since they do not have a direct object focus. A recognition of the language limitations undergirding empirical knowledge demystifies it and renders unconditional acceptance less attractive. More importantly, acknowledging language limitations legitimizes the development of multiple language representations for similar phenomena. The development of multiple representations for the same phenomena supports the holistic notion that the experiences of humans across contexts and time differ. In addition to alter-

ing expectations for empirics as a knowledge form, holism mandates some changes in approaches to empirical knowledge development.

Traditional experimental research as a process for creating empirical knowledge proves difficult to reconcile with the tenets of holism. Indeed, it can be argued that assumptions undergirding traditional scientific methods are incompatible with holism. Experiments require narrowing the research focus and stripping away contextual factors interfering with manipulation of independent variables. In short, in experimental research the focus is on isolated parts. Most devastating to holism, traditional scientific methods assume that the empirical reality being observed is static or slow to change and can be observed by a detached knower.

Regardless of arguments that traditional science can never be holistic, there are some methodological choices to be made that are significant to knowledge development for holistic practice. First, "holistic empirics" requires that the part be studied in relation to the whole—not the part in relation to another part. This point is critical, for in holism the whole is not the additive or linear sum of parts. Rather, the whole determines the parts and their characteristic ways of behaving (Kitchener, 1982). Secondly, variables should be operationalized as "holistically" as possible. In research that requires isolation and definition of variables for observation, variables isolated for study may be those easy to observe or those for which there is a convenient measure. When measures of convenience are used, they may not represent the variable well. If the study of parts in relation to the whole is to become possible in research, ways must be created to capture meaningfully and express the characteristics of both parts and whole. Concept clarification techniques, particularly concept analysis, has great potential for elucidating meaning of "holistic" variables. Through application of concept analysis techniques, presently used indicators of organismic behavior are confirmed and new indicators are created.

When empirics is viewed as only one form of knowledge that must be integrated with other knowledge patterns to promote holistic health outcomes, the mandate to create outcome variables for experimental research that reflect total organismic behavior can be challenged. Rather than "whole organism variables," "part of person" variables that reflect holistic health, such as acceptance of change, self-awareness, or self-responsibility, may be more appropriate. To the extent that "whole organism behavior" expresses holistic health, it is important in the pursuit of significant empirics. However, utilizing "whole person variables" in research may be less useful to practice than utilizing "part of person variables" that are clearly related to holistic health.

A third suggestion to facilitate traditional empirics more consistent with holism is to account for factors affecting function of the whole organism. Such factors should be described and interpreted in relation to experimental research findings. Variables affecting organismic function may also be left to occur naturally so that underlying empirical patterns can emerge during study. Such an experimental environment may approximate reality more closely and result in a more useful research product.

It merits mention that all forms of empirical knowledge are needed to facilitate holistic practice. Schultz (1987) has argued that a holistic view of humans requires methods that are both qualitative and quantitative. Descriptions—factual and phenomenological—historical analyses, and multiple other empirically based interpretations of reality will broaden our understanding of holistic nursing care. Focusing efforts for empirical knowledge development on traditional scientific approaches severely limits the spectrum of empirical events about which knowledge accrues.

Changing or refocusing our view of empirics, that is, broadening, demystifying, and placing it on equal footing with other knowledge patterns, removes the urgency to make empirics a complete knowledge pattern. Refocusing our view allows us to consider how ethical, personal, and esthetic knowledge—the three remaining knowledge patterns—are vital to holistic nursing practice (Carper, 1978).

INTEGRATION OF EMPIRICS WITH OTHER KNOWLEDGE PATTERNS

Health, in the holistic view, is an expression of integrated wholeness. Clearly the absence of illness or disease is not an indication of health. The healthy person is one who changes with life's challenges and takes initiative to be responsible for herself or himself. Healthy persons have a sense of meaning and purpose in life. A holistic care provider promotes these characteristics in clients (Cmich, 1984; Gross, 1980). One of the first things notable from this formidable summary of holistic health indicators is that none of these "features" can be given to or conferred on another person. Nor are they features nursing will necessarily be able to recognize as present, given their normative and abstract nature and considering the time span clients are cared for in many nursing care contexts.

Asserting the promotion of holistic health as a focus for nursing raises the fundamental and difficult question: What do we do? To answer, it is the enhancement of freedom and choice that heightens self-awareness and one's experience of harmony and integration that underpins holistic health (Lemko, 1981). Freedom and choice as holistic health goals for nurses do not summarily negate nursing's curative dependent role, but rather include cure. Freedom and choice as health goals provide an option when cure, in the traditional sense, is not a possibility. Promoting choice and freedom requires that nurses teach, consult, care, collaborate, and advocate, to name a few traditional descriptors of nursing's role. It is not just what is done that makes care holistic, but it is also the intent with which care is approached.

The assertion that empirics must be integrated with other knowledge patterns implies that all are vital to enhancing choice and freedom in clients. Moreover, integration of diverse knowledge patterns mandates a focus on whole and parts "all at once." When empirics is "let go of" as a way to control health-related goals and subsequently integrated with ethical, personal, and esthetic knowledge, the holistic health ideals of freedom and choice can emerge. It follows that an understanding of the remaining knowledge patterns and their effect on holistic health needs clarification.

Ethical Knowledge

Ethics relates to matters of duty, rights, obligations, and moral imperatives. Ethics is invoked when it is necessary to make a decision about a deliberate voluntary action that is subject to the judgment "right" or "wrong" (Carper, 1978). Although ethical knowledge is communicable through language symbols it is not public, verifiable, and common in that legitimate disagreements can exist over whether or not the same course of action is ethical or unethical.

Ethical knowledge is useful for clarifying values and in advocating for clients and family. When one is considering what is "good" ethical knowledge, it is necessary to abandon the security felt in the realm of empirics. In ethics, repeatable sensory experiences, however broadly interpreted, do not render knowledge "good." Rather, in ethics, the question is whether the ethical knowledge is just, and dialogue—not research—is relied on for the answer. Although ethical knowledge can be expressed structurally in language as codes, standards, and normative-ethical theories, it also is expressed in descriptions of ethical decision making (Chinn & Jacobs, 1987; Jacobs-Kramer & Chinn, 1988). Integrating empirics with ethics implies, for example, that clients and families have choices regarding treatment options. Moreover, there is a collaborative understanding of the nature of the choices available. When ethical knowledge is ignored in practice, "choices" are forced on individuals, independent of or against their will. Thus what clients would have chosen and its outcome remains unknown. Although empirical predictions about what will follow from a given ethical decision can be made, for example, administering "heroic" measures to keep a client alive, whether or not such measures ought to be instituted is a different decision. Ideally, ethics will provide information about what ought to be done, which is not to imply comfort with any ought, while empirics provides information that allows for prediction of events likely to follow multiple courses of action. In the example cited, the two knowledge patterns must be knowledgeably integrated if freedom and choice and therefore health, on behalf of the client and family, is to be promoted.

Personal Knowledge

The personal knowledge pattern, named by Carper (1978), is awareness of self and others in relationship. It involves encountering and actualizing the self. Personal knowledge cannot be structured, as can empirics and ethics, and is expressed as the self. Personal knowledge accrues by focusing and attending to oneself in relation with others and is rendered good to the extent that one's authentic and disclosed selves are congruent. Not only is personal knowledge to be cultivated in the health care provider, but also in the client. Personal knowledge is the basis of personal authenticity, that is, being what one honestly is (Chinn & Jacobs, 1987; Jacobs-Kramer & Chinn, 1988).

Personal knowledge as a basis for authenticity is central to choice and freedom. Personal knowledge imparts comfort with risk taking, inherent in choosing freely. When humans are congruent, that is, acting authentically, pretenses leading to discomfort with self begin to dissipate. For nurses as care givers, pursuing personal knowledge strengthens the ability to assume a collaborative stance with a person in moving toward holistic health, particularly in inhospitable contexts. In a broad sense, personal knowledge moves nurse and client toward increasing self-awareness, which also enhances freedom and choice.

Esthetic Knowledge

Esthetics, the final knowledge pattern, is knowledge by subjective acquaintance. Whereas empirical knowledge involves the abstraction of generalities, esthetic knowing requires abstracting particulars. According to Carper (1978), this knowledge pattern represents an immediate knowing that is based on the gathering of specific and unique particulars into a balanced and unified whole, integrating those particulars and acting in relation to projected outcomes.

It is proposed that esthetics as a knowledge pattern is the synthesis of all other patterns—the expression of the total knowledge spectrum integrated into practice. Esthetics embodies and expresses the particulars or those aspects of care that are so situation-dependent that they cannot be known until the nurse is actually in the care situation. Although in a clinical encounter, esthetic knowledge is available from past nursing experience, during the actual encounter that knowledge is integrated with other knowledge patterns to form new patterns of engaging with clients, interpreting contexts and situations, and envisioning outcomes. To illustrate, imagine a nurse who on arriving to work assumes responsibility for an acutely ill person. Recall the earlier example of a client with overwhelming sepsis who is gravely ill. The nurse, before entering the person's room "knows" that he or she is in need of "rest," and the nurse intends to dim the lights in the room and attempt to reduce noise to provide a restful environment (empirics). The nurse also "knows" what actions would jeopardize the client's life and are to be avoided (ethics).

When the nurse enters the room, however, the client's body, clothing, and bed linens are found to be soiled with drying blood from a gastric hemorrhage, which occurred just before shift change. The nurse, although empirically "knowing" how critical the client's need for rest is, senses the personal distress felt by the client from an unesthetic physical state. As the nurse interacts with the patient, a sense of physical and emotional distress is communicated more fully (personal and esthetic knowledge). Thus rather than dim the lights and close the door to reduce noise, the nurse slowly and calmly bathes the client and changes the linens, allowing sufficient time for rest so as not to compromise unduly the client's energy. The nurse "knows" (esthetics) that ultimately the act of bathing and cleaning the immediate environment will calm the client. Thus the nurse recognized and integrated the particulars of this situation: the client's need for rest, distress communicated from soiled bedclothes and the person's soiled body, and a sense of the energy reserves of the client. The nurse changed a preconceived plan projecting that calm and rest would be the outcome for the client.

Esthetic knowledge finds expression in the art-act of nursing and, it is the art-act of nursing that is a proper focus for examining holistic nursing practice. Simply stated nursings' art-acts are what expert nurses "do" for and with clients. It includes not only what is done, but also the processes used in engaging with clients in care situations. Valid "holistic" empirics, just ethics, and coherent personal selves as separate knowledge patterns are not to be undervalued; however, achievement of the "final" practice goal must evolve from an examination of the art-act that integrates all patterns in practice (Jacobs-Kramer & Chinn, 1988). This emphasis on examining the art-act as the enfoldment of multiple knowledge patterns moves nursing away from its historical quest for structured knowledge about health.

Practitioners who are cognizant of integrating personal, ethical, and empirical knowledge esthetically are better able to approach the holistic health goal of enhancing choice and freedom, for themselves as well as for clients. Such practitioners are freed from the constraints of considering only one knowledge pattern as credible. Other patterns can be brought into consciousness and viewed as interacting with empirics to promote choice and freedom. A holistic care focus also challenges practitioners with the near impossibility of practicing holistically within hierarchical health-care settings. Attempts to realize a holistic care focus, with its mandate to integrate multiple knowledge patterns in enhancing choice and freedom, removes the blinders from our eyes. In seeing the vision, old ways of practice become more intolerable and means are found to facilitate holistic care. Restructuring the deeper social realities that limit realization of the ideal will take time. Recognizing this, it is suggested that nurses retain the vision of holistic nursing, doing *what* we can, *where* we can, *when* we can. Thus rather than being overwhelmed with the difficulty of maintaining a focus on holistic care, the efforts of countless nurses will unfold the vision into reality.

REFERENCES

Carper, B. A. (1978). Fundamental patterns of knowing in nursing. *Advances in Nursing Science, 1,* 13–23.

Chinn, P. L., & Jacobs, M. K. (1987). *Theory and nursing: A systematic approach* (2nd ed.). St. Louis: C. V. Mosby.

Cmich, D. E. (1984). Theoretical perspectives of holistic health. *Journal of School Health, 54,* 32–34.

Edlin, G., & Golanty, E. (1982). *Health and wellness: A holistic approach*. Boston, Science Books.

Freund, P. E. S. (1984). Reclaiming the body from social domination: Holistic medicine's limit and potential. *Psychology and Social Theory, 4,* 15–24.

Gross, S. J. (1980). The holistic health movement. *Personnel and Guidance Journal, 59,* 96–100.

Jacobs-Kramer, M. K., & Chinn, P. L. (1988). Perspectives on knowing: A model of nursing knowledge. *Scholarly Inquiry for Nursing Practice: An International Journal, 2,* 129–139.

Kitchener, R. F. (1982). Holism and the organismic model in developmental psychology. *Human Development, 25,* 233–249.

Lemko, A. (1981). Of holism, freedom, and the creative meaning of opposites. *ReVISION, 4*(1), 78–87.

Rogers, M. E. (1970). *The theoretical basis of nursing*. Philadelphia, F. A. Davis.

Schultz, P. R. (1987). Toward holistic inquiry in nursing: A proposal for synthesis of patterns and methods. *Scholarly Inquiry for Nursing Practice: An International Journal, 1,* 135–146.

Woodhouse, M. B. (1981). Holism and the foundations of morality. *ReVISION, 4*(2), 78–87.

✳ EDITOR'S QUESTIONS FOR DISCUSSION ✳

What are the tenets of holism and possible implications for developing nursing knowledge? What implications would the tenets of holism have for the conceptualization of health? How does Kramer's conceptualization of health as a dynamic process compare with that inherent in Lyon's thesis (Chapter 34)? Is it necessarily true that one cannot generate knowledge and at the same time answer important questions? If no, why have important questions not been addressed or answered in the development of nursing knowledge and nursing science?

Provide some examples whereby a liberal view of empiricism as suggested in this chapter would help the development of nursing knowledge. What are the potential conflicts between scientific empiricism and holism as approaches in knowledge development? How can the potential problems or issues be resolved? How can holistic practice benefit from considerations related to empirical knowledge development? Does Kramer's statement regarding what makes empirics "empirics" a reflection of the evolutionary or revolutionary process of knowledge develop-

ment as addressed by Sarah Fry (Chapter 28)? How does Kramer's usage of the term empirics compare with Menke's (Chapter 27) use? To what extent is Carper's use and definition of "empirics" justifiable? How does the term differ from or relate to empiricism? Discuss the extent parts have been addressed in relation to wholes in science. Discuss whether or not confusion is evident between "holistic practice" and the way knowledge is developed. Is scientific knowledge in and of itself sufficient to approach patients holistically? Provide examples whereby what is done in nursing practice does not necessarily make care holistic, but the intent in which care is approached is holistic. Should empirics be "let go of" as a way to control health-related goals? What other kinds of knowledge are necessary for nursing to develop a complete or whole knowledge for holistic practice? What examples are offered by Fowler (Chapter 4), Brown and Davis (Chapter 38), and Flynn and Davis (Chapter 39) that pertain to the integration of holism, empiricism, and ethics?

33

Conceptual Models and Rules for Nursing Practice

Jacqueline Fawcett, Ph.D., R.N., F.A.A.N.

The purpose of this chapter is to present a discussion of conceptual models and their implications for nursing practice. Three rules for nursing practice are identified and developed for the nursing models formulated by Dorothea Orem (1985) and Callista Roy (1984). The chapter continues with a discussion of theories and the need for the development of conceptual-theoretical systems of nursing knowledge.

CONCEPTUAL MODELS

The term *conceptual model*, and synonomous terms such as conceptual framework, conceptual system, paradigm, and disciplinary matrix, refer to global ideas about the individuals, groups, situations, and events of interest to a discipline. Conceptual models are made up of concepts, which are words describing mental images of phenomena, and propositions, which are statements about the concepts. A conceptual model, therefore, is defined as a set of concepts and the propositions that integrate them into a meaningful configuration (Lippitt, 1973; Nye & Berardo, 1981).

The concepts of a conceptual model are highly abstract and general. Thus they are not directly observed in the real world, nor are they limited to any specific individual, group, situation, or event. Adaptation is an example of a conceptual model concept. It can refer to all types of individuals and groups in a wide variety of situations.

The propositions of a conceptual model also are very abstract and general. Therefore they are not amenable to direct empirical observation or test. Some propositions provide the foundation for further development of the model; these are the basic assumptions of the model. An example of this kind of proposition is: People are rational beings. Other propositions are broad definitions of conceptual model concepts. Adaptation, for example, might be defined as the ability to adjust to changing situations. Because conceptual model concepts are so abstract, not all of them are defined, and those that are defined have rather loose definitions. Definitional propositions for conceptual model concepts, therefore, do not and cannot state how the concepts are observed or measured.

Still other propositions state the relationships between conceptual model concepts. This kind of proposition is exemplified by the following statement: Nursing intervention is directed toward management of environmental stressors.

This chapter is adapted from portions of Chapters 1, 7, and 9 of Fawcett, J. (1989). *Analysis and evaluation of conceptual models of nursing* (2nd ed.). Philadelphia: F.A. Davis.

The concepts and propositions of each conceptual model often are stated in a distinctive vocabulary. One model, for example, uses the terms adaptation and stress, and another uses the terms stability and forces. Furthermore the meaning of each term usually is connected to the particular focus of the model. Thus the same or similar terms may have different meanings in different conceptual models. For example, stressor may be defined as a negative stimulus in one model and as a positive, growth-promoting force in another.

USES OF CONCEPTUAL MODELS

A conceptual model provides a distinctive frame of reference for its adherents, telling them what to look at and speculate about. Most importantly, a conceptual model determines how the world is viewed and what aspects of that world are to be taken into account (Redman, 1974; Rogers, 1973). Conceptual models thus have the "basic purpose of focusing, ruling some things in as relevant, and ruling others out due to their lesser importance" (Williams 1979, p. 96). For example, one conceptual model may focus on interventions designed to help the person adapt to stressors, and another may emphasize the person's capacity for self-care.

The utility of conceptual models comes from the structure that they provide for thinking, for observations, and for interpreting what is seen. Conceptual models also provide a systematic structure and rationale for activities. Furthermore they give direction to the search for relevant questions about phenomena, and they point out solutions to practical problems. Conceptual models also provide general criteria for knowing when a problem has been solved. These features of conceptual models are illustrated in the following example. Suppose that a conceptual model focuses on adaptation of the person to external stressors, and it proposes that management of the stressor that is most obvious to the person leads to adaptation. Here, a relevant question might be: What is the most obvious stressor in a given situation? Anyone interested in solutions to problems in adaptation would focus on the various ways of managing stressors, and one would look for manifestations of adaptation when seeking to determine if the problem has been solved.

CONCEPTUAL MODELS OF NURSING

Conceptual models of nursing present distinctive perspectives of the phenomena of interest to the discipline of nursing. These phenomena are capsulized by four central concepts: person, environment, health, and nursing (Fawcett, 1984). "Person" refers to the recipient of nursing actions, who may be an individual, a family, a community, or a group. "Environment" refers to the recipient's significant others and surroundings, as well as to the setting in which nursing actions occur. "Health" refers to the wellness or illness state of the recipient of nursing actions. "Nursing" refers to the actions taken by nurses on behalf of or in conjunction with the recipient.

Conceptual models of nursing provide explicit orientations, not only for nurses but also for the general public. They identify the purpose and scope of nursing and provide frameworks for objective records of the effects of nursing care. Johnson (1987) explained: "Conceptual models specify for nurses and society the mission and boundaries of the profession. They clarify the realm of nursing responsibility and accountability, and they allow the practitioner and/or the profession to document services and outcomes" (pp. 196–197).

In summary, a conceptual model is composed of abstract and general concepts and propositions. These global ideas and statements constitute a view of the phenomena of interest to a discipline. Each conceptual model treats the relevant phenomena in a distinctive manner. Conceptual models of nursing present different perspectives of the person, the environment, health, and nursing.

CONCEPTUAL MODELS OF NURSING AND RULES FOR PRACTICE

A fully developed conceptual model of nursing guides all aspects of clinical nursing practice. The model tells the clinician what to look at when interacting with patients and how to interpret observations. It also tells the clinician how to plan interventions in a general manner and provides global criteria for evaluation of intervention outcomes. Three rules have been formulated to specify the domain of nursing practice and nursing processes encompassed by any given conceptual model. These rules represent an extension of Laudan's notion (1981) of the rules or norms of research traditions and Schlotfeldt's discussion (1975) of how a conceptual model influences research to the realm of nursing practice. More specifically, Laudan's and Schlotfeldt's ideas were adapted for nursing practice and restated in the language of nursing practice. The nursing practice rules are:

1. The first rule identifies the purposes to be fullfilled by nursing practice, as well as the general nature of the clinical problems to be considered.
2. The second rule identifies the settings in which nursing practice occurs and the characteristics of legitimate recipients of nursing care.
3. The third rule identifies the nursing process to be employed and the technologies to be used, including assessment format, diagnostic labels, intervention typology, and evaluation methods.

The rules for practice provide an outline of the content of a conceptual model of nursing that is relevant for clinical practice. They amplify, rather than replace, a systematic analysis of the historical evolution, concepts and propositions, and areas of major emphasis of a conceptual model. Furthermore they provide information that facilitates evaluation of the utility of a conceptual model for nursing practice. In particular, specification of rules permits an answer to the following question: "Is the practitioner able to make pertinent observations, decide that a nursing problem exists, and prescribe and execute a course of action which achieves the goal specified?" (Johnson, 1987, p. 197). Readers who are interested in the results of analysis and evaluation of conceptual models are referred to works by Fawcett (1989), Fitzpatrick and Whall (1989), George (1985), and Marriner (1986).

Rudimentary rules for practice have been presented for several conceptual models of nursing elsewhere (Fawcett, 1989). The next section of this chapter presents an expansion of that work for Orem's (1985) Self-Care Framework and Roy's (1984) Adaptation Model.

OREM'S SELF-CARE FRAMEWORK

Rules for nursing practice are evident in Orem's (1985) Self-Care Framework. She presented detailed lists of directives for nursing practice within the following five sets: (a) initial period of contact between nursing and patient; (b) continuing nurse-patient contacts; (c) the quality of interpersonal situations with patients; (d) the production of nursing; and (e) relationships of the nurse with other nurses and other health care providers. It is clear from these directives and the content of the conceptual framework that for Orem the first rule of nursing practice states that nursing practice is directed toward and contributes to facilitation and enhancement of patients' abilities to care for themselves. The first rule goes on to state that the clinical problems of interest are the patients' therapeutic self-care demands from their universal, developmental, and health deviation self-care requisites; self-care agency; and self-care deficits.

The second rule of nursing practice for Orem indicates that nursing care may be carried out in various settings, including but not limited to ambulatory clinics; acute care, critical care, obstetrical, psychiatric, and rehabilitation units; nursing homes; college health programs; and hospices. Furthermore Orem (1985) stated that nursing care may occur at three levels of prevention: primary, secondary, and tertiary. Universal self-care and developmental self-care, when therapeutic, constitute the primary level of prevention. Nursing care at this level includes assisting the patient to learn self-care practices that "maintain and promote health and development and [that] prevent specific diseases" (Orem, 1985, p. 192). Health-deviation self-care, when therapeutic, constitutes the secondary or tertiary level of prevention. Nursing care at these levels focuses on helping the patient learn self-care practices that "regulate and prevent adverse effects of the disease, prevent complicating diseases, prevent prolonged disability, or adapt or adjust functioning to overcome or compensate for the adverse effects of permanent or prolonged disfigurement or dysfunction" (Orem, 1985, p. 194). Legitimate recipients of nursing care are persons whose therapeutic self-care demand exceeds their self-care agency, that is, people who have self-care deficits.

The third rule of nursing practice for Orem specifies a nursing process encompassing three steps: (a) diagnosis and prescription, (b) designing and planning, and (c) producing care to regulate therapeutic self-care demand and self-care agency. The first step focuses on determining why the person needs nursing care. This requires assessment of basic conditioning factors, such as age, gender, health state, developmental state, sociocultural orientation, health care system variables, family system elements, and patterns of living; calculation of the person's therapeutic self-care demand; assessment of self-care agency; and identification of the person's self-care deficit. The nursing diagnosis in Orem's conceptual framework is stated with regard to the "existent level of self-care agency for meeting current and emergent demands and potential for continuing development or redevelopment of self-care agency" (Taylor, 1985).

The second step of the nursing process starts with the design of a system of nursing assistance. A nursing system "is a dynamic action system constituted from series and sequences of actions, produced by nurses as they engage in the diagnostic, prescriptive, and regulatory operations of nursing practice" (Orem & Taylor, 1986, p. 53). Orem (1985) identified three types of regulatory nursing systems: (a) wholly compensatory, (b) partly compensatory, and (c) supportive-educative. The choice of a nursing system is based on the answer to the question: Who can or should perform self-care actions? The wholly compensatory nursing system is selected when the patient cannot or should not perform any self-care actions, and thus the nurse must perform them. The partly compensatory nursing system is selected when the patient can perform some, but not all, self-care actions. The supportive-educative nursing system is selected when the patient can and should perform all self-care actions.

The selection of the appropriate nursing system is followed by selection of appropriate method(s) of helping or assistance. Orem (1985) identified the following five methods that a person can use to give help or assistance to others: (a) acting for or doing for another; (b) guiding another; (c) supporting another physically or psychologically; (d) providing an environment that promotes personal development; and (e) teaching another.

The planning component of the second step of the nursing process requires "specification of the time, place, environmental conditions, and equipment and supplies [as well as] the number and qualifications of nurses or others necessary . . . to produce a designed nursing system or a portion thereof, to evaluate effects, and to make needed adjustments" (Orem, 1985, p. 237). The plan specifies the organization and timing of tasks to be performed, allocates task performance to nurse or patient, and identifies methods to be used by nurses to help the patient.

The final step of the nursing process encompasses the provision of direct nursing care and decisions regarding the continuation of direct care in its present form or changing the form. Regulatory nursing systems are produced "when nurses interact with patients and take consistent action to meet their prescribed therapeutic self-care demands and to regulate the exercise or development of their capabilities for self-care" (Orem, 1985, p. 237).

ROY'S ADAPTATION MODEL

Rules for practice are inherent in Roy's (1984) Adaptation Model. The first rule of nursing practice is capsulized in Roy's statement (1987) about the influence of her conceptual model on nursing practice. She commented:

> As a practice discipline, nursing focuses on nursing's function of promoting adaptation, that is, nursing diagnoses, interventions, and outcomes for persons or groups. Nursing as a practice discipline can be seen from the point of view of the role of the nurse. Model-based practice helps look at how

nursing models are taught. It sheds light on the content of nursing. Implementing the model of nursing care in whole health care systems will require another area of expertise, both in implementation and in evaluation of the outcomes. Some of the outcomes are important in relation to what the model does for nursing, such as increasing autonomy, accountability, and professionalism in general, and in changing relationships with other disciplines. (p. 44)

Clinical problems include all ineffective responses to focal, contextual, and residual stimuli within the physiological, self-concept, role function, and interdependence adaptive modes.

The second rule of nursing practice for Roy indicates that nursing practice is appropriate in many different settings. Legitimate recipients of nursing care are individuals, families, groups, communities, and society. Recipients may be sick or well and may or may not be adapting positively.

The third rule of nursing practice for Roy puts forth a detailed nursing process. The first step is assessment of behaviors or first-level assessment. This step involves collection of data regarding the person's internal and external behavior. Behavior of particular interest to the nurse is "the person's responses to environmental changes that require further adaptive responses" (Roy, 1984, p. 46). The methods of assessment are identified as direct observation of behavior; objective measurement of behavior using appropriate tools, such as paper and pencil instruments and measures of physiological parameters; and interviewing to obtain subjective reports (Roy, 1984). Once the data are collected, the nurse must judge whether the behavior "is of concern to the nurse and/or to the person" (Roy, 1984, p. 49). Furthermore, "the nurse determines, in collaboration with the person, whether the behavior is adaptive or ineffective" (Roy, 1984, p. 49). Judgments are based on comparison of the person's behavior with known norms signifying adaptation. In areas where norms have not been established, general signs of adaptation difficulty are used as a basis for comparison. These signs, according to Roy (1984), are "identified as pronounced regulator activity with

cognator ineffectiveness" (p. 50). Some manifestations of pronounced regulator activity are increase in heart rate or blood pressure, tension, excitement, or loss of appetite. Manifestations of cognator ineffectiveness include faulty perceptual/information processing, ineffective learning, poor judgment, and inappropriate affect.

Roy (1984) maintained that the person should actively participate in the judgment about the effectiveness of behavior. She stated:

> The person is often the best judge of whether or not behavior is effective in coping with a given stimulus. . . . The nurse should always take the person's observations of his or her own behavior into account in making a judgment about whether the behavior is adaptive or ineffective. The range of adaptive responses is wide. Norms are broad and circumstances change the judgment about whether a behavior is adaptive or ineffective. (p. 50)

The second step of the nursing process, assessment of influencing factors or second-level assessment, involves assessment of the factors that influence the behaviors of concern to the nurse and the person. Ineffective behaviors are of interest because the nurse wants to change these to adaptive behaviors, and adaptive behaviors are of interest because the nurse wants to maintain or enhance them. Furthermore, "in situations where all presenting behaviors appear adaptive, it may be necessary to carry out second-level assessment to identify potential threats to that adaptation" (K. Des Rosiers, cited in Roy, 1984, p. 51). This step of the nursing process requires the nurse to prioritize the behaviors to be assessed. Roy (1984) based her priorities on the goals of the adaptive system (survival, growth, reproduction, and mastery) and offered the following hierarchy of importance for assessment of behaviors:

> (a) those that threaten the survival of the individual, family, group, or community; (b) those that affect the growth of the individual, family, group, or community; (c) those that affect the continuation of the human race or of society; (d) those that affect the attainment of full potential for the individual or group. (p. 58)

Once priorities have been established, second-level assessment involves identification of the focal, contextual, and residual stimuli that influence the behaviors of interest and contribute to adaptive or ineffective responses. Roy (1984) pointed out that the nurse can presume the influence of residual stimuli from theoretical knowledge and intuitive hunches. Residual stimuli become focal or contextual stimuli when their effects can be validated. She also advocated continued participation of the person in second-level assessment (Roy, 1984). She suggested using Orlando's deliberative nursing process (1961) to validate the relevant stimuli with the person. Thus the nurse should share her or his ideas of influencing factors with the person and receive confirmation or discuss the person's perception of the situation until agreement is reached.

The third step of the nursing process is nursing diagnosis, defined as "the nurse's interpretation of the assessment data that have been compiled" (Roy, 1984, p. 55). Three approaches to nursing diagnosis were given by Roy (1984). One method is to cluster the behaviors and influencing factors within each of the adaptive modes and to name each cluster with a label from a beginning typology of adaptation problems identified by Roy (1984). The second method is to again cluster the behaviors and influencing factors within each adaptive mode and to simply state the diagnosis as the behavior of concern with the most relevant influencing factors. This method "allows for the incompleteness of the typology of problems, and . . . it provides more specific indications for nursing intervention" (Roy, 1984, p. 56). The third method is to summarize all behaviors across adaptive modes that are affected by the same stimuli. Roy (1984) maintained that this method "recognizes the holistic functioning of the person and the interrelatedness of the adaptive modes" (pp. 56–57). Roy (1984) pointed out that nursing diagnosis may be used for both adaptive and ineffective behaviors. She also noted that labels approved by the North American Nursing Diagnoses Association may be used "as they relate to developments within the adaptive modes of the Roy model" (p. 57). Regard-less of the method and labels used, diagnoses are placed in a hierarchy of importance, using the priorities identified in the section on second-level assessment.

The fourth step of the nursing process is goal setting. The goal for nursing care is established from the behavioral description of the person's situation developed through first- and second-level assessments and nursing diagnosis. Goals are stated as behavioral outcomes of nursing intervention.

The fifth step of the nursing process is intervention or selection of approaches. This step involves management of stimuli that were identified as influencing factors to achieve the stated goals for nursing care. Management encompasses increasing, decreasing, maintaining, removing, or otherwise altering or changing relevant focal and/or contextual stimuli (Andrews & Roy, 1986). The focal stimulus is selected for management whenever possible because it is the primary influence on the behaviors of interest. If it is not possible to alter the focal stimulus, contextual stimuli are to be managed to raise the adaptation level. Roy (1984) advocated using the nursing judgment method outlined by McDonald and Harms (1966) as a basis for selection of which stimuli to change. Roy explained that the McDonald and Harms method

> is a way of listing possible approaches, then selecting the approach with the highest probability of achieving the valued goal. Combining this method with the Roy Adaptation Model, we can say that the various stimuli affecting patient behaviors are listed. Then the consequences of dealing with each stimuli are outlined. The probability of each consequence is determined. In addition, the values of the outcomes of the approach are judged. The approach with the highest probability of reaching the valued goal can then be selected. (1984, p. 60)

The sixth and final step of the nursing process is evaluation of the effectiveness of nursing intervention. The criterion for effectiveness of nursing intervention is whether the desired goal was attained, that is, whether the person exhibited adaptive behavior after the nursing intervention was performed.

The end result of this step is an update of the nursing care plan.

CONCEPTUAL MODELS AND THEORIES

The rules for nursing practice specified in the two conceptual models included in this chapter provide only general guidelines for nursing practice. The specifics of nursing assessment, diagnosis, intervention, and evaluation must come from middle-range theories, which are sets of concepts and propositions that are more specific and concrete than those of a conceptual model. Although the conceptual model may, for example, direct the clinician to look for certain categories of problems in adaptation, middle-range theories are needed to describe, explain, and predict manifestations of actual or potential problems of adaptation in particular situations. Similarly, middle-range theories are needed to direct the particular nursing interventions needed in such situations.

It is important to point out that a conceptual model is not a theory, nor is a theory a conceptual model. Conceptual models and theories are distinguished by the level of abstraction. More specifically, a conceptual model is an abstract and general set of concepts and propositions. A middle-range theory, in contrast, deals with one or more relatively specific and concrete concepts and propositions. Conceptual models are only broad outlines that must be specified further by relevant and logically congruent theories before action can occur. Thus all pragmatic activities of members of a discipline are finally directed by conceptual-theoretical systems of knowledge. The content of the three rules for nursing practice for each conceptual model, therefore, must be linked with appropriate theories before nursing practice actually can be undertaken. For example, a conceptual model may identify physiological needs as an assessment parameter, but it does not explain differences between normal and pathological functions of body systems in any detail. Such differences are spelled out in detail in more specific and concrete theories of physiology and pathophysiology.

SUMMARY

The construction of conceptual-theoretical systems of knowledge for nursing practice is guided by the content of three rules that encompass the domain of nursing practice and nursing processes inherent in a conceptual model of nursing. Theories are then linked with the conceptual model content and nursing practice ensues.

REFERENCES

Andrews, H. A., & Roy, C. (1986). *Essentials of the Roy adaptation model*. Norwalk, CT: Appleton-Century-Crofts.

Fawcett, J. (1984). The metaparadigm of nursing. Current status and future refinements. *Image*, 16, 84–87.

Fawcett, J. (1989). *Analysis and evaluation of conceptual models of nursing* (2nd ed.). Philadelphia: F. A. Davis.

Fitzpatrick, J.J., & Whall, A.L. (1989). *Conceptual models of nursing. Analysis and application.* (2nd ed.). Norwalk, CT: Appleton and Lange.

George, J. (Ed.). (1985). *Nursing theories: The base for professional nursing practice* (2nd ed.). Englewood Cliffs, NJ: Prentice-Hall.

Johnson, D.E. (1987). Guest editorial: Evaluating conceptual models for use in critical care nursing practice. *Dimensions of Critical Care Nursing*, 6, 195–197.

Laudan, L. (1981). A problem-solving approach to scientific progress. In I. Hacking (Ed.), *Scientific revolutions* (pp. 144–155). Fair Lawn, NJ: Oxford University Press.

Lippitt, G.L. (1973). *Visualizing change: Model building and the change process*. Fairfax, VA: NTL Learning Resources.

Marriner, A. (1986). *Nursing theorists and their work*. St. Louis: C.V. Mosby.

McDonald, F.J. & Harms, M. (1966). Theoretical model for an experimental curriculum. *Nursing Outlook, 14*(8), 48-51.

Nye, F.I., & Berardo, F.N. (Eds.). (1981). *Emerging conceptual frameworks in family analysis*. New York: Macmillan.

Orem, D.E. (1985). *Nursing: Concepts of practice* (3rd ed.). New York: McGraw-Hill.

Orem D.E., & Taylor, S.G. (1986). Orem's general theory of nursing. In P. Winstead-Fry (Ed.), *Case studies in nursing theory* (pp. 37–71). New York: National League for Nursing.

Orlando, I.J. (1961). *The dynamic nurse-patient relationship*. New York: Putnam.

Redman, B.K. (1974). Why develop a conceptual framework? *Journal of Nursing Education, 13*(3), 2–10.

Rogers, C.G. (1973). Conceptual models as guides to clinical nursing specialization. *Journal of Nursing Education, 12*(4), 2–6.

Roy, C. (1984). *Introduction to nursing: An adaptation model* (2nd ed.). Englewood Cliffs, NJ: Prentice-Hall.

Roy, C. (1987). Roy's adaptation model. In R.R. Parse, *Nursing science: Major paradigms, theories, and critiques* (pp. 35–45). Philadelphia: W.B. Saunders.

Schlotfeldt, R.M. (1975). The need for a conceptual framework. In P. J. Verhonick (Ed.), *Nursing Research I* (pp. 1–24). Boston: Little, Brown.

Taylor, S.G. (1985, August). *Dorothea Orem's framework*. Paper presented at conference on Nursing Theory in Action, Edmonton, Alberta, Canada (Cassette recording).

Williams, C.A. (1979). The nature and development of conceptual frameworks. In F.S. Downs & J.W. Fleming, *Issues in nursing research* (pp. 89–106). New York: Appleton-Century-Crofts.

✳ EDITOR'S QUESTIONS FOR DISCUSSION ✳

What is the purpose of conceptual models? What is the relationship between conceptional frameworks, models, and theories? How might the same and similar terms used in a conceptual model have different meaning for different models? To what extent does Newman illustrate an example of this in Chapter 30? What does Fawcett mean by rules for practice?

Can Fawcett's rules for practice be applied to any other proposed frameworks, models, or theories in nursing? May Fawcett's rules of practice be a means for bridging the gap between traditional science and application to practice? What relationship or application might there be between Fawcett's rules for practice and the development of diagnostic categories for nursing and the nursing diagnosis movement? What are the differences in how the rules are applied between the frameworks of Orem and the adaptation model by Roy? Does Fawcett actually apply her three rules for practice to the various frameworks or does she look at the various frameworks and models to determine whether or not the three rules of practice exist within a framework? Of the two nursing models (Orem and Roy) examples, which approach is inductive and which one is deductive? Does the fact that there are different numbers and steps involved in applying Fawcett's rule three to different models raise questions regarding the validity of the rules for practice?

34

Getting Back On Track:
Nursing's autonomous scope of practice

Brenda Lyon, D.N.S., R.N.

Some of you will say, "We've never been off track; in fact, the practice of nursing is right on track!" However, I believe that the necessity of using the modifier "autonomous" to speak of *nursing* practice at this point in our evolution tells an important story. It reflects that as a discipline we have for too long been sidetracked in our focus. None of nursing's foremost leaders in the past felt the need to use such words when defining the focus of nursing or its unique practice focus. Yet today it is necessary to clarify, in some manner, that when speaking of *nursing* practice we are not referring to the practice of medicine.

Over 130 years have passed since Nightingale (1859/1969) gave us direction by essentially defining nursing in the context of treating the person, not the disease. She said that she used the word nursing

> for want of a better. It has been limited to signify little more than the administration of medicines and the application of poultices. It ought to signify the proper use of fresh air, light, warmth, cleanliness, quiet and the proper selection and administration of diet—all at the least expense of vital power to the patient. (p. 8)

Furthermore she purported that the purpose of nursing "is to put the patient in the best condition for nature and act upon him" (p. 133). Despite the direction given to us by Nightingale, "we do not yet know exactly what nursing is" (Downs, 1988, p. 19).

Is it that the essence of nursing has not been defined, or is it that the real nature of nursing is too often adulterated for a variety of seemingly justifiable, although spurious, reasons? I believe it is the latter.

The adulteration of nursing and the resulting lack of consensus within the discipline on what we are about is our most serious and pressing, yet least attended to, problem. Lacking consensus, we lack unified direction in resolving our problems in both the educational and practice arenas. We get off track because we are not sure of what we are, and to compensate we try to be everything to everybody and pretend that all nurses have the same competencies in practice. Not having a clear and distinct identity, we often look like and feel like nobodies or, at best, substitutes for other health team members. By losing sight of who we are and what nursing is, we create an unnecessary sense of inadequacy and experience a paucity of pride in the discipline. Because we want more respect than we get and we want more status than we have, we often fight the wrong battles. We fight for prescription writing privileges and for third-party reimbursement for substitutive services, when the answer to what we need—an identity—lies in getting back on track.

The purpose of this chapter is twofold. One purpose is to discuss why we lack consensus on what nursing is, and thus get off the track of nursing's unique or autonomous scope of practice. Another purpose is to identify parameters of our autonomous scope of practice.

A LACK OF CONSENSUS

Why is it that we lack consensus on what nursing is? There are three underlying reasons that deserve particular attention. First, nursing's goal is to promote health (Nightingale, 1859/1969; *American Nurses' Association*, 1980), but what is health to nursing? Although health means more to nursing than the absence of disease (Newman, 1986), what is the "more" that we are uniquely concerned with as nurses? "A discipline is characterized by its distinct way of viewing phenomena" (Carnevali, 1984, p. 12). Yet nursing does not have a prevailing definition of health that reflects nursing's unique focus. Second, we tend to confuse autonomous action with the setting in which the practice takes place or the act of judgment. Thereby we erroneously believe that, when a nurse practices outside a bureaucratic setting or makes a judgment regarding the medical condition of a patient, the nurse is engaged in autonomous practice. Third, we do not agree on phenomena that are of unique concern to nursing, which makes us vulnerable to adopting knowledge from other disciplines (e.g., medicine) as nursing knowledge. Many in our discipline believe that there is nothing to know about nursing and that the answer to advancing nursing is learning more about medicine. The consequence is that knowledge development in nursing is hindered and we obscure nursing's unique contribution to society.

Definition of Health

With respect to a concept of health that reflects nursing's concern, Nightingale (1893/1949) asserted that "health is not only to be well but to be able to use well every power we have" (p. 6). Nightingale's definition focuses on how the person feels as well as his or her functional ability; it does not identify the absence of disease as an attribute of health. Very different from Nightingale's concept of health, medicine defines health as the absence of disease and measures health in terms of morbidity and mortality rates (Chapman, 1981; Thomas, 1981). There have been many attempts at moving away from medicine's concept of health. Dubos (1981) asserted that "health transcends biological fitness. It is primarily a measure of such person's ability to do what he wants to do and become what he wants to become; [it] implies an individual's success in functioning—" (p. 6). Like Nightingale and Dubos, many others have included how a person feels and the person's functional ability in a definition of health (Keller, 1981).

The definition of health in the social policy statement of the American Nurses' Association (ANA) is an example of an attempt to have a non-disease-related definition for nursing. Health is defined as "a dynamic state of being in which the developmental and behavioral potential of an individual is realized to the fullest extent possible" (ANA, 1980, p. 5). The ANA definition, like many others, is problematic, however, in that health is defined as an idealistic end point. A person who has not realized full potential does not have health.

Despite the existence of many nonmedical definitions of health, it is medicine's definition of health that "has pervaded most of our thinking" (Newman, 1986). Thus the prevailing practical concept of health is the absence of disease. Newman's proposed new paradigm of health (1986) evidences current dissatisfaction with the dichotomy between health and disease as well as with illness and health. She proposes that health is a dynamic manifestation of person-environment interaction and is a synthesis of disease and nondisease involving transformations conceptualized as expanding consciousness. The definition encompasses both the human experience of illness and the human experience of wellness.

It is common to equate illness and disease (Millstein & Irwin, 1987). Yet Nightingale (1859/1969) observed that illness and suffering "are very often not symptoms of the disease at all, but of something quite different" (p. 8). Viewing illness in the same manner, Kleinman (1981) purported that "the experience of a biological disorder is distinct from the disorder itself . . . patients with the same disease—a heart ailment, for instance—may experience different illness" (p. 19). However, in nursing we commonly conceive of illness in the same manner that medicine does and consequently view treating the disease as treating the illness. Likewise when a patient is ill, but no disease is found, there is a tendency to think that there is no justifiable reason for the illness.

It is imperative that we develop a definition of health that captures our unique focus and that can be operationalized. Such a definition might be: *health is the dynamic subjective quality of person-environment interaction that is expressed in a person's composite evaluation of the somatic sense of self and functional ability*. Somatic sense, as used here, encompasses both physical sensations and emotions; functional ability encompasses all functional abilities, for example, self-care abilities and cognitive and learning abilities. Emotions are considered somatic because they are feelings that have physical sensation as well as cognitive components. The composite evaluation of somatic sense and functional ability represents a subjective manifestation of the whole that falls within one of two quality domains: illness or wellness. Both illness and wellness are health conditions that can be experienced in the presence or absence of disease. The overall goals of nursing care would then be stated as: (a) promotion of wellness; (b) prevention of illness; and (c) resolution or cure of illness.

Illness, consistent with the proposed definition of health, would be defined as a dynamic subjective condition that is characterized by the experience of uncomfortable or unpleasant somatic sensations, or the inability to function at an optimal level, or both. Consistent with the proposed definition of health, the goal of nursing care for a person who is ill is to assist the person in eliminating or decreasing uncomfortable or unpleasant somatic sensations and to assist the person in reaching full functional potential.

Wellness is also a dynamic subjective condition. It is characterized by the experience of comfortable or pleasant somatic sensations accompanied by optimal functional ability. Nursing's goal in working with well persons is to assist them in maintaining wellness.

Defining health in the proposed manner makes illness and wellness, not disease, the target conditions to which nursing care is directed. When we confuse medicine's definition of health with a nursing-oriented definition of health, we get off track and focus on the diagnosis and treatment of disease.

Autonomy

Autonomy is universally recognized as a main attribute of a profession (Cogan, 1953; Flexner, 1915; Hughes, 1963; Parson, 1954; Wilensky, 1964). Autonomous practice is *self-directed* diagnosis and treatment. Self-directed means self-determined and controlled action that does not require authorization from another—simply put, it means ownership.

We often confuse the definition of autonomy with the setting in which the practice occurs and with the ability to make judgments. The confusion of autonomy with setting is captured in the following quote: "Whether perceived autonomy (of nurses) is a product of the work setting and its organizational features or whether nurses who possess greater independence choose to work in more autonomous settings remains to be determined" (Wood, Tiedje, & Abraham, 1986, p. 132). Nurse practitioners who function in satellite clinics are said to be functioning autonomously (Selby, 1986). The classification is erroneous. Regardless of setting, for each *medical* problem the nurse *treats*, the authority to do so must be delegated in some manner by a physician. Our focus on setting, however, is understandable since nurses are predominantly employed in a hospital setting where authority over working conditions and standards still primarily rests with administrators, doctors, and trustees. Furthermore it is not uncommon for the hospital or physicians, or both to assume authority over the diagnosis and treatment of phenomena that fall within nursing's unique domain. It is here where we need to continue to exert considerable effort in attaining control over our practice.

Another important factor that contributed to our confusion between "setting" and autonomous nursing action is the fact that the nurse practitioner revolution occurred as a response to the post-Vietnam-era shortage of primary care physicians. Nurses felt a responsibility to help in meeting society's need for primary medical care and moved in to fill the gap, often in satellite clinics. The provision of medical care was camouflaged by such phrases as, "extended or expanded scope of nursing practice." Because nurses were practicing outside the usual bureaucratic setting of a hospital, nurses were said to be practicing nursing autonomously.

The meaning of autonomy is also frequently confused with the ability to make judgments. For example, when a coronary care nurse makes a judgment regarding the presence of a cardiac arrhythmia, such a judgment is often viewed as an example of autonomous practice. Yet the nurse either refers the problem to a physician or treats the arrhythmia in a manner consistent with protocol established by a physician.

Both setting and the ability to make judgments are irrelevant when defining nursing's autonomous scope of practice. Regardless of where the nurse is practicing or what judgment the nurse is capable of making, if the nurse uses therapeutics for problems that legally require authorization from a physician, then the activity does not fall within nursing's autonomous scope of practice.

The practice of medicine has been traditionally and legally defined as the diagnosis and treatment of disease (Murchison & Nichols, 1970; Thomas, 1981). Acts of medical treatment can be classified into three general categories: (a) administration or prescription of medications; (b) surgical procedures (including breaking the skin); and (c) mechanical and electrical procedures applied to manipulate an internal pathology, for example, traction for a fracture and defibrillation for a life-threatening arrhythmia.

Nurses frequently and necessarily judge the medical condition of a patient and act on those judgments by the authority granted through delegation from a physician. The delegation occurs in many forms: policy, standing orders, protocols, or specific medical orders for a patient. The right of the physician to delegate acts that, if performed without authorization would constitute the unauthorized practice of medicine, is generally recognized. The registered nurse can and enters the treatment sphere of medicine on the proper delegation of such acts by a physician. In fact nursing, unlike any other discipline, has a social mandate for two scopes of practice: the medical scope that requires authorization to initiate treatment, and the autonomous nursing scope that does not require authorization. It is important to emphasize that a nurse's judgments about the medical condition of a patient and the medical treatment needed *are not devalued here*. Nurses have well-developed judgment abilities in the medical realm. We just need to call the judgments medical judgments because the treatment is medical and requires *medical* authorization. The distinction between medical and nursing judgment (diagnosis) is based on who bears primary responsibility for the action that is required in response to the diagnosis (Murchison & Nichols, 1970). Basic to the distinction and to the adjective used to describe the judgment is who can, in a self-directed manner, treat the problem. That is the basis for autonomous practice in any discipline. Autonomous nursing practice is the diagnosis and treatment of phenomena that nurses have the self-directed authority to treat.

Phenomena of Concern to Nursing

Nursing has experienced serious challenges from other disciplines and policymakers. Often the challenges occur because nursing does not have a well-recognized unique body of knowledge and purpose. For example, Freidson (1970) classified nursing as a lower-level medical profession, because most of what nurses learn in their educational programs is determined by the parameters of medical phenomena. He identified the dilemma of nursing as "to escape subordination to medical authority, it must find some area of work over which it can claim and maintain a monopoly" (p. 66). To have control over an area of practice, it is imperative that we articulate and study the phenomena that are of unique concern to nurses.

What phenomena are of unique concern to nursing? Definitions of nursing since Nightingale (1859/ 1969) have attempted to specify nursing's unique scope of practice, thereby identifying the domain boundaries of phenomena that are of unique concern to nursing. One hundred years after Nightingale defined nursing, Henderson (1964) defined nursing as

> primarily assisting the individual (sick or well) in the performance of those activities contributing to health, or its recovery (or to a peaceful death) that he would perform unaided if he had the strength, will, or knowledge. It is likewise the unique contribution of nursing to help the individual to be independent of such assistance as soon as possible. (p. 62)

From 1859 through the 1970s the prevailing notions (Abdellah, 1969; Henderson, 1964; McManus, 1950; Nightingale, 1859/1969; Orem, 1980; Wiedenbach, 1964) about the essence of nursing carried the same unifying theme, that is, assisting a person—sick or well—in the performance of self-care activities so that he or she could realize maximum health potential. However, domain debates about what phenomena could appropriately be considered the targets of nursing care began in the 1960s. The debates have centered on whether disease and its symptom manifestations could be considered nursing diagnoses, or whether nursing diagnoses target phenomena that require nursing treatment in addition to or instead of medical treatment (Durand & Prince, 1966; Kim & Moritz, 1981; Levine, 1966; Rothberg, 1967). Contemporary definitions of nursing diagnosis are characterized by the theme that the diagnosis identifies a problem or potential problem (phenomenon) *that a nurse can treat*. (Campbell, 1978; Carpenito, 1987; Gordon, 1987). On the surface, the definition appears clear enough until nurse practitioners or intensive care nurses say, "I have the authority to implement medical treatments; therefore when I diagnose the presence of a problematic cardiac arrhythmia or otitis media, it is a nursing diagnosis." Different interpretations of the phrase, "a nurse can treat" form the foundation for contemporary debates. The phrase could mean that which the nurse has the knowledge and skill to do or that which the nurse has the self-directed authority to do. When the former interpretation is used, the diagnosis of a medical condition falls

within the domain of nursing diagnosis if the nurse has the knowledge and skill to make the diagnosis. When the latter interpretation is used, only those health-related phenomena that have contributing factors or etiologies that nurses have the self-directed authority to treat would be considered nursing diagnoses.

The former interpretation caught on in the 1970s in the midst of the nurse practitioner movement. In part, the inclusion of medical problems and etiologies in nursing diagnoses can be explained by the fact that we had not articulated the phenomena of concern to nursing, nor articulated clear and generalizable exemplars of nursing per se. Thus we were vulnerable to considering medical knowledge the sine qua non of nursing knowledge. The track the departure took had been suggested earlier by Levine (1966). Because of concerns about the legal ramifications of using medical terms and the term *diagnosis*, she suggested that the term *trophicognosis* be used. Trophicognosis would mean the diagnosis of "disease and its manifestations . . . without using the formal language of the medical diagnosis" (Levine, 1966, p. 58).

During the nurse practitioner revolution of the 1970s, with our emphasis on extended and expanded roles, state nurses' associations (SNA) were diligently working to impact the statutory definitions of registered nursing practice. In particular, many SNAs proposed new statutory language that incorporated nursing diagnosis. Typically the legislation that was successful attempted to distinguish between medical and nursing diagnoses. The distinctions were characteristically not clear, and Bullough (1975) suggested "that the only operational definition of a nursing diagnosis and care plan that would hold up over time and empirical study would be a diagnosis and care plan done by a nurse, as distinguished from one done by a physician" (p. 162). Thus a nursing diagnosis becomes any judgment that the nurse has the knowledge to make. Such an operationalization is consistent with Levine's (1966) trophicognosis. In other words, a nursing diagnosis can be a diagnosis of a disease or medical problem; it just cannot look like one. Such an orientation has seemingly greatly influenced the work of the National Conference Group on Nursing Diagnosis (NCGDN), now called the North American Nursing Diagnosis Association (NANDA). Many of the diagnostic labels approved by the NCGDN that continue to be approved by NANDA represent trophicognoses. An example of numerous such diagnoses in the current group of NANDA-approved diagnoses is decreased cardiac output due to electrical or mechanical problems (in the heart) (Guzzetta & Dossey, 1983).

A similar application of the trophicognosis idea is use of the term *collaborative* to modify a nursing diagnosis (Carpenito, 1987; Kim, 1985). Collaborative nursing diagnoses are diagnoses that require physician's orders to treat. Kim (1985) argued that, since nurses are accountable for their actions when implementing treatments ordered by physicians, judgments about pathophysiological phenomena should be called nursing diagnoses.

Pain experienced postoperatively is a common example of a collaborative diagnosis, when pain relief not only requires nursing measures but also the administration of a medication for pain relief. It is argued here that there are different types of pain as well as different contributing factors to the pain experience. Examples of contributing factors that *can intensify* postoperative pain are improper positioning or alignment, anxiety, coughing without splinting, and cognitive focus on the pain. Each of these etiological factors are amenable to nursing treatment. Additionally each factor could serve as a descriptor of the pain phenomenon being treated by means of nursing treatments, for example, positional pain, anxiety-related pain, nonsplinting pain, and attentional pain.

Pain is a phenomenon that can have many contributing factors, including both medical-related and nursing-related etiologies. Nursing, as a learned discipline, must identify and study those etiologies that are amenable to nursing treatments. However, focusing primarily on the etiologies amenable to medical treatment by means of a "collaborative" diagnosis diverts our attention away from furthering nursing knowledge for patient or client benefit.

As discussed earlier, in addition to the phenomena that are amenable to nursing treatments, nurses make judgments about the presence of phenomena

as well as treat phenomena that require medical treatment by means of delegated authority. However, it is the phenomena that nurses autonomously treat and the treatment armamentaria of nursing that define the essence of nursing and the parameters of nursing's unique scope of practice.

PARAMETERS OF NURSING'S AUTONOMOUS SCOPE OF PRACTICE

For the purpose of this chapter, nursing is defined as the diagnosis and treatment of actual or potential health conditions. Health conditions are defined as dynamic, subjective manifestations of illness or wellness. Examples of such manifestations include lowered self-esteem, feeling different or abnormal, fatigue, pain and discomfort, negative or troublesome emotions, impaired social relationships, role strain, and inadequate self-care or functional abilities (e.g., nutrition, rest/sleep/activity, skin care, ventilation, circulation, elimination, inability to concentrate or problem-solve). Manifestations of wellness would include such phenomena as sense of vigor, hardiness, positive emotional tone or mood states, and optimal self-care or functional ability.

The health conditions or phenomena that nurses are uniquely concerned with are amenable to nursing treatments. Nursing treatments are self-care activities that a nurse either assists in or performs for a patient or client. Nursing treatments may be categorized as follows: (a) hygiene-related activities; (b) nutrition-related activities; (c) elimination-related activities; (d) comfort-related activities; (e) rest- or activity-related activities; (f) learning and development – related activities; (g) safety-related activities; (h) sense of normalcy – related activities; (i) interaction-related activities; (j) coping-related activities; and (k) daily living – related activities (Lyon, 1983). Each category of autonomous nursing treatments is very broad in scope and thereby encompasses many specific types of actions. Each category includes teaching and counseling activities as well as specific motor activities on the part of the nurse. For example, hygiene-related activities include teaching, counseling, and assisting actions as well as "doing-for" activities in skin care (e.g., relief of pressure, cleansing), mouth care, and eye care. Rest- and activity-related activities include relevant teaching and counseling on such matters as sleep, activity progression, and pacing of activity. "Doing-for" activities include actions that enable implementation of sleep rituals, environmental manipulation to alter sensory overload or underload problems, reducing sleep interruptions, and activity progression. Nutrition-related activities encompass such diverse activities as feeding techniques, enchancement of appetite, and use of muscular facilitation techniques to facilitate swallowing.

Nursing treatments are actions that a nurse can self-initiate to promote wellness, prevent illness, or resolve or cure illness. Nursing's treatment domain encompasses self-care-related activities directed at maintaining, promoting or altering somatic sensations and functional ability.

CONCLUSION

The uniqueness of every profession lies in the special contribution that profession makes to society and specifically in what the respective provider diagnoses and treats. A physician diagnoses and treats disease; a nurse diagnoses and treats illness, or diagnoses and assists patients or clients in the maintenance of wellness. It is imperative, both for scientific advancement of the discipline and professional identity, that nursing define its unique focus. Twenty years ago Abdellah (1969) asserted that "fundamental to the development of a nursing science is the nurse's ability to make a nursing diagnosis and prescribe nurse actions or strategies that will result in specific responses in the patient" (p. 391). As Vredevoe (1984) purported, a "science is defined most clearly by the dependent variables that it manipulates" (p. 90). To advance the science of nursing, and to promote the professional identity of nurses and the worth of nursing we must be clear on what nursing is about. We must get back on track.

REFERENCES

Abdellah, F.G. (1969). The nature of nursing science. *Nursing Research, 18,* 390–393.

American Nurses' Association (ANA). (1980). *Nursing: A social policy statement.* Kansas City, MO: Author.

Bullough, G. (Ed.). (1975). *The law and the expanding nursing role.* New York: Appleton-Century-Crofts.

Campbell, C. (1978). *Nursing diagnosis and interventions in nursing practice.* New York: John Wiley & Sons.

Carnevali, D.L. (1984). Nursing diagnosis: An evolutionary view. *Topics in Clinical Nursing, 5,* 10–20.

Carpenito, L.J. (1987). *Nursing diagnosis: Application to clinical practice.* Philadelphia: J. B. Lippincott.

Chapman, J.S. (1981). Health and medicine. In P.R. Lee, N. Brown, & I. Red (Eds.), *The nation's health* (pp. 14–17). San Francisco: Boyd & Fraser Publishing Co.

Cogan, M. (1953). Toward a definition of profession. *Harvard Educational Review, 23,* 33–50.

Downs, F.S. (1988). Doctoral education: Our claim to the future. *Nursing Outlook, 36,* 18–20.

Dubos, R. (1981). Health and creative adaptation. In P. R. Lee, N. Brown, & I. Red (Eds.), *The nation's health* (pp. 6–13). San Francisco: Boyd & Fraser Publishing Co.

Durand, M., & Prince, R. (1966). Nursing diagnosis: Process and decisions. *Nursing Forum, 5,* 50–64.

Flexner, A. (1915). Is social work a profession? *Proceedings of the National Conference of Charities and Corrections.* Chicago: Hildermann Printing Co.

Freidson, E. (1970). *Professional dominance.* Chicago: Aldine.

Gordon, M. (1987). *Nursing diagnosis: Process and application.* New York: McGraw-Hill.

Guzzetta, C.E., & Dossey, B.M. (1983). Nursing diagnosis: Framework, process, and problems. *Heart and Lung, 12,* 282–291.

Henderson, V.. (1964). The nature of nursing. *American Journal of Nursing, 64,* 62–68.

Hughes, E.C. (1963). Professions. *Daedalus, 92:*655–668.

Keller, M. (1981). Toward a definition of health. *Advances in Nursing Science, 4,* 43–64.

Kim, M.J. (1985). Without collaboration, what's left? *American Journal of Nursing,* March, 281–285.

Kim, M.J., & Moritz, D.A. (Eds.). (1981). *Classification of nursing diagnoses: Proceedings of the 3rd and 4th National Conferences.* New York: McGraw-Hill.

Kleinman, A. (1981). The failure of Western medicine. In P.R. Lee, N. Brown, & I. Red (Eds.), *The nation's health* (pp. 18–20). San Francisco: Boyd & Fraser Publishing Co.

Levine, M.E. (1966). Trophicognosis: An alternative to nursing diagnosis. In American Nurses' Association, *Exploring progress in medical-surgical nursing practice: Vol. 2* (pp. 23–27). Kansas City, MO: American Nurses' Association.

Lyon, B.L. (1983). *Nursing practice: An exemplification of the statutory definition*. Birmingham, AL: Pathway Press.

McManus, L. (1950). Assumptions of functions in nursing. In *Regional planning for nursing and nursing education* (pp. 54–55). New York: Bureau of Publications, Teachers College, Columbia University.

Millstein, S.G., & Irwin, C.E. (1987). Concepts of health and illness: Different constructs or variations on a theme? *Health Psychology, 6*, 515–524.

Murchison, I., & Nichols, T. (1970). *Legal foundations of nursing practice*. London: Macmillan.

Newman, M. (1986). *Health as expanding consciousness*. St. Louis: C. V. Mosby.

Nightingale, F. (1969). *Notes on nursing*. New York: Dover Publications. (Original work published 1859)

Nightingale, F. (1949). Sick nursing and health nursing. In I. Hampton. (Ed.), *Nursing of the sick* (pp. 1–12). New York: McGraw-Hill. (Original work published in 1893)

Orem, D.E. (1980). *Nursing: Concepts of practice* (2nd ed.). New York: McGraw-Hill.

Parson, T. (1954). The professions and social structure. In *Essays in sociological theory* (pp. 54–83). Glencoe, IL: Free Press.

Rothberg, J.S. (1967). Why nursing diagnosis? *American Journal of Nursing, 67*, 1040–1042.

Selby, T.L. (1986, March 1). Nurse practitioners show nursing's promise. *The American Nurse*, 18(3)1.

Thomas, L. (1981). On the science and technology of medicine. In P.R. Lee, N. Brown, & I. Red (Eds.), *The nation's health* (pp. 485–492). San Francisco: Boyd & Fraser Publishing Co.

Vredevoe, D.L. (1984). Curology: A basic science related to nursing. *Image, 16*, 89–92.

Wiedenbach, E. (1964). *Clinical nursing: A helping art*. New York: Springer Publishing.

Wilensky, H.L. (1964). The professionalization of everyone? *American Journal of Sociology, 70*, 137–158.

Wood, J.E., Tiedje, L.B., & Abraham, I.L. (1986). Practicing autonomously: A comparison of nurses. *Public Health Nursing, 3*, 130–139.

✳ EDITOR'S QUESTIONS FOR DISCUSSION ✳

How important is it to the development of nursing as a profession to have a unified definition of nursing? What is nursing's autonomous scope of practice? Provide specific examples in professional nursing practice. Discuss at what point and how knowledge adopted from other disciplines may or may not become nursing knowledge. What is your definition of health? How is it differentiated from illness, disease, and wellness? To what extent is illness and wellness, not disease, the target conditions for nursing care? Provide specific examples in an acute care setting in which the autonomous independent nursing role, the dependent role, and interdependent nursing role are all performed by a nurse for holistic care of the patient. How can potential role conflicts be presented and resolved? How appropriate is it to define and discuss the professional nursing role as one role with no distinct parts or types versus multiple aspects or types of one role? Are there circumstances or settings in which one type of nursing practice is more appropriate than another, or should there be only one type of nursing practice?

What is the difference between a nurse's making a medical judgment and making a medical diagnosis? Who bears the ultimate responsibility for making a medical judgment, or a medical diagnosis, or both? Compare Chapter 35 by Soares O'Hearn with this chapter. To what extent is the content by each author supported by the other? How does Lyon differ from NANDA and Soares O'Hearn in her classification and use of nursing diagnoses? Which approach to classification is the most restrictive? Which approach has the most relevance for developing nursing knowledge and professional practice?

35

Nursing Diagnosis:

A phenomenological structural description and multidimensional taxonomy or typological redefinition

Carol A. Soares O'Hearn, Ph.D., R.N.

The structural description of nursing's phenomena of concern is critical to the scope of nursing practice. The act of describing a nursing phenomenon presupposes a classification schema by which a new phenomenon can be identified. The method of phenomenological description is used[1] to describe the features of nursing diagnosis. Phenomenological description offers a method for describing the rules for constituting new phenomena, as well as for investigating or reexamining known classified objects (Soares, 1975, 1978; Soares O'Hearn, 1987a).

Descriptive analyses are made of the structural definition of actual and potential nursing diagnoses. An actual diagnosis is commonly written as a two-part statement that describes a presenting problem and its etiology (Carpenito, 1983; Gordon, 1982; Little & Carnevali, 1976; Marriner, 1975; Mundinger & Jauron, 1975; Soares, 1978; Yura & Walsh, 1973). An example is Fatigue related to Sleep Pattern Disturbance. A potential nursing diagnosis is not a presenting phenomenon because it has not occurred. Therefore, the problem and etiology format is not used. Instead, a potential diagnosis is written as a potential problem with its presenting risk factors as the defining characteristics. An example is Potential for Injury (falls): weakness, poor vision, balancing difficulties, reduced large or small muscle coordination (McLane, 1987). No etiology is written, precisely because the phenomenon has not occurred (Carpenito, 1987; Gordon, 1987b; Kim, McFarland, & McLane, 1987).

A structural analysis of nursing diagnosis necessitates examining nursing phenomena that fit a problem/etiological or a potential problem: risk factor format.[2] In addition, the examiner must be open to

---

The editor acknowledges Brenda Lyon, D.N.S., R.N., Associate Professor and Chairperson, Department of Nursing of Adults with Biodissonance, School of Nursing, Indiana University, Indianapolis, Indiana, for the review, comments, and questions on a draft of this chapter.

[1]For a more detailed explanation of the phenomenological method the reader is referred to Soares O'Hearn, C. A. (1987a). Phenomenology for theory development in nursing. *Proceedings of the Fourth Nursing Science Colloquium*. Boston: Boston University.

---

[2] The slash will be used in this chapter to replace "due to, related to, or associated to." The slash should be read to mean "influenced by" when the diagnosis is in the present time. In those diagnoses that describe future states the colon will be used instead of the slash. The colon has the same meaning as "influenced by."

looking at those phenomena that do not fit these formats. Rules for constituting phenomena can be identified by examining instances of negation (Spiegelberg, 1965). Negative criticism has been levied against the concept of nursing diagnosis (Porter, 1986; Rash, 1987; Shamansky & Yanni, 1983). One criticism is that by focusing on problems rather than wellness, nursing diagnosis portrays a limited perspective of health.

PURPOSE

The purpose of this chapter is to demonstrate how two structural definitions of nursing diagnoses (presenting problem/etiology and potential problem: risk factors) can be expanded into a multidimensional structural taxonomy or typology of nursing diagnoses. This proffered taxonomy or typology reflects the expanding scope of nursing practice and is grounded in an enhanced view of nursing's area of concern. This multidimensional taxonomy or typology of the structural definitions of nursing diagnosis is derived from the analysis of (a) actual nursing diagnoses, clinically identified in a research study focusing on wellness and illness diagnoses among the elderly in varied settings (Soares O'Hearn 1987b); (b) those diagnoses submitted to and accepted by the North American Nursing Diagnosis Association (NANDA, 1988); (c) those diagnoses rejected by NANDA; and (d) the language used to support or oppose proposed nursing diagnoses, by participants in the Diagnostic Review Sessions at the 1986 and 1988 NANDA biennial conferences on classification of nursing diagnoses.

The North American Nursing Diagnosis Association, the American Nurses' Association, and Classification

NANDA was formed for the purpose of developing, refining, and promoting a nursing diagnosis taxonomy for general use (NANDA, 1988). As of 1986, accepted nursing diagnoses were classified alphabetically. The NANDA Taxonomy Committee (McLane, 1987) proposed nine human response patterns as the organizing structure for diagnostic categories in a document entitled *NANDA Taxonomy I*. Accepted diagnoses were grouped into the nine patterns: exchanging, communicating, relating, valuing, choosing, moving, perceiving, knowing, and feeling (McLane, 1987).

The American Nurses' Association (ANA) is also concerned with classifying nursing diagnoses. Boards of both associations approved the NANDA-ANA Collaborative Model for Classification of Nursing Phenomena (NANDA, 1988). Through this model the ANA Board recognizes the ANA Practice Council's use of NANDA for development, review, and approval of nursing diagnoses (NANDA, 1988). The use of human response patterns as organizing domains is consistent with the ANA (1980) definition of nursing in its social policy statement, "Nursing is the diagnosis and treatment of human responses to actual or potential health problems" (p. 9).

The social policy statement (ANA, 1980) also clearly identifies the parallel relationships between (a) the defining characteristics of nursing practice, (b) the nursing process, and (c) the standards of nursing practice. Within the scope of practice are the dimensions of observing, judging, planning, acting, and evaluating. *All* of these, then, are essential features of practice and need to be incorporated into the definition of nursing. The present definition merely focuses on diagnosis (judging) and treatment (acting). An expanded definition would encompass all the features of practice, that is, the nursing process. All the dimensions of the nursing process need (a) to be identified as essential to nursing's area of concern, (b) to have their respective diagnostic structural definitions explicated, and (c) to be analyzed to develop a broader definition of nursing.

NURSING DIAGNOSIS: PROBLEM/ETIOLOGY STATEMENT

Nursing's close alliance with medicine has often led to the interpretation of the term *nursing diagnosis*, as a problem, to be equated to a medical problem, that is, somehow tied in with disease or pathology. Although concern has been expressed regarding the labeling of nursing's phenomena of concern as "Problem," as particularistic negative states, the term *problem* has been intrinsically tied to the structural definition of nursing diagnosis. In 1966 Soares[3] identified the two-part statement: Presenting Problem and Etiological Problem as the structural definition of nursing diagnosis. Gordon (1982) expanded this format to three components: the state-of-the-patient or health problem (P), the etiology of the problem (E), and the signs and symptoms (S). These components are referred to as the PES format. The etiological component was further subdivided by Carpenito (1983), who delineated contributory factors, situational factors, and maturational factors.

The NANDA Diagnostic Review Committee's criteria (McLane, 1987) for submitting a proposed nursing diagnosis include (a) the diagnostic category as the label for the term being submitted, (b) the major and minor defining characteristics, and (c) related factors as optional (the term *etiology*, meaning causal, is replaced by the term *related factors*). Since NANDA's classification of nursing diagnoses consists of diagnostic categories, it is possible to equate a diagnosis as being a mere diagnostic category (label) or problem.

Writers in the nursing diagnosis literature seem to support the structural definition of a nursing diag-

---

[3]The two-part format was taught by the author in a course entitled Dimensions of Nursing Practice from 1966 to 1968 in Boston University's School of Nursing for the RN Baccalaureate Program and from 1968 to 1969 for the Graduate Medical Surgical Program in the course Theory and Process.

TABLE 35-1
Nursing diagnosis: two-part statement

Left *H*and Side of the Statement		Right *H*and Side of the Statement
LHSOS		RHSOS
Problem	related to	Etiology
Fatigue		Sleep Pattern Disturbance

nosis as being (a) the Problem, or, as one is apt to say, the left-hand side of a two-part statement (LHSOS), and (b) an Etiology or a right-hand side of statement (RHSOS). This format is found in Carpenito (1983), Gordon (1982), Little and Carnevali (1976), Marriner (1975), Soares (1978), Yura and Walsh (1973), and in most texts referring to nursing diagnosis. Table 35-1, Nursing Diagnosis: Two-Part Statement depicts this format.

A classification of nursing diagnosis was developed by Soares (1978) that identified multiple types of problem/etiological statements. At that time Soares stated:

> This format may be necessary until nurses examine their practice and begin to collect a number of the problem-etiology statements and to analyze them comparatively in order to isolate repetitive patterns of problem-etiologies. Once these repetitive patterns are isolated, nurses can begin to categorize these "syndromes" into diagnostic labels. (p. 227)

It is now possible to describe the structural definition of these problem/etiology patterns as one diagnostic category label.

Category Label: Concept and Construct Formation

The procedure for specifying meaning or definition differs for concepts and constructs (Kaplan, 1964, p. 73). Some diagnostic categories are concept labels that can be defined by clustering phenomena, that is, observable empirical signs and symptoms or characteristics. In defining a concept, the term being defined is mutually replaceable with a set of synonymous terms (Kaplan, 1964, p. 73). For example, the NANDA diagnostic category or concept label, Stress Incontinence (Gordon, 1987a, p. 114) is synonymous with its clustered set of defining characteristics: dribbling with increased abdominal pressure, urinary frequency (more than every 2 hours). These synonymous terms are directly observable phenomena.

The NANDA Diagnostic Review Committee (DRC) guidelines (Gordon, 1987b) are stipulated in concept formation requirements, namely, defining characteristics or empirical phenomena. Thus the diagnostic category label, qua concept, is defined by its presenting phenomena or empirical manifestations. To date, for the most part, these guidelines have been pragmatic. Unsurprisingly the majority of category labels identified by NANDA are concepts. However, analysis of the structural components of nursing diagnoses reveals two major types of conceptual entities.

Type 1: definitional concept

One type of conceptual entity is identified with existant clinical manifestations (characteristics) and can be defined in terms of these same defining characteristics. These are lower order concepts in that they are closely related to the objective, sensory, perceptual, experiential world. The concepts are definitional because their defining empirical factors provide for the operational definition of the diagnostic category. Examples of these factors are (a) defining characteristics (signs and symptoms); (b) indicating factors; (c) risk factors; (d) growth or maturational factors; and (e) strength factors.

Type 2: attributional or theoretical construct

The second type of conceptual entity describes or points to the phenomena that assist, aid, help, or somehow influence bringing about the definitional concept or diagnostic category. These are higher order concepts and are indirectly observable inasmuch as they are removed from being known in direct experience. They are not immediately perceived and are therefore abstract or theoretical. These concepts are attributional constructs because they identify the theoretical or influencing factors[4] that account for the emergence of the definitional concept or diagnostic category. These construct labels are made up of concept clusters. An example would be Anxiety (construct) (Kim, McFarland, & McLane, 1987) specified as: fear (concept), worry (concept), dis-

tress (concept), and so on. Each of these clustered concepts can be further defined in terms of their synonymous presenting phenomena or characteristics.

The procedure for specifying constructs, unlike concepts, is not in the defining of equivalent directly observable terms. The definitions of constructs are specified from within a theory. This suggests that nursing diagnostic categories, qua constructs, are specified in terms of their (theoretical) explanatory or predictive accounts rather than in terms of descriptors. Examples of specifying factors are (a) etiological factors; (b) unresolved problem clusters; (c) contributory factors; (d) related factors; (e) associated factors; and (f) situational factors.

Nursing Diagnosis: Problem Category Concept Types

Two concept types of problem nursing diagnoses have been described: presenting and potential. These two are:

Concept Type 1. Presenting Problem category, qua concept (the Diagnostic Category), defined in terms of empirical phenomena characteristics.

Concept Type 2. Potential Problem category, qua concept, identified by its empirical risk factors.

In addition to types of Problem Concept Categories there are also types of Problem Construct Categories. Each category type is discussed in the following sections.

Nursing Diagnosis: Problem Category Construct Types

Four types of single nursing diagnostic categories are derived from two-part statements of nursing diagnoses. These four are:

Construct Type 1. Presenting Problem modified by its relational factor(s).

Construct Type 2. Relational Factor specified by presenting problems.

Construct Type 3. Potential Consequence: risk factors are unresolved presenting problem(s).

---

[4]Influencing factor was suggested by Fitzpatrick (1987) in lieu of etiology. I find the term *influencing* conceptually useful and retain etiological factors as one subtype of influencing factor.

Construct Type 4. Potential Consequence: risk factor identified as a common relational factor specified as a cluster of presenting problems.

Construct Type 1. Presenting problem modified by its relational factor(s)

Construct Type 1 can be derived from those diagnoses in which the LHSOS is a presenting problem and the RHSOS has a number of relational factors that also are presenting problems. For example, the diagnostic category Decisional Conflict[5] (see Table 35-2, Decisional Conflict: Diagnostic Category and Related Factors) as a presenting problem (LHSOS) may have one or five relational factors (RHSOS). Each relational factor also is a presenting problem.

In this example there is one presenting problem with multiple related factors across domains (Soares, 1978). The diagnostic category (Decisional Conflict) can have one to five related factors. The specificity of the diagnostic category is in the type of relational factor. Therefore, it is suggested that these kinds of diagnostic categories be restructured to bring the relational factor (RHSOS) as a modifier into the diagnostic category (LHSOS). In this case, the diagnostic category (LHSOS) would become (specify) Decisional Conflict. Instead of one presenting problem with five related factors, there are five types of Decisional Conflict specified by relational factors. Thus the diagnostic category Decisional Conflict becomes Relational Type Decisional Conflict. The specified relational types are:

1. Altered Sensory Perception
2. Lack of Information
3. Lack of Trust
4. Situational Depression
5. Values Conflict

A two-part statement, a presenting-problem LHSOS and another presenting problem as a RHSOS, has become one diagnostic category. The RHSOS has made the LHSOS more specific by defining it as

---

[5]This diagnosis is used within this chapter as a construct, as it was discussed in the Diagnostic Review Sessions at the Eighth NANDA Conference. However, NANDA has accepted the label but redefined it as a concept.

TABLE 35-2
Decisional conflict: diagnostic category and related factors

LHSOS	RHSOS
Diagnostic Category (Presenting Problem) Decisional Conflict	Related Factors (Presenting Problem) Altered Sensory Perception Lack of Information Lack of Trust Situational Depression Values Conflict

a type of decisional conflict. For example, the former Decisional Conflict related to Altered Sensory Perception is transformed into Sensory Perceptional Decisional Conflict. In another example, Decisional Conflict related to Lack of Information becomes Informational Decisional Conflict.

Thus certain problem/etiological statements can be restructured into one specified category label using the transpositional rule. The transpositional rule is: When the conditions of a two-part statement (LHSOS Presenting Problem/RHSOS Relational Factor) exist, transpose the position of the relational factor to the position of modifier of the presenting problem in order to construct a one-category label. Thus Decisional Conflict related to Altered Sensory Perception becomes Sensory Perceptional Decisional Conflict. For taxonomic purposes, these restructured categories are more representative of nursing diagnoses than the present category labels.

Construct Type 2. Relational factor specified by presenting problems

The second type of construct is similar to Construct Type 1. Both are derived from presenting problem/presenting problem statements. Both have one problem on one side of the equation and a number of problems on the other. In Construct Type 1 there was one presenting problem LHSOS and a number of relational factors (RHSOS) (see box, Decisional Conflict). In Type 2 there are a number of presenting problems (LHSOS) and one relational factor (RHSOS) (Fig. 35-1).

In the example in Figure 35-1 there are 10 LH-

Potential Consequences	Presenting Problems	Common Etiology

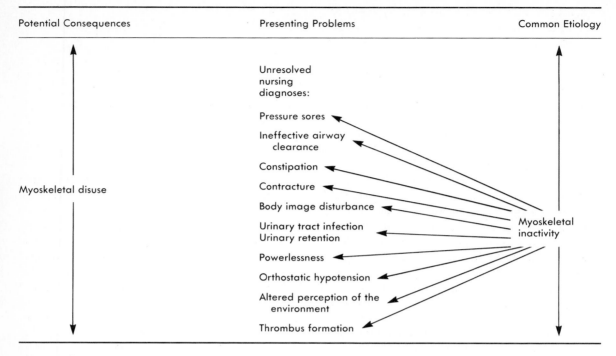

FIGURE 35-1

Nursing diagnoses: potential for myoskeletal disuse.

SOS presenting problems related to 1 RHSOS etiological factor. Following the transpositional rule for Construct Type 1, as previously indicated, the RHSOS relational factor shifts to become the modifier for the LHSOS presenting problems. An example is Myoskeletal Inactivity Constipation, or simply Inactivity Constipation.

The cluster of 10 Construct Type 1 categories in the nursing diagnosis Potential for Myoskeletal Disuse[5] (Esposito, Tracey, & McCourt, 1989), Figure 35-1 all contain the same modifier, namely, the former RHSOS etiological factor: Myoskeletal Inactivity. It is here suggested that this etiological modifying factor be redefined as the LHSOS priority presenting concern. The clustered 10 presenting problems then become the specifying terms for Myoskeletal Inactivity, as the priority problem of concern. Myoskeletal Inactivity, qua construct, is not defined in terms of empirical phenomena or characteristics.

It is specified in terms of its clustered presenting effects or problems. This does not negate the use of the category Myoskeletal Inactivity as a concept problem Type 1 category. In this latter case, Myoskeletal Inactivity would be defined in terms of empirical characteristics: nonmovement of the muscular skeletal structure of the body.

Present analysis suggests that when a diagnostic category is used as an influencing, etiological, or relational factor, and is transposed to become the priority presenting concern, it is defined in terms of its associated cluster of problems. When the same diagnostic label is the presenting category associated with another relational factor, then it is specified by the relational factor and defined in empirical terms.

Another example of a Construct Type 2 category is Powerlessness. The presenting concept category of Powerlessness is defined empirically as verbal expressions of having no control or influence over situations, verbal expressions of having no control or influence over outcome, and so forth (Kim et al., 1987). However, when the construct of Powerlessness as a common etiological factor to a number of associated problems is the focus of concern, it is specified in terms of its associated problems: Sleep Pattern Disturbance, Situational Depression (Translocation Syndrome—nursing home), Social Isolation (withdrawal), and Hopelessness.[6]

Construct Type 3. Potential consequence: risk factors—unresolved presenting problem(s)

As in the preceding examples a potential problem, qua concept, is specified in terms of its empirical risk factors. In the case of a Construct Type 3 potential consequence, its risk factors are specified in terms of one or more unresolved Construct Type 1 nursing diagnoses. An example is the nursing diagnosis Potential for Malnutrition: (risk factor) Self-Care Deficit (feeding level 2) related to Fatigue. In this example, the risk factor is an unresolved nursing diagnosis: Self-Care Deficit (feeding level 2) related to Fatigue. To transform this LHSOS: RHSOS diagnosis to a Type 1 Construct category, the LHSOS is modified by the RHSOS so that it becomes: Fatigue Self-Care Deficit (feeding level 2).

In another example the diagnosis Ineffective Breast Feeding (related to) Interrupted Breast Feeding, becomes a risk factor for the larger concept Potential for Nutritional Deficit. Nutritional Deficit would be the consequence of the unresolved or uncompensated nursing diagnosis, namely, Ineffective Breast Feeding (related to) Interrupted Breast Feeding. This latter diagnosis can become a one-category construct-type nursing diagnosis by following the transpositional rule for the related factor (RHSOS). The specified problem would read: Interrupted Ineffective Breast Feeding. For classification purposes, Interrupted Breast Feeding specifies only one type of Ineffective Breast Feeding. For clinical purposes, the use of the more specific type is more helpful in determining interventions.

---

[6]The specifications of the construct Powerlessness have been identified clinically by the author but are unpublished.

Construct Type 4. Potential consequence: risk factor specified by an unresolved common etiological factor to a cluster of nursing diagnoses

In the discussion of a Construct Type 2 category, the example of Myoskeletal Inactivity as the common etiological problem to 10 presenting problems was described. The potential consequence of an unresolved Construct Type 2 category is an example of Construct Type 4. The example is Potential Myoskeletal Disuse (Potential Consequence): (risk factor) Myoskeletal Inactivity specified by the 10 associated presenting problems, that is, pressure sores, etc. (see Figure 35-1).

In these examples risk factors are not at the direct observable level of signs and symptoms. The risk factors are already categorized into indirectly observable concepts. Interventions with this type of diagnosis parallel potential problems, for example, the unresolved nursing diagnoses are equated to the risk factors in a potential problem. In these examples the interventional category could be either other unresolved nursing diagnoses (Construct Type 3) or a common etiological factor that runs through several unresolved nursing diagnoses (Construct Type 4).

For Potential Myoskeletal Disuse, the risk factor Myoskeletal Inactivity is a construct interventional factor. It is specified in terms of 10 associated presenting problems: pressure sores, constipation, etc. However, the category label could also be a concept presenting problem, which then would be defined in terms of the empirical phenomenon: the inability to move.

Thus a category label can be classified as a presenting concept defined by its empirical presenting phenomena. The same label as etiological problem would be specified in terms of its clustered associated presenting nursing problems.

Nursing Diagnosis: Medically Associated Categories

Diagnostic reasoning has been described as clustering signs and symptoms into a conceptual inference or problem (Gordon, 1982). The term *problem* can have varying levels of conceptual meaning, depending on who is making the judgment and the situational context in which it is made. In medically associated nursing diagnostic categories the nurse identifies biophysical symptoms as a nursing diagnosis. The nurse is not diagnosing disease but a manifestation of such a process or its signs and symptoms, the presenting phenomena. A nurse's medically related diagnostic categories (signs and symptoms) can become the defining characteristics for a physician's medical diagnosis. In examining Figures 35-2 and 35-3 differentiating levels of diagnoses begin to emerge.

In the example of medical diagnosis (Fig. 35-2), Neoplasm of the Oral Cavity, three of the medically defining characteristics are NANDA nursing diagnostic categories, that is, Impaired Oral Mucous Membranes, Malnutrition, and Pain.

For the NANDA nursing diagnostic category, Impaired Oral Mucous Membranes (Kim et al., 1987, p. 59), the list of defining characteristics includes signs and symptoms, that is, oral pain, unhealing oral lesions, coated tongue, leukoplakia (Fig. 35-3). The nurse does not "treat" these signs and symptoms in terms of their etiological causes. The nurse intervenes to alleviate these present conditions, for example, through mouth care. In addition, the nurse anticipates potential consequences, such as Potential for Malnutrition, through ensuring adequate nutritional intake.

The ability to treat or intervene in clinical phenomena per se does not delineate an individual's scope of practice. Many physicians, for example, can identify and confirm a medical diagnosis but must refer to other health professionals for treatment. The ability to identify a possible diagnosis also is insufficient for defining one's scope of practice.

The skill that differentiates between the scope of a physician's and a nurse's practice is the ability to validate or confirm indirect pathological inferences. The control of the interventions for these validated inferences must fall within the scope of the respective individual's professional practice. In the case of the neoplasm, the confirming histological evidence is within the scope of medical practice. The control of indirect evidence, such as lung sounds, varies. For example, the use of physical assessment skills has enabled nurses to confirm such indirect observables as rales and wheezing. Consequently, through the implementation of specified protocols some nurses have expanded their nursing practice. In the realm of medical treatment of disease the physician is concerned with treating the causes of the disease, whereas the nurse intervenes to ease the presenting phenomena (signs and symptoms), not to cure but to comfort.

Typification can be made of medically associated

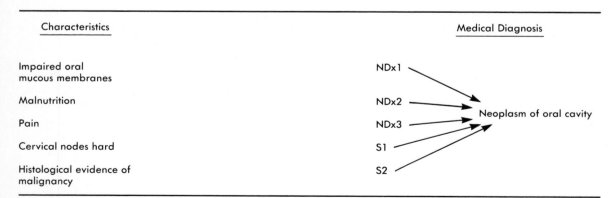

Characteristics		Medical Diagnosis
Impaired oral mucous membranes	NDx1	
Malnutrition	NDx2	Neoplasm of oral cavity
Pain	NDx3	
Cervical nodes hard	S1	
Histological evidence of malignancy	S2	

Note: NDx = Nursing diagnosis label for clustered signs and symptoms (see Figure 35-3) S = additional signs and symptoms the physician confirms.

FIGURE 35-2

Medical diagnosis: construct disease label.

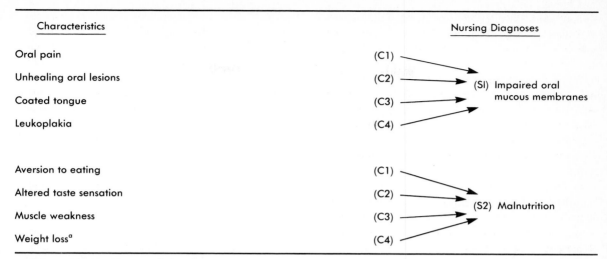

Characteristics		Nursing Diagnoses
Oral pain	(C1)	
Unhealing oral lesions	(C2)	(Sl) Impaired oral
Coated tongue	(C3)	mucous membranes
Leukoplakia	(C4)	
Aversion to eating	(C1)	
Altered taste sensation	(C2)	(S2) Malnutrition
Muscle weakness	(C3)	
Weight loss[a]	(C4)	

Note: C = Characteristic; S = Sign or symptom.
      [a]Loss = 20% less than ideal weight.

FIGURE 35-3

Nursing diagnosis: concept categories—signs and symptoms as problems.

nursing diagnostic categories. The transpositional rule is the same as for a Construct Type 1 category. It is suggested that when a nursing diagnosis is the *consequence* of a medical diagnosis, biophysical or psychosocial, the medical diagnosis becomes the associated factor following the nursing diagnosis. The medical diagnosis specifies the associated context of the nursing diagnosis. Examples of this are Malnutrition (Neoplasm Oral Cavity), Malnutrition (Bulemia), Malnutrition (Depression), and Malnutrition (Alcoholism). Nursing diagnoses as medical consequences can be classified as Type 1 (medically associated) Concept categories. They are defined in terms of empirical phenomena. Having examined the structural definition of "problem" type of statements, this discussion now shifts to address wellness diagnoses.

Nursing Diagnosis: Wellness Categories

Five types of structural definitions for wellness diagnoses are offered: Developmental, Wellness, Health Management, Health Maintenance, and Health Promotion. Many persons do not adhere to or support a Problem/Etiological statement format for a wellness diagnosis. They do not attend to "problems" in the sense of illness or deviations from the norm. Problem, however, does not necessarily have to have a negative connotation. A mathematical problem does not conjure images of negative states. Inventors, creators, artists, writers, all deal with problems. None of their acts are interpreted in terms of illness, disease, or pathophysiology. To solve problems is to be alive, to be creatively participating in the unfolding process of growth and development.

Type 1a. Potential developmental diagnoses. The format for a wellness diagnosis as a future state follows that of Potential Problem: Risk Factors present. That is, the developmental diagnosis format is: Potential for Growth or Development (specify): Growth Factors Present.

A clinical example of a potential developmental state with growth factors present is reflected in the potential state of accepting the maternal role in the category label: Maternal Role Readiness.[7] The pre-

---

[7]This unpublished diagnosis was identified by a Stonehill College (Massachusetts) RN Baccalaureate graduate, Sharon Hill.

senting growth factors are: actively seeking information about family planning, verbalizing wanting to start a family, and sharing the desire with significant other.

Type 1b. Actual developmental diagnoses.
An example of an actualized developmental diagnosis with indicating factors present is: Physical and Social Boundary Redefinition (Acceptance).[8] Indicating factors are: verbalizes being able to maintain social or family contact via phone and letters, verbalizes acceptance of physical limitations and loss of previous roles and status, verbalizes meaning in limitation as time for self-growth, verbalizes letting go of wants beyond physical ability.

In addition to developmental diagnoses there are four other types of wellness diagnoses as phenomena of concern with influencing factors. These are as follows.

Type 2. Wellness levels (specify levels).   These diagnoses identify levels of wellness. Their influencing factors are described in definitional concepts as indicating factors.

Type 3. Health management diagnoses (specify).   These diagnoses identify the ability to make decisions and to plan and manage one's health-related activities. Influencing factors can be described as definitional concepts or in construct types as self-management factors and supporting resource factors.

Type 4. Health maintenance diagnoses (abilities).   These diagnoses include all of the health practices used to maintain health states. Influencing factors are defined in concept terms as supportive factors and strength factors.

Type 5. Health promotion diagnoses (specify — structural, functional, and developmental).
These diagnoses project future health promotion goals. They can pertain to a structural category, functional health, and optimum development. Influencing factors can be described in concept or construct terms as high-level wellness goals, health-seeking factors, strength factors, and ability factors.

---

[8]This wellness diagnosis was adopted with permission from one identified by two Stonehill College RN Baccalaureate graduates, C. Bonin and V. Hodder, in their research analysis of clinical assessment data among the well elderly in conjunction with their coursework.

Nursing Diagnosis Taxonomy or Typology

Nursing diagnoses can be classified according to different types of phenomena of concern. The phenomena can be (a) problem or wellness categories, (b) presenting or potential, and (c) concept or construct. A classification of domain categories can be made from concept and construct category types. These domains reflect the essential features of nursing practice: assessment, judgment, planning and management, intervention, and goal or outcomes. The five Nursing Diagnosis Domains are as follows.

Type 1. Assessment domain diagnoses.   These include all of the actual phenomena — signs and symptoms or concrete manifestations — that nurses identify and in which they intervene. For most nurses this type of information is assessment data. However, under physicians' protocols, some nurses such as clinical specialists and nurses with expanded roles intervene in these phenomena directly. Others are referred for collaborative treatment. The capacities identified in NANDA Typology I (McLane, 1987) applied to this domain would be: Perceiving (Sensing), Exchanging (Energy), and Moving (Physical).

Type 2. Judgment domain diagnoses.   This type of domain diagnosis includes the human responses to judgments about actual or potential health phenomena (or Type 1 Domain). Human capacities characterizing this domain are: Perceiving (Feeling), Perceiving (Knowing), and Choosing.

Type 3. Planning and management domain diagnoses.   This would include all of the management categories that patients or clients use to organize their lives: health maintenance, home management, health promotional activities, and other similar categories. This allows for the many health-facilitating wellness types of diagnoses, which in themselves are not human responses to problems, but are still intervened in by nurses. It also includes categories describing a consequence of a human response to a health problem. The human capacities characterizing this domain are Communicating and Relating.

Type 4. Intervention domain diagnoses.   This includes all of those diagnoses commonly referred to as etiological. This allows for the inclusion in the Taxonomy diagnoses that are not human responses (phenomena) but are influencing the emergence of a human response, namely, the theoretical or influencing factors. This would include all Construct Type 1 and Type 2 categories. I characterize the capacities for this domain as Willing and Acting.

Type 5. Goal or outcome domain diagnoses. This would include all of those diagnoses pertaining to valued "states" or goals. Future-oriented diagnoses such as high-level wellness would be included here. It could also include potential consequence

categories Construct Type 3 and Type 4. To the human capacity of Valuing, the author added Hoping in this domain.

These five domains are the organizing structure for outlining a multidimensional taxonomy or typology of nursing diagnosis (see Table 35-3, Taxonomy or Typology of Structural Definitions of Nursing Diagnosis). Human capacities describing each domain include Perceiving (Sensing), Exchanging (Energy), and Moving (Physical); Perceiving (Feeling), Per-

TABLE 35-3

Taxonomy or typology of structural definitions of nursing diagnosis

Type 1. Assessment Domain diagnoses

Parameter Capacities: Perceiving (Sensing), Exchanging (Energy), Moving (Physical)

Phenomena of Concern	*Influencing Factors*
A. Wellness (Actual, Structural, Development Level)	1. Indicating Factors

B. Presenting Problem (Actual Structural, Functional, Developmental Signs and Symptoms) Secondary to Medical, Surgical, or Psychiatric Diagnoses	1. Associated Medical, Surgical or Psychiatric Diagnoses
	   a. Possible Indicator of
	   b. Co-occurring with
	   c. Secondary to

C. Potential Problem (Developmental, Structural, Functional)	1. Risk Factors

Type 2. Judgment Domain diagnoses

Parameter Capacities: Perceiving (Feeling), Perceiving (Knowing) and Choosing

Phenomena of Concern	*Influencing Factors*
A. Development (Actual Function)	1. Indicting Ability Factors
B. Potential Development (Function)	1. Growth Factors 2. Maturational Factors
C. Presenting Problems (Developmental, Structural, Functional, Consequential) *Not* Secondary to Medical, Surgical, or Psychiatric Diagnoses	1. Related Factors 2. Contributory Factors 3. Situational Factors 4. Etiological Factors 5. Other Presenting Problems
D. Potential Consequences (Developmental, Structural, Functional)	1. Unsolved Nursing Diagnoses 2. Common Etiological or Related Factors (to a Cluster of Unresolved Nursing Diagnoses)
E. Nonpresenting Problems* (Actual)	1. Compensating Factors

*This category was brought to my attention by H. S. Kim and B. Bartlett of the University of Rhode Island.

TABLE 35-3

Taxonomy or typology of structural definitions of nursing diagnosis—cont'd.

Type 3. Planning and Management Domain diagnoses

Parameter Capacities: Communicating and Relating

Phenomena of Concern	*Influencing Factors*

A. Health Management (Actual)	1. Facilitating Factors
	   a. Self-Management Factors
	   b. Supporting Resource Factors

B. Health Management (Ineffective)	1. Inhibiting Factors
	   a. Dependency Factors
	   b. Nonsupporting Factors

Type 4. Intervention Domain diagnoses

Parameter Capacities: Willing and Acting

Phenomena of Concern	*Influencing Factors*

A. Health Maintenance Abilities	1. Facilitating Factors
	   a. Supporting Factors
	   b. Strength Coping Factors

B. Etiological Factors	1. Presenting Problems
	   a. Structural
	   b. Functional
	   c. Developmental

Type 5. Goal or Outcome Domain diagnoses

Parameter Capacities: Valuing and Hoping

Phenomena of Concern	*Influencing Factors*
A. Health Promotion Developmental, "Structural Functional"; High-Level Wellness Goals	1. Health-Seeking Factors 2. Strength and Abilities Factors
B. Health Promotion Outcome Goals (Secondary to Problem Diagnoses)	1. Self-Healing Factors 2. Strength and Abilities Factors

ceiving (Knowing), and Choosing; Communicating and Relating; Willing and Acting; and Valuing and Hoping. Components of the structural diagnoses are given within each domain. Diagnoses include both a phenomenon of concern and an influencing or interventional factor.

SUMMARY

In exploring various structural definitions of nursing diagnosis the following suggestions are offered:

1. That the Problem/Etiology/Signs and Symptoms PES structural definition of a nursing diagnosis be seen as only one subtype of structural diagnosis.
2. That multiple structural definitions of nursing diagnosis subtypes be recognized.
3. That the definition of a nursing diagnosis reflect all situated practices and specialities.
4. That the general structural definition shift focus from a negative to a neutral term.

Based on these suggestions, the following structural definition for a general nursing diagnosis is offered.

Phenomena of Concern (Influencing Factor)

With this format, phenomena of concern can be problem or wellness states. Presenting Problem becomes a subtype of Phenomena of Concern. In the same manner, developmental stages or wellness states can be phenomena of concern. In addition, further subtypes can be defined by the transpositioning of influencing factors as modifiers of phenomena of concern. Etiological Problems then become a subtype of Influencing Factor. So also risk factors, growth factors, facilitating factors, self-management factors, contribution factors, maturational factors, etc., all can be seen to be subtypes of Influencing Factors. Thus Phenomena of Concern (Influencing Factor) can be a structural definition sufficiently broad to include all subtype examples. In addition, reexamining nursing diagnosis within the framework of nursing process expands the potential for incorporating diagnoses from assessment to outcome or goal types. This would more accurately reflect the diverse types of phenomena being described within the scope of nursing practice.

REFERENCES

American Nurses' Association (ANA). (1980). *Nursing: A social policy statement*. Kansas City: Author.

Carpenito, L. (1983). *Nursing diagnosis: Application to clinical practice*. New York: J. B. Lippincott.

Carpenito, L. (1987). *Nursing diagnosis: Application to clinical practice* (2nd ed.). New York: J. B. Lippincott.

Esposito, M., Tracey, C., & McCourt, A. (1989). Nursing diagnosis: Potential for disuse syndrome. In R. Carroll-Johnson (Ed.), *Classification of Nursing Diagnoses*. Proceedings of the Eighth Conference (pp. 464-468). Philadelphia: J.B. Lippincott.

Fitzpatrick, J.(1987). Etiology: Conceptual concerns. In A. McLane (Ed.), *Classification of nursing diagnoses*. Proceedings of the Seventh Conference (pp. 61–64). St. Louis: C. V. Mosby.

Gordon, M. (1982). *Nursing diagnosis: Process and application*. New York: McGraw-Hill.

Gordon, M. (1987a). *Manual of nursing diagnosis 1986–1987*. New York: McGraw-Hill.

Gordon, M. (1987b). *Nursing diagnosis: process and application* (2nd ed.). New York: McGraw-Hill.

Kaplan, A. (1964). *The conduct of inquiry*. New York: McGraw-Hill. Kim, M., McFarland, G., & McLane, A. (1987). *Pocket guide to nursing diagnoses* (2nd ed.). St. Louis: C. V. Mosby.

Little, D., & Carnevali, D. (1976). *Nursing care planning*. Philadelphia: J. B. Lippincott.

Marriner, A. (1975). *The nursing process*. St. Louis: C. V. Mosby.

McLane, A. (Ed.). (1987). *Classification of nursing diagnoses*. *Proceedings of the Seventh Conference*. St. Louis: C. V. Mosby.

Mundinger, M., & Jauron, G. (1975). Developing a nursing diagnosis. *Nursing Outlook, 23*, 94–98.

North American Nursing Diagnosis Association (NANDA). (1988, March). *Report of the president* (biennial business meeting book of reports, pp. 6–11). St. Louis: Author.

Porter, E. (1986). Critical analysis of NANDA nursing diagnosis Taxonomy I. *Image, 18*, 136–139.

Rash, R. (1987). The nature of taxonomy. *Image, 19*, 147–149.

Shamansky, S., & Yanni C. (1983). In opposition to nursing diagnosis: A minority opinion. *Image, 15*, 47–50.

Soares, C. (1975, March). *Ethnoscience and phenomenology as methods for isolating categories of nursing diagnoses*. Paper presented at the task force meeting of the First National Conference on Classification of Nursing Diagnosis, St. Louis, Mo.

Soares, C. (1978). Nursing and medical diagnoses: A comparison of variant and essential features. In N. Chaska (Ed.), *The nursing profession: Views through the mist* (pp. 198–204). New York: McGraw-Hill.

Soares O'Hearn, C. (1987a). Phenomenology: Strategies for theory development in nursing. In C. Bridges & N. Wells (Eds.), *Proceedings of the Fourth Nursing Science Colloquium: Strategies for theory development in nursing* (pp. 31–47). Boston: Boston University.

Soares-O'Hearn, C., (1987b). The relation between a structural-functional health/illness pattern (S.H.I.P.) tool and the generating of nursing diagnoses: A qualitative and quantitative study. In A. McLane (Ed.), *Classification of nursing diagnoses*. Proceedings of the Seventh Conference (pp. 352–359). St. Louis: C. V. Mosby.

Spiegelberg, H. (1965). *The phenomenological movement: A historical introduction* (2nd ed.). The Hague: Martinus Nijhoff.

Yura, H., & Walsh, M. (1973). *The nursing process: Assessing, planning, implementing, evaluating*. New York: Appleton-Century-Crofts.

✳   EDITOR'S QUESTIONS FOR DISCUSSION   ✳

Present arguments for and against the development of nursing diagnosis for professional practice and advancing the scientific knowledge base for nursing. Specifically, how does nursing diagnosis differ from a medical diagnosis? To what extent does one have to make a medical judgment before making a nursing diagnosis? What differentiates medical and nursing inferences? Are patient condition inferences that are validated by a nurse a medical diagnosis or a nursing diagnosis? Are interventions that are specified by a physician and carried out by a nurse medical acts or nursing acts? Whose legal right is it to define whether an intervention is medical or nursing? Discuss the statement that whether or not the control of the intervention is within a particular profession determines whether one is practicing medicine or nursing. What are the differences between the levels of nursing practice in being able to confirm a diagnosis? Is there a difference in nursing levels in making a nursing diagnosis or the extent that a medical judgment is made?

Discuss the extent to which some symptoms are multicausal and have some contributing factors that are treatable by nursing interventions. Discuss the knowable risk factors that the nurse attempts to alter in order to prevent a problem for a vulnerable person. What is the role of the professional nurse in terms of the prevention of potential problems that may render a need for medical intervention? How is legitimization established for nursing diagnoses? How do unpublished nursing diagnoses become accepted by NANDA and the profession? Compare the method explicated by Soares O'Hearn for constructing and utilizing nursing diagnoses with the methods and classifications indicated by other nursing leaders and authors.

36

Nurses' and Physicians' Expectations and Perceptions of Staff Nurse Role Performance as Influenced by Status Consistency

Norma L. Chaska, Ph.D., R.N., F.A.A.N.
Diana Clark, M.H.A., R.N.
Suzanne M. Rogers, M.S.N., R.N.
Carol A. Deets, Ed.D., R.N.

Coordination within and between professional groups requires knowledge about participants in terms of their behavior in a particular role-interaction situation. If a set of expectations is internally consistent within and between two professional groups, relatively little conflict should occur. The development of guidelines for action and interaction should be a simple and straightforward task because of this agreement.

The interface between the medical and nursing professions has become a common topic for discussion and focus in the health care scene (Mechanic & Aiken, 1982). There is even consensus that interfac-

ing is a critical issue in defining the responsibility of the staff nurse role (McClure & Nelson, 1982). However, in the articulation of these responsibilities there is confusion and blurring of the staff nurse role by one or both of the professions.

Determining views of both physicians and nurses regarding interdisciplinary and professional role expectations and performance is essential. In addition, it is important to ascertain how the status of a person as a professional plays a role in these perceptions because of the discrepant status accorded the two professions. Data are needed for clarification of roles and for systematic reflection before decisions about practice are made that involve the economic, ethical, political, legal, and professional realm.

PURPOSE OF THE STUDY

The purposes of this study were (1) to determine if nurses and physicians differ in their expectations

This research was funded and supported by the Department of Medical Research and the Division of Patient Care Services, Methodist Hospital of Indiana, Inc., Indianapolis, Indiana. The principal investigator acknowledges the assistance of Judith A. Barrett, R.N., former Senior Vice President Patient Care Services and Daniel M. Newman, M.D., former President of the Medical Staff, for facilitating access to the study population.

and perceptions of the staff nurse role, and (2) to determine if status consistency influences role expectations. Inherent in this study was the assumption that role modifications consciously take place as interactions occur among professionals. For example, a nurse or physician may choose to depart from (or adhere to) the anticipated performance of a role partner. If there is agreement on what the expected performance will look like, the reaction to the departure will be minor. On the other hand, if there is no agreement on expected behavior, there will be reactions to differences in expectations *and* to the departure from the expected. Confusion results from this lack of agreement, negatively influencing future interactions. It is critical that health professionals have some agreement about role definitions and expectations; otherwise, high-quality care of patients is at risk.

CONCEPTUAL FRAMEWORK

Conceptually this study incorporates aspects of role theory and the theory of status consistency. Role theory concepts predict how actors will perform in a given role, or under what circumstances certain types of behaviors can be expected (Conway, 1978). The behavior of the individual is shaped by the demands and rules of others, by their sanctions for his or her conforming and nonconforming behavior, and by the person's own understanding and conceptions of what his or her behavior should be (Thomas & Biddle, 1979).

The theory of status consistency holds that each person occupies a particular status configuration determined by his or her location on dimensions such as occupation, education, and income (Chaska, 1978; Jackson & Curtis, 1972; Lenski, 1954). When individuals hold a view of other individuals in terms of their status, this view is termed a status set. Geschwender (1967) first explained how status sets function in the social system. Not only do status sets influence an individual's development of behavioral expectations, but they also influence expectations for the person in a role and for the behavior of all persons with whom that person interacts in the social structure. For example, a person who ranks high in

education, position, *and* income may be expected to have certain behavioral patterns, whereas a person who ranks high in education but low in position and income may have a very different set of behavioral patterns. In the former case the person would be considered high status consistent. Physicians might be an example of those likely to hold that status set. In the latter case, an inconsistent status is apparent and may likely be held by staff nurses.

In this study status consistency was conceptualized in terms of *type* and *degree*. Type of status consistency was an objective measure of the respondent's rank on the dimensions of position, education, and income. Degree of status consistency was a subjective measure of the subject's rank using these same dimensions.

The following hypotheses were generated for this study:

1. Nurses have higher expectations and perceptions than physicians for the characteristics/responsibilities that pertain to the independent aspect of the staff nurse role.
2. Nurses have higher expectations and perceptions than physicians for the characteristics/responsibilities that pertain to the dependent aspect of the staff nurse role.
3. Nurses have higher expectations and perceptions than physicians for the characteristics/responsibilities that pertain to the interdependent aspect of the staff nurse role.
4. High status consistent nurses (type and degree) have higher expectations and perceptions of the staff nurse role than low status consistent and status inconsistent nurses.
5. Status inconsistent nurses (type and degree) have higher expectations and perceptions of the staff nurse role than low status consistent nurses.

REVIEW OF THE LITERATURE

This study is similar to and an expansion of a study by Chaska (1978). She identified differential expectations and perceptions of role performance among nurses related to status consistency and status inconsistency. A significant relationship was found between expectations and perceptions of role behavior and status consistency. Furthermore, statistically significant differences were found between role expectations and perceptions scores, with expectations being higher than perceptions for all nursing roles. In the original study of 303 nurses, the focus was on 12 nursing roles (practitioners, specialists, administrators, and others), whereas the present research was concerned only with the staff nurse role.

Although studies on the role concept of nurses have been reported in the literature, few studies have examined components of role expectations. Weiss and Davis (1985) examined aspects of collaborative practice. They indicated that interactive behaviors, assertion of the nurse's professional expertise, and communication were major components of collaboration. Numerous items in their scales parallel the items developed for this study. Their findings suggested that the average staff nurse is ill-prepared for collaborative practice with physicians and experiences difficulty in a collegial role. The nurse's initiation of an active interchange with physicians to communicate clearly what nursing can contribute was clearly seen as an important factor in collaboration.

In another study, Kinney (1985) examined the relationships of three personality variables to role concepts. Findings indicated that assertiveness was associated with both feminine and masculine attributes. Assertiveness is assumed to be an inherent attribute of an independent nursing role. Nurses who are unable to view nursing and the role expectations within nursing as a complex undertaking are less able to recognize that different situations require different roles and behaviors.

Role diffusion, particularly in the area of professional responsibility, has been identified as a major issue (Singleton & Nail, 1984). Staff nurses are seen as the facilitator in the delivery of care, the link with the physician, and the provider of nursing care that complements the medical regimen. As a result there are overlapping and gray areas of responsibility. Role clarity and expectations in the staff nurse role are viewed as essential if autonomy in professional nursing practice can become a reality. Ideas sug-

gested by Singleton and Nail (1984) were utilized as items in the development of this study's scales.

Taunton and Otteman (1986) reported that components of role expectations were explored for staff nurses. The way they operationally defined the staff nurse role was not clear. The findings provided evidence that studies conducted by researchers in the past have not reflected the real diversity of expectations among the staff nurses' roles. The authors emphasized the effects of staff nurse expectations and the expectations of others about staff nurses on patient care but also on the work environment.

Prescott and Bowen's work (1985) provided another dimension in understanding staff nurse role expectations and perceptions. They examined the perspectives of physicians and nurses on interaction between the two groups. The method utilized by Prescott and Bowen was similar to the present study in that both Likert-type scales and semistructured interviews were used to collect data. However, disagreements between physicians and nurses regarding patient care was the predominant focus of their study. Some of their items, namely, physician's orders, calling physicians, and the domain of nursing practice, were similar to items employed in this study. Their findings indicated little evidence of collaborative practice and lend further support to the fact that the absence of a clearly defined, distinct domain of nursing and thus the staff nurse role is related to lack of effective collaboration between physicians and nurses.

Physicians may have differing expectations and evaluations of staff nurses among themselves just as staff nurses have among themselves (Chaska, 1978). To the extent that there is significant disagreement about role definitions between physicians and staff nurses (as well as among nurses and physicians themselves), their working relationships in providing health care as a cooperative professional community are in jeopardy.

Both theoretical formulations and growing empirical evidence point to the interrelatedness of role expectations and perceptions and high-quality patient care. The present study addresses the interplay between components of role expectations held by two professional groups, which are critical in professional nursing practice and the fostering of cooperative roles to benefit patient care.

DEFINITION OF TERMS

The following definitions were used for this study and are defined conceptually and then operationally.

Expectations are the anticipated performances of self and/or others in terms of some idealized norm. In this study they are represented as a summed score to a series of expected staff nurse behaviors.

Perceptions are the view of self or others' performances past or present relative to an idealized norm. Operationally they are a summed score reflecting the actual extent that the behaviors occur.

Status refers to an individual's place within a system of social ranking and in this study is measured on a three-dimensional scale consisting of education, position, and income. Operationally for nurses, education was defined as high (baccalaureate degree), medium (diploma), and low (associate degree); position was defined as high (manager and above) and low (staff); income was defined as high ($23,000 and above), medium ($15,001 to $22,900), and low (below $15,000). For physicians, education and position were assumed high with salary defined as low (less than $60,000), medium ($60,100 to 90,999), and high ($91,000 plus).

Type of status consistency refers to an *order* of ranking held by an individual in regard to their education, position, and income. Type is classified as either status consistent or status inconsistent. Operationally, status consistency occurred when a person had a high *or* low rank on all three dimensions of status: education, position, and income; status inconsistency occurred when a person had a combination of high *and* low rankings on the status dimensions.

Degree of status consistency reflects an individual's beliefs about the consistency among salary received, educational preparation, and job responsibilities. Operationally, it was a summed score representing consistency in educational preparation for job responsibilities and salary received.

METHODOLOGY
Sample

A random sample of staff nurses and physicians was drawn from the medical-surgical unit rosters of a large Midwestern hospital. Intensive care units were excluded because there is some evidence that ICU staff nurses are different from medical-surgical staff nurses.

Data were also collected from a number of persons who volunteered (nonrandom group). An open invitation was issued to nurses and physicians through a personal letter signed by medical staff and nursing administration representatives, as well as by the principal researcher (NLC). The volunteers responded to this open invitation.

From the random sample of staff nurses, 58 agreed to participate and 22 nurses volunteered. From the random sample of physicians, 30 participated and an additional 20 volunteered. The data analyses revealed that the random and nonrandom groups were comparable. Thus the responses from both groups were combined for a total sample of 80 staff nurses and 50 physicians.

Subjects Rights'

A cover letter that explained the project's purpose, how anonymity was ensured, and what was expected of the participant was approved by both the university and hospital institutional review boards. Because of the sensitive nature of the study, a coding system was employed that eliminated the need for names.

Instrument Development

Based on the research literature, specific behaviors were identified that were attributed to the staff nurse role. Sources that addressed the three dimensions of the staff nurse role were considered. The independent, dependent, and interdependent aspects of the role were identified in the nursing process, autonomous practice, and collaborative relationships. Generated items were categorized into four groups: behaviors of the staff nurse in the role, qualities of the staff nurse in the role, behaviors of the physician in relation to the staff nurse role, and qualities of the physician in regard to the staff nurse role. Twenty scales were developed that addressed decision making, assessment, planning, teaching, interacting with physicians, skills, legal responsibilities, and other direct and indirect care activities.

A pilot study was conducted on the first version of the instrument, which contained 167 items. In addition, there were 23 items pertaining to demographic and organizational variables. The purpose of the pilot study was to test item clarity and content validity of the items. Fifteen doctoral nursing students and nurse administrators participated. They indicated if the item was part of the staff nurse role and to which of the 20 scales the item belonged. The criterion for retaining an item was at least 70% agreement by participants. The final instrument reflected revisions based on the pilot study and consisted of demographic items plus 166 Likert-type items designed to measure expectations and perceptions toward the independent, dependent, and interdependent aspects of the staff nurse role.

The same set of items was employed for both expectations and perceptions, so it was very important that the respondents understood their tasks. First, the subjects were asked to respond to the set of items in terms of the their expectations, and then the subjects were asked to respond to them in terms of their perceptions. Expectations were assessed in terms of importance (very important to very unimportant) to the staff nurse role. The perceptions were measured in terms of behaviors and qualities actually occurring "to a maximum degree" to those occurring "to a minimum degree." Explicit directions were designed to focus the attention of the respondents on their task.

Demographic variables included more general variables such as age, sex, and type and length of present employment. Variables relating to the professional realm included type of basic educational program, amount of continuing academic prepara-

tion, subscriptions to professional journals, year of graduation from a basic nursing program or medical school, name of the school and state where the education program was completed, physicians' average number of patient admissions per year, number of years admitting patients at this institution, and type of medical specialty.

Procedure

The instrument was administered individually to enhance independence of data among respondents. Data collection occurred over a 4-month period. Staff nurses in the random sample were approached at all three shifts of duty. If the nurse could not complete the instrument during the tour of duty, she or he mailed it to the investigator. The collection of data from the nonrandom group of nurses and physicians was done by making appointments. Times were set aside to allow respondents an opportunity to talk with the investigator regarding the study and to provide additional information beyond that requested in the questionnaire if they desired. From the initial query to the random sample group concerning participation in the study, only four staff nurses and seven physicians specifically indicated that they did not wish to participate.

Analyses

Factor analysis techniques were employed to assess construct validity of the scales. The one-way analysis of variance (ANOVA) techniques were used to test the hypotheses. The .01 probability level was chosen because of the differences in sample size.

FINDINGS
Demographic Data for the Samples

The mean age of the staff nurses was 37, with a range from 21 to 63 years. Sixty-seven (83.75%) of the nurses in the sample indicated that they were employed full-time, and 11 (16.25%) part-time. The mean years of full-time employment was 5.51, with the mean total number of years employed at the hospital being 4.55. Forty-two (52.5%) of the nurses had been employed at only one hospital during their career. The mean income reported was $21,800 per year based on validated salary data for 1983–1984. Forty-eight (60%) indicated that they were married, 16 (20%) were single, and 15 (20%) were divorced or separated.

Of the 80 nurses in the sample, 32 (40%) were graduated from a hospital diploma program, 27 (33.8%) from an associate degree program, and 19 (23.8%) from a baccalaureate degree program. Of the total sample, 30 (37.5%) had additional education beyond their basic program. Ten nurses each had accumulated additional credits toward a bachelor's degree, earned a baccalaureate degree, or earned credits toward a master's degree in nursing. Forty (50%) of the nurses graduated before 1973, with 64 (80%) graduating from programs in the same state and 31 (39.7%) graduating from programs within the same university. Thirty-six (45%) of the nurses participated in continuing education programs the previous year, 52 (65.1%) subscribed to professional journals, and 5 (5.3%) belonged to the American Nurses' Association.

The mean age of the staff physicians was 46; 43 were married, 1 was single, and 3 were divorced. The mean number of years that physicians admitted patients to this hospital was 14.6, with the mean number of admissions per year being 160 patients. Of the 50 physicians, 25 specialized in internal medicine, 16 were surgeons, and 9 represented the area of family practice or other specialized fields. All physicians were board eligible/certified. Thirty-nine (78%) belonged to the American Medical Association; 26 (52%) were in private practice, and 21 (42%) were in a group practice. Thirty-five (70%) of the physicians graduated from the same medical school, with 33 (66%) completing their residency and 29 (58%) completing specialty preparation in the same state as their medical school. The median income reported was $95,000.

Scales

As a test of construct validity, a factor analysis employing an alpha method with varimax rotation was computed for the items with expectation re-

sponses. The same analysis was repeated for the items when the subjects' responded in terms of perceptions. Results indicated that there were 14 factors rather than the expected 20. If an item loading was above .4 on a factor, the item was included as part of the scale that was represented by the factor. For the most part the factor structure for the items in terms of expectations was the same as for items when responses were in terms of perceptions.

The last 3 of the 14 factors accounted for only 2% or less of the variance each. Only two or three items loaded on each of these factors. Thus only the 11 more viable factors were employed in the remainder of the analyses.

Factors were identified based on the theme represented by the higher weighted items. The Organization scale, which only measured perceptions, was the only one to contain the same items before and after analysis. The other items tended to form scales that reflected broader topics or content than the originally conceptualized scales. The theme for each factor is summarized by its title: Assessment, Collaboration, Current Role, Judgment, Liaison, Medical/Technical, M.D. Communication, M.D. Legal, M.D. Understanding of R.N. Role, and R.N. Communication.

In order to test the hypotheses, decisions had to be made about which scales represented the different staff nurse roles. The revised scales Assessment, Judgment, and Current Role seemed to reflect aspects of the independent nursing role. The dependent aspects of the role seemed to by typified by the Medical/Technical scale, and the physician's role vis-à-vis nurse viewed in the M.D. Communication, M.D. Legal, and M.D. Understanding of R.N. Role scales. The interdependent aspects of the role were identified as the R.N. Communication, Liaison, and Collaboration scales. In all, the evidence for construct validity was less than desired but since the ideas that were inherent in the 20 pilot study scales were still in the new scales, just in a more summary form, the final 11 scales were employed for hypotheses testing (see Table 36-1 for examples of scale items).

The 11 independent scales were analyzed for internal-consistency reliability using Cronbach's al-

TABLE 36-1
Item examples for each scale

SCALE NAME	SCALE ITEMS
1. Assessment	Focus on identification of patient's existing problems manageable to a nursing regimen.
	Identify the patient's need for nursing care including preventive, restorative, and maintenance/health promotion activities.
2. Medical/Technical	Devote the majority of time to carrying out physician orders.
	Devote the majority of time to taking vital signs of the patient.
3. Judgment	Delegate tasks that do not require professional judgment to unlicensed personnel.
	Use appropriate nursing judgment in the completion of physician orders.
4. R.N. Communication	Communicate to the physician the nursing evaluation of patient status.
	Question physician orders that appear inappropriate.
5. Liaison	Act as a resource person for professional and nonprofessional nursing.
	Act as liaison between physician and health care team.
6. Current Role	Ability to make independent nursing decisions.
	Has knowledge of the professional responsibility for delegated medical activities.
7. Organization (for role perceptions only)	The majority of the staff nurse time is primarily devoted to carrying out the functions outlined in the job description.
	Policies, rules, and procedures inhibit physician-nurse collaboration.
8. M.D. Communication	Communicate the status of patient's condition to nursing staff.
	Listen to nurses' recommendations, assessments, and observations in patient care.
9. M.D. Legal	Countersign verbal and altered physician protocols or standing orders.
	Return calls from nursing staff on a timely basis.
10. M.D. Understand R.N. Role	Has different expectations for performance in practice of the staff nurse based on academic preparation.
	Clearly define the difference between nursing and medical responsibilities. Clearly define the difference between a nursing regimen/activities and medical regimen/activities.
11. Collaboration	Provide appropriate assistance to physicians in carrying out procedures.
	Collaborate with physicians before making alterations to protocols, physicians' orders.
	Demonstrate managerial skills of the nursing unit.

TABLE 36-2
Summary of expectations scales analyses for R.N.s and M.D.s

EXPECTATION SCALES	TOTAL NO. OF ITEMS	RESPONSE RANGE	SAMPLE	MEAN	SD	ALPHA
1. Assessment	19	VI = 19	R.N.	35.79	9.11	.89
		N = 47				
		VUI = 95	M.D.	40.77	10.13	.84
2. Medical/Technical	8	VI = 8	R.N.	23.14	5.29	.80
		N = 24				
		VUI = 40	M.D.	25.50	5.36	.69
3. Judgment	11	VI = 11	R.N.	21.01	5.58	.80
		N = 33				
		VUI = 55	M.D.	24.69	6.01	.68
4. R.N. Communication	14	VI = 14	R.N.	25.80	6.33	.83
		N = 33				
		VUI = 70	M.D.	29.04	6.58	.73
5. Liaison	9	VI = 9	R.N.	15.49	4.43	.81
		N = 27				
		VUI = 45	M.D.	21.90	7.03	.83
6. Current Role	16	VI = 16	R.N.	24.99	5.96	.85
		N = 48				
		VUI = 80	M.D.	24.77	5.73	.78
8. M.D. Communication	15	VI = 15	R.N.	22.78	6.78	.91
		N = 45				
		VUI = 75	M.D.	23.08	5.98	.83
9. M.D. Legal	9	VI = 9	R.N.	12.85	3.70	.83
		N = 27				
		VUI = 45	M.D.	13.52	3.79	.66
10. M.D. Understand R.N. Role	7	VI = 7	R.N.	17.47	4.65	.72
		N = 21				
		VUI = 35	M.D.	15.04	4.88	.72
11. Collaboration	15	VI = 15	R.N.	32.41	6.06	.74
		N = 45				
		VUI = 75	M.D.	28.36	6.11	.71

VI = Very Important, N = Neutral, VUI = Very Unimportant

TABLE 36-3
Summary of perceptions scales analyses for R.N.s and M.D.s

PERCEPTIONS SCALES	TOTAL NO. OF ITEMS	RESPONSE RANGE		SAMPLE	MEAN	SD	ALPHA
1. Assessment	19	MAX =	19	R.N.	52.00	10.17	.86
		MIDPT =	57				
		MIN =	95	M.D.	47.86	9.51	.83
2. Medical/Technical	8	MAX =	8	R.N.	23.16	4.02	.56
		MIDPT =	24				
		MIN =	40	M.D.	22.36	4.23	.58
3. Judgment	11	MAX =	11	R.N.	26.99	6.19	.80
		MIDPT =	33				
		MIN =	55	M.D.	26.10	5.70	.74
4. R.N. Communication	14	MAX =	14	R.N.	32.29	5.83	.74
		MIDPT =	42				
		MIN =	70	M.D.	32.46	6.94	.80
5. Liaison	9	MAX =	9	R.N.	20.95	5.25	.80
		MIDPT =	42				
		MIN =	70	M.D.	23.60	4.98	.72
6. Current Role	16	MAX =	16	R.N.	31.90	6.61	.82
		MIDPT =	48				
		MIN =	80	M.D.	33.12	6.77	.81
7. Organization	22	SA =	22	R.N.	60.90	7.49	.61
		MIDPT =	66				
		SDis =	110	M.D.	56.44	7.69	.56
8. M.D. Communication	15	MAX =	15	R.N.	43.78	7.76	.85
		MIDPT =	45				
		MIN =	75	M.D.	36.58	7.98	.88
9. M.D. Legal	9	MAX =	9	R.N.	24.34	4.86	.76
		MIDPT =	27				
		MIN =	45	M.D.	18.98	5.42	.81
10. M.D. Understand R.N. Role	7	MAX =	7	R.N.	22.24	4.33	.78
		MIDPT =	21				
		MIN =	35	M.D.	16.76	4.35	.69
11. Collaboration	15	MAX =	15	R.N.	32.41	6.06	.74
		MIDPT =	45				
		MIN =	75	M.D.	33.46	6.79	.77

MAX, Maximum, MIDPT, Midpoint, MIN, Minimum, SA, Strongly agree, SDIS, Strongly disagree.

pha. The nurse sample was separated from the physician sample for these analyses (Tables 36-2 and 36-3). Expectation scales reliabilities for the nurses ranged from .72 for M.D. Understanding of R.N. Role to .91 for M.D. Communication. The reliabilities for the physician sample tended to be lower probably because of the smaller sample size. Although the lower reliabilities (.56) are modest, they are acceptable for research efforts.

There are two important factors to note when interpreting these data. First, there are 11 perception scales and only 10 expectation scales. There is no Organization scale for expectations. Second, responses were scored with 1 equaling the most positive score. On the expectation scales, the lower the score the more important the behaviors. For the perception scales the lower the score the greater the extent to which nurses actually performed the behaviors.

Intervening Variables

A series of one-way ANOVAs were computed to identify if any of the possible intervening variables included in the study were related to the differences in expectation and perception scores for the nurses or physicians. For nurses the Medical/Technical expectation scale demonstrated significant differences owing to type of basic education program. Baccalaureate graduates held the highest expectations in contrast to diploma graduates, who held the lowest ones. Income influenced expectations for the two Communication scales and the M.D. Legal scale, as well as perceptions of the Medical/Technical scale. No pattern was discernible, with the low salary group significantly different for one variable and the middle and highest groups significantly different for other variables. For the physicians, The Collaboration expectation scale differed because of specialty; the R.N. Communication expectation scale differed because of number of patients admitted per year; and the M.D. Legal scale differed owing to number of years a physician had been admitting patients.

For the interval intervening variables such as age, Pearson correlations were computed for each scale. For the nurses, age and the expectations for the M.D. Communication scale (.18), and perceptions of the Medical/Technical (.20) and M.D. Legal scales (−.21) were significant. For the physicians, significant relationships were found for age and expectations for R.N. Communication (−.25), Current Role (−.30), Medical/Technical (.26), Liaison (.30), and for the perception scale of M.D. Legal (−.42).

Although there were several scales that were influenced by the intervening variables, there was no trend indicating that the intervening variables were systematically influencing the dependent variables. Based on these findings, no attempt was made to control for these variables in further analyses.

Hypotheses Testing

The one-way analysis of variance technique was employed to test hypotheses 1 through 4 (see list of hypotheses under Conceptual Framework). These results are summarized in Tables 36-4 and 36-5. For hypothesis 1, two of the six scales resulted in significant differences at the .01 level. Expectation scores for Assessment and Judgment differed as predicted; however, there were no significant differences for the Current Role expectation scores. For perceptions, there were no significant differences for any of the scales. Overall the hypothesis was not supported.

For hypothesis 2 concerning the dependent role, there are mixed findings. For the four expectation scales only the M.D. Understanding of R.N. role was significantly different. On the other hand, all of the perception scales are significantly different except for the Medical/Technical scale. For each of the significantly different scales the physicians rated themselves higher than the nurses rated the physicians. Since only four of the possible eight tests produced significant differences, the hypothesis was not supported.

For hypothesis 3, which addressed the collaborative nature of the staff nurse role, two of the three scales on expectations (R.N. Communication and Liaison) produced significant differences. For perceptions, the only scale with significant differences was the Liaison scale. Again only three of the six possible tests produced significant findings; thus hypothesis 3 was not supported.

TABLE 36-4
One-way ANOVA comparing R.N. and M.D. role expectations of importance toward selected activities of 10 scales

SCALE	DF	SS	F RATIO	P
1. Assessment	1	888.12	9.81	.002
	128	11592.11		
2. Medical/Technical	1	62.39	2.76	.099
	128	2851.69		
3. Judgment	1	413.86	12.54	.0006
	128	4225.87		
4. R.N. Communication	1	323.00	7.82	.006
	128	5290.72		
5. Liaison	1	1265.24	40.75	.000
	128	3974.49		
6. Current Role	1	1.88	0.055	.82
	128	4418.61		
7. Organization	No scale available			
8. M.D. Communication	1	3.71	0.098	.76
	128	4848.01		
9. M.D. Legal	1	15.40	1.024	.031
	128	1925.37		
10. M.D. Understand R.N. Role	1	182.44	8.120	.005
	128	2875.87		
11. Collaboration	1	22.10	0.642	.42
	128	4405.51		

Before testing hypotheses 4 and 5, the nurses had to be grouped according to their type of status consistency. Three groups were created: high status consistent, status inconsistent, and low status consistent. All subjects who did not qualify as high status consistent (high education, high position, and high salary) or low status consistent (low education, low position, and low salary) were placed in the inconsistent category. Seventy-one of the 80 nurses were classified as inconsistent. They tended to have a high education, low income, and low position or a low education, moderate income, and low position. There were so few nurses who were either high status consistent or low status consistent that it was not possible to test the type aspect of hypotheses 4 and 5.

Degree of status consistency was a summed score of three items in which the nurse was asked to indicate from 1 to 7 how consistent she or he perceived her or his salary/education and job responsibilities. These scores ranged from 7 to 21. The lowest possible score was 3, midpoint was 12, and the highest score was 21. Either a high or low extreme score represented an inconsistent status, with the midpoint representing consistent status. Frequency distribution scattergrams of the degree of status consistency variable were inspected for a bimodal distribution, which is what would have been found if inconsistent subjects differed from consistent subjects. None was in evidence; thus hypotheses 4 and 5 were not supported.

These results were most disappointing because of the interest in the status consistency variable. Alternative methods of conceptualizing both type and degree of status consistency are being considered. Explication of these methods and their rationale will be in a forthcoming publication.

TABLE 36-5
One-way ANOVA comparing R.N. and M.D. role perceptions toward selected activities

SCALES	df	SS	F RATIO	P
1. Assessment	1	527.37	5.35	.02
	128	12618.02		
2. Medical/Technical	1	38.77	2.807	.10
	128	1768.00		
3. Judgment	1	24.24	0.672	.41
	128	4617.49		
4. R.N. Communication	1	35.39	0.808	.37
	128	5607.41		
5. Liaison	1	216.08	8.126	.005
	128	3403.80		
6. Current Role	1	231.85	5.035	.03
	128	5894.03		
7. Organization	1	121.24	2.069	.15
	128	7501.87		
8. M.D. Communication	1	1231.92	23.900	.00
	128	6597.81		
9. M.D. Legal	1	913.92	34.562	.00
	128	3384.70		
10. M.D. Understand R.N. Role	1	923.17	34.562	.00
	128	2405.61		
11. Collaboration	1	20.10	0.581	.40
	128	4103.41		

DISCUSSION

Although in the sample two thirds of the nurses were employed on medical-surgical nursing units, the total number of baccalaureate graduates in the sample is low in proportion to the number of associate degree and diploma graduates employed on these units. Furthermore the nurse sample ($N = 80$) reflects an older, more experienced, and stable nursing staff, which may not be typical of other large institutions. The physician sample ($N = 50$) is not reflective of the total (over 300) practicing on these units.

Independent Aspects of Role

The hypotheses reflect current beliefs about the nursing role, namely, that there are three types of functions inherent in the role: independent, dependent, and interdependent. Surprisingly the staff nurses did not differ significantly from the physicians for perceptions of the independent role function. Assessment skills were slightly higher than the scale midpoint with Judgment one standard deviation above the midpoint and Current Role two standard deviations above it. In other words, the physicians and nurses agreed that the extent or amount to which assessment was conducted—independent judgments were made and the nurse role performed—was not that high. This finding is particularly important, given that there were significant differences between staff nurses and physicians regarding expectations in independent functions concerning assessment, judgment, and carrying out the current, independent role being advocated for the staff nurse.

Encouragingly the staff nurses placed significantly more importance on the Assessment and

Judgment expectations than the physicians, whereas both groups agreed that the Current Role is important. However, the question should be raised as to what degree the significantly higher expectations than perceptions of actual practice for the Assessment and Judgment scales indicate dissatisfaction? The literature indicates that there is a strong relationship between autonomous nursing practice, professionalism, and job satisfaction. While there is more consensus about what the functions of the staff nurse should be and are in this sample than previous authors have indicated (Chaska, 1978; Singleton & Nail, 1984; Taunton & Otteman, 1986), this may be due to the lack of perceived need and acknowledgment of autonomy for professional nursing practice in this setting.

Dependent Aspects of Role

For the perception scales, M.D. Communication, M.D. Legal, and M.D. Understanding of R.N. Role, the physicians' means were more positive, that is, skills and behaviors were rated as being performed more frequently than nurses indicated. The significant differences regarding perceptions in actual practice for the activities in the M.D. Communication and M.D. Legal scales may be an indication of the source of misunderstanding for the professional nurse role. The physicians significantly rated themselves higher not only on expectations in the M.D. Understanding of R.N. Role scale, but also in actual practice, thus increasing the discrepant findings between the two samples. Further exploration of these data will be presented in a future publication.

For the Medical/Technical scale, the nurses and physicians agreed that both perceptions and expectations were near the midpoint of the scale. The fact that there were no differences in perceptions of actual practice regarding the activities in the Medical/Technical scale may support the conclusion that the role activities in the scale are being performed at a level acceptable to physicians. This situation may reflect the role confusion cited in other studies (Kinney, 1985; Prescott & Bowen, 1985; Singleton & Nail, 1984; Taunton & Otteman, 1986). Current and

potential conflict or confusion about dependent role activities by the staff nurse seems highly probable.

Interdependent Aspects of Role

In viewing the data pertaining to the interdependent role of the nurses, the findings for the activities in the Liaison scale are relevant for further exploration of the differences found in the M.D. Understanding of R.N. Role scale (hypothesis 2). The interface or bridge may be unclear between nurses and physicians on the legal ramifications of their roles. The findings for the Liaison scale indicate that critical interfacing functions and responsibilities may be in jeopardy or are not being carried out. This is further substantiated by the fact that there were no significant differences regarding the activities in the Collaboration scale, which is opposite to the findings of Weiss and Davis (1985). Activities in the Collaborative scale pertain specifically to those that directly help assist the physician or assist in the plan of patient care, whereas activities in the Liaison scale more directly focus on coordinating functions of the nurse. The interfacing of roles is implicit to coordination.

Status Consistency

Perhaps the most distressing finding in this study is that 71 of the 80 nurses were classified as status inconsistent. As distressing is the fact that they tended to have a high education, low income, and low position *or* a low education, moderate income, and low position. On the other hand, these data simply reflect the reality that hospitals do not provide salary increments based on educational preparation. The added reality is that longevity in a position is rewarded by increased salary even if the quality of the work does not improve.

According to the literature there is a strong relationship between role expectations and job satisfaction. If the discrepancies between physician and nurse role perceptions and expectations lead to confusion and/or conflict, the likelihood of job satisfaction will decrease. Intraprofessional conflicts may also become a problem when the higher educated nurses realize that less educated nurses are receiving higher salaries. Since job satisfaction is a major component of any retention effort, attention to role perceptions and expectations of staff provides important information that could allow effective intervention before actual conflict.

CONCLUSION

The findings of this study support the conclusion that there are differences in expectations and perceptions of role behavior between nurses and physicians, particularly in the independent, dependent, and interdependent aspects of the staff nurse role. These differences suggest confusion in roles and potential problems in promoting a cooperative climate. Confusion regarding roles needs to be openly acknowledged, discussed, and resolved if physicians and nurses are to work as an *effective* team in providing care.

The chief contribution of the present study may be its affirmation that the staff nurse role is unclear within as well as between the professional staff nurse and physician groups. Potential problematic areas for a consistent set of expectations were identified. A tool with evidence of acceptable reliability and minimal validity was developed. Additional work is needed in the development of this tool. Since data collection occurred immediately after a major change in nursing administration, this study should be replicated in other large institutions in diverse areas of the country to determine if differences are institution-specific or generalizable. Responses by these subjects may reflect assessment of previous nursing administration's effects on nursing practice, as well as anticipation for future desired change. The implications are great not only for effective collaboration with other professional groups, but essentially for the provision of high-quality care.

REFERENCES

Chaska, N. (1978). Status consistency and nurses' expectations and perceptions of role performance. *Nursing Research.* 27, 356–364.

Conway, M. (1978). Theoretical approaches to the study of roles. In M. Herdy, & M. Conway (Eds.), *Role theory: Perspectives for health professionals* (pp. 17–27). New York: Appleton-Century-Crofts.

Geschwender, J. A. (1967). Continuities in theories of status consistency and cognitive dissonance. *Social Forces,* 46, 160–171.

Jackson, E. F., & Curtis, R. F. (1972). Effects of vertical mobility and status inconsistency: A body of negative evidence. *American Sociological Review,* 37, 7011–7013.

Kinney, C. K. D. (1985). A re-examination of nursing role conceptions. *Nursing Research,* 34, 170–176.

Lenski, G. (1954). Social participation and status crystallization. *American Sociological Review,* 19, 405–413.

McClure, M. L., & Nelson, M. J. (1982). Trends in hospital nursing. In L. Aiken (Ed.), *Nursing in the 1980's: Crises, opportunities, challenges,* (pp. 59–73). Philadelphia: J. B. Lippincott.

Mechanic, D., & Aiken, L. (1982). Sounding board: A cooperative agenda for medicine and nursing. *New England Journal of Medicine,* 3, 747–750.

Prescott, P. A., & Bowen, S. (1985). Physician-nurse relationships. *Annals of Internal Medicine,* 103, 127–133.

Singleton, E. K., & Nail, F. C. (1984). Role clarification: A prerequisite to autonomy. *The Journal of Nursing Administration,* 10, 17–22.

Taunton, R. L., & Otteman, D. (1986). The multiple dimensions of staff nurse role conception. *The Journal of Nursing Administration,* 16, 31–37.

Thomas, E. J., & Biddle, B. (1979). The nature and history of role theory. In E. J. Thomas & B. Biddle (Eds.), *Role theory: Concepts and research* (pp. 3–19). New York: Robert E. Krieger Publishing Co.

Weiss, S., & Davis, H. P. (1985). Validity and reliability of the collaborative practice scales. *Nursing Research,* 34, 299–304.

⁎   **EDITOR'S QUESTIONS FOR DISCUSSION**   ⁎

Discuss the strengths and the limitations of this study from the aspects of design, methodology, and data analysis. What other alternative methods might be suggested for the development of scales or measures of role performance? What other intervening variables might account for the findings? What alternative explanations might be offered in interpreting the findings? Discuss the implications of the findings for the various nursing roles and the development of nursing as a profession, facilitating communication and understanding of the nursing role among physicians, and the development of professional nursing practice. Discuss strategies by which the professional staff nurse role may more clearly be defined in the practice setting for staff nurses.

37

Critical Care Nursing:
Perspectives and challenges

Kathleen Dracup, D.N.Sc., R.N., F.A.A.N.
Celine Marsden, M.N., R.N.

Critical care nursing is in a state of rapid evolution. As a specialization, it was affected by the patterns of health care delivery and reimbursement policies established in the 1950s and 1960s, the development of technology to support the severely ill patient, and the traditional socialization of nurses and physicians to gender roles. However, two of the most important forces in the early development of critical care nursing were the organizational patterns of American hospitals and the development of technology as a force toward specialization.

HISTORICAL VIEWS
Hospital Structure

Unlike other nursing specializations that are practiced in a community setting, critical care nursing was (and still is) practiced exclusively within hospitals. Hospitals are modeled on a military paradigm. Many of the phrases familiar to nurses and physicians in acute care settings reflect this para-

digm, for example, "doctors' orders," "chief of staff," "chain of command," and "house officers." In the past, certain uniforms were required of the different professions and of students within that profession. Each uniform indicated the status of the person wearing it within the system. For example, female student nurses wore plain white caps. Upon graduation, nurses wore caps with one stripe. When a female nurse was promoted to an administrative position, she was given an extra stripe to wear on her cap, similar to promotion from private to sergeant. Short white coats and white pants (for males) and white skirts (for females) were mandatory for medical students and physicians-in-training, while faculty and attending physicians could be identified by knee-length white laboratory coats.

The nursing care provided in critical care units also reflected a military structure, with the physician at the top of the decision-making hierarchy. Physicians gave medical orders that were implemented by nurses, but physicians, by law, held ultimate authority and responsibility for all the care given to the hospitalized patient. Decisions about the care that patients received were made exclusively by physicians, and hospital committees that dealt with clinical practice issues were usually restricted to physician membership.

This paper was presented with the support of the National Institutes of Health, Heart, Lung, and Blood Institute (RO1-HL32171-04).

lic health nursing, but it was no longer considered a specialty. Rather, public health preparation became the hallmark of baccalaureate nursing education.

The brief period in which public health nursing was considered a separate clinical specialty did, however, establish the collegiate setting as a possible training arena for specialty practice. The precedent became important at a later date when collegiate nursing education expanded.

FACTORS INFLUENCING THE CURRENT NURSING SPECIALTY MOVEMENT

The current advanced specialty movement builds on the older, more informal models of specialization, but it is marked by some major changes: (a) educational preparation has been upgraded; (b) there is a clear trend in the direction of graduate level preparation; (c) certification by professional organizations has emerged as an important credential; and (d) the certification has been recognized by state lawmakers. Several factors have helped to bring about these changes.

Educational reform was a key prerequisite to the advanced specialties. The struggle to change the basic educational system from the hospital apprenticeship model to a collegiate model was slow, but by the year 1965 13.7% of the new graduates were from baccalaureate programs, 2.6% were from associate degree programs, and 83.7% were from diploma programs (American Nurses' Association, 1967). The baccalaureate group, although small by current standards, was large enough to provide a pool of nurses who could enter graduate programs. The first formal educational programs for clinical nurse specialists and nurse practitioners were started in 1965. By 1984 the pool of collegiate graduates had grown significantly with 29.5% of the new graduates finishing with baccalaureate degrees and 55.3% with associate of arts degrees, while only 15% were diploma graduates (Rosenfeld, 1985). The upgrading of the nursing educational system had supported the development of the advanced nursing specialties.

The movement was facilitated by the Nurse Training Act, which was enacted in 1964 under Title VIII of the Public Health Service Act (Kalisch &

Kalisch, 1978). This legislation was aimed at strengthening nursing education. In response to this opportunity many schools of nursing established master's degree programs, or expanded existing programs, and made clinical specialization the focus of the new curricula.

The women's movement was an important factor in the rapid expansion of midwifery and to a lesser extent the other nursing specialties. The movement helped to break down the strict sex role barriers that defined medicine as men's work and nursing as women's work. For midwifery, the movement also furnished clients. There has long been a group of women who were angry with or fearful of the male-dominated medical establishment. The women's movement allowed those women to express openly their anger, to engage in self-care, and to seek alternative sources of obstetrical and gynecological care (Boston Women's Health Collective, 1976). Some women sought underground lay midwives, but others found that nurse-midwives could furnish the much wanted support along with technical competence.

The advanced specialty movement in nursing has also been stimulated by the rapid expansion of medical science and technology. Health care providers need to know more in order to be competent. Since it is impossible to know everything about everything, it is reasonable to break down the span of needed knowledge into nursing specialties. In medicine the specialization process has advanced much further than it has in nursing. At the beginning of this century most doctors were general practitioners. Now specialists outnumber generalists by almost five to one. Moreover the medical specialty process has proceeded to the second generation with the development of pediatric cardiologists. This advanced degree of medical specialization is fragmenting patient care and distancing physicians from their clients. Consequently there is a void that is being filled by the first-generation advanced nursing specialties.

CERTIFICATION

The American Nurses' Association (ANA) started its certification program in 1973, establishing two levels of certification to support the development of nursing specialties (ANA, 1987). The first level is the ordinary clinician. ANA uses the title "Registered Nurse Certified." In order to be certified at this level the individual must document an appropriate educational program and pass a test. Some of the specialties also require work experience in the specialty, although the trend is in the direction of certification at entry into the specialty. The second level of certification uses the title "Registered Nurse Certified Specialist," which is more broadly known as the clinical nurse specialist. Master's degree preparation is necessary to qualify at this level. Table 45-2 shows the types and levels of clinical specialists and clinicians who are certified by the ANA.

There are a variety of other nursing professional organizations that certify their members. Twenty-eight specialty organizations belong to the National Federation of Specialty Nursing Organizations (NF-SNO)—see accompanying box. A few of the smaller groups leave certification to the ANA and serve their members by publishing a journal or holding national meetings, which provide continuing education for the membership. However, the larger specialty groups carry more responsibilities. For example, the American Association of Critical-Care Nurses, which includes more than 50,000 members, holds conventions, publishes a journal, offers coursework, gives examinations, and certifies specialists in the field.

The education of the various clinical specialists represented by the NFSNO is in a period of transition. The old hospital postgraduate courses have been replaced with either hospital in-service programs, continuing education certificate programs, a bachelor's degree, or a master's degree. A clear trend in the direction of the master's degree for the more complex specialties can be seen.

NURSE PRACTITIONERS

The first formal educational program for nurse practitioners was established in 1965 in Colorado. It was set up as a 4-month certificate course (Silver, Ford & Day, 1968). The content was complex and new to nurses. Most of the early nurse practitioner programs were started outside of schools of nursing because many nurse educators of that era questioned the validity of the role. These educators perceived

TABLE 45-2
Certification of specialists by the American Nurses' Association

NURSE	GENERALIST LEVEL REGISTERED NURSE CERTIFIED (RNC)	CLINICAL SPECIAL LEVEL REGISTERED NURSE CERTIFIED SPECIALIST (RNCS)
Medical surgical	X	X
Gerontological	X	
Gerontological nurse practitioner	X	
Adult nurse practitioner	X	
Child and adolescent	X	X
Pediatric nurse practitioner	X	
School nurse practitioner	X	
Maternal and child health	X	
High-risk perinatal	X	
Family nurse practitioner	X	
Community health	X	
Adult psychiatric mental health	X	X
Child and adolescent psychiatric mental health	X	X

From American Nurses' Association. (1987). *The career credential, professional certification: 1987 certification catalog*. Kansas City, MO: Author.

National Federation of Specialty Nursing Organizations
American Association of Critical-Care Nurses (AACN)
American Association of Neuroscience Nurses (AANN)
American Association of Nurse Anesthetists (AANA)
American Association of Occupational Health Nurses (AAOHN)
American Association of Spinal Cord Injury Nurses (AASCIN)
American College of Nurse-Midwives (ACNM)
American Nephrology Nurses' Association (ANNA)
American Public Health Association (APHA) Nursing Section
American Society of Ophthalmic Registered Nurses, Inc. (ASORN)
American Society of Plastic and Reconstructive Surgical Nurses, Inc. (ASPRSN)
American Society of Post Anesthesia Nurses (ASPAN)
American Urological Association, Allied (AUAA)
Association for Practitioners in Infection Control (APIC)
Association of Pediatric Oncology Nurses (APON)
Association of Rehabilitation Nurses (ARN)
Emergency Nurses Association (ENA)
International Association for Enterostomal Therapy, Inc. (IAET)
Intravenous Nursing Society (INS)
National Association of Orthopaedic Nurses (NAON)
National Association of Pediatric Nurse Associates and Practitioners (NAPNAP)
National Association of School Nurses, Inc. (NASN)
National Flight Nurses Association (NFNA)
National Nurses Society on Addictions (NNSA)
Nurse Consultants Association, Inc. (NCA)
The Nurses' Association of the American College of Obstetricians and Gynecologists (NAACOG)
Oncology Nursing Society (ONS)
Society of Gastrointestinal Assistants, Inc. (SGA)
Society of Otolaryngology and Head-Neck Nurses, Inc. (SOHN)

From National Federation of Specialty Nursing Organizations. Member Organizations and Participants, July 21, 1987.

the health care team as divided into workers who focused on care, and those whose job it was to cure. Nursing was thought of as the caring profession. It followed that nurses should be interested primarily in the social and psychological problems that accompany illness, rather than in treating the actual illness. Nurses were described as maternal, expressive, supportive, and feminine while physicians were described as paternal, instrumental, masculine, and cure-oriented (ANA, 1965; Johnson, 1974; Kreuter, 1957; Rogers, 1964). The nurse practitioner role combined the care and cure elements, so it did not fit the format. Probably the most outspoken of the educators who did not favor nurse practitioners was Martha Rogers. She perceived the development of the nurse practitioner role as a ploy by physicians to lead nurses into "paying obeisance to an obsolete hierarchy" (Rogers, 1972, p. 42). She wanted nursing to be an independent profession and felt that the nurse practitioner movement was a step backward. She argued that those who became nurse practitioners left the nursing profession.

Educators who accepted this way of thinking were, naturally, unwilling to accept nurse practitioner programs in their schools. Consequently the lack of acceptance by educators was a powerful barrier to the early institutionalization of the educational programs within the mainstream of nursing education. Nevertheless, there were a few university nursing schools that were willing to set up nurse practitioner programs at the master's level. Gradually the fears and hostility lessened; the educational pattern was upgraded and switched from the certificate to the master's level. Women's health is now the only practitioner field left with any appreciable number of certificate programs. The master's degree programs are the norm in all other nurse practitioner specialties (Geolot, 1987; Sultz, Henry, Kinyon, Buck, & Bullough, 1983a, 1983b).

The nurse practitioner movement is now almost 25 years old and there are more than 15,000 nurse practitioners in practice. Six major nurse practitioner specialties have now emerged: pediatric, adult, geriatric, women's health care, and family health care nurse practitioners are the major specialties in the field. (U.S. Congress, 1986).

Certification varies by specialty. ANA certifies adult, family, gerontological, pediatric, and school nurse practitioners. However, 80% of the pediatric nurse practitioners who are certified have achieved that status through the National Board of Pediatric Nurse Practitioners/Associates rather than through the ANA (Dickenson-Hazard, 1988). Obstetrical-gynecological nurse practitioners are certified by the Nurses' Association of the American College of Obstetricians and Gynecologists (NAACOG, 1984). Each of these certifying bodies requires registered nurse licensure, graduation from a recognized nurse practitioner program, and the successful completion of a certifying examination.

NURSE-MIDWIFERY

Traditionally, assisting with the birth process was considered a field for women and midwifery was a time-honored profession learned by apprenticeship (Leavitt, 1986). Obstetrics developed a medical specialty in the 19th century and other physicians added deliveries to their functions. Deliveries were moved from the home to the hospital, where analgesics and anesthesia were used, and promises of "painless childbirth" were made.

With the advent of the trained nurse most European countries developed nurse-midwifery as a specialty. Often a collaborative agreement was made, whereby nurse-midwives handled the normal deliveries and obstetricians took over for the problem cases. Nurse-midwifery was much slower to develop in the United States and the specialty has had to struggle for its existence (Litoff, 1978).

The first American nurse-midwifery training program was established in connection with the Maternity Center of New York City in 1932 (Tom, 1982). Unfortunately, many of the graduates of the program were prevented from practicing as midwives. They had to content themselves with serving as teachers or working in hospital maternity units. Nurse-midwives encountered the least opposition in the rural areas. Their best-known trailblazer was Mary Breckenridge of Kentucky. She established a service for mothers and children, which eventually came to

be called the Frontier Nursing Service. Adopting the rule that if a husband could reach the nurse at the center, the nurse could make it back to the mother, nurses traveled on horseback and foot to the isolated hill residences (Breckenridge, 1952).

While the Frontier Nursing Service became a recognized outpost of expanded nursing function, nurse-midwives continued to be much less welcome in areas where there were more physicians. Such exclusion continued, despite the fact that research evidence indicated that lives could be saved by nurse-midwives. A landmark study carried out from 1960 to 1963 provided this evidence (Levy, Wilkinson, & Marine, 1971). The demonstration project employed two nurse-midwives to manage normal deliveries at the Madera County Hospital in rural California. They gave prenatal care, attended labor and delivery, and managed the care of the mothers and infants in the postpartum period. They were successful in breaking down cultural barriers between the patients and health care providers. The number of women seeking prenatal care and other preventive services increased significantly. Even more important was the fact that, during the span of the project, prematurity and neonatal mortality rates among the patient population fell significantly. Yet, when the project sponsors sought to institutionalize the practice and secure a change in the state law, which would have allowed nurse-midwives to continue practicing, they were unsuccessful because of opposition from the California Medical Association (CMA). When the CMA opposition forced the cancellation of the project, the neonatal mortality rate went from the project rate of 10.3 per 1000 live births to 32.1 per 1000 live births (Levy et al., 1971).

Because of the positive record of both nurse-midwives and nurse practitioners in caring for women from all social strata, including the socially and economically high-risk population, the Institute of Medicine recommended:

> More reliance should be placed on nurse-midwives and nurse practitioners to increase access to prenatal care for hard-to-reach, often high-risk groups. Maternity programs designed to serve socio-

46

Discharge Planning and Continuity of Care

Evelyn G. Hartigan, Ed.D., R.N.

During the 1980s a major shift in the provision of health care occurred; acute care that in the past was provided solely in hospitals moved to some acute care being provided in alternative sites (Fig. 46-1). Some acute care in other settings was provided as a result of early discharge from a hospital. This shift was brought about primarily by the effects of technological advances; limited and often decreased resources (manpower, money, supplies); increased numbers of elderly and handicapped; a more active, participative third-party payor; and a more knowledgeable, cost-conscious consumer. As a result, the efficient use of resources demanded a systematic approach to health care with built-in mechanisms to assure accountability for the achievement and evaluation of care outcomes. One response to this demand has been the emphasis placed on the need for discharge planning in all agencies providing health care—hospitals, nursing homes, extended care facilities, and ambulatory settings—by the government, accrediting bodies, and third-party payors. This chapter reviews the definitions of continuum of care and discharge planning, Medicare and Joint Commission on Accreditation of Healthcare Organizations (JCAHO) major requirements, third-party payor's role in determining the quality of health care, program components and components requiring special nursing attention, and lastly, current unresolved issues and problems related to the continuum of care.

DEFINITIONS

Discharge planning is a component of a broader system, namely, continuum of care. Continuum of care has been defined as "an integrated, client-centered system of care composed of both services and integrating mechanisms that guides and tracks clients over time through a comprehensive array of health, mental health, and social services spanning all levels of intensity of care" (Evashwick & Weiss, 1987, p. 23). Historically the definition of discharge planning was limited to the patient's being referred to services required after hospitalization. The social worker was the primary health care provider involved and referrals were made, for the most part, to clinics and intermediate or chronic care agencies. The Prospective Payment System (PPS) in 1983, with its demand for efficient use of resources, broadened the function and scope of discharge planning. Hartigan and Brown offered a broader definition of discharge planning in keeping with changing societal and economic factors:

Discharge planning, which helps to ensure continuity of care, helps sick and well persons and their

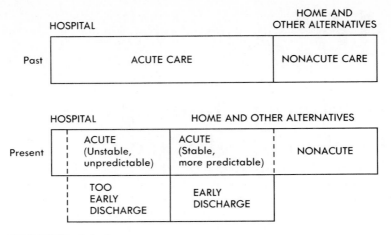

FIGURE 46-1
Discharge planning.

families find the best solutions to their health problems, at the right time, from the appropriate source, at the best price, and on a continuous basis for the required period of time. (1985, p. 9)

MEDICARE AND JOINT COMMISSION ON ACCREDITATION OF HEALTHCARE ORGANIZATIONS (JCAHO) REQUIREMENTS

Despite the many recommendations for discharge planning by government and other groups, there are no readily available blueprints to guide the health care provider charged with the planning, implementation, and evaluation of a program. However, health care providers are *required* to develop a program even though the requirements are not always clear or all-inclusive. The Health Care Financing Administration (HCFA, 1986) has issued for Medicare providers "Conditions for Participation" relating to discharge planning. The conditions came about as a result of the Omnibus Budget Reconciliation Act of 1986. The standard requires a hospital to have an ongoing discharge planning program and plan, which have provisions for follow-up care that are consistent with available resources within the agency and community. The discharge plan must meet the medically related needs of the patient and make available social work, and psychological and educational services. Other major requirements are:

1. Discharge planning needs must be identified at an early stage of hospitalization or in HCFA language, "in a timely manner." Most hospitals have developed high-risk tools to be used on admission, or preadmission when possible, to identify patients most likely to require posthospitalization services. It is anticipated that the HCFA will develop a high-risk tool for use by participating hospitals. A physician, patient, or patient representative may request discharge planning evaluation even though the patient may not have been categorized by the hospital as high risk.

2. The discharge planning evaluation, in addition to including a patient's likely need for postdischarge care, must be included in the patient's medical record and discussed with the patient or the patient's representative.

3. The evaluation and discharge plan must be developed by, or under the supervision of, a registered nurse, social worker, or other qualified person.

The JCAHO, in January 1988, incorporated new discharge planning standards. These standards parallel to a great degree the HCFA Conditions for Participation. The JCAHO also requires that discharge

lic health nursing, but it was no longer considered a specialty. Rather, public health preparation became the hallmark of baccalaureate nursing education.

The brief period in which public health nursing was considered a separate clinical specialty did, however, establish the collegiate setting as a possible training arena for specialty practice. The precedent became important at a later date when collegiate nursing education expanded.

FACTORS INFLUENCING THE CURRENT NURSING SPECIALTY MOVEMENT

The current advanced specialty movement builds on the older, more informal models of specialization, but it is marked by some major changes: (a) educational preparation has been upgraded; (b) there is a clear trend in the direction of graduate level preparation; (c) certification by professional organizations has emerged as an important credential; and (d) the certification has been recognized by state lawmakers. Several factors have helped to bring about these changes.

Educational reform was a key prerequisite to the advanced specialties. The struggle to change the basic educational system from the hospital apprenticeship model to a collegiate model was slow, but by the year 1965 13.7% of the new graduates were from baccalaureate programs, 2.6% were from associate degree programs, and 83.7% were from diploma programs (American Nurses' Association, 1967). The baccalaureate group, although small by current standards, was large enough to provide a pool of nurses who could enter graduate programs. The first formal educational programs for clinical nurse specialists and nurse practitioners were started in 1965. By 1984 the pool of collegiate graduates had grown significantly with 29.5% of the new graduates finishing with baccalaureate degrees and 55.3% with associate of arts degrees, while only 15% were diploma graduates (Rosenfeld, 1985). The upgrading of the nursing educational system had supported the development of the advanced nursing specialties.

The movement was facilitated by the Nurse Training Act, which was enacted in 1964 under Title VIII of the Public Health Service Act (Kalisch &

Kalisch, 1978). This legislation was aimed at strengthening nursing education. In response to this opportunity many schools of nursing established master's degree programs, or expanded existing programs, and made clinical specialization the focus of the new curricula.

The women's movement was an important factor in the rapid expansion of midwifery and to a lesser extent the other nursing specialties. The movement helped to break down the strict sex role barriers that defined medicine as men's work and nursing as women's work. For midwifery, the movement also furnished clients. There has long been a group of women who were angry with or fearful of the male-dominated medical establishment. The women's movement allowed those women to express openly their anger, to engage in self-care, and to seek alternative sources of obstetrical and gynecological care (Boston Women's Health Collective, 1976). Some women sought underground lay midwives, but others found that nurse-midwives could furnish the much wanted support along with technical competence.

The advanced specialty movement in nursing has also been stimulated by the rapid expansion of medical science and technology. Health care providers need to know more in order to be competent. Since it is impossible to know everything about everything, it is reasonable to break down the span of needed knowledge into nursing specialties. In medicine the specialization process has advanced much further than it has in nursing. At the beginning of this century most doctors were general practitioners. Now specialists outnumber generalists by almost five to one. Moreover the medical specialty process has proceeded to the second generation with the development of pediatric cardiologists. This advanced degree of medical specialization is fragmenting patient care and distancing physicians from their clients. Consequently there is a void that is being filled by the first-generation advanced nursing specialties.

CERTIFICATION

The American Nurses' Association (ANA) started its certification program in 1973, establishing two levels of certification to support the development of nursing specialties (ANA, 1987). The first level is the ordinary clinician. ANA uses the title "Registered Nurse Certified." In order to be certified at this level the individual must document an appropriate educational program and pass a test. Some of the specialties also require work experience in the specialty, although the trend is in the direction of certification at entry into the specialty. The second level of certification uses the title "Registered Nurse Certified Specialist," which is more broadly known as the clinical nurse specialist. Master's degree preparation is necessary to qualify at this level. Table 45-2 shows the types and levels of clinical specialists and clinicians who are certified by the ANA.

There are a variety of other nursing professional organizations that certify their members. Twenty-eight specialty organizations belong to the National Federation of Specialty Nursing Organizations (NFSNO)—see accompanying box. A few of the smaller groups leave certification to the ANA and serve their members by publishing a journal or holding national meetings, which provide continuing education for the membership. However, the larger specialty groups carry more responsibilities. For example, the

American Association of Critical-Care Nurses, which includes more than 50,000 members, holds conventions, publishes a journal, offers coursework, gives examinations, and certifies specialists in the field.

The education of the various clinical specialists represented by the NFSNO is in a period of transition. The old hospital postgraduate courses have been replaced with either hospital in-service programs, continuing education certificate programs, a bachelor's degree, or a master's degree. A clear trend in the direction of the master's degree for the more complex specialties can be seen.

NURSE PRACTITIONERS

The first formal educational program for nurse practitioners was established in 1965 in Colorado. It was set up as a 4-month certificate course (Silver, Ford & Day, 1968). The content was complex and new to nurses. Most of the early nurse practitioner programs were started outside of schools of nursing because many nurse educators of that era questioned the validity of the role. These educators perceived

TABLE 45-2
Certification of specialists by the American Nurses' Association

NURSE	GENERALIST LEVEL REGISTERED NURSE CERTIFIED (RNC)	CLINICAL SPECIAL LEVEL REGISTERED NURSE CERTIFIED SPECIALIST (RNCS)
Medical surgical	X	X
Gerontological	X	
Gerontological nurse practitioner	X	
Adult nurse practitioner	X	
Child and adolescent	X	X
Pediatric nurse practitioner	X	
School nurse practitioner	X	
Maternal and child health	X	
High-risk perinatal	X	
Family nurse practitioner	X	
Community health	X	
Adult psychiatric mental health	X	X
Child and adolescent psychiatric mental health	X	X

From American Nurses' Association. (1987). *The career credential, professional certification: 1987 certification catalog*. Kansas City, MO: Author.

their ethical and legal responsibilities in caring for acutely ill patients with irreversible and irrevocable disease.

STRATEGIES FOR HUMANIZING CRITICAL CARE

When nurses work in a humanizing atmosphere, as an autonomous professional supported by peers and administration, working collaboratively with other disciplines, they are better able to reduce the dehumanization of patients and families. Howard (1975) has proposed the following "necessary and sufficient" conditions for humanized health care: (a) patients, and their caregivers, must be recognized as possessing inherent worth, irreplaceability, and holistic selves; (b) they must be granted freedom of action, equality, and shared decision-making; and (c) they must be treated with empathy and positive affect, rather than neutrality. Critical care nurses have made great strides in humanizing critical care. Among team members, nurses often have the greatest insight into the individual needs of patients and families. Critical care nurses can take the lead in further humanizing the intensive care unit by striving for (a) a holistic approach to the individual patient and family; (b) collaborative decision-making; and (c) a more flexible and humane environment.

Holism

The concept of holistic care has always been part of nursing's value system. Today it means treating the patient, not as an accumulation of nursing or medical diagnoses, but as a unique individual, irreplaceable to his or her significant others and part of a past and present that is valuable. Holism also demands that the patient be treated with affect, rather than neutrality (Howard, 1975). Although professionals need professional reserve, this must not mean detachment, which may be interpreted by the patient and family as lack of concern and care. Interactions with patients and families lose their meaning if they are based on neutrality rather than empathy. Empathy humanizes both the patient and the nurse. To continue providing empathetic care in the

critical care setting nurses need ongoing education, as well as reinforcement and support from supervisors who understand the importance of humanized care.

Collaborative Decision-Making

The hierarchical model of decision making in critical care is dysfunctional and outmoded (Walton & Donen, 1986). The team approach, although sometimes criticized as cumbersome (Fagerhaugh et al., 1980), is the only justifiably sound means to make decisions in critical care today. Interaction and coordination that evolve from a team approach to care has been shown to improve significantly patient outcomes (Knaus, Draper, Wagner, & Zimmerman, 1986).

Today nurses, educated appropriately for the responsibility they assume, must be accountable for the care they give. Institutional mechanisms, such as shared governance, and a philosophy of collaborative practice will provide nurses with the autonomy and the support they need to participate fully in the decision-making process. A collaborative model also includes the patient and family.

Patients have the right to self-determination, even when caregivers do not agree with the choices that patients make. This right is based in the ethical principle of autonomy, which holds that persons have the right to decide on the course of action for their own lives. Humanizing critical care means finding mechanisms that uphold patient autonomy. For example, informed consent for either a clinical treatment or participation in a research study must be a collaborative process, not a ritual of signing a consent form. Part of this process involves a willingness on the part of caregivers to share with patients and families the uncertainty about outcome that is always present in critical illness. Many caregivers believe that this will undermine patient and family confidence, but in reality it provides a realistic view of the illness situation and mitigates against unrealistic expectations.

Often in critical care, too little is known too late about the values and wishes of patients regarding treatment. Asking patients about their views and preferences early in the disease course can prevent conflicts later, when issues about withholding and withdrawing treatment arise.

Flexible Environment

Nurses need to support one another in establishing a healing environment for patients suffering from catastrophic illness. They must seek ways to provide more flexibility in their daily routines and in their interactions with patients. Some of this flexibility will be achieved when nurses delegate tasks that are more properly done by others (e.g., ward clerks, housekeepers, and technicians) and when clinical data are computerized for better efficiency.

A flexible environment requires effective head nurse leadership (Duxbury, Armstrong, Drew, & Henley, 1984). Head nurses need to provide structures to support the nursing staff, such as psychiatric liaison rounds and continuing education classes. They need to encourage staff to set their own goals for professional development and performance, rather than follow proscribed guidelines from a personnel office. Finally they need to achieve consensus in the policies and procedures of the unit.

A humanized environment must be flexible enough to take individual patient and family needs into account. Methods of humanizing care in the ICU include flexible visiting hours, allowing patient choices regarding routine care, and involving the family in patient care. A more subtle factor is the atmosphere created in the critical care unit. Norman Cousins, the noted proponent of humanistic medical care, wrote about his experience in intensive care (1983). He reflected on the fact that the critical care environment itself does not allow the patient to forget at any time that he or she is critically ill. Without the intervention of caregivers, feelings of panic, which may exacerbate any illness, are a real possibility. He described the qualities of the nurses who cared for him and prevented such feelings from overwhelming him: "Their knowledge, their compassionate understanding and care, and their total support were powerful healing forces" (p. 48).

The nurse's responsibility for creating a healing environment has its roots in the earliest conceptions of nursing. Nightingale (1859) said that "what nursing has to do . . . is put the patient in the best condition for nature to act upon him" (p. 33). She meant that a person who is ill needs an environment conducive to health: clean, free of unnecessary noise, with sufficient air and light. This environment would also include the introduction of supportive family and friends, which would be conducive to the well-being of the patient. The caregiver was to be observant and attentive to the patients' needs. Nightingale's recommendations are still relevant to nurses today as they create healing environments for the critically ill.

REFERENCES

Aiken, L. (1987). The nurse shortage: Myth or reality? *New England Journal of Medicine, 317,* 641–646.

Allan, J. D., & Hall, B. A. (1988). Challenging the focus on technology: A critique of the medical model in a changing health care system. *Advances in Nursing Science, 10,* (3) 22–34.

American Nurses' Association (ANA). (1975). *Human Rights Guidelines for Nurses in Clinical and Other Research.* Kansas City, MO: Author.

American Nurses' Association (ANA). (1985). *Code for Nurses with Interpretive Statements.* Kansas City, MO: Author.

Astbury, J., & Yu, V. Y. H. (1982). Determinants of stress for staff in a neonatal intensive care unit. *Archives of Disease in Childhood, 57,* 108–111.

Bailey, J. T., Steffen, S. M., & Grout, J. W. (1980). The stress audit: Identifying the stressors of ICU nursing. *Journal of Nursing Education, 19* (Suppl. 6), 15–25.

Bandman, E. L. (1985). Our toughest questions—ethical quandries in high tech nursing. *Nursing and Health Care, 6,* 483–487.

Barger-Lux, M. J., & Heaney, R. P. (1986). For better and worse: The technological imperative in health care. *Social Science and Medicine, 22,* 1313–1320.

Brubakken, K., & Ball, M. (1983). Factors affecting job satisfaction of critical care nurses. *Heart Lung, 12,* 430–431.

Cousins, N. (1983). *The healing heart.* New York: W. W. Norton.

Dear, M. R., Weisman, C. S., Alexander C. S., & Chase, G. A. (1982). The effect of the intensive care nursing role on job satisfaction and turnover. *Heart Lung, 11,* 560–565.

Duxbury, M. L., & Thiessen, V. (1979). Staff nurse turnover in neonatal intensive care units. *Journal of Advanced Nursing, 4,* 591–602.

Duxbury, M. L., Armstrong, G. D., Drew, D. J., & Henley, S. J. (1984). Head nurse leadership style with staff nurse burnout and job satisfaction in neonatal intensive care units. *Nursing Research, 33,* 97–101.

Englehardt, T., & Rie, M. A. (1986). Intensive care units, scarce resources, and conflicting principles of justice. *Journal of the American Medical Association, 255,* 1159–1164.

Fagerhaugh, S., Strauss, A., Suczek, B., & Wiener, C. (1980). The impact of technology on patients, providers, and care patterns. *Nursing Outlook, 28,* 666–672.

Feller, I., Tholen, D., & Cornell, R. G. (1980). Improvements in burn care, 1965 to 1979. *Journal of the American Medical Association, 244,* 2074–2078.

Fuchs, V. R. (1968). The growing demand for medical care. *New England Journal of Medicine, 279,* 190–193.

Hagey, R. S., & McDonough, P. (1984). The problem of professional labeling. *Nursing Outlook, 32,* 151–157.

Hartshorn, J. (1988). President's message: It's up to you. *Focus on Critical Care, 15,* 67–69.

Hasting's Center. (1987). *Guidelines on the termination of life-sustaining treatment and the care of the dying.* New York: Author.

Hay, D., & Oaken, D. (1972). The psychological stresses of intensive care unit nursing. *Psychosomatic Medicine, 24,* 109–118.

Hilberman, M. (1975). The evolution of intensive care units. *Critical Care Medicine, 3,* 159–165.

Holland, J., Sgroi, S. M., Marwit, S. J., & Solkoff, N. (1973). ICU syndrome: Fact or fancy. *International Journal of Psychiatric Medicine, 4,* 241–249.

Howard, J. (1975). Humanization and dehumanization of health care. In Jan Howard & Anselm Strauss (Eds.). *Humanizing Health Care* (pp. 57–102). New York: John Wiley & Sons.

Huckabay, L., & Jagla, B. (1979). Nurses' stress factors in the intensive care unit. *Journal of Nursing Administration, 9,* 21–26.

Jacobson, S. P. (1978). Stressful situations for neonatal intensive care nurses. *American Journal of Maternal Child Nursing, 3,* 144–150.

Jacobson, S. P. (1983). Stresses and coping strategies of neonatal intensive care unit nurses. *Research in Nursing and Health, 6,* 33–40.

Jameton, A. (1984). *Nursing practice: The ethical issues.* Englewood Cliffs, NJ: Prentice-Hall.

Keane, A., Ducette, J., & Adler, D. (1985). Stress in ICU and non-ICU nurses. *Nursing Research, 34,* 231–236.

Killip T., & Kimball, J. T. (1967). Treatment of myocardial infarction in a coronary care unit: A two-year experience with 250 patients. *American Journal of Cardiology, 20,* 457–464.

Kirchhoff, K. T. (1982). Visiting policies for patients with myocardial infarction: A national survey. *Heart Lung, 11,* 571–576.

Knaus, W. A., Draper, E. A., Wagner, D. P., & Zimmerman J. E. (1986). An evaluation of outcome from intensive care in major centers. *Annals of Internal Medicine, 104,* 410–418.

Lester D., & Brower, E. R. (1981). Stress and job satisfaction in a sample of pediatric intensive care nurses. *Psychological Reports, 48,* 738.

Maloney, J. (1982). Job stress and its consequences on a group of intensive care and non-intensive care nurses. *Advances in Nursing Science, 4,* (2), 31–42.

Martino, J. H., & McIntosh, N. J. (1985). Effects of patient characteristics and technology on job satisfaction and stress of intensive care unit and non-intensive care unit nurses. *Heart Lung, 14,* 300–301.

Mohl, P. C., Denny, N. R., Mote, T. A., & Coldwater, C. (1982). Hospital unit stressors that affect nurses: Primary task vs. social factors. *Psychosomatics, 23,* 366–374.

Mundt, M. M. (1985). A descriptive study of intensive care unit staff nurses' perceptions of stress in their work environment. *Heart Lung, 14,* 301–302.

Nightingale, F. (1859). *Notes on nursing, what it is and what it is not.* London: Harrison Sons.

Norbeck, J. S. (1985). Types and sources of social support for managing job stress in critical care nursing. *Nursing Research, 34,* 225–230.

President's Commission for the Study of Ethical Problems in Medicine and Biomedical and Behavioral Research. (1983). *Deciding to forego life-sustaining treatment.* Washington DC: U.S. Government Printing Office.

Raymond, J. (1982). Medicine as patriarchal religion. *The Journal of Medicine and Philosophy, 7,* 197–216.

Steffen, S. M. (1980). Perceptions of stress: 1800 nurses tell their stories. In K. E. Claus & J. T. Bailey (Eds.), *Living with stress and promoting well-being* (pp. 38–58). St. Louis: C. V. Mosby.

Stehle, J. L. (1981). Critical care nursing stress: The findings revisited. *Nursing Research, 30,* 182–186.

Walton, D. N., & Donen, N. (1986). Ethical decision-making and the critical care team. *Critical Care Clinics, 2,* 101–109.

Woeliner, D. S. (1988). Flexible visiting hours in the adult critical care unit. *Focus on Critical Care, 15,* 66–69.

✳ EDITOR'S QUESTIONS FOR DISCUSSION ✳

How can a professional nurse maintain simultaneously an autonomous role in professional nursing practice while collaborating with physicians? Define and explicate specific situations in which there may be "gray areas" or an overlap between biomedical and nursing models of practice. To what extent are the so-called gray areas of practice in an ICU unit actually situations that call for interdependence in professional practice? Is the nurse who follows medical protocols in an ICU unit making a medical judgment rather than a medical diagnosis when she or he initiates the protocol, or is the nurse making or using a nursing diagnosis? Is it not more a matter of semantics than the nursing role when a nurse differentiates among a nursing assessment, nursing diagnosis, medical assessment, medical judgment, and a medical diagnosis? How can a collaborative practice model provide nurses with the autonomy and the support they need to participate fully in the decision-making process of care?

What qualifications academically and experientially should a professional nurse have for being an ICU nurse? What is the basis of the interpersonal conflicts that often exist in ICU care? Discuss the role of technology as it has influenced professional practice in ICU units. Discuss the four concepts related to dehumanization and indicate specific strategies that could be implemented to prevent dehumanization in ICU care. How can ethical and legal responsibilities be more clearly defined and understood regarding ICU care? How can some of the stress related to ethical dilemmas faced by ICU nurses be reduced? Discuss strategies for reducing institutional constraints for right courses of action being followed in an ICU unit. What principles suggested in the chapters by Brown and Davis (Chapter 38) and Flynn and Davis (Chapter 39), as well as those by Fowler (Chapter 4), Murphy (Chapter 5), and Driscoll (Chapter 40), may be applied to reduce stress in ICU units? Discuss the role of the professional nurse on a clinical practice committee in a hospital.

38

The Ethics of Refusing to Provide Care

Johnna Sue Brown, M.S., R.N.

Anne J. Davis, Ph.D., R.N., F.A.A.N.

With recent advancements in biomedical knowledge and technology, nurses confront new clinical realities in their practice. Some of these advances can be positive for both patient and nurse, while others can and raise questions including ethical ones. Conflicts arise for nurses when their values and obligations are potentially compromised because of a specific patient care assignment. Such conflicts have led to nurses' asking questions about whether or not they can and should refuse a patient assignment on personal or professional grounds (Creighton, 1986).

Numerous lawsuits in which nurses brought actions for damages against their employer have pushed this issue into the public arena (Blum, 1984; Tammelleo, 1981). While law and ethics differ, legal cases elucidate the ethical issues in refusal situations. The basic ethical question for consideration here is: Under what conditions is it morally permissible for nurses to refuse a patient care assignment? In this chapter this question is explored from the perspective of the nurse's right to refuse to provide care.

RIGHTS, DUTIES, AND RESPONSIBILITIES

Fagin (1975) proposed a list of rights for nurses and said that there had historically been the right not to do or act. She called for nurses to obtain the right to do. Because the focus was on the right to do, the list does not include refusal behavior. A few years later, another author (Bennett, 1982) addressed nurses' rights and included the right and obligation to refuse any patient assignment when they did not have the necessary skills needed to accomplish the assignment. However, such a right is not absolute. It does not include the right to refuse to float or to accept additional patients when confronted with understaffing (Bennett, 1982, p. 88).

The *Code for Nurses*, developed by the International Council of Nurses, reviews the primary obligation of nurses to those people who require nursing care. Because this code focuses on patients and society, it does not mention any specific rights for nurses (ICN, 1973). The American Nurses' Association *Code for Nurses* (1976) emphasizes nurses' obligations to clients within the context of rights and responsibilities for both the nurse and the client (Mappes & Zembaty, 1986, p. 119). Specifically, in Section 1.4 of the 1976 ANA Code for Nurses entitled "The Nature of Health Problems," we find the idea that nurses' personal attitudes or beliefs should not limit their concern for human dignity and the provision of quality nursing care. However, this section continues by saying that if personally opposed to the delivery of care in a particular case because of the nature of the health problem or procedure to be used, nurses are justified in refusing to participate. Advanced notice of a refusal to participate is necessary to allow for other appropriate arrangements to be made (ANA, 1976). In the updated revised ANA *Code for Nurses* (1985) several sections address the nurse's refusal of an assignment. Section 1.4 referred to above has been changed and now reads: "If ethically opposed to interventions in a particular case because of the procedures to be used, the nurse is justified in refusing to participate" (ANA, 1985, pp. 3–4). The phrase, "the nature of the illness" as part of this refusal has been deleted. In addition to this change, more detail has been provided indicating the appropriate measures to take when refusing an assignment (ANA, 1985). Refusal in those cases when the nurse lacks competence or is inadequately prepared to carry out specific functions is regarded not only as a right but as a responsibility to safeguard clients. While such codes of ethics are necessary and important, it can happen that the ethical principles expressed in them conflict with an individual's moral beliefs. Therefore, such codes cannot substitute for analysis of an issue using ethical theories (Munson, 1979).

Several writers have discussed the nurse's role and conflicts among rights, duties, and responsibilities that create ethical dilemmas for nurses (Bandman, 1984; Fagin, 1975; Sellin, 1986; Smith & Davis, 1980). Each nurse is entitled to basic human rights that include the right to speak freely, and the right to act in accord with one's personal values and ethical code. With these rights go certain ethical and legal responsibilities to the patient and the employing institution. Traditionally nurses' duties and responsibilities have been stressed far more than their rights. In any discussion of refusal to provide patient care, it becomes necessary to examine rights, duties, and responsibilities and the possible tension among them.

While such tensions have become more apparent recently, especially when discussing refusal of nursing care for the abortion patient and the patient with acquired immunodeficiency syndrome (AIDS), nevertheless refusal of an assignment as an ethical concern can be traced back to the 1920s (Melosh, 1982). At that time most nurses freelanced in private-duty positions. Such an arrangement permitted them to evade unappealing work situations. According to one survey, 61% of nurses routinely refused certain cases by listing their restrictions with the registrar. We have no data of refusals that were under the guise of being off duty (Melosh, 1982, p. 80).

By the 1940s and World War II private duty became obsolete owing to numerous factors including insurance for hospital care. The nurse's relationship with the patient and the hospital underwent a fundamental structural change that had an impact on the rights and duties of nurses.

The legal and ethical systems share similarities, but they also differ. A law is generally understood to be a body of enacted or customary rules recognized by a community as binding. Laws may or may not reflect a moral view. Ethics focuses on moral problems and their treatment and tends to be more individually determined (Smith, 1983).

From a legal perspective, Creighton (1986) discusses the dilemma found in a nurse's refusal to accept a patient care assignment. She points to the court's warning against confusing reliance on professional ethics with reliance on personal beliefs and values. Nurses should reflect on the legal dimensions before they refuse to give care.

The Warthen case has been cited in discussing what nurses should do if they want to stop treating a patient. In this case, the appellate opinion states that nurses cannot use their "personal morals" to prevent an employer from "pursuing its business" (Tammelleo, 1986b, p. 59). The message inherent in this decision is that a nurse can refuse to participate in a procedure, but in doing so she or he may be fired (Tammelleo, 1986a). Some states have "conscience statutes" to protect health care personnel who do not want to participate in abortions or sterilizations. In the last analysis, however, for most situations nurses cannot rely on the courts for protection when they refuse to treat a patient on ethical grounds.

Another point of view justifies nurses' refusal to follow a doctor's orders based on spiritual principle. Lass (1985) advocates conscientious objection for nurses based on their religious-moral views. Yet another point of view advocates the principle of obey and grieve. That is, the nurse follows an order even when she or he questions it and worries about it later (Refusing an Assignment, 1986).

Since staff shortages are a major reason for nurses' refusal of assignments, some state nurses' associations have undertaken devices to focus attention on this problem. For example, the New York State Nurses' Association has developed a Protest Assignment form that nurses complete and submit when confronted with a situation in which refusal is indicated. The association follows up on these protests and if the problem persists, they alert the appropriate governing or accrediting agency to the situation (Mallison, 1987).

The Maryland Hospital Association is investigating the issue of unsafe assignments for nurses, while both the North Carolina and Michigan Nurses' Associations have developed guidelines for nurses in accepting or rejecting a work assignment (Mallison, 1987, p. 151).

California has also recognized the issue of unsafe staffing assignments. The California Board of Registered Nurses (1987b) has taken the position that nurses should not assume responsibility for care they are not competent to provide. If this occurs, both the nurse giving the care and the nurse making the assignment may be disciplined by the Board for incompetence or gross negligence, or both—even if the patient was not harmed. This position sanctions the right of the nurse to refuse an assignment based on competency.

The California Board of Registered Nurses has also discussed actions the nurse should take when questioning the appropriateness of an order or when the legal authority for the order is unclear (1987a). If a nurse believes the order is not in the best interest of the patient, the nurse must become the patient's advocate by challenging and, if appropriate, changing the order. Nursing supervisors and administrators are expected to support the nurse in this situation.

Childress (1985) discusses the moral issues raised by illegal actions in health care and presents a framework for their moral justification. Conscientious objection, the illegal action that encompasses refusal actions, has been defined as a public, nonviolent, and submissive violation of the law based on personal-moral, often religious-moral, convictions and is intended primarily to witness those principles or values.

Childress (1985) includes several relevant moral considerations to examine in determining whether to obey or to violate the law. These include the prima facie obligation to obey the law in a relatively just political order, the end of the action, the availability of legal channels, the probable positive and negative consequences of the action, and the nature of the disobedience. Even within a just legal system there are times when individual cases warrant the violation of the law based on one's moral convictions.

Refusals to cooperate in employment situations are similar to conscientious objection or civil disobedience because noncooperation violates the employer's policies or one's conditions of employment and protests are based on issues of conscience. Nurses who object to an assignment should not be required to accept the assignment, not because they might provide bad care, but because they should not be required to cooperate in what they regard as wrong or against their moral convictions (Jameton, 1984). In conclusion, Childress (1985) states that "to be responsible is, in part, to answer for one's actions, and answering includes giving reasons, that is, attempting to justify those actions by appealing to the moral principles, rules, and values that support the actions" (p. 81). These situations arise frequently in nursing and have compelled an examination of nurses' decision-making processes for ethical dilemmas in refusal of an assignment.

Readers of a nursing journal were asked to respond to a situation in which a medical and surgical staff nurse is told she must leave her unit to work in the intensive care unit (ICU), where she would be responsible for four acutely ill patients, and would take charge duty because the one other nurse there is a new graduate. After telling the supervisor she is unprepared to work in the ICU, the supervisor responds by telling her she has no choice and must do the best she can under the circumstances.

The poll sought answers to the following questions:

1. Should you refuse to take charge duty in the ICU or to work there at all?
2. Should you accept charge duty as the supervisor ordered, just doing the best you can?

Of the 113 nurses who responded, 51% said they would refuse the ICU assignment because it is unethical to jeopardize patients' safety. The 47% who said they would accept the assignment believed they had an ethical duty to consider the patients' welfare first and while inexperienced, they would be better than no nurse at all. When asked about taking charge in the ICU, 82% said they would not undertake this responsibility. Many of the respondents indicated that they had left hospital nursing because of similar ethical dilemmas. The 16% who said they would take charge cited the ethical duty to the patients as their reason (Staff, 1986).

Little systematic study of nurses' rights and obligations in refusing a patient care assignment can be found in the literature. What can be found centers on legal issues, not on moral and ethical ones. The literature reviewed above cites several reasons for refusal of an assignment. These reasons include conscientious objection, competency, patient advocacy, and personal values. However, the literature reveals arguments both for and against a nurse's refusing a patient care assignment.

ARGUMENTS FOR AND AGAINST REFUSAL

According to Brown's analysis (1987), these arguments can be reduced to four fundamental positions, two in opposition to nurses' rights of refusal and two in support of these rights. The two arguments against refusal of an assignment are (1) refusal as abandonment, and (2) refusal as insubordination. The arguments for refusal of an assignment are (1) refusal as protection of a patient against inappropriate treat-

ment or harm, and (2) refusal as protection of a nurse from harm. These arguments are discussed briefly.

A major argument against nurses' rights to refuse to give care equates refusal with abandonment of the patient (Bennett, 1982; Tammelleo, 1985). Since patient abandonment is morally impermissible, then so is refusal of an assignment. The ANA *Code for Nurses* (1985) states clearly that if a patient's life is in jeopardy the nurse has an obligation to give care to protect the patient's safety. The nurse may withdraw only when care can be given by someone else. Sellin (1986) argues that the duty to the patient outweighs the nurse's personal values and beliefs. Therefore, if refusal would present a real danger to the patient, the nurse cannot ethically do so since such an action would constitute abandonment.

Would refusal of assignment in an emergency situation constitute abandonment of the patient? Yes, it would and therefore refusal cannot be ethically justified. The risk to the patient of not receiving emergency care is too serious to be overridden by the nurse's moral values. The nurse has a moral duty to assist unless or until another nurse can become responsible for the patient. This situation is very straightforward. But what about a nurse who refuses to give care to a patient with a communicable or infectious disease? This issue has arisen recently with AIDS patients. One study found that the majority of nurses questioned said they would want to be transferred off a ward if it had AIDS patients (Blumenfield, Smith, Milazzo, Seropian, & Wormser, 1987). If there are instances when the nurse cannot be protected from the physical risk posed by the patient's illness, refusal does not constitute abandonment. The usual likelihood, though, is that nurses can be protected from this risk. Hospitals have policies and procedures so that the risk to the nurse is reduced if not completely eliminated. Refusal of assignment on the grounds of risk, when risk is minimal and commensurate with professional expectations regarding tolerable levels of exposure, does constitute patient abandonment and is not permissible. However, if the nurse cannot be reasonably protected, refusal of assignment does not constitute patient abandonment.

The second argument based on court rulings essentially says that a nurse cannot refuse an assignment and cannot refuse to follow physicians' orders because such behavior is insubordination. Not only is this not an ethical argument, but it is an inaccurate legal one as well. The basic assumption underlying the argument is that nurses only follow orders and do so without question. The reality is that nurses have an ethical and legal duty to question. Nevertheless, in the everyday practice world, refusal viewed as insubordination is often a reality. However, there is no way this argument can be sustained ethically. One of the most stringent positions about refusal says that nurses must provide treatment in an emergency but in other situations they have limited ethical rights to refuse (Tammelleo, 1986a). Another position is that refusal can be justified if the action or treatment is illegal. None of these arguments take into account the nursing role of patient advocate (ANA, 1980, 1985).

The above discussion indicates that two arguments oppose a nurse's refusal of an assignment. Of these two, the abandonment of the patient argument has merit since such an action cannot be ethically justified. Refusal as insubordination, although used in clinical situations, cannot be upheld when the nurse is acting ethically to safeguard or prevent harm. Nurses' rights are not absolute, but neither are physicians' or institutional rights.

The arguments that support the nurse's refusal of an assignment include refusal as protection of a patient against inappropriate treatment or harm, and refusal as protection of a nurse from harm. The protection of the patient argument takes three forms: (1) refusal to provide a specific intervention based on patient refusal of that intervention; (2) refusal on grounds of prevention of harm to the patient by others; and (3) refusal based on prevention of harm when a nurse lacks the necessary skills to intervene. The nursing profession has viewed this function of the patient advocacy role as an ethical duty for many years. In some states, it is now required by law as well (California Board of Registered Nurses, 1987a). Essentially, some of the traditional values of nursing have gained increased importance in the face of advanced knowledge and technology. These values include respect for patient autonomy, patient advo-

cacy, and nurse accountability (Fry, 1987). Each of these three forms of the argument are discussed briefly.

If a patient refuses intervention, the nurse has a duty to uphold this refusal. Such a duty is grounded in the ethical principle of autonomy, which means that the autonomous, self-determining patient has the right to make this independent choice. If the patient is unable to be self-determining, the nurse still has the responsibility to protect the patient from harm and to preserve the patient's rights. This argument has some limitations. Patient autonomy would be wrongly preserved by the nurse if the patient were allowed to do harm to others. Also the nurse must be certain that the patient is fully informed and has freely consented. It is wrong for the nurse to respect patient autonomy when the patient has made an ill-informed or coerced decision. Under these circumstances, the decision is not autonomous.

In a discussion of the second argument, refusal as protection from harm from others, the ANA *Code for Nurses* (1985) states that the nurse must protect the patient from intentional harm as well as unintentional, nonmalicious harm. Patients cannot possibly evaluate the complex treatment regimens prescribed. They must be protected from incompetence and error as well as neglect, illegal practices, or even abuse. Refusal on these grounds can be ethically justified.

The third argument, refusal as protection from harm that occurs because of lack of skill, means that the patient must be protected from nurses who lack specific technical skills. The ANA *Code for Nurses* (1985) is clear on this point. Nurses must determine the scope of their practice in light of their education, knowledge, competence, and extent of experience. If a nurse concludes that she or he lacks competence or is inadequately prepared to carry out a specific function, there is a responsibility to refuse and seek alternative sources of care. If there are no others to care for the patient, then refusal becomes abandonment. In this case there may be potential for causing harm, but to have no nursing care may cause even more harm.

Another basis of nurse refusal of assignment is an assignment that has potential to harm the nurse. This argument is controversial, causes conflict between nurses and their employing agency, and is of the greatest concern to nurses (Creighton, 1982; Horsley, 1987; Jameton, 1987). This argument arises from the principle of duties to self. An examination of these duties to self will help determine if the rights arising from them, including refusing an assignment, has an acceptable ethical foundation. The principle of duties to self has been divided into (a) integrity, (b) identity, and (c) self-regarding duties (Jameton, 1987).

Integrity or integration of the self is stressed when one is divided by personal and professional concerns and faces a conflict in duties to self. The question of integrity and dedication is the balance between the limits of the nurse's obligation to take personal risks in taking care of the patient, and the nurse's duties to care for the "risky" patient. The ANA Committee on Ethics (1986) asks at what point does it cease to be a nurse's duty to undergo risk for the benefit of the patient. Is the risk to the nurse in providing care greater than the benefit received by the patient? If so, then taking care of the patient is a superrogatory act or moral option rather than a moral obligation. A problem arises in using this argument when the underlying issue is one of prejudice toward the patient or toward the disease process. These are not legitimate grounds for refusing an assignment.

Another aspect of this duty to self concerns psychological, religious, or moral risks to the nurse. The ideal of service and providing care to those in need has been a main historical theme in nursing. Service, however, is an ideal, not an absolute. According to the ANA Committee on Ethics (1986), the profession cannot morally demand the sacrifice of the nurse's well-being, physical or psychological, or the nurse's life, for the benefit of the patient. Nurses may refuse an assignment on the basis of physical risk to self when strong evidence supports this request. They may also refuse an assignment on religious-moral or psychological grounds when those objections have been made known in advance.

Refusal is protection of the nurse's identity as a moral professional. The duty to self is to uphold one's moral values, which includes upholding standards of professional practice. To condone poor practice assaults the nurse's moral identity. A strong professional identity requires that a nurse take ap-

propriate actions to protect the patient from unsafe practices, not simply to protect the patient (beneficence), but also to preserve the moral identity of the nurse.

This argument has weaknesses. If nurses frequently refuse assignments on grounds of protection of their moral identity without strong justification, the agency could face difficulties in fulfilling its duties to the patients. Staff conflicts could arise as well. Nurses must undertake a critical, objective, and honest examination of personal values to determine to what extent participation in procedures will affect their personal life. A nurse may permissibly refuse a patient care assignment on the grounds of moral identity only in nonemergency, adequately staffed situations when no conflict with coworkers arises.

A third set of duties to self is that of self-regarding duties or those that primarily affect oneself. By establishing personal competence with others, one's own place in the institution is defined. Maintaining those competencies requires virtues that are mainly personal and self-regarding. To maintain and improve competence, one must be an objective and honest judge of personal abilities and limitations. Just as individual nurses take responsibility for judging their own quality of care, so they also should judge when they think the level of nursing care has fallen below an acceptable level (Jameton, 1987). In the principle of duties to self, competence, as a self-regarding duty, is a strong argument on which to base a refusal of assignment.

It is important morally to treat oneself with care. This means treating oneself as an autonomous individual and not placing oneself in degrading or dangerous situations, not depriving oneself unduly, and not forcing oneself to obey meaningless demands (Jameton, 1987).

SUMMARY

This chapter concludes that nurses may morally refuse a patient care assignment if, and only if, certain conditions are met. In evaluating the ethical arguments for and against refusal, it is concluded that:

1. A nurse has a moral right to refuse to partici-

pate in specific medical and nursing orders and assignments on the grounds of preservation of patient autonomy insofar as the patient is truly autonomous and the patient's actions will not harm others.

2. A nurse has a moral right to refuse specific medical and nursing orders and assignments on the grounds of protection of the patient from incompetence or errors, as well as on the grounds of neglect, illegal practice, or even abuse.

3. A nurse has a moral right to refuse an assignment or task as protection of the patient against inappropriate treatment. This can be a decision made by the patient or a decision made by the nurse acting as patient advocate.

4. A nurse has a moral right to refuse specific medical and nursing orders and assignments on the grounds of physical risk to self when strong evidence supports the existence of more than minimal risk.

5. A nurse has a moral right to refuse specific medical and nursing orders and assignments on religious-moral or psychological grounds when those objections have been made known in advance. In addition, no emergency can exist nor can the patient be placed in jeopardy by the refusal.

6. A nurse has a moral right to refuse specific medical and nursing orders and assignments on the grounds of lack of competence in order to uphold personal-professional standards of practice when no emergency situation exists, when the agency has adequate staffing to care for the patient, and when it does not create a conflict with coworkers.

Along with these rights come some duties and responsibilities. Clearly the nurse may not leave or abandon the patient if the patient's life is in jeopardy. There are times when the rights of the patient are so strong that refusing an assignment is ethically unacceptable. In addition, if a nurse does not wish to participate in a treatment or assignment while on duty, adequate notice must be given so that there is time to locate another nurse to handle the assignment. If a nurse has strong objections to a certain treatment or procedure, this should be stated at the time of employment and followed with a written notice.

In summary, nurses have a strong ethical obligation to patients by virtue of their professional status and role. They also have the right to remain true to their own moral and religious beliefs. Therefore, nurses' ethical decision-making process, concerning refusal of a patient care assignment, should be flexible enough to accommodate these beliefs without compromising the legitimate rights of patients and the highest standards of professional care.

REFERENCES

American Nurses' Association (ANA). (1976). *Code for nurses with interpretative statements*. Kansas City, MO: Author.

American Nurses' Association (ANA). (1980). *Nursing: A social policy statement*. Kansas City, MO: Author.

American Nurses' Association (ANA). (1985). *Code for nurses with interpretative statements*. Kansas City, MO: Author

American Nurses' Association Committee on Ethics. (1986). *Statement regarding risk vs. responsibility in providing nursing care*. Kansas City, MO: Author.

Bandman, B. (1984). The role and justification of rights in nursing. *Medicine and Law, 3,* 77–87.

Bennett, H. M. (1982). A bill of rights for nurses. *Critical Care Nurse, 2*(6), 88.

Blum, J. D. (1984). The code of nurses and wrongful discharge. *Nursing Forum, 21,* 149–151.

Blumenfield, M., Smith, P. J., Milazzo, J., Seropian, S., & Wormser, G. P. (1987). Survey of attitudes of nurses working with AIDS patients. *General Hospital Psychiatry, 9,* 58–63.

Brown, J. S. (1987). *Ethical issues in nurses' rights to refuse patient care assignments*. Unpublished master's thesis, California State University, Los Angeles.

California Board of Registered Nurses. (1987a). Board adopts new policy on implementation of orders by RNs. *The BRN Report, 5*(1), 6.

California Board of Registered Nurses. (1987b). Nurses' floating to another area. *The BRN Report, 5*(1), 1.

Childress, J. F. (1985). Civil disobedience, conscientious objection and evasive noncompliance: A framework for the analysis and assessment of illegal actions in health care. *Journal of Medicine and Philosophy, 10* (1), 63–83.

Creighton, H. (1982). Refusing to participate in abortions. *Nursing Management, 13*(4), 27–28.

Creighton, H. (1986). When can a nurse refuse to give care? *Nursing Management, 17*(3), 16–20.

Fagin, C. (1975). Nurses' rights. *American Journal of Nursing, 75,* 82–85.

Fry, S. T. (1987). Autonomy, advocacy, and accountability: Ethics at the bedside. In M. D. M. Fowler & J. Levine-Ariff (Eds.), *Ethics at the bedside: A source book for the critical care nurse* (pp. 39–49). Philadelphia: J. B. Lippincott.

Horsley, J. E. (1987, May). Can you refuse to assist in abortions? *RN,* 65–66.

International Council of Nurses (ICN). (1973). *Code for nurses.* Geneva: Imprimerines Populaires.

Jameton, A. (1984). *Nursing practice: The ethical issues.* Englewood Cliffs, N.J.: Prentice-Hall.

Jameton, A. (1987). Duties to self. In M. D. M. Fowler & J. Levine-Ariff (Eds.), *Ethics at the bedside: A source book for the critical care nurse* (pp. 115–135). Philadelphia: J. B. Lippincott.

Lass, R. (1985). Orders with kingdom consequences. *Journal of Christian Nursing, 2*(3), 3.

Mallison, M. B. (1987). Protesting your assignment. *American Journal of Nursing, 87*(2), 151.

Mappes, T. A., & Zembaty, J. S. (1986). *Biomedical ethics.* New York: McGraw-Hill.

Melosh, B. (1982). *The physician's hand: Work culture and conflict in American nursing.* Philadelphia: Temple University Press.

Munson, R. (1979). *Interventions and reflection: Basic issues in medical ethics.* Belmont, CA: Wadsworth Publishing.

Refusing an assignment. (1986). *RNABC News, 18*(3), 8–9.

Sellin, S. C. (1986). The ethics of refusal: Nurses' rights and responsibilities. *Perioperative Nursing Quarterly, 2*(2), 31–34.

Smith, J. D. (1983). The relationship between rights and responsibilities in health care: A dilemma for nurses. *Journal of Advanced Nursing, 8,* 437–440.

Smith, S. J., & Davis, A. J. (1980). Ethical dilemmas: Conflicts among rights, duties, and obligations. *American Journal of Nursing, 80,* 1463–1466.

Staff. (1986). What our readers said about refusing to work in an intensive care unit. *Nursing Life, 6*(2), 41–42.

Tammelleo, A. D. (1981). Nurse refused to assist in abortion: Demoted. *Regan Report on Nursing Law, 22,* 4.

Tammelleo, A.D. (1985). Nurse refuses to treat: Moral, ethical, legal dilemma. *Regan Report on Nursing Law, 25* (11), 1.

Tammelleo, A. D. (1986a, June). If you want to stop treating a patient. *RN,* 59–60.

Tammelleo, A. D. (1986b). Nurse refuses to "float": Sunk. *Regan Report on Nursing Law, 24*(7), 1.

✳   **EDITOR'S QUESTIONS FOR DISCUSSION**   ✳

Under what circumstances is it morally permissible for nurses to refuse patient care assignments? How can a nurse present the fact that she does not have the necessary skills to do a task to a supervisor without reprisal? What legal grounds may support a nurse who refuses an assignment based on competency? Discuss some examples of refusing to treat a patient on the basis of ethical grounds, rather than relying on personal beliefs and values. Under what conditions may a nurse intervene in patient care regardless of the consent of the patient? How might a nurse objectively determine the extent that participation and procedures of care may effect her or his personal or moral life?

Discuss the processes that a nurse may use in questioning the appropriateness of a physician's order, challenging it, or changing it. How are the processes the same or different in questioning the appropriateness of a staff nurse's act, or nursing diagnosis, or the directive of a team leader or a nursing supervisor? How can many of the issues regarding ethical decisions in patient care be raised for discussion and cleared at the time of the staff nurse's employment? How may a staff nurse's job description be an advocate for the nurse as well as the patient in resolving ethical dilemmas?

39

Decisions to Forego Life-Sustaining Treatment:
Nursing considerations

Patricia A.R. Flynn, M.S., R.N.
Anne J. Davis, Ph.D., R.N., F.A.A.N.

This chapter deals with foregoing life-sustaining treatment decisions for adults. Many have struggled with the growing concern that it may be inappropriate to apply technological capabilities to the fullest extent in all cases and without limitation. However, in order not to treat, someone must give the directive and someone must carry it out. Increased awareness of patients' rights to be treated in accordance with their own decisions and expectations is a recent development. The use of heroic measures to sustain life can be justified only by fidelity to the patient's right to elect or decline the benefits of medical technology. The role of the nurse as participant in decision making, as patient advocate, and as the caregiver once decisions to withdraw or withhold treatment are made is crucial in this process.

Life-sustaining treatment includes all health care interventions that lengthen the patient's life. When these interventions are a matter of choice, a salient question is—who decides? Two general categories of patients, the competent patient and the patient unable to make his or her own health care decisions, have been identified. Competence is broadly defined as the capacity to understand and appreciate the nature and consequences of one's actions.

THE PATIENT WHO IS COMPETENT

Patients, competent to determine the course of their therapy, may refuse any and all interventions proposed by others as long as their refusals do not seriously harm or impose unfair burdens on others (President's Commission for the Study of Ethical Problems in Medicine and Biomedical Research, 1982). The patient's right to make these decisions is clearly stated in a 1891 U.S. Supreme Court decision that says:

> No right is held more sacred, or is more carefully guarded, by common law, than the right of every individual to the possession and control of his own person, free from all restraint or interference by others, unless by clear and unquestionable authority of law. (*Union Pacific Railway v. Botsford*, 1891)

The work by P. Flynn was supported in part by a research training grant in gerontological nursing (AGDO 130) funded by the National Institute on Aging, Jeanie Kayser-Jones, Ph.D., Program Director.

More recently a patient's rights to control bodily has been embodied in the doctrine of informed consent. In the case of *Natanson v. Kline* (1960), the judge stated that:

Anglo American law starts with the premise of thorough-going self-determination. It follows that each man is considered to be master of his own body, and he may, if he be of sound mind, expressly prohibit the performance of life-saving surgery, or other medical treatment. A doctor might well believe that an operation or form of treatment is desirable or necessary, but the law does not permit him to substitute his own judgment for that of the patient by any form of artifice or deception.

Competent patients are at liberty to make their own medical treatment decisions; incompetent individuals are not. Since ethically and legally the competent patient has the right to make this decision, there should be little question about such a patient's refusing treatment. However, cases continue to enter the courts.

For example, Kathleen Farrell, a competent 37-year-old woman with amyotrophic lateral sclerosis, requested that her ventilator be turned off. No treatment would benefit her. Her physician refused her request, so her husband sought court authorization to order that treatment be ceased. The court granted his request, but deferred the order until the request could be reviewed by a higher court. Mrs. Farrell died connected to the ventilator before the appeal was heard. The court ruled that treatment could be terminated since the patient clearly wanted it to happen (Annas, 1987). A relatively straightforward situation of a competent patient's making her wishes known took a court decision to compel the physicians to honor the patient's wishes.

The President's Commission (1983) established that informed decisions by competent patients regarding choices about life-sustaining treatment should be respected, enhanced, and promoted by health care professionals. While there should be a presumption in favor of sustaining life, the right of competent patients to reject even life-sustaining treatments should be recognized.

Serious problems arise in discerning patients' wishes concerning how they view the situation and their desire to be treated or not, because of incomplete knowledge, uncertainty of treatment outcomes, and the diversity of personal values and objectives of both patients and practitioners. In a pluralistic society we cannot impose a single moral vision on either patients or practitioners.

The informed consent doctrine provides a firm basis for the legal and ethical recognition of the competent, terminally ill person's prerogative to resist life-preserving medical treatment. The doctrine of informed consent entitles patients to be informed about the plan and the course of their prospective medical treatment, as well as allowing patients to withhold consent, when they do not view the prospective treatment to be in their best interest. Fundamentally, informed consent rests on respect for the individual, and for each individual's capacity and right to both define his or her own goals, and to make choices designed to achieve these goals. However, in defining informed consent (and its exceptions) the law has tempered this right of self-determination with respect for other values, such as the promotion of well-being in the context of an expert-layperson relationship (Capron, 1986; President's Commission, 1982). Nevertheless, the competent patient's wishes must prevail. Although doctors and nurses find it difficult to reject the demands of family members when they differ with the patient, this is clearly required by the respect-for-persons moral principle (Macklin, 1987, p. 54).

THE PATIENT WHO IS INCOMPETENT

What should guide those who must decide for a patient who cannot decide? If the terminally ill patient's ability to make decisions becomes diminished, the treatment team must increasingly rely on the prestated or presumed wishes of the person. Nurses need to think about what means might be used to determine a patient's wishes. A statement, written before the person experiences diminished capacity to make decisions, can be helpful in indicating the patient's preferences about terminal decisions.

Arrangements for surrogate decision-making need

to be available when patients are unable to make decisions by themselves. When others make decisions, they should be those that the patient would have made or, if the patient's wishes are not known, the decisions must be made in the patient's best interest. Neither caregivers nor family members may seize the opportunity of the patient's unresponsiveness to do what they think is best for a patient who recently and clearly expressed his or her own wishes about the level of treatment. Although an unconscious person lacks autonomy, if that same person, while conscious, recently exercised autonomy and stated preferences about medical treatment, those wishes must be accepted (Macklin, 1987).

Another aid to decision making when the patient cannot participate is a proxy designated in advance by the patient to speak on his or her behalf. In some states this option has been provided by law as part of the state's living will legislation or, as in California, as an amendment to the durable power of attorney statute, which extends the authorization to health care decisions (Keene, 1983). While not a flawless mechanism for projecting a patient's wishes into a period of future incapacity, a proxy designate has the advantage of initiating discussions with patients about their wishes before such decisions are needed.

TREATMENT DECISIONS

Life-sustaining measures extend on a continuum from respirators and dialysis, through antibiotics, intravenous glucose and water, to food and drink. A number of treatment distinctions concerning these have been made. One distinction, between omission and commission of a particular act or use or nonuse of a particular treatment, is neither always obvious nor obvious to all, especially if judged only by the results (Kass, 1980). A legal difference between actively doing something and not doing anything has been established, but a vigorous debate about whether ethical differences exist is under way. The matter of actively killing rather than allowing someone to die refers to the moral principle that says it is not right to kill an innocent human being even when it might result in more good than harm. Those in favor of active euthanasia seek to change this princi-

ple. In health care today we can ethically justify allowing people to die, but only in certain circumstances. We avoid killing directly but will allow someone to die.

Another distinction, extraordinary or ordinary treatment, originated in the Roman Catholic tradition as a way of differentiating optional treatment from treatment that was obligatory for medical professionals to offer and for patients to accept (Lynn & Childress, 1983; McCartney, 1980). This distinction refers to a treatment as being only customary and unusual. Sometimes this difference relates to the particular circumstances of each patient, so that ordinary treatment for one person is extraordinary treatment for another. To clarify the distinction, Pope Pius XII said that we are normally obliged to use only ordinary means to preserve life, and that a more strict obligation would prove too burdensome to most people (McCartney, 1980).

Treatment criteria can also be categorized in numerous ways, including simple or complex, natural or artificial, usual or unusual, invasive or noninvasive, reasonable chance of success or futile, proportionate or disproportionate balance of burdens and benefits, inexpensive or costly. An examination of these criteria shows that most of them are not morally relevant in distinguishing optional from obligatory medical treatments (Lynn, 1986).

In determining whether or not to provide a treatment to a particular patient, the question becomes whether or not the treatment will provide sufficient advantages to make it worthwhile for the patient to endure the hardships that would attend the therapy (Lynn & Childress, 1983 p. 21). One cannot make an a priori decision that a treatment is ordinary or extraordinary, but must examine the particular situation and people involved. The President's Commission (1983) adopted the criteria that treatments are expendable, if they are useless or the burdens exceed the benefit.

WITHHOLDING OR WITHDRAWING TREATMENT

While in theory no moral difference appears between withholding a treatment and withdrawing it, health professionals have inordinate difficulty withdrawing treatment once it has begun. The difference between the ease of withholding a treatment and the difficulty of withdrawing it once started provides a psychological explanation of certain actions, but it does not justify them (Lynn, 1986). This difficulty may lead to an irrational decision process. For example, if hospital policy states that treatments can be withheld or omitted but once started not withdrawn, then a distinct motivation to refuse to start procedures exists. This might lead to *not* treating a patient even when that treatment would benefit the person. A better health care policy than to deny possibly useful treatment is to permit treatment to begin even with reservation about its efficacy and then withdraw it when it is no longer useful or if the patient no longer wants the treatment to continue.

The President's Commission (1983) maintains that neither law nor public policy should make a difference in moral seriousness between stopping and not starting treatment. Furthermore, unless a special expectation of continued treatment has been created, it ought to be no more significant, morally or legally, to cease a treatment for a patient than not to start the same treatment for that patient (Capron, 1986).

INTENTION

One further distinction in decisions to forego life-sustaining treatments is the differentiation between intended and unintended death. Sometimes one option is "doing evil to achieve good" (McCormick & Ramsey, 1978). "Evil" consequences of actions are morally permissible provided that (1) the action itself is good (or indifferent); (2) the intention of the agent is for good; (3) the "evil" effect of the action is not intended; (4) the "evil" and the good effect must be equally immediate causally; and (5) there must be a proportionally grave reason for allowing the "evil" to occur (McCormick & Ramsey, 1978). Thus the doctrine of double effect says that it is always wrong to do intentionally a bad act for the sake of good consequences that will ensue, but that it may be permissible to do a good act in the knowledge that bad consequences will follow.

An example of the double effect principle might arise when giving morphine to a patient with compromised respiration. The action of giving the morphine is good because it is intended to reduce pain and not to slow or stop respiration. Both pain reduction and respiratory compromise are equally immediate causally. The proportionally grave reason to allow the "evil" is that the pain reduction is so needed that the benefit outweighs the possible deleterious effect of the morphine (Davis, 1987).

The doctrine of double effect holds that killings are wrong only if we intend them. Is the role of intention adequate when determining an act's wrongness or rightness? Some hold that the morality of an action can be distinguished from the blameworthiness of the actor, and that someone can do the right act out of a bad intention. Likewise, one can do the wrong thing out of a good motive. Someone who actually kills for mercy may be an example. Others argue that if we know with certainty that an indirect "evil" will result, the good intentions of the actor should not matter (Veatch & Fry, 1987). The American Nurses' Association *Code for Nurses* (1985) states that nurses have a duty to prevent and relieve suffering commonly associated with the dying process. The nurse may provide interventions to relieve symptoms in the dying client even when the interventions entail substantial risks of hastening death (ANA, 1985). This statement distinguishes between direct and indirect killing and acknowledges that it is ethical to risk the killing of a patient, if one does not intend to kill, but to prevent and relieve suffering during the dying process.

WITHHOLDING OR WITHDRAWING FOOD AND FLUIDS

We do not tend to view withholding or withdrawing food and water from a patient with the same objectivity that we might have in discontinuing chemotherapy or dialysis treatments. If a competent patient has the right to forego any life-sustaining treatment, this includes food and water. With incompetent patients, the surrogate's decision should reproduce what the patient would have wanted if competent. If the preferences are not known, the surrogate will assess the benefits and burdens to the patient.

A competent patient's decision regarding whether or not to accept the provision of food and water by medical means such as tube feeding or intravenous alimentation raises questions about the practitioners who must participate in the process (Lynn & Childress, 1983).

What should guide those who must decide about nutrition for a patient who cannot decide? Standards for other medical decisions say: one should decide as the incompetent person would have if he or she were competent, when that is possible to determine, and advance that person's interests in a more generalized sense when individual preferences cannot be known (Lynn & Childress, 1983).

A California court found that artificial feeding does not differ from any other life support measure and may be withdrawn when its administration brings no hope of recovery (*Barber v. Superior Court of California*, 1983). Some see no reason to apply a different standard of decision making about treatment decisions to feeding and hydration. The question for them becomes, Is it ever in the patient's interests to become malnourished and dehydrated, rather than to receive treatment (Lynn & Childress, 1983).

When may a procedure that might improve nutrition and hydration for a patient be foregone? Only when the procedure and the resulting improvement in nutrition and hydration do not offer the patient a net benefit over what he or she would otherwise have faced. Some such circumstances are: (1) the procedures that would be required are so unlikely to achieve improved nutritional and fluid levels that they could correctly be considered futile; (2) the improvement in nutritional and fluid balance, although achievable, could be of no benefit to the patient; (3) the burdens of receiving the treatment may outweigh the benefit (Lynn & Childress, 1983).

The American Nurses' Association *Guidelines on Withdrawing or Withholding Food and Fluid* (1987) establish that in most circumstances nurses have no moral permission to withhold or withdraw food or fluid and should not be involved in doing so. In a few circumstances such as those occasions when patients would clearly be more harmed by receiving than by withholding feeding, permissibility allows

nurses to withhold food and fluid. The basic ethical question becomes whether life, under certain conditions, might be a greater burden or harm than death. The *Guidelines* further say that the wishes of competent adults who refuse food and fluid should usually be respected. Morally and legally, nurses should honor the refusal of competent patients.

When providing food and water to a patient becomes an impossible or futile task, does it place an intolerable burden on the patient to provide them? When death is imminent, ineffective procedures that attempt to deliver nutrition and hydration may directly cause suffering and offer no benefit for the patient. Such procedures may be tried, but cannot be considered mandatory (Lynn & Childress, 1983). In these cases feeding a person might become a disproportionate burden. Normal nutritional status could be restored but not without a harsh burden for the patient. Treatment then becomes futile in a broad sense since the patient will not actually benefit from improved nutrition or hydration (Lynn & Childress, 1983). There may be no possibility of benefit for patients who are permanently unconscious, are in a persistent vegetative state, or are in preterminal comas.

SLIPPERY SLOPE ARGUMENTS

The slippery slope or wedge argument assumes that, once allowed in specific circumstances, an action will occur in other circumstances or that once something is allowed to occur it becomes a mandate. There are a number of situations when the slippery slope argument could present problems.

In foregoing food and water, Callahan (1986) agrees that discontinuation of feeding under some circumstances is not always morally wrong but is always repulsive and repugnant even when in the patient's own good and under legitimate circumstances. Using the slippery slope argument he focuses on the symbolic nature of feeding and the emotions evoked by not feeding. He fears that the symbol of feeding, if not respected, might lead us to callousness in feeding people generally and the poor in particular. Our commitment to feed the poor will be eroded if we, as a society, tolerate withholding or withdrawing nutrition without revulsion. Is there, though, any logical connection between withholding and withdrawing treatment and allowing the poor to starve? It seems perfectly possible for society to allow a patient to discontinue an intravenous line and still to continue to feed the poor.

Callahan (1986) believes that if our society defines discontinuation of medical nutrition and hydration as a right, it will eventually define this discontinuation as a duty. This slippery slope argument from may to must, from permissible to required, may become a more serious problem under economic pressures. Given the demographic trends in society of more chronically ill, physically marginal, and elderly people, the denial of food and fluids might become the nontreatment of choice (Callahan, 1983).

Weisbard and Siegler (1986) see the danger that, once the determination to forego food and fluid has been made, even if for humanitarian reasons, death is the desired outcome. The decision makers will become increasingly less troubled by the choice of means employed to achieve that outcome. The line between allowing to die and actively killing can be elusive, and these writers are skeptical about logical or psychological distinctions between these alternatives proving viable. They believe that if our society is to retain the prohibition against active killing, the wavering line demarcating permissible allowings to die must exclude death by avoidable starvation. Their interest exceeds concern for the outcome for a patient, and includes a fear for the reverberations of these decisions on family members, health care professionals, and societal values, all of which will survive the patient's death. These larger concerns draw on historical data that show how easily we disvalue the lives of the unproductive.

The possibility of harm increases when the medical and ethical legitimation of withholding treatments, in this case food and fluids, converges with cost-containment strategies that may well impose significant financial penalties on the prolonged care of the impaired elderly (Weisbard & Siegler, 1986). A societal focus on the use of living wills or durable power of attorney for health care as strategies toward cost control, rather than patient's self-determination, becomes the issue (Weisbard & Siegler, 1986).

Childress (1986) recognizes a moral presumption in favor of life-sustaining medical treatment in accord with the patient's interests and preferences, and this moral presumption must be rebutted before treatment, including food and fluid, can be withheld or withdrawn.

NURSING IMPLICATIONS

The basic moral fabric of the professions, including the basic issues of trust and safety, remain important in these distinctions just discussed. The preservation and maintenance of nursing's ethical integrity is a compelling avowal. The primary commitment of nurses to the patient requires contemporary nursing ethics to focus on nurses as patient advocates. Then how can we both do what the patient requests and what our conscience may dictate in those cases of nonconcordance of these values? Whose interest must we serve first?

The American Nurses' Association *Code for Nurses* mandates respect for human dignity and support of the patient's rights to self-determination as cardinal components of nursing practice (ANA, 1985). In the event that patients are unable to decide, the nurse advocates for them by pursuing their best interests rather than simply following the medical position.

Nurses are entitled to resist providing any treatment that they believe to be wrong. However, one must make a distinction between treatment that the nurse believes damaging to the person's best interests and treatment to which the nurse has a conscientious objection. Nurses have a duty not to allow their judgment about what is in the patient's best interests to be influenced by their own personal beliefs, when they would be counter to the patient's expressed wishes.

If the nurse, caring for a patient who requests cessation of treatment, believes the request to be against the patient's best interests, what should the she or he do? If adequate staff is available, then another nurse may be assigned to the patient. Is that an appropriate outcome? If the nurse cannot provide care or take part in it because of her or his own principles, what responsibility does the nurse have and to whom? Must one tell the patient? The nurse in all cases must ensure that the patient receives care, for to abandon a patient is unethical and causes harm.

Suppose a staff member asked the nurse to implement a decision that the nurse believes to be morally wrong (Theis, 1986). The complexity of situations in which nurses disagree with the moral appropriateness of a given order, and the conflict between what nurses think ought to be done and what they are expected to do, has been discussed (Theis, 1986). Nurses experience difficulty in exercising conscience because of the multiple obligations they have to their patient, the physician, and the hospital (Davis & Aroskar, 1983).

The ANA Committee on Ethics' guidelines (1987) on withdrawing or withholding food and fluid underline the professional obligation to provide nourishment to the sick who can be helped by it. When the patient can clearly be helped by the nourishment, no one doubts the obligation to provide it. What about the nourishment that does not nourish? These guidelines detail circumstances in which nurses should withhold food and fluid because the patient would clearly be harmed by receiving them. Such action is morally permissible and indeed morally obligatory. The ethical difficulty ensues when uncertainty remains on whether nourishment benefits or harms.

Is it morally permissible for the nurse to honor the refusal of food and fluid by competent patients? The view of the nurse as patient advocate would certainly seem to support this view of respect for patient self-determination or autonomy. The ethics code for nurses ordinarily supports this opinion.

The nurse must legally omit a treatment that might hasten death, but what if the nurse finds such action morally objectionable? Does the nurse have the right to challenge the omission and to withdraw from any commitment to patient care? How and when can nurses decide they are justified in either going along with or refusing to accept the decision to treat or to refuse treatment including food and fluid?

The nurse not only plays a role in determining whether life support measures are a burden for a patient that outweigh their benefit, but also must continue to provide care while these treatment decisions are being considered. Input from the nursing staff

that the care given imposes continued suffering, pain, or indignity becomes a major factor in withholding and withdrawing treatment decisions (Groh, 1987).

Suppose that the nurse has not participated in the decision to withdraw support but receives the order to discontinue a ventilator. It is the nurse, finally alone after all is done and everybody else has gone, who wonders if enough or too much was done (Groh, 1987).

The ANA *Code for Nurses* (1985) affirms the patient's right to self-determination in relation to treatment decisions. Traditionally nursing ethics advances and supports the concept of patient autonomy and agrees that no patient should be forced to undergo procedures that will increase suffering when he or she wishes to avoid this by foregoing life-sustaining treatments (President's Commission, 1983).

SUMMARY

Once a patient makes a decision to refuse treatment or discontinue it, the issue of nursing care still exists. Nurses cannot assume that patients want all of the nursing care that we might wish to provide but must evaluate each situation (California Nurses' Association, 1987). The fully informed patient who wishes to refuse treatment has a moral right to do so, and the nurse and the physician are morally bound to accept the patient's directive. Neither nurses nor any other health care staff have the right to treat patients against their will. As patient advocates, nurses have a greater responsibility than other members of the treatment team to see that the patient's wishes are honored. In instances when the patient's rights or welfare is jeopardized, nursing must take a united, proactive, and firm stance (California Nurses' Association, 1987).

Comfort measures including pain relief and hydration and nutrition are clinically and morally acceptable. Everything done for the dying patient should meet only the test of whether it will make the patient more comfortable and whether it will honor his or her wishes.

Many believe that acceptance of the patient's choice to forego treatment reflects concern for individual self-determination, bodily integrity, avoidance of suffering, and empathy with an individual's effort to shape his or her dying process, rather than deprecation of life's values. Courts that concur with a patient's decision are impelled by profound respect for individual autonomy as an integral part of human dignity, and not by any disregard or disdain for the value or sanctity of life (Cantor, 1987).

With the support of nursing administration, personal variations in moral convictions can be addressed in the moral discourse at the unit level. Nurses should never be compelled to violate their own moral principles in order to comply with treatment orders. For example, if a particular nurse is unable to extubate a patient whose life is sustained by a ventilator, the nurse should be relieved of this burden, without prejudice. Nurses have no obligation to provide useless treatment, but they always have an obligation to provide care. Easing of pain, relief of suffering, and supportive and comforting care are necessary and morally required, especially in the presence of incurable and progressive illness. Nurses have the privilege and the responsibility to comfort, always.

REFERENCES

American Nurses' Association (ANA). (1985). *Code for nurses with interpretive statements*. Kansas City, MO: Author.

American Nurses' Association Committee on Ethics. (1987). *Guidelines on withdrawing or withholding food and fluid*. Kansas City, MO: Author.

Annas, G. J. (1987). In thunder, lightning, or in rain: What three doctors can do. *Hastings Center Report, 17* (5), 28–30.

Barber v. Superior Court of California, 195 Cal. Rptr. 484, 147 Cal. App. 3d 1006 (1983).

California Nurses' Association. (1987). *Statement on the nurse's role in withholding and withdrawing life-sustaining treatment*. San Francisco: Author.

Callahan, D. (1983). On feeding the dying. *Hastings Center Report, 5*(13), 22.

Callahan, D. (1986). Public policy and the cessation of nutrition. In J. Lynn (Ed.), *By no extraordinary means: The choice to forego life-sustaining food and water* (pp. 61–66). Bloomington: Indiana University Press.

Cantor, N. L. (1987). *Legal frontiers of death and dying*. Bloomington: Indiana University Press.

Capron, A. (1986). Historical overview: Law and public perceptions. In J. Lynn (Ed.), *By no extraordinary means: The choice to forego life-sustaining food and water* (pp. 16–20). Bloomington, Indiana University Press.

Childress, J. (1986). When is it morally justifiable to discontinue medical nutrition and hydration? In J. Lynn (Ed.), *By no extraordinary means: The choice to forego life-sustaining food and water* (pp. 63-83). Bloomington: Indiana University Press.

Davis, A. J. (1987). The boundaries of intervention: Issues in the noninfliction of harm. In M. D. Fowler, J. Levine-Ariff, and American Association of Critical Care Nurses (Eds.), *Ethics at the bedside: A source book for the critical care nurse* (pp. 50–61). Philadelphia: J. B. Lippincott.

Davis, A. J., & Aroskar, M. (1983). *Ethical dilemmas and nursing practice*. Norwalk, CT: Appleton-Century-Crofts.

Groh, D. H. (1987). Treatment or torture: Why critical care? In M. D. Fowler, J. Levine-Ariff, and American Association of Critical Care Nurses (Eds.), *Ethics at the bedside: A source book for the critical care nurse* (pp. 1–23). Philadelphia: J. B. Lippincott.

Kass, L. R. (1980). Ethical dilemmas in the care of the ill. *Journal of the American Medical Association, 244,* 1946–1949.

Keene, S. B. (1983). Durable power of attorney for health care. [SB 762 (Keene) Ch. 1204 Stats 1983].

Lynn, J. (Ed.) (1986). *By no extraordinary means: The choice to forego life-sustaining food and water*. Bloomington: Indiana University Press.

Lynn, J., & Childress, J. (1983). Must patients always be given food and water? *Hastings Center Report, 5*(13), 17–21.

McCartney, J. J. (1980). The development of the doctrine of ordinary and extraordinary means of preserving life in Catholic moral theology before the Karen Quinlan case. *Linacre Quarterly, 47,* 215–220.

McCormick, R., & Ramsey, P. (Eds.). (1978). *Doing evil to achieve good: Moral choice in conflict situations*. Chicago: Loyola University Press.

Macklin, R. (1987). *Mortal choices: Bioethics in today's world*. New York: Pantheon Books.

Natanson v. Kline, 186 Kan. 393, 350 P.2d 1093 (1960).

The President's Commission for the Study of Ethical Problems in Medicine and Biomedical Research. (1982).

Making health care decisions. Washington, DC: U.S. Government Printing Office.

The President's Commission for the Study of Ethical Problems in Medicine and Biomedical Research. (1983). *Deciding to forego life-sustaining treatment*. Washington, DC: U.S. Government Printing Office.

Theis, E. C. (1986). Ethical issues: A nursing perspective. *New England Journal of Medicine, 315*, 1222–1224.

Union Pacific Railway v. Botsford, 141 U.S. 250, 251 (1891).

Veatch, R. M., & Fry, S. T. (1987). *Case studies in nursing ethics*. Philadelphia: J. B. Lippincott.

Weisbard, A. J., & Siegler, M. (1986). On killing patients with kindness: An appeal for caution. In J. Lynn (Ed.), *By no extraordinary means: The choice to forego life-sustaining food and water* (pp. 108–116). Bloomington: Indiana University Press.

✳ EDITOR'S QUESTIONS FOR DISCUSSION ✳

What options does a nurse have as a patient advocate when a patient requests that his or her treatment be discontinued and a physician refuses to honor the request? Discuss the nurse's role in patients' informed consent regarding treatment, as well as the withdrawal of treatment. Provide examples of the multiple obligations nurses have to their patients, physicians, and the hospital that might be in conflict simultaneously. Discuss whether or not it is more significant ethically to cease a treatment for a patient than to choose not to start a treatment for the patient. What is the basic principle that must be rebutted before treatment, including food and fluid, can be withheld or withdrawn? Discuss the ANA's guidelines on withholding or withdrawing food and fluid in relation to the nurse's role. Why should or should not nurses be involved in such decision making? What other guidelines might be followed in deciding the extent of nurses' participation in the decision to withdraw or withhold food and fluid?

Can a nurse participate or have an ethical responsibility in only one portion of a decision to withdraw care or must she or he have been involved in the entire decision-making process and final act to withdraw care to have an ethical obligation? For example, must the nurse have been involved in the decision to discontinue a ventilator as well as performing the actual act, for an ethical obligation to ensue, or is it ethically possible for the nurse to be involved in the decision and either just follow or not follow the medical orders to discontinue a ventilator, or ethically not be involved with the decision and either just follow or not follow the medical orders for an ethical obligation? Why do nurses have a greater responsibility than any other member of the health care team to see that a patient's wishes are honored?

40

Legal Considerations in the Refusal of Life-Sustaining Measures

Kathleen M. Driscoll, J.D., M.S., R.N.

OVERVIEW

"Since, man, through his ingenuity, has created a new state of human existence—minimal human life sustained by man-made life supports—it must now devise and fashion rules and parameters for that existence" (*Leach v. Akron General Medical Center*, 1980 at 52). Can the existence made possible by respirators, cardiopulmonary resuscitation, and artificial feeding be declined? By whom? For what reasons? Which of these measures can be refused? In what settings? At what times? How? The court in *Leach* (1980) aptly identified the task.

Since the 1976 New Jersey decision *In Re Quinlan*, the law has consistently recognized the right to refuse life-sustaining measures in both case and statutory law. In doing so, courts have invoked the common law right to be free of intrusion upon one's body, absent consent, and both an implicit federal constitutional right to privacy and the express right to privacy granted by many state constitutions. Legislatures have supported case law by enacting statutes defining brain death, legalizing living wills, and providing for durable powers of attorney. How such rights can apply to children has been debated and

addressed. Individual practitioners and bioethicists have written extensively on the right of treatment refusal. Professional associations and task forces have voiced their collective positions (American Medical Association, 1986; Hastings Center, 1987; President's Commission for the Study of Ethical Problems in Medicine and Biomedical and Behavioral Research, 1983). Within health care institutions committees have deliberated how best to achieve moral good for patients while operating within the societal ethics reflected by law.

Because nurses have intimate contact with patients for extended periods of time, they are ideally situated to remind patients of the right to refuse life-sustaining measures, to provide through documentation in the patient's record the clear and convincing standard of evidence required to honor the patient's refusal (*Leach*, 1980) and to support then those choices.

This chapter primarily discusses the law as it applies to refusal of life-sustaining measures by adults, including case law and statutory law. A brief discussion of the law as it applies to refusal of life-sustaining measures by children, and of the law as it potentially applies to hospital ethics committees then follows.

THE LAW AND ADULTS
Case Law
The issue of competency

Who may refuse life-sustaining measures? Case law discusses four categories of persons: (a) persons whose decision-making capability remains intact; (b) persons who have expressed their wishes in a living will, specific oral directives, or conversation with relatives or friends; (c) persons who when capable never made a clear statement about their wishes; and (d) persons always incapable of making decisions.

The terms *competent* and *capable* are frequently used interchangeably in discussing refusal of life-sustaining measures. Competency, in its pure sense, refers to legal competency, that is, the ability to make decisions for oneself instead of those decisions being made by a natural guardian such as a parent or a legal guardian appointed by a probate court. Persons in a coma or unable to communicate because of a stroke may be incapable of decision making but not be declared legally incompetent. A minor child may be legally incompetent but be capable of decision making. Parents should consider the wishes of their child in making health care decisions. A legal guardian should respect wishes communicated by the ward.

Competent persons Courts first dealt with a competent person's wishes in *Satz v. Perlmutter* (1978). Mr. Perlmutter suffered from amyotrophic lateral sclerosis (ALS) and wished to have the respirator that sustained his life removed. Family agreed, but physicians and the hospital were reluctant to take the action because of fears of criminal and civil liability. The court honored Mr. Perlmutter's wishes.

California first considered refusal of life-sustaining measures by a competent person in the case of Elizabeth Bouvia. A quadriplegic because of cerebral palsy, and also suffering from increasingly painful rheumatoid arthritis, in 1983 she first sought court approval of her desire to have the nasogastric tube supplying her nutrition removed. The hospital caring for her fought her wishes and won at the trial level (*Bouvia v. County of Riverside*, 1983). Ms. Bouvia abandoned a legal appeal and eventually left the adversary facility, living with friends or being cared for in nursing homes until further deterioration of her status required another hospitalization in 1986. By this time totally incapable of feeding herself, she again refused insertion of a nasogastric tube. This time the court was prepared to honor her request (*Bouvia v. Superior Court*, 1986).

In the interim, between Bouvia's 1983 and 1986 actions, the same California court had dealt with two significant cases addressing refusal of life-sustaining measures (*Barber v. Superior Court*, 1983 and *Bartling v. Superior Court*, 1984). In both, patients' wishes to be removed from life-sustaining measures—for Mr. Herbert in *Barber*, a respirator and intravenous fluids, and for Mr. Bartling, a respirator—had been upheld. *Barber* had particular significance because it exonerated two physicians charged with murder. Thus by the 1986 *Bouvia* case the court could comment:

> Although alert, bright, sensitive, perhaps even brave and feisty, she must lie immobile, unable to exist except through physical acts of other. Her mind and spirit may be free to take great flights but she herself is imprisoned and must lie physically helpless subject to the ignominy, embarrassment, humiliation and dehumanizing aspects created by her helplessness. We do not believe it is the policy of this State that all and every life must be preserved against the will of the sufferer. It is incongruous, if not monstrous, for medical practitioners to assert their right to preserve a life that someone else must live. (*Bouvia v. Superior Court*, 1986 at 305).

More recently the New Jersey Supreme Court honored the wishes of two women suffering from ALS who remained competent—a 37-year-old woman seeking removal from a respirator (*In Re Farrell*, 1987) and a 55-year-old woman who refused insertion of a nasogastric tube (*In Re Requena*, 1986).

Persons with express wishes prior to incompetency The first court to honor clear prior express wishes regarding use of life-sustaining measures was in New York. There the religious superior of a Catholic brother acted as spokesperson for Brother Fox who had suffered a cardiac arrest and was being maintained on a respirator (*In Re Eichner*, 1981). Brother Fox had clearly indicated his desire not to have his life sustained under such conditions. The court quoting the seminal informed consent case, *Schloendorff v. Society of New York Hospital* (1914) extended the right of "every human being of adult years and sound mind . . . to determine what shall be done with his own body" to individuals no longer capable of expressing their wishes but who had previously done so (*Schloendorff*, at 93). Courts in New York have reiterated and courts in California, Delaware, Florida, Maine, New Jersey, and Ohio have followed with decisions at either appellate or high court levels permitting assertion of prior expressed wishes by another (*Severns v. Wilmington Medical Center*, 1980; *John F. Kennedy Memorial Hospital v. Bludworth*, 1984; *Leach v. Shapiro*, 1984; *In Re Gardner*, 1987; *In Re Peter*, 1987).

Persons lacking express wishes prior to incompetency Because of lack of certitude about patient desires, situations in which individuals have not previously expressed their wishes have been more troublesome for courts. Nancy Ellen Jobes was 31 years old and in a persistent vegetative state. The Supreme Court of New Jersey considered authorizing her husband to direct removal of the jejunostomy tube artificially supplying her nutrition. In 1980, Mrs. Jobes had sustained a severe loss of oxygen to the brain during surgery to remove her dead fetus, after she suffered injuries in an automobile accident. Before that time, she had worked as a certified laboratory technologist and had commented on several occasions that she would not want to live in a state similar to that of Karen Ann Quinlan. The court found that her comments did not specifically express wishes regarding treatment in her present situation. It acknowledged that her comments evidenced her values and combined with exercise of judgment on her behalf by a caring family member—her husband—provided assurance that her best interests would be considered (*In Re Jobes*, 1987).

Uncertainty about a person's wishes in the actual situation that triggers consideration of removal of life-sustaining measures is a continuing problem for jurists in cases lacking clear prior expressed wishes. The New Jersey Supreme Court approached the problem of uncertainty in *In Re Conroy* (1985) by developing a series of three tests to help assure surrogates that they are decision making as the person might desire and in the person's best interest.

The first, the subjective test, is used when persons have prior expressed wishes communicated clearly in oral expressions or written directives, such as a living will or through a durable power of attorney. The two additional tests directly address the problem of uncertainty. The first, the limited-objective test, couples some trustworthy evidence that the patient would have refused treatment with the decision maker's judgment that the burdens of the patient's continued life with the treatment outweigh the benefits. The second, the pure-objective test, permits declining treatment when "the net burdens of the patient's life with the treatment . . . clearly and markedly outweigh the benefits that the patient derives from life" (*In Re Conroy*, 1985 at 1232).

The *Conroy* court specifically identifies pain and suffering as burdens of treatment and specifically declines "to authorize decision making based on assessments of the personal worth or social utility of another's life, or the value of that life to others" (*Conroy* at 1233). Justice Handler, in his concurring opinion in *Jobes*, notes that the lack of societal consensus regarding a "best interests" standard delimits the worth of even the carefully articulated tests of *Conroy*.

The court in *Conroy* dealt with withdrawal of a nasogastric tube. A best interests standard was used by the Arizona Supreme Court in *Rasmussen by Mitchell v. Fleming* (1987), again to accord the right to refuse medical treatment to the patient's guardian, including removal of a nasogastric tube. Had *Conroy* preceded *In Re Conservatorship of Torres* (1984), a limited-objective test might have been used to determine Torres' best interests. Torres had stated no specific desires regarding use of life-sustaining measures, but he had indicated unwillingness to wear a pacemaker. This evidence, coupled with a burdens over benefits determination, could have served to permit his conservator (guardian) to act on his behalf to withdraw the respirator on which he had been placed following a cardiopulmonary arrest. A similar analysis could have been applied in *Foody v. Manchester Memorial Hospital* (1984) for a 42-year-old woman suffering from multiple sclerosis who was in an "awake but unaware" state after aspirating and developing a respiratory arrest.

Persons always incapable of expressing wishes. Few cases deal with persons who have always been incapable of making their own decisions. Courts in Washington, New York, and Massachusetts have dealt with the issue. All accord such individuals the right to refuse treatment, with a surrogate decision maker using a substituted judgment standard. This standard requires that the surrogate choose—not as the majority of persons nor as the surrogate might choose—but as the incompetent, given the circumstances, would choose. The pure-objective test of *Conroy* lends needed perspective to decision making in these circumstances.

Situations addressed have included (a) a 42-year-old individual, blind and mentally retarded since birth, on a respirator (*In Re Guardianship of Hamlin*, 1984); (b) a 67-year-old mentally retarded long-term resident of a state institution suffering from treatable but inevitably fatal leukemia (*Superintendent of Belchertown v. Saikewicz*, 1977); and (c) a 52-year-old profoundly retarded man with cancer of the bladder (*In Re Storar*, 1981). Only in the last situation was the person treated. This occurred when staff of the state institution where Storar resided opposed the decision of his legal guardian, his mother. She refused continued blood transfusions after her son's cancer became terminal. New York's highest court ordered continued transfusions because they resulted in his having the physical strength and energy to engage in his usual activities and did not involve excessive pain.

The four state interests

The *Saikewicz* case (1977) enunciated four state interests that must be outweighed by the individual's interests when refusing medical treatment. The four are (a) the preservation of life; (b) the protection of innocent third parties; (c) the prevention of suicide; and (d) maintaining the ethical integrity of the medical profession.

The preservation of life can be outweighed by the individual's fundamental constitutional right to privacy, which includes the right of self-determination or the common law right to refuse treatment. The

protection of third parties asks whether the individual's interest outweighs responsibilities that individual may have, for example, to care for minor children. This has not been an issue in any of the cases addressing use of life-sustaining measures. The prevention of suicide has been raised, particularly in the dissents in cases involving refusal of nourishment. No court has used this interest as justification for refusing to honor an individual's wishes. Instead, courts have stated that suicide is not an issue because the individual is not setting in motion the means of producing death. It is the disease process, over which the individual has not control, that is the initiating agent. Maintenance of the ethical integrity of the medical profession has not kept courts from honoring the individual's rights. It has, however, required moving individuals to institutions where individual and institutional values coincide. This was necessary for Karen Ann Quinlan to be removed from the respirator.

One court required that an institution honor a patient's wishes without transfer despite conflict with hospital policy. In a moving opinion the court in *In Re Requena* (1986) found the individual's reliance on and trust in hospital staff, who had cared for her for a year and a half, to outweigh the hospital's policy against withholding nourishment. The court may have been influenced by the hospital's hasty generation of a policy when this ALS patient indicated that she did not want a nasogastric tube.

Types of measures refused, site and timing of refusals

Which measures can be refused? Case law has dealt with the following: (a) cardiopulmonary resuscitation (*In Re Dinnerstein*, 1978); (b) cancer chemotherapy *(Saikewicz)*; (c) respirators *(Quinlan; Eichner; Hamlin; Farrell)*; (d) amputation of a gangrenous extremity (*Lane v. Candura*, 1978); (e) dialysis (*In Re Spring*, 1980); and (f) artificial feeding (*In Re Conroy; Brophy v. New England Sinai Hospital*, 1986; *Delio v. Westchester County Hospital*, 1987; *In Re Guardianship of Grant*, 1987; *In Re Gardner*, 1987). Courts have frequently addressed the withdrawal of respirators and generated little public outcry. The question of withdrawing hydration and nutrition has generated much debate (Capron, 1984; Meilaender, 1984). No state high court addressed the issue until *Conroy* in 1985. Then the New Jersey Court took the opportunity to equate artificial feeding with other medical procedures and to assert that these measures could also be refused.

In December 1987, the Maine Supreme Court permitted removal of a nasogastric tube despite a provision in the Maine living will statute that forbade honoring directives to withdraw nutrition or hydration. The Court stated that the legislature could not override Maine common law supportive of Gardner's right of self-determination in matters of health care (*In Re Gardner*). Courts in Florida (*Corbett v. D'Alessandro*, 1986) and Colorado (*In Re Rodas*, 1987) have acted similarly.

Life-sustaining measures may be refused by patients in hospitals *(In Re Requena)*, nursing homes (*In Re Conroy; In Re Peter by Johanning*, 1987; *In Re Jobes*) and at home (*In Re Farrell*).

Life-sustaining measures may be refused at any time as long as none of the four state interests previously mentioned outweigh the individual's right to self-determination. Whether a person must be terminally ill to assert that right has been at issue. The response has been in the negative (*Bartling*, 1984; *Bouvia*, 1986). Only *Conroy* differed—holding that an incompetent person with a life expectancy of more than a year could not refuse treatment. Situations where the individual has been in a persistent vegetative state have most frequently posed this question because such persons may continue to exist for long periods of time (Cranford, 1988). In answer, several courts, although with strong dissents, have specified that persons in persistent vegetative states may refuse treatment (*Bouvia*, 1986; *Brophy; Jobes; Delio v. Westchester County Hospital*, 1987).

Procedures for refusing life-sustaining measures

Lastly, how may persons refuse life-sustaining measures? Massachusetts continues unique in requiring court approval for refusal of treatment by persons incapable of making decisions for themselves (*Saikewicz*, 1977; *In Re Spring*, 1980). *In Re Dinnerstein* remains the exception to this rule and

provides that without court approval "do not resuscitate orders" may be written for persons of advanced age, in an essentially vegetative state, and suffering irreversible and terminal illness. The Supreme Court of Washington initially required judicial intervention for persons incapable of treatment decisions with no close family members (*In Re Welfare of Colyer*, 1983). The Court modified its position in *In Re Hamlin* (1984) requiring judicial intervention only when guardians and physicians could not agree on a course of treatment.

In *Quinlan* the New Jersey Supreme Court provided that with concurrence of physician, guardian, family, and a hospital ethics committee acting as a consultative body, the respirator could be withdrawn. The court in *Conroy* dealt with a nursing home setting and provided that the process for withholding or withdrawing treatment from the incompetent person include (a) documentation of the patient's condition furnished by the attending physician and nurses; (b) concurrence regarding the patient's medical condition and prognosis by two physicians unaffiliated with the nursing home appointed by the New Jersey ombudsman's office or a court; (c) good faith belief of the patient's guardian, the attending physician, and the ombudsman that one of the legal tests is satisfied; and (d) concurrence of the patient's family or next of kin if either the limited-objective or pure-objective tests is being used.

In *In Re Peter by Johanning* (1987) the New Jersey Supreme Court refined its opinion in *Conroy* stating that the limited life expectancy test did not apply to elderly patients in persistent vegetative states, nor did the limited-objective and pure-objective tests. Instead, like *Quinlan*, the court emphasized prognosis as the critical deciding factor. The *Jobes* decision deleted the role of the ombudsman for nonelderly patients with caring family or friends. For persons at home the court in *Farrell* required that two nonattending physicians assess the person as competent to refuse life-sustaining measures, and as making the decision uncoerced and fully informed of the alternatives, risks, and outcomes.

Overall, case law favors approaching courts only when agreement cannot be reached among patient, family, physician, and health care facility. Existing case law also assures that civil and criminal liability for the health care provider is not an issue when a decision to withdraw or withhold life-sustaining measures is made in good faith.

Two recent cases in the highest courts of Missouri and New York mark an important turning point in case law development in the right to refuse life-sustaining measures. In both cases the courts found that incompetent persons not terminally ill had not clearly and convincingly expressed their wish to refuse life-sustaining measures when competent (*Cruzan v. Harmon*, 1988; *In Re Westchester County Medical Center*, 1988). Clear and convincing evidence is the highest evidentiary standard in civil cases. It contrasts with the lower standard, more common in civil cases, of preponderance of the evidence. Both cases signal that individuals should express wishes about use of life-sustaining measures at moments when their expressed wishes can later be determined to be clear and dispassionate. Furthermore those wishes, if not put in writing, should be reaffirmed at regular intervals when life experiences, such as the loss of a loved one, are not influencing factors.

Other legal actions involving the refusal of life-sustaining measures

Leach v. Shapiro (1984), an Ohio appellate case, reminds physicians that an obligation extends to surrogates to inform them of patient prognosis. Fulfilling the obligation permits family and other surrogates the opportunity for considered decisions in relation to use of life-sustaining measures. Nondisclosure may lead to an action in fraud independent of malpractice. When life-sustaining measures continue against patient or surrogate wishes, actions for pain, suffering, and mental anguish may also result.

Statutory Law

Brain death statutes, living will laws, and durable power of attorney statutes are relevant to legal considerations in use of life-sustaining measures. These are discussed below.

Brain death statutes

Traditional definitions of death no longer sufficed when the development of life support systems permitted continued respiratory and cardiac functions in the absence of brainstem function. However, maintenance of perfusion and respiration was useful to increase the chances of success with the concurrently developing technology of organ transplantation. In 1968, a committee of Harvard University faculty developed a definition of brain death that became the standard of medical practice (Report of the Ad Hoc Committee of the Harvard Medical School to Examine the Definition of Brain Death, 1968). Gradually states added brain death to the traditional statutory definitions of death—cessation of respiratory and cardiac function. Use of life-sustaining measures when a person meets the criteria for brain death is thus a contradiction in terms. It is not sustaining life, but often merely extending the duration of time that organs remain suitable for transplant.

Further revision of legal definitions of death looms in the future. Defining death to include persons without neocortical functions has been suggested (Smith, 1986). Proposals to amend the definition of death to permit access to anencephalic infants for organ transplants have occurred in California and New Jersey (Capron, 1987) and also in Ohio (House Bill 718, 1988).

Living wills

Although living will bills have been introduced in all state legislatures, the Society for the Right to Die reports that by the end of 1987 statutes existed in only 38 states and the District of Columbia. Statutes are lacking in twelve states: Kentucky, Massachusetts, Michigan, Minnesota, Nebraska, New Jersey, New York, North Dakota, Ohio, Pennsylvania, Rhode Island, and South Dakota (Society for the Right to Die, 1987b).

Statutes generally include a number of provisions: (a) recognition of advance directives; (b) immunity from legal liability for caregivers who honor directives; (c) suggested forms for drawing declarations; (d) definition of relevant terms; (e) procedures for executing declarations including witnessing and revocation methods; (f) an unlimited term of effectiveness; (g) a requirement that the declaration be made part of the person's medical record; (h) a requirement that physicians unwilling to honor a declaration make an effort to transfer or permit transfer of the patient, and often a penalty for violation; and (i) indication that the declaration is one way to effectuate individual rights but is not the exclusive approach (Society for the Right to Die, 1987b). The laws are known by a variety of names, such as natural death act, medical treatment decision act, life-prolonging procedure act, life-sustaining procedures act, and withdrawal of lifesaving mechanisms act (Society for the Right to Die, 1987b).

Variations in state living will laws prompted the Conference of Commissioners on Uniform State Laws to develop and approve in 1985 the Uniform Rights of the Terminally Ill Act. The act lacks two useful provisions: (a) the appointment of a proxy to act on behalf of the person executing the living will and (b) procedures for decision making on behalf of incompetent patients who have not made their wishes known (Society for the Right to Die, 1987b).

Durable powers of attorney

Because all states do not have living will statutes, because provisions of statutes vary, and because individuals may not have anticipated the circumstances or choice of procedures that may set in motion the terms of their living will, living wills are not ideal instruments. In all states the living will serves as evidence that the person has contemplated death and indicated an aversion to an artificially prolonged existence when there is no hope of recovery. The execution of a durable power of attorney as a complement to a living will, or the appointment of a proxy decision maker as one of the terms of a living will, reduces opportunities for dispute among caregivers and family.

Durable powers of attorney effectively authorize another person, an agent or a proxy, to make decisions and act on behalf of another even when the authorizing person—the principal—has become unable to make decisions. Ordinary powers of attorney cease effectiveness with the incapacity of the principal. Persons designated as proxies by individuals are viewed as more likely than court appointed guardians to exercise the wishes of the appointing person. This is because the proxy generally is a good friend or relative of the appointing person.

The Society for the Right to Die reports that all 50 states and the District of Columbia now have durable power of attorney statutes. Eight statutes clearly address medical treatment decisions and five of them speak specifically to withholding or withdrawing life support. Five additional statutes authorize consent but do not address refusal of treatment. In cases addressing refusal of life-sustaining measures, courts in Colorado and New Jersey have specifically recognized durable powers of attorney (Society for the Right to Die, 1987a).

THE LAW AND CHILDREN

Since the Indiana *Baby Doe* case in 1982, extensive discussion of the rights of handicapped infants has occurred (Nolan, 1987). Legally, however, rights of infants hinge on the 1984 amendments to the federal Child Abuse Prevention and Treatment Act. These call for "appropriate nutrition, hydration, and medication" to all infants with life-threatening conditions. In the judgment of the treating physician'(s) reasonable medical judgment, other treatments may be withheld when:

> (A) the infant is chronically and irreversibly comatose; (B) the provision of such treatment would (i) merely prolong dying, (ii) not be effective in ameliorating or correcting all of the infant's life-threatening conditions, or (iii) otherwise be futile in terms of the survival of the infant; or (C) the provision of such treatment would be virtually futile in terms of the survival of the infant and the treatment itself under such circumstances would be inhumane. (Child Abuse Prevention and Treatment Act, § 5102(3) (1984).

The amendments required states to have programs or procedures in place by October 9, 1985, in order to receive continued federal funding for child abuse programs (§ 5103 (b) (2) (K)).

Courts have consistently viewed treatment for children beyond infancy as necessary when treatment for a life-threatening condition offers opportunity for survival. Consistent with the provisions of federal and state child abuse statutes, parents and legal guardians have been prosecuted for neglect when a child's medical needs were ignored.

ETHICS COMMITTEES

The first mention of an ethics committee occurred with the *Quinlan* mandate that a hospital ethics committee determine Karen Ann Quinlan's prognosis. The work of ethics committees has never become the flourishing business once anticipated. When institutional ethics committees exist, potential liability for the work of ethics committees is present for both institutions and committee members.

When the ethics committee performs only an educational function the risk of suit is minimal. It remains minimal when policy development is the ethics committee's function. Facilities need to be aware, however, that policies set the standard of care. When standards are not followed, potential for actions in negligence is posed. Prospective case review produces potential for actions in negligence, invasion of privacy, the unauthorized practice of medicine, and failure to report suspected cases of abuse and neglect. Retrospective case review, while posing threats for actions in negligence and defamation and presenting difficult decisions for individuals required to report neglect, may overall present less threat. Both members and informants of such committees frequently may have immunity from civil suit if ethics committees are constituted as peer review committees. Statutes providing such protection are known as peer review laws. They prohibit legal adversaries from obtaining committee records during the pretrial discovery phase of a suit (Brooks, 1985).

CONCLUSION

The law regards withdrawing and withholding of life-sustaining measures as equivalent. To permit withholding and forbid withdrawing would be inconsistent with standards of medical practice. This is because initial administration of life-sustaining measures affords time for accurate medical diagnosis as well as time to accustom a family to the probable loss of a loved one.

Health care facilities need policies and procedures for informed decision making in this sensitive area. Supporting law cannot be ignored in framing facility guidelines for use of life-sustaining measures. Sufficient flexibility to assure that the values both of individuals and institution can be recognized and must be maintained in the development and implementation of policies and procedures addressing refusal of life-sustaining measures.

Facility policy and procedures should include five essential components: (a) recognition of patient autonomy, (b) provision for surrogate decision making, (c) documentation of medical judgments regarding prognosis and discussions with patient, family, and surrogate decision makers, (d) approaches to resolution of conflict among decision participants, and (e) provision for periodic renewal of orders following reevaluation of patient status. Affirmation that other care will not be diminished when withdrawal or withholding of life-sustaining measures occurs acknowledges the caregiver's continued commitment to patients.

Other health care providers acknowledge their respect for the perspective nurses bring to the decision-making process in the care of the dying and the permanently unconscious patient. As nursing increasingly turns to activate its power in the patient care domain, nurses need to know the law in relation to life-sustaining measures. Nurses can then exert their professional influence on institutional ethics committees, on policy and procedure committees, and in individual patient situations.

REFERENCES

American Medical Association, Current Opinions of the Council of Ethical and Judicial Affairs. (1986). Withholding or withdrawing life prolonging medical treatment. Chicago: Author.

Barber v. Superior Court, 147 Cal. App. 3d 1006, 195 Cal. Rptr. 484 (Ct. App. 1983).

Bartling v. Superior Court, 163 Cal. App. 3d 186, 209 Cal. Rptr. 220 (Ct. App. 1984).

Bouvia v. County of Riverside, No. 159780 (Cal. Super. Ct. Riverside County Dec. 16, 1983) (Hews J.).

Bouvia v. Superior Court (Glenchur), 179 Cal. App. 3d

1127, 225 Cal. Rptr. 297 (Ct. App. 1986), *review denied* (Cal. June 5, 1986).

Brooks, T. A. (1985, October). *Ethics committees: Legal issues under alternative formats*. Presentation at a program on critical care decision making in hospitals of the Forum Committee on Health Law of the American Bar Association, Washington, D.C.

Brophy v. New England Sinai Hospital, Inc., 398 Mass. 417, 497 N.E. 2d 626 (1986).

Capron, A. M. (1984). Ironies and tensions in feeding the dying. *Hastings Center Report, 14*(5), 32–35.

Capron, A. M. (1987). Anencephalic donors: Separate the dead from the dying. *Hastings Center Report, 17* (1), 5–9.

Child Abuse Prevention and Treatment Act, § 5102(3) and 5103 (b) (2) (K) (1984).

In re Colyer, 99 Wash. 2d 114, 660 P.2d 738 (1983), *overruled in part, In re Guardianship of Hamlin*, 102 Wash. 2d 810, 689 P. 2d 1372 (1984).

In re Conroy, 98 N.J. 321, 486 A.2d 1209 (1985).

Corbett v. D'Alessandro, 487 So.2d 368 (Fla. Dist. Ct. App.), *review denied*, 492 So.2d 1331 (Fla. 1986).

Cranford, R. E. (1988). The persistent vegetative state: The medical reality (getting the facts straight). *Hasting Center Report, 18* (2), 27–32.

Cruzan v. Harmon, No. 70813 (Mo. Sup. Ct. Nov. 16 1988), 57 LW 2325.

Delio v. Westchester County Hospital, 516 N.Y.S.2d 677 (A.D. 2 Dept. 1987).

In re Dinnerstein, 6 Mass. App. 466, 380 N.E.2d 134 (Ct. App. 1978).

In re Eichner (*In re* Storar), 52 N.Y.2d 363, 420 N.E.2d 64, 438 N.Y.S.2d 266, *cert. denied*, 454 U.S. 858 (1981).

In re Farrell, 108 N.J. 335, 529 A.2d 404 (1987).

Foody v. Manchester Memorial Hospital, 40 Conn. Supp. 127, 482 A.2d 713 (Super. Ct. 1984).

In re Gardner, 534 A.2d 947 (Maine 1987).

In re Guardianship of Grant, 109 Wash. 2d 545, 747 P.2d 445 (Wash. 1987).

In re Guardianship of Hamlin, 102 Wash. 2d 810, 689 P.2d 1372 (1984).

Hastings Center. (1987). *Guidelines on the termination of life-sustaining treatment*. Briarcliff Manor, NY: Author.

In re Jobes, 108 N.J. 394, 529 A.2d 434 (1987).

John F. Kennedy Memorial Hospital v. Bludworth, 452 So.2d 921 (Fla. 1984).

Lane v. Candura, 6 Mass. App. 377, 376 N.E.2d 1232 (1978).

Leach v. Akron General Medical Center, 68 Ohio Misc. 1, 426 N.E.2d 809 (Com. Pl. 1980).

Leach v. Shapiro, 13 Ohio App. 3d 393, 469 N.E.2d 1047 (Ct. App. 1984).

Meilaender, G. (1984). On removing food and water: Against the stream. *Hastings Center Report, 14*(6), 11–13.

Nolan, K. (1987). Imperiled newborns. *Hastings Center Report, 17* (6), 5–32.

Ohio House Bill 718 (1988).

In re Peter by Johanning, 108 N.J. 365, 529 A.2d 419 (1987).

President's Commission for the Study of Ethical Problems in Medicine and Biomedical and Behavioral Research. (1983). *Deciding to forego life-sustaining treatment*. Washington DC: U.S. Government Printing Office.

In re Quinlan, 70 N.J. 10, 355 A.2d 647, *cert. denied sub nom Garger v. New Jersey*, 429 U.S. 922 (1976), *overruled in part, In re Conroy*, 98 N.J. 321, 486 A.2d 1209 (1985).

In re Rasmussen by Mitchell v. Fleming, 154 Ariz. 207, 742 P.2d 674 (1987).

Report of the Ad Hoc Committee of the Harvard Medical School to Examine the Definition of Brain Death. (1968). A definition of irreversible coma. *Journal of the American Medical Association, 205*(6), 85–88.

In re Requena, 213 N.J. Super. 475, 517 A.2d 886 (Super. Ct. Ch. Div.), *aff'd*, 213 N.J. Super. 443, 517 A.2d 869 (Super. Ct. App. Div. 1986) (per curiam).

In re Rodas, No. 86PR139 (Colo. Dist. Ct. Mesa County Jan. 22, 1987) (Buss, J.).

Satz v. Perlmutter, 362 So.2d 160 (Fla. Dist. Ct. App. 1978), *aff'd*, 379 So.2d 359 (Fla. 1980).

Schloendorff v. Society of New York Hospital, 211 N.Y. 125, 105 N.E. 92 (1914).

Severns v. Wilmington Medical Center, Inc., 421 A.2d 1334 (Del. 1980).

Smith, D. R. (1986). Legal recognition of neocortical death. *Cornell Law Review, 71*, 850–888.

Society for the Right to Die. (1987a). *What you should know about durable power of attorney*. New York: Author.

Society for the Right to Die. (1987b). *Handbook of living will laws* (1987 ed.). New York: Author.

In re Spring, 380 Mass. 629, 405 N.E.2d 115 (1980).

In re Storar, 52 N.Y.2d 363, 420 N.E.2d 64, 438 N.Y.S.2d 266, *cert. denied*, 454 U.S. 858 (1981).

Superintendent of Belchertown State School v. Saikewicz, 373 Mass. 728, 370 N.E.2d 417 (1977).

In re Conservatorship of Torres, 357 N.W.2d 332 (Minn. 1984).

In re Westchester County Medical Center, 72 N.Y. 2d 517, 531 N.E.2d 607 (N.Y. 1988).

✳   **EDITOR'S QUESTIONS FOR DISCUSSION**   ✳

Compare the principles as indicated by Brown and Davis (Chapter 38) and Flynn and Davis (Chapter 39) with the legal considerations indicated by Driscoll. What contradictions appear to exist between some of the rulings indicated in the cases cited by Driscoll and the ethical principles previously presented? Is letting someone die always killing? Is there any difference between allowing a patient to die by withholding treatment and causing a patient to die by ceasing treatment? What are the criteria for brain dead and the legal definition of death at this time? What problems does the whole brain dead donor rule pose for patients, families, and professionals? How might the dilemmas concerning organ donors be addressed and resolved?

What is the role of a nurse in relation to a pa-

tient formulating a living will or the communication of a durable power of attorney? How enforceable and useful is a living will and a durable power of attorney? Who may be indicated as a durable power of attorney? Discuss what the professional nurse has to offer in relation to the decision-making process for the care of the dying and the permanently unconscious patient. What should be the role of the professional nurse in the decision process? What arguments can be presented for recognizing a fifth state interest in refusing medical treatment, that is, maintaining the ethical integrity of the nursing profession? Discuss whether or not there is such a thing as ethical integrity of the nursing profession, and how does it manifest itself through a legal framework?

41

The Emerging Role of the Oncology Clinical Nursing Specialist

Joyce M. Yasko, Ph.D., R.N., F.A.A.N.
Linda A. Dudjak, M.S.N., R.N., O.C.N.S.

The role of the oncology clinical nursing specialist has been in existence since 1970, when graduates of the University of Pittsburgh School of Nursing, the first master's degree program in oncology nursing, entered the health care system. In the past 18 years, many changes have occurred. The knowledge and practice of cancer nursing has expanded, a revolution has occurred in the health care system as it converted from a service to a business orientation, and the health care delivery system is more consumer-oriented today then it was in 1970. Through these dynamic and often turbulent times, the educational preparation and the role definition of the oncology clinical nursing specialist has remained as it was conceptualized in 1970. In a review of the literature, the same definition continues to emerge: that of the combined role of clinician, educator, consultant, and researcher, with some definitions including the role of administrator. The "all things to all people at all times" conceptualization of the role of the oncology clinical nursing specialist was difficult to understand and implement initially, and remains even more difficult in the present health care system that is being driven by

cost and measurable outcomes. This chapter addresses the emerging role of the oncology clinical nursing specialist and the trends in health care and cancer care that currently or potentially influence the role of the oncology clinical nursing specialist in the future.

CONCEPTUALIZATION OF THE ROLE OF THE ONCOLOGY CLINICAL NURSING SPECIALIST

We have never subscribed to the traditional conceptualization of the role of the oncology clinical nursing specialist (OCNS). We could never fully comprehend how one person could be functioning in all of these roles—clinician, educator, consultant, researcher, and administrator simultaneously. So since our graduate school days, we took what we had learned and set about developing our own conceptualization of the role of the OCNS. We came to the conclusion that the role of the OCNS has four major responsibilities:

1. Advancing the practice of oncology nursing.
2. Educating nurses and health professionals,

persons with cancer and their families, and the public about cancer and cancer care.

3. Providing and/or directing the provision of nursing care for persons with cancer and their families.

4. Developing, implementing, and evaluating health care programs, resources, and services for persons with cancer and their families in a variety of clinical settings.

With these four broad categories, we could further delineate and include all of the components of advanced nursing practice and more clearly communicate to other health care professionals, patients, and families, and the public the answer to those often-asked questions: What is an oncology clinical nursing specialist? What does an oncology clinical nursing specialist do? Behavioral outcomes are the communicator of the worth and value of the OCNS role to the health care system and therefore the four role responsibilities are described in behavioral outcomes.

Advance the Practice of Oncology Nursing

To advance the practice of oncology nursing, the OCNS must have a firm foundation in the theory and practice of nursing. This includes an advanced knowledge of the biology of cancer, cancer prevention and early detection, cancer diagnosis and treatment, and management of symptoms related to cancer and cancer care. The OCNS must have a clear perception of the role of an oncology nurse, that is, to assess, monitor, prioritize, plan, intervene, and evaluate to meet physical, psychological, sociocultural, and economic needs of the patient and family; to provide health teaching and health counseling; and to refer patient and family to appropriate resources. She or he must also be able to implement in practice principles of change theory, teaching and learning theory, role theory, and organizational theory, and must be attuned to the impact of the changing health care trends and issues (Chambers, Dangel, German, Tropodi, & Jaeger, 1987). By applying this knowledge base, the OCNS can advance the practice of oncology nursing, through the following behavioral outcomes:

- Develop, implement, and evaluate standards of care, policies, procedures, and quality assurance parameters to enhance the nursing care of persons with cancer and their family members.

- Identify researchable questions and hypotheses, and collaborate with others to design, implement, and evaluate cancer nursing research studies. The ultimate goal is to have oncology nursing practice grounded in research findings rather than anecdodal reports.

- Implement research findings in oncology nursing practice through analysis of the methods and findings of research studies. The OCNS analyzes research studies and determines which findings are worthy of incorporating into oncology nursing practice.

- Advocate the role of the oncology nurse in identifying and meeting the needs of persons with cancer and the members of their family. The OCNS identifies the resources needed, defines the role of the oncology nurse in meeting the health care needs of patients and families, and communicates this information within and outside the health care agency. The worth and value of the oncology nurse must be recognized by the providers, payors, and consumers of cancer care.

- Present and publish findings learned through research or clinical practice, or both. The OCNS must contribute to the body of knowledge that constitutes the foundation of the practice of oncology nursing.

- Consult with nurses and health professionals to assist them in providing an optimal level of care, solving clinical problems, and designing new models of care and health care delivery.

Educate Nurses, Health Care Professionals, Patients and Families, and the Public

Behavioral outcomes for the responsibility of educating nurses, health care professionals, patients and families, and the public about cancer and cancer care include:

- Identify learning needs and design, implement, and evaluate educational programs to meet the identified needs. Utilize all teachable moments to facilitate the integration of this role responsibility into the daily practice of the OCNS. Develop and evaluate written, audio, and audiovisual educational resources.

- Function as a role model and teach by demonstrating expertise in cancer care.

Provide Nursing Care

The responsibility of providing and/or directing the provision of nursing care for persons with cancer and their families includes behavioral outcomes throughout the process of cancer prevention, early detection, diagnosis, treatment, rehabilitation, and palliation. The OCNS will ensure that the following outcomes are achieved for all patients with cancer and their family members:

- Assess, monitor, and document the physical, psychological, pathophysiological, sociocultural, and economic dimensions of each patient and family.
- Intervene to achieve and maintain optimal lifestyle patterns in the following areas:
  - Nutritional status
  - Sleep and rest status
  - Coping status
  - Elimination status
  - Level of comfort
  - Sexual and reproductive status
  - Exercise and mobility status
- Prevent and minimize symptoms related to cancer and cancer treatment.
- Prevent and minimize complications related to cancer and cancer treatment.
- Provide health teaching to prepare patients and families for self-care.
- Provide psychological support and counsel to facilitate the process of coping with the diagnosis and treatment of cancer.
- Coordinate all aspects of care to ensure that the needs of patients and families are met in a cost-efficient and cost-effective manner in the hospital, outpatient facilities, and the home.
- Refer patients and families to cancer care resources within the health care agency and the community.

- Advocate for patients and families to ensure that their needs are met.
- Implement the medical diagnosis and treatment plan.

The most cost-effective implementation method for this aspect of role responsibility is to have the OCNS function as a case manager for a selected population of persons with cancer and allow the OCNS to direct others (oncology nurses, practical nurses, nursing assistants) to implement the plan of care. It is the systems or models that are developed and implemented in the health care system that are the lasting, stable components of this role responsibility.

Develop, Implement, and Evaluate Cancer Care Programs, Resources, and Services

The last role responsibility is to develop, implement, and evaluate cancer care programs, resources, and services in a variety of clinical settings (hospital, outpatient, community, home). Behavioral outcomes for this responsibility include:

- Identify and document the need for cancer care programs or new models and systems of health care delivery.
- Develop the program proposals within the confines of health care policy, legislation, and reimbursement.
- Collaborate with others to generate revisions for program development and implementation.
- Market the program to the appropriate audience(s).
- Advocate for the employing agency to ensure a positive image and financial stability.

PHILOSOPHICAL FOUNDATION FOR ROLE IMPLEMENTATION

To accomplish the OCNS role responsibilities, practice must be based on four philosophical beliefs:
1. Positive self-concept
2. Belief in the pursuit of lifelong learning
3. Commitment to assume responsibility for achieving and maintaining one's own level of competence
4. Commitment to obtain and provide mentorship

Self-Concept

The OCNS must have a positive self-concept of who she or he is, believe in the importance of the OCNS role in the care of persons with cancer and their families receive, as well as in the effectiveness and efficiency of the health care delivery system. One must have a strong sense of self if the role responsibilities of the OCNS are to be fulfilled, since most of what is accomplished occurs through changes others are willing to make. When facilitating changes in the practice of health care professionals and the functioning of health care systems, a strong belief in self, timing, and tenacity are factors that often make the critical difference between success and failure.

Lifelong Learning

Subscribing to the philosophical belief of lifelong learning serves to influence the OCNS to never be satisfied with what is, but to be always exploring what can be. This philosophical belief will also facilitate the OCNS in learning new information about the biology of cancer, the role of the immune system in the initiation and progression of cancer, the treatment of cancer utilizing biological response modifiers (agents that are components of the immune system and are used to stimulate and augment the immune system), methods to manage symptoms related to cancer and cancer treatment, innovative ways to ensure documentation and preparation for self-care, current information about the cost of health care services as well as the reimbursement policies of third-party payors, and models for efficient and effective health care delivery. A knowledge explosion is occurring in cancer care and in health care delivery, and the role of the OCNS is needed to pave the way for cancer care of the future.

Competence

Assuming the responsibility for achieving and maintaining one's own level of competence is a philosophical belief that can facilitate a more positive perception of the professional nurse. Traditionally nurses have believed that it was the responsibility of their employer or their professional organiza-

tions to make sure that they were competent in their practice. This attitude is unprofessional. Assuming the responsibility for achieving and maintaining one's own level of competence is the first step in assuming the responsibility for one's practice. To facilitate the process of changing the attitude that their employer "owes" them educational opportunities, which many nurses subscribe to, a strategy termed "gaps and contracts" has been utilized with success (Donovan, Wolpert, & Yasko, 1981).

This strategy requires that nurses attending continuing education programs do so with the understanding that they "owe" their employer something on their return, especially if they have had their expenses paid or have received the day off with pay, or both. Participants are asked to identify gaps between their present practice and what they are learning in the educational programs. The participants are then asked to prioritize the gaps they have identified and to develop a contract, explaining the changes they are going to implement in their own practice or in the practice of their agency. The contract includes the methods that they will utilize, the time frame required, the resources needed, and the anticipated cost. This contract is to be communicated to the participant's supervisor for input and approval. This strategic plan communicates to the participant that changes in practice must occur as a result of attending educational programs, and that they owe the agency something for the expenditure that allowed them to attend the educational program. It also gives the employing agency an incentive to send participants to educational programs. Achieving and maintaining one's own level of competence can also eliminate or minimize the experience of feeling incompetent in the work arena.

Mentoring

The fourth philosophical belief is that of mentorship, both obtaining a mentor for one's own career development and providing mentorship for the advancement of the careers of others. Nursing is a practice profession; much of what is known about the care of persons with cancer and their family members has been learned through testing various methods in practice. It is this knowledge base that must be taught to those that come to the practice of oncology nursing without either the knowledge or experience that they should have. Each generation of oncology nurses must achieve what the present generation of oncology nurses achieved sooner and with far fewer "battle scars" than the present generation experienced.

Nurses have been socialized to stand alone and not to depend on the support and counsel of their professional colleagues. They were socialized by being initiated into the profession of nursing by colleagues who subscribed to the philosophy of "it was tough for me; it is going to be tough for you and I am going to see to it that it is." Mentorship, teaching other nurses what you have learned, is the most effective way to advance the practice of oncology nursing. Mentors do not compete with their mentees. They understand that the goal of mentorship is that the mentee will go beyond where the mentor can take them. Mentors get their satisfaction out of watching these mentees grow, develop, and become. They take satisfaction in seeing their mentees take their place as advancers of the practice of nursing. Everyone needs a mentor regardless of where they are in their professional career—student, new graduate, new to the practice of oncology nursing, new head nurses, new oncology clinical nursing specialist, new faculty member, new dean, or new vice president for nursing. One will outgrow a specific mentor but never the need for mentorship.

Mentor and mentee relationships are developed and nurtured; they rarely, if ever, just happen. The first step is to recognize the worth and value of a mentor, to select persons who you believe can effectively serve in this role and who possess the skills that you need to learn, and to seek their interest in serving as your mentor. You should then establish some ground rules so that communication can be open and honest and both parties will be aware of time constraints. You should then present your mentor with issues or problems for which you need help, hear the feedback the mentor provides, utilize the advice of the mentor, and then provide your mentor with feedback about what was positive and negative about the advice that was given. In other words, mentorship is a give-and-take relationship that is satisfying to both participants. Being mentored is the

best way to learn how to become a mentor and to participate actively in the advancement of nursing practice.

FACTORS INFLUENCING ROLE IMPLEMENTATION AND THE CHALLENGES PROVIDED

Many factors, economic, political, technological, and social, are influencing or have the potential to influence the implementation of the role of the OCNS in today's health care system (Yasko, 1985). The major influencing factors are (a) escalating health care costs, (b) nursing shortage, (c) need for advanced level of political and administrative skills, and (d) consumerism.

Health Care Costs

Escalating costs compounded by an increase in cost restraints by third-party payors have reduced the frequency and length of hospitalization for all types of illness and medical procedures; diagnostic and therapeutic procedures are occurring in the outpatient setting whenever possible. This is particularly true of cancer care when it is estimated that 90% of all cancer care will be delivered in the outpatient or home setting in the near future. Concepts such as same-day surgery, short-stay admissions, and preadmission testing have become major components of health care facilities of all sizes. Consumers and health care professionals alike recognize that third-party payors will not reimburse the costs associated with inpatient care—if the same services can be provided as an outpatient. It is also known that the most reimbursement one can expect to receive from a third-party payor is 80% of the total cost of the health care; reimbursement denials, delays, and partial payments are commonplace in today's health care system. The awareness among health care consumers that a rising percentage of health care costs must be absorbed by the consumers, rather than by the payor, has precipitated a reluctance to seek care and a tendency to minimize time within the health care environment when the need becomes acute (Yasko & Fleck, 1984).

Because patients and families are remaining for

shorter periods of time in the health care system because patients who are hospitalized are acutely ill and because the acuity of illness of patients being treated in outpatient facilities is increasing, many challenges to the implementation of the role of the OCNS occur:

- Documentation methods must improve in content and format to ensure continuity of care and reimbursement of health care services provided.
- Methods to identify patient and family self-care needs must be designed.
- New methods and models of health teaching that are cost- and time-efficient must be developed to ensure that patients and families are prepared to care for themselves in their home environment.
- Referral to community cancer care resources must be more timely and more comprehensive in nature, and more cancer care community resources must be developed to meet newly identified needs.
- Health care delivery systems, based on present and anticipated reimbursement systems, must be developed to ensure an optimal level of care at the lowest possible cost while making certain that "touch" and caring remain dominant themes as our health care system converts to "big business and "high tech."

Nursing Shortage

A second major factor influencing the implementation of the role of the OCNS is the nursing shortage. This health care delivery crisis is predicted to intensify significantly over the next decade and its resolution remains as tenuous as the forces that molded its appearance. Accomplishing more with less is the resounding theme of nursing departments of hospitals, outpatient facilities, and home health care agencies. The OCNS must take the leadership role in meeting the challenges presented to the nursing profession and must prepare nurses to:

- Change the practice patterns of professional nursing to ensure individualized, prioritized care. Nurses have been socialized to assess patients and their family for all needs, actual and

potential, and then attempt to develop care plans to meet all of the identified needs. This is an expensive (in time and resources) and impossible feat and will not be tolerated in today's health care system. Rather, nurses need to be taught how to identify and prioritize needs and to develop, in collaboration with the other members of the health care team and the patient and family, a patient-family care plan (not a nursing care plan) to meet the identified high-priority care needs. This plan must be based on the patient and family economic resources, belief systems, intellectual and physical capabilities, and available support systems; they must receive a written copy of the plan to use as a reference in their home environment. Time and money do not exist for the delivery of generic, ritualistic, nonprioritized nursing care.
- Change the nursing care delivery system to a case management model in which the OCNS or oncology nurse manages a caseload of patients utilizing a primary nursing model that includes nurse extenders (technical nurses, licensed practical nurses, nursing assistants), to ensure that the patient-family care plan is fully implemented. Nurses must take responsibility for their own practice and for the nursing care delivered by a particular health care agency. The case management and primary nursing model is an excellent model to facilitate this process.
- Develop, implement, and systematically evaluate cancer care standards, policies, procedures, and quality assurance outcomes that are "state of the art" and cost-effective.

Political and Administrative Skills

Owing to budgetary constraints of health care systems compounded by the nursing shortage, an advanced level of political and administrative skills will be needed.

- The desired level of care and clinical expertise that ensured employment of the OCNS in the traditional health care setting may well become inadequate to justify the OCNS position, in terms of philosophy as well as cost. The need for quantifiable evidence of significant contribution to organizational goals, in terms of revenue, improved care, enhanced competition, and similar goals, will equal and may exceed the altruistic value of expert clinical practice and professional accomplishment (Hamric, 1985; Malone, 1986). Herein lies another demand for the OCNS to demonstrate competency in (a) the development of systems of care, (b) design and implementation of nursing research, (c) innovative program development, (d) creative marketing strategies, and (e) documentation of the positive impact of activities (1–4) on fiscal solvency (Hoffman & Fonteyn, 1986).

- Another significant trend in the economics of health care systems is the growth of multiinstitution and multifacility centers that offer the economic advantage of shared resources and shared expertise as well as enhanced recruitment potential. This concept requires a sophisticated understanding of complex organizational systems and a high level of expertise in communication, collaboration, and negotiation.

The OCNS must not only work effectively within a given administrative structure, but operate as a major actuator in the development and evolution of that structure to maintain a power base necessary to achieve organizational and professional nursing goals (McDougall, 1987). The competitive and increasingly bureaucratic health care industry will create new opportunities as well as new challenges for the OCNS to combine advanced education and clinical expertise with sophisticated political, administrative, and economic savvy.

Consumerism

Consumerism is a trend that will have a great impact on the implementation of the role of the OCNS of the future. As consumers pay more "out of pocket" costs for health care, and as health care agencies and physicians compete for patient-consumers, the role of consumer has become stronger in the health care system. Consumers are making more demands on the health care system and health care administrators; providers are responding by ensuring that amenities are available in the

health care system and that the health care system is consumer-oriented. Changes in health care delivery that are influenced by consumers are esthetically pleasing health care environments that:

- Are located in easy-access geographical areas with convenient low-cost transportation and parking.
- Have available within the health care setting such amenities as an open kitchen area; resources to provide distraction and pleasure, such as current reading materials; television, radio, audiotapes, videotapes; comfortable waiting rooms; private patient and family consultation rooms.
- Contain all needed services and resources: diagnostic services, comprehensive treatment (surgery, radiotherapy, chemotherapy, biotherapy) services, rehabilitation and palliation services, within the health care setting.
- Have service hours that are more amiable to a rehabilitative focus. If over 50% of patients with cancer will be cured of their disease, and approximately one half of the 49% of patients who are not cured of their disease will experience long term-control of the disease with a high quality of life, then our cancer care delivery services must allow these individuals to receive their treatment and care while remaining in the mainstream of life. This means that outpatient cancer care services must have extended hours (early morning, evening, weekends) to allow persons with cancer to remain in the work force.
- Are designed to meet patient and family needs. In a recent study (Houts, Yasko, Kahn, Schelzel, & Marconi, 1986) it was learned that the unmet needs identified by patients and families within 1 year of the diagnosis of cancer all fell within the nursing domain: (a) coping with the diagnosis of cancer; (b) help with the technological aspects of cancer (assistance with ports, pumps and catheters, ostomy care, and so on); (c) help with maintaining the nutritional status; (d) help with maintaining physical stamina; and finally (e) help with maintaining the activities of daily living. Many persons with cancer are not

eligible for health care services because they are not acutely ill enough to be hospitalized, and if they are not homebound or do not require skilled nursing care, they are not sick enough to receive home care. Most persons with cancer receive care in their physician's office or an outpatient facility. Since the unmet needs fall within the nursing domain, if nurses are not available to practice nursing (not as a physician extender or office manager), the patient and family do not have access to a nurse to assist them in learning what they need to know in order to achieve self-care. The consumers of health care have created a demand; and the nursing profession, under the leadership of clinical nursing specialists, must respond to this demand or it will be met by another available or newly created health care professional.

These are only four factors that are or have the potential to influence the emerging role of the OCNS. Other factors include (a) the knowledge explosion in cancer and cancer care; (b) the inclusion of acute care nursing in oncology nursing practice as oncology nurses learn to care for the acute care needs of patients receiving biological response modifiers; (c) the widespread use of technological devices in cancer care (pumps, ports, catheters, and the like); (d) the abundance of physicians and, in particular, medical oncologists who are competing for patients and also competing for a broader range of cancer care roles and functions; and (e) the acquired immunodeficiency syndrome (AIDS) epidemic that is sweeping the country, which has the potential to take needed resources away from cancer care and to expand the practice of oncology nursing to include the care of patients with AIDS. By being aware of the trends and issues facing oncology nursing, the OCNS can plan strategies and programs that are proactive in nature and designed to meet the demands of health care consumers (Hodges, Poteet, & Edland, 1985).

PRACTICE AREAS FOR THE EMERGING ROLE OF THE OCNS

The role of the OCNS is versatile and a definite asset to many health care arenas in which access to

persons with cancer and their families is a reality. When reviewing the possibilities for functioning in the role of the OCNS, it is important to keep in mind the major role responsibilities: advancing the practice of oncology nursing; educating patients and families, health professionals, and the public about cancer, cancer care, and the role of the oncology nurse; providing or directing the provision of nursing care for persons with cancer and their families; and developing, implementing, and evaluating programs, resources, and services for persons with cancer and their family members in a variety of clinical settings. The OCNS focuses on persons with cancer and their family members and implements the conceptualization of the role in a variety of clinical settings, often with a title that does not include the words oncology clinical nursing specialist. Possible clinical settings for role implementation include:

- Hospital (unit or hospital-based)
- Home health care agency
- Hospice programs
- Outpatient facility
- Physician's office
- Extended care facilities (rehabilitative hospitals, nursing homes, and the like)
- Private practice — client- or contract-generated. The private practitioner can obtain fees for services provided for the patient and family. In some states this fee is third-party reimbursable, while in others it is self-pay. The private practitioners can also develop contracts with health care agencies for services rendered.

The role of the oncology nursing specialist is versatile and dynamic. This role is the safeguard for the advancement of oncology nursing in practice settings in the future.

REFERENCES

Chambers, J. K., Dangel, R. B., German, K., Tropodi, V., & Jaeger, C. (1987). Clinical nurse specialist collaboration: Development of a generic job description and standards of performance. *Clinical Nurse Specialist*, *1*(3), 124–127.

Donovan, M., Wolpert, P., & Yasko, J. (1981). Gaps and contracts. *Nursing Outlook*, *29*, 467–471.

Hamric, A. B. (1985). Clinical nurse specialist role evaluation. *Oncology Nurse Forum, 12*(2), 62–66.

Hodges, L. C., Poteet, G. W., & Edland, B. J. (1985). Teaching clinical nurse specialists to lead and to succeed. *Nursing and Health Care, 6*, 193–196.

Hoffman, S. E., & Fonteyn, M. E. (1986). Marketing the clinical nurse specialist. *Nursing Economics, 4*, 140–144.

Houts, P. S., Yasko, J. M., Kahn, S. B., Schelzel, G.W., & Marconi, K. M. (1986). Unmet psychological, social, economic needs of persons with cancer in Pennsylvania. *Cancer, 58*, 2355–2361.

Malone, B. L. (1986). Evaluation of the clinical nurse specialist. *American Journal of Nursing, 86*, 1375–1377.

McDougall, G. J. (1987). The role of the clinical nurse specialist consultant in organizational development. *Clinical Nurse Specialist, 1*(3), 133–139.

Topham, D. L. (1987). Role theory in relation to roles of the clinical nurse specialist. *Clinical Nurse Specialist, 1*(2), 81–84.

Yasko, J. M. (1985). The predicted effect of recent health care trends on the role of the oncology clinical nursing specialist. *Oncology Nursing Forum, 12*(2), 58–61.

Yasko, J. M., Fleck, A. E. (1984). Prospective payment (DRG's): What will be the impact on cancer care? *Oncology Nursing Forum, 11*(3), 63–72.

✳   **EDITOR'S QUESTIONS FOR DISCUSSION**   ✳

In comparing this chapter with Chapter 43 by Whitney, what is the difference in the role of the clinical nurse specialist and the nurse practitioner? In providing nursing care, how does the clinical nurse specialist prevent and minimize symptoms in a way that is different from that of the nurse practitioner's role? What empirical evidence is there that the two roles are different or the same? Should or should not the academic preparation be different for the clinical nurse specialist and the nurse practitioner roles? What are the driving forces and restraining forces that exist for combining the clinical specialist and nurse practitioner roles? What is the difference between case management, primary nursing, and primary care? Should the roles be different for the clinical nurse specialist and the nurse practitioner in primary and tertiary care and, if so, how? Debate the pros and cons of whether or not the clinical specialist and nurse practitioner roles should be combined, the basis for their practice, the academic preparation, their functions, the appropriate type of specialty practice, and their settings for practice.

42

Aged and the Nursing Profession

Sr. Rose Therese Bahr, A.S.C., Ph.D., R.N., F.A.A.N.

As more elderly Americans live longer, gerontological nursing will assume an increasingly important role in the nursing profession. This chapter exhibits the demography of the aging population in America, with special attention to the years 1990 to 2050 and the influence of this phenomenon on American society; standards of gerontological nursing practice as guidelines for delivery of quality nursing care to older adults in various health care facilities; and the future roles of gerontological nurse generalist and specialist as turning points related to the increasing demographical statistics of older adults in America.

ORIGIN OF THE GERONTOLOGICAL NURSING SPECIALTY

Gerontological nursing is an emerging specialty within the profession of nursing. The term *gerontological nursing* is defined as

> that branch of nursing concerned with assessment of the health needs of older adults, planning and implementing health care to meet these needs, and evaluating the effectiveness of such care. . . . Gerontological nursing strives to identify and use the strengths of older adults and assists them to use those strengths to maximize independence. (American Nurses' Association, 1976, p. 3)

A turning point within the nursing profession came in 1966 at the national convention of the American Nurses' Association (ANA) in San Francisco, with the establishment of an organizational unit within the ANA giving visibility to those nurses interested in the care of older adults. This unit was called the Council of Geriatric Nursing. The emphasis at that time was on sick and debilitated elderly, hence the word *geriatric* in the title. In 1973, the name was changed to the Division of Gerontological Nursing, to reflect the nursing model focus on wellness and quality of life for older adults seeking nursing care. In 1985, with restructuring of the ANA, the unit's name was changed from "Division" to "Council."

One of the first tasks undertaken by the Council of Gerontological Nursing was to project guidelines for nursing care delivery to older Americans. Why was this task so important? This was so because the demographics of America reflected a drastic change. A steady increase in the numbers of elderly adults is continually being traced by demographers. This change has great implications for the nursing profession.

DEMOGRAPHICS: THE GROWING NUMBERS OF OLDER ADULTS IN AMERICA

In 1900, 1 in 10 Americans was 55 years and over, and 1 in 25 was 65 years and over. By 1988, 1 in 5 was at least 55 years old, and 1 in 8 was at least 65 years (*Aging America*, 1988). The older population grew twice as fast as the rest of the population in the last decade. The 85 and older age-group is growing especially rapidly. This "old-old" population is expected to increase seven times by the middle of the 21st century. The elderly population is growing older. In 1980, 39% of the elderly population was age 75 and older. By the year 2000, half of the elderly population is projected to be 75+ (*Aging America*, 1988).

Future trends and projections in terms of the aging population in America reveal a steady increase of aged individuals. The median age of the American population in 1990 will be 33 years of age, and in the year 2050 it will be 42 years. Demographers indicate that, if current fertility rates and immigration levels remain stable, the only age-groups to experience significant growth in the 21st century will be those past 55 years. The increase is expected to occur in two stages. Through the year 2000, the proportion of the population 55 years and older is expected to remain relatively stable, at just over 1:5 (22%). By 2010, because of the maturation of the baby boom population, the proportion of older Americans is projected to rise dramatically; more than one-fourth of the total United States population is expected to be 55 years old, and 1 in 7 Americans will be 65 years old. By 2050, 1 in 3 persons is expected to be 55 years or older, and 1 in 5 will be 65+ (*Aging America*, 1988). Figure 42-1 is the projection of the population 55 years and over by age for the years 1900 to 2050.

The impact of these demographics is profound in terms of economic, social, and political issues and of changes in housing and architectural design to accommodate the increased numbers of aging persons. For example, one of the current major legislative debates involves catastrophic insurance for long-term care. This legislation addresses the political issue surrounding older adults who suffer from chronic illnesses and need skilled nursing care for 24-hour coverage by professional nurses in long-term care facilities without experiencing great financial burden. This debate continues to elucidate the high costs of long-term care, and at this writing, it appears that the development of such an insurance package will not be accomplished readily.

Likewise, other effects of increasing numbers of older adults in America will place demands on society to accommodate this change, and similarly, difficulties at resolution will be experienced. Societal attitude reflects the view that older adults have lived their lives and therefore should not be allocated scarce resources. The motto seems to be "pro-youth, anti-aged!" A contemporary controversy revolves around the issue of where the more important needs reside—with the young or with the old. Nurses need to become more involved in these political debates as advocates of the older adult, a growing clientele who will seek nursing care in the future.

A significant problem emerging from the growth in numbers of older adults is the projected impact on health care delivery. All types of health care facilities (e.g., hospitals; nursing homes; home health care agencies; community-based programs, such as wellness clinics for seniors in low-income high-rise housing units for older adults) are gradually implementing more services for older adults (*Aging America*, 1988). Statistics show that between 55% to 65% of all hospital admissions for acute illnesses, surgeries, and chronic illness complications are individuals in the older age-group (*Aging America*, 1988). Older adults present a challenge to nursing care because of their unique health needs, which change with each decade of life. Consequently nursing care plans must reflect the changes in the physical, psychological, sociological, and spiritual dimensions of the older adult, which are highly complex and challenging from a nursing perspective. Professional nurses realize that gerontological nursing is emerging as a specialty in its own right with its own scope and standards of nursing practice.

STANDARDS OF GERONTOLOGICAL NURSING PRACTICE: GUIDELINES FOR QUALITY CARE OF OLDER ADULTS IN HEALTH CARE FACILITIES

Gerontological nursing practice standards are defined as guidelines that describe contemporary nurs-

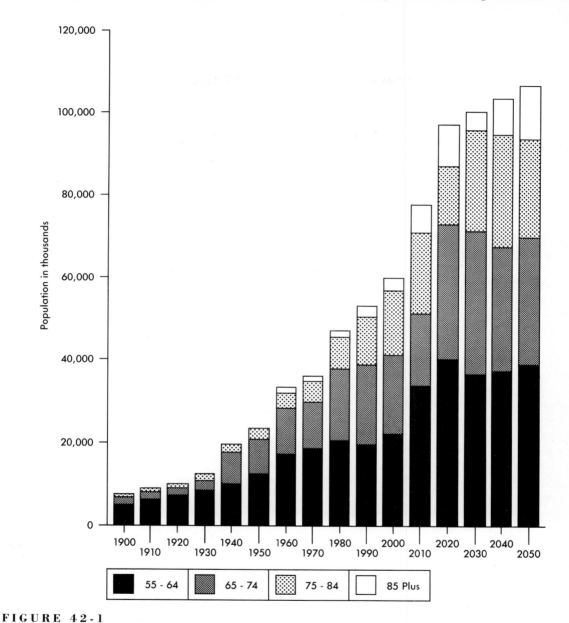

FIGURE 42·1

Population 55 years and over by age: 1900–2050. (Source: U.S. Census of Population, 1890–1980 and projections of the population of the United States: 1983–2080. *Current Population Reports* [Series P-25, No. 952 middle series].)

ing practice in the provision of quality care to older adults in a variety of settings, for example, hospitals, long-term care facilities, community programs, and at home. These standards delineate the necessity for nursing care beyond the regulatory statutes promulgated by state agencies or the state's nurse practice act. These latter documents are primarily legislated for protection of the general public and are not directed toward the level of quality of care that professional nurses provide for older adults. Standards of practice are measures utilized to gauge the quality of care provided to aging and aged persons; and they may be used in quality assurance programs or in evaluative programs effecting measurement of nursing outcomes of care offered in various settings (ANA, 1988). Standards may also serve as a resource for development of assessment tools, to be utilized by professional nurses in comprehensive data collection about aging individuals seeking nursing care (ANA, 1988). The standards of gerontological nursing practice embody concepts included in a document portraying professional nursing in the 20th century, developed by the ANA in 1980 and titled, *Nursing: A Social Policy Statement*. This document stipulates that professional nursing encompasses four dimensions inherent within each person: physical, psychological, sociological, and spiritual. These dimensions weave a holistic orientation to quality nursing care and dictate nursing interventions necessary to address each dimension for inclusion in the nursing care plan.

The nursing process is a systematic and scientific format employed when providing quality nursing care. The steps of the nursing process include data collection and assessment, nursing diagnosis, planning, implementation, and evaluation (Yura & Walsh, 1983). Data collection and assessment is a systematic process with continuous input of information from the aging person and significant others regarding the status of the person seeking nursing care. Sources of information for this initial step are the social and family history of the aging individual regarding health status, both past and present (Ebersole & Hess, 1985). Nursing diagnosis is the identification of the major problem facing the aging individual; it is derived, in conjunction with the older

adult and significant others, from an analysis of the health status data.

Planning of nursing care is the next logical step in which the older adult, his or her family and significant others, and the nurse establish priorities of mutually derived goals and nursing approaches for the achievement of these goals. Implementation of these measures incorporates the active participation of the older person in health promotion and health maintenance activities for restoration of health to its optimal functioning. Evaluation of the outcomes of the nursing actions identifies the progress made toward the determined goals and is a task accomplished by the older adult, family or significant other, and the nurse. Continual reassessment, reordering of priorities, and evaluation of outcomes is integral to quality nursing care for older individuals whose health status in each of the four dimensions may change quickly, demanding active and immediate response for additional nursing actions. Gerontological nursing is a challenging specialty in nursing; the specialty requires in-depth knowledge, clinical competency, and clinical decision-making expertise, warranted by the complexities of the aging process and demonstrated uniquely by each aging person (Gress & Bahr, 1984). The nursing process, then, is a basic framework—both interpersonal and dynamic—for the provision of quality care to aging persons in varying degrees of health and in every setting in which they seek nursing care (Ebersole & Hess, 1985).

Standards of Practice

In early 1987, the American Nurses' Association Council of Gerontological Nursing appointed a Task Force to revise and update the scope and standards of gerontological nursing (ANA, 1976). The revisions made by the Task Force, of which I was a member, were submitted to gerontological nurses throughout the United States for critique and additional input, to define the current state-of-the-art of contemporary gerontological nursing practice. The revisions were incorporated into the final draft and the document was published in January 1988 under the title *Scope and Standards of Gerontological Nurs-*

ing Practice (ANA, 1988). There are 11 standards, complete with a rationale, structure criteria, process criteria, and outcome criteria for each standard. Each of the standards with its rationale are presented below (ANA, 1988, pp. 3–18):

Standard I. Organization of gerontological nursing services

All gerontological nursing services are planned, organized, and directed by a nurse executive. The nurse executive has baccalaureate or Master's preparation and has experience in gerontological nursing and administration of long-term care services or acute care services for older clients.

Rationale: The nurse executive uses administrative knowledge to plan and direct nursing services delivered in an environment where nursing is an integral component of the gerontological interdisciplinary team and may be the discipline with responsibility for the coordination of services. . . . In all gerontological settings (day care, home care, ambulatory care, retirement homes and communities, adult homes, health-related facilities, intermediate care and extended care facilities, skilled care nursing homes, and community-based social program), the nurse executive assures appropriate services, adequately coordinated to meet the multiplicity of conditions and needs of the older population.

Standard II. Theory

The nurse participates in the generation and testing of theory as a basis for clinical decisions. The nurse uses theoretical concepts as a basis for the effective practice for gerontological nursing.

Rationale: Theoretical concepts from nursing and other disciplines are an essential source of knowledge for professional nursing practice. Theories help organize and interpret isolated information obtained from clients and families. Theoretical concepts provide a framework for assessing, intervening, and evaluating care to clients, as well as providing the rationale for nursing care to other health professionals. Furthermore, the testing of theory in practice settings is essential for the development of the discipline of nursing.

Standard III. Data collection

The health status of the older person is regularly assessed in a comprehensive, accurate, and systematic manner. The information obtained during the health assessment is accessible to and shared with appropriate members of interdisciplinary health care team, including the older person and the family.

Rationale: The information obtained from the older person, the family, and the interdisciplinary team, in addition to nursing judgments based on knowledge of gerontological nursing, is used to develop a comprehensive plan of care. This plan incorporates the older person's perceived needs and goals.

Standard IV. Nursing diagnosis

The nurse uses health assessment data to determine nursing diagnoses.

Rationale: Nursing diagnosis is an integral part of the assessment process. Each person, having a unique perception of health and well-being, responds to aging in a unique way. The basis for nursing intervention rests on the identification of those diagnoses that flow from gerontological nursing theory and scientific knowledge.

Standard V. Planning and continuity of care

The nurse develops the plan of care in conjunction with the older person and appropriate others. Mutual goals, priorities, nursing approaches, and measures in the care plan address the therapeutic, preventive, restorative, and rehabilitative needs of the older person. The care plan helps the older person attain and maintain the highest level of health, well-being, and quality of life achievable, as well as a peaceful death. The plan of care facilitates continuity of care over time as the client moves to various care settings, and is revised as necessary.

Rationale: Planning guides nursing interventions and facilitates the achievement of desired outcomes. Plans are based on nursing diagnoses and contain goals and interventions with specific time frames for accomplishment.

Goals are a determination of the results to be achieved and are derived from the nursing diagnosis. Goals are directed toward maximizing the older person's state of well-being, health, and achievable independence in all activities of daily living. Goals are based on knowledge of the client's status, the desired outcomes, and current research findings to increase the probability of helping the client achieve maximum well-being.

Standard VI. Intervention

The nurse, guided by the plan of care, intervenes to provide care to restore the older person's functional capabilities and to prevent complications and excess disability. Nursing interventions are derived from nursing diagnoses and are based on gerontological nursing theory.

Rationale: The nurse implements a plan of care in collaboration with the client, the family, and the interdisciplinary team. The nurse provides direct and indirect care, using the concepts of health promotion, maintenance, and rehabilitation or restoration. The nurse educates and counsels the family to facilitate their provision of care to the older person. The nurse teaches, supervises, and evaluates care givers outside the health professions and assures that their care is supportive and ethical and demonstrates respect for the client's dignity.

Standard VII. Evaluation

The nurse continually evaluates the client's and family's responses to interventions in order to determine progress toward goal attainment and to revise the data base, nursing diagnoses, and plan of care.

Rationale: Nursing practice is a dynamic process that responds to alterations in data, diagnoses, or care plans. Evaluation of the quality of care is an essential component. The effectiveness of nursing care depends on the continuing reassessment of the client's and family's health needs and appropriate revision of the plan of care.

Standard VIII. Interdisciplinary collaboration

The nurse collaborates with other members of the health care team in the various settings in which care is given to the older person. The team meets regularly to evaluate the effectiveness of the care plan for the client and family and to adjust the plan of care to accommodate changing needs.

Rationale: The complex nature of comprehensive care to elderly clients and their family members requires expertise from a number of different health care professions. A multidisciplinary approach is optimal for planning, carrying out, and evaluating care of older adults and their families.

Standard IX. Research

The nurse participates in research designed to generate an organized body of gerontological nursing knowledge, disseminates research findings, and uses them in practice.

Rationale: The improvement of the practice of gerontological nursing and the future of health care for older persons depend on the availability and utilization of an adequate knowledge base for gerontological nursing practice.

Standard X. Ethics

The nurse uses the Code for Nurses established by the American Nurses' Association as a guide for ethical decision-making in practice.

Rationale: The nurse is responsible for providing health care to individuals in settings where decisions about health care are jointly made with the client, family, and physician when appropriate. The nurse determines with the client and family the appropriate setting for care during acute and chronic illnesses. Nurses and other care providers are prepared by education and experience to provide the care needed by the older person.

The Code for Nurses provides the parameters within which the nurse makes ethical decisions. Special ethical concerns in gerontological nursing care include informed consent; admission to a health care facility with collaboration of the client, family, nurse and physician; emergency interventions; nutrition and hydration; pain management; the need for self-determination by the client; treatment termination; quality-of-life issues; confidentiality; surrogate decision-making; nontraditional treatment modalities; fair distribution of scarce resources; and economic decision-making.

Standard XI. Professional development

The nurse assumes responsibility for professional development and contributes to the professional growth of interdisciplinary team members. The nurse participates in peer review and other means of evaluation to assure the quality of nursing practice.

Rationale: Scientific, cultural, societal, and political changes require a commitment from the nurse to the continual pursuit of knowledge to enhance professional growth. Peer evaluation of nursing practice, professional education, and participation in collaborative educational programs serve as mechanisms to ensure quality care.

Clarification of Standard V is warranted, because of its problematic presentation in the original document. The first sentence of this standard may be restated as follows: (The nurse, in conjunction with the older person and appropriate others, develops the plan of care, mutual goals, priorities, and nursing approaches; and measures in the care plan address the therapeutic, preventive, restorative, and rehabilitative needs of the older person.)

Supporting Criteria: Structure, Process, Outcome

As noted earlier, each standard of practice is designed with its own set of structure, process, and outcome criteria (ANA, 1988). Structure criteria delineate the mechanisms that are to be in place to accomplish the standard's expectations. Process criteria list nursing actions required to accomplish the standard of practice and guide the nurse in implementing the standard. Finally, identified outcome criteria enable the nurse to evaluate excellence in nursing interventions or actions in the care of older persons.

Example of structure criteria for Standard III (data collection).   (ANA, 1988, p. 6):

1. A data collection method is used in the setting; the method provides for—
   (a) Systematic and complete collection of data.
   (b) Frequent updating of records.
   (c) Retrievability of data from the record-keeping system.
   (d) Confidentiality when appropriate.
2. The health status information is obtained from—

(a) The older adult, family, or significant other.
(b) Members of the health care team.
(c) Health records.

3. A record-keeping system based on the nursing process is used in the setting; the system provides for concise, comprehensive, accurate, and continual recording.

Example of process criteria for Standard III (data collection).   (ANA, 1988, p. 7): The nurse generalist—

1. Collects and records assessment data including the following:
   (a) Physical, psychosocial, cultural and spiritual status
   (b) Response to the aging
   (c) Functional status
   (d) Response to acute and/or chronic illness
   (e) Past and current lifestyle
   (f) Communication pattern
   (g) Individual coping pattern
   (h) Available and accessible human and material resources
   (i) Perception and satisfaction with health status
   (j) Health goals
   (k) Knowledge and receptivity to health care

Example of outcome criteria for Standard III (data collection).   (ANA, 1988, p. 7):

1. The individual, the family and members of the health care team can participate in the data collection process.
2. The health status information is—
   (a) Current, accessible, and accurate.
   (b) Kept confidential, as appropriate.
   (c) Shared with care givers, interdisciplinary team members, the individual, and the family, as appropriate.
3. The data base is complete.
4. Mechanisms for data collection are evaluated and revised on a regular basis.

Efficacy of Standards of Practice

The standards of gerontological nursing practice set the tone for quality care in long-term care facilities, hospitals, and community-based nursing services to older adults. Moreover, these standards represent criteria with legal implications, for they are used by the legal profession to measure the quality of care when a litigation process begins. Full implementation of these standards will promote a high level of satisfaction for both the professional nurse and the elderly client. For the older adult, care needs are met; for the nurse, the satisfaction of providing these needs in accordance with professional standards of care are rewarding. Standards of practice are essential for guiding quality care in facilities ministering to the health care needs of older adults, and further, they provide clarification of the roles and functions required for professional gerontological nursing practice.

NURSING ROLES: FUTURE NEEDS RELATED TO DEMOGRAPHICS OF AGING IN AMERICA

Nursing roles in gerontological nursing fall into two categories: generalist and specialist. The generalist is the nurse who possesses the bachelor of science in nursing (BSN) degree. The nurse generalist

> provides care primarily to individuals and families and participates in the planning, implementation, and evaluation of nursing care. The generalist draws on the expertise of the specialist. If a specialist is not available in the practice setting, the generalist may assume some aspects of the role of the specialist; but the use of a consultant is recommended. (ANA, 1988, p. 1)

The generalist preparation requires content on aging in the curriculum that focuses on the normal changes of aging, common illnesses experienced by the aging individual, health maintenance and health promotion of older adults, community services available for elderly residing in the community, and clinical experiences involving health care needs of aging persons. The nursing process and its problem-solving methodology should be mastered by the generalist in gerontological nursing. In the future, the role of the generalist may move from the institution to the home, with nurse employment in home health care agencies and home nursing care.

The specialist encompasses the comprehensive level of skills, competencies, and knowledge needed to perform at the advanced level of practice. The nurse specialist

> may perform all functions of the nurse generalist. In addition, the specialist possesses substantial, clinical experience with individuals, families, and groups; expertise in the formulation of health and social policy; and demonstrated proficiency in planning, implementing and evaluating health programs. (ANA, 1988, pp. 1–2)

Specialist preparation requires content on advanced aging research, theory building and testing, managerial skills, teaching and learning methods, clinical expertise in providing and managing the care of complex problems in acutely ill or terminally ill aged, and complicated chronic illnesses and neurological conditions requiring advanced scientific knowledge. In addition, specialist preparation requires knowledge on the consultation process, political acuity, health and social policy formulation, program planning, evaluation, and research.

SUMMARY

The future for gerontological nursing is based on the projection of an increasing population of aged individuals. Projection of aged persons in America arises as a major phenomenon in the 1990 to 2050 period with ever-increasing numbers in the old-old age-group, 85 to 100 years of age. The health needs of these aged individuals will be met by qualified professional nurses who are prepared at the BSN and MSN level with expertise in gerontological nursing. The major thrust of this preparation will be knowledge of and implementation of the standards of gerontological nursing practice, which promote quality care to aging persons in all settings.

REFERENCES

Aging America, 1987–1988 Edition. (1988). Washington, DC: American Association of Retired Persons and U.S. Department of Health and Human Services.

American Nurses' Association (ANA), Division of Gerontological Nursing. (1976). *Standards of gerontological nursing practice*. Kansas City, MO: Author.

American Nurses' Association. (1980). *Nursing: A social policy statement*. Kansas City, MO: Author.

American Nurses' Association (ANA), Council of Gerontological Nursing. (1988). *Scope and standards of gerontological nursing practice*. Kansas City, MO: Author.

Ebersole, P., & Hess, P. (1985). *Toward healthy aging:*

Human needs and human responses. (2nd ed.) St. Louis, MO: C. V. Mosby.

Gress, L., & Bahr, R. T. (1984). *The aging person: A holistic perspective*. St. Louis, MO: C. V. Mosby.

Yura, H., & Walsh, M. B. (1983). *The nursing process: Assessing, planning, implementing, evaluating* (4th ed.). Norwalk, CT: Appleton-Century-Crofts.

✳ **EDITOR'S QUESTIONS FOR DISCUSSION** ✳

How can nursing as a profession best prepare practitioners for the increasing care of the elderly at a professional level? What data are available indicating the types of services and care more frequently demanded by the average elderly consumer? Should all students be required to have experience in gerontological nursing practice? What curriculum implications are there for various nursing programs regarding the increasing elderly population? How can curriculum be developed effectively for a specialized area so that maximum use of qualified faculty and resources occur? Discuss strategies by which interdisciplinary programs may be planned with various subdisciplines of nursing for such specialty areas as gerontology. What guidelines might be offered for interdisciplinary planning approaches for nursing education? How may accountability be established for the content and quality of a interdisciplinary program?

43

Nurse Practitioners:
Mirrors of the past, windows of the future

Fay W. Whitney, Ph.D., R.N., C.R.N.P., F.A.A.N.

Nine years of watching the percent of the gross national product (GNP) devoted to health care cost rise from 8% and $100 billion in 1978 (Aiken, 1978, p. 274) to 11.4% and $500 billion in 1987 (Ginzberg, 1987) may have made the American citizen cynical and wary. John Q. Public is overwhelmed by the continuously escalating costs, increasing regulations, decreasing subsidy, and the quickly changing availability of goods and services within the health care industry. If a person is among the 37 million people without any health care coverage (Roemer, 1988), he or she faces a future in which financial ruin looms as an unknown part of the process of aging, or as the sequela of a catastrophic illness. The costs of health and illness are becoming painfully clear, but measures of the value of health care are more elusive.

There are enormous forces forging the shape of present and future health care delivery. In a fiscal environment in which private and public payors of health care costs are becoming less sanguine about the ability to finance health care as a right, competition has openly entered the marketplace. In the once quiet monopoly of the health care industry, a cacophony of bids and prices can now be heard.

As the government has attempted to shift the decisions for health care services closer to the populations served, we have learned that merely legislating access to services has not necessarily made them available (Roemer, 1988). Major changes in payment policies for Medicare and Medicaid populations have heightened present recognition of the enormous fiscal commitment the public has made in the name of health, without decreasing the projected deficit. The rising costs of goods, spurred by continued development of sophisticated technology, show no downward trends. Dramatic changes in demographics have occurred, and will continue to occur. Fewer earners and more use of services by the dependent, sick, and elderly cannot help but add to the financial burden of health care in the future.

As providers, nurses could give in to the despair arising from the increased expectations of the public and the constraints imposed by limited resources. Nurses, however, are at a turning point where neither we nor the public will be well served by despair or cynicism. In the past 20 years, nurse practitioners have learned the cost and value of sound, effective nursing care delivered to people, who have come to expect that they will be cared for appropriately. The success of nurse practitioners has not been accidental. This chapter reflects on what has been accomplished, looks at present dilemmas, and projects the roles that may be played by nurse practitioners who are willing to risk small costs for added value in the future. Although there may be different definitions of the term *nurse practitioner*, for the purpose of this chapter nurse practitioner means a nurse who has had a course of study that includes principles of health assessment, management of acute and chronic illness, health promotion, prevention of disease and illness, community-based nursing care, and advanced practice nursing roles in programs designed to produce primary care providers who carry a caseload of individual clients and families.

A MIRROR OF THE PAST

Looking in a mirror of the past, images are reflected of major accomplishments in nursing that were greatly influenced by nurse practitioners. Four of their accomplishments are briefly addressed.

A Public Image of Advanced Practice

In the 1970s and 1980s, nurse practitioners armed themselves with additional skills. These included skills in physicial assessment and decision making, management of acute and chronic illness, health promotion, and illness prevention. Nurse practitioners became highly visible as community-based, direct providers. It was clear that their practice embodied the broader concepts of primary care: comprehensive, continuous, family-centered, self-actualizing care. The public became aware that nurses who had additional education could provide a high level of nursing intervention and management from which they and their families could directly benefit. This positive image gave the public a view of advanced practice that came to include hospital and community-based nurses.

Growth in the Ability to Influence Policy

To develop and protect their practices, nurse practitioners gained valuable skills in legislative maneuvering and political action. Nurse midwives and anesthetists had preceded nurse practitioners in this activity, and later other nursing groups joined in legislative activity. Nurse practitioners, however, were, and continue to be, a formidable group of politically active nurses. Their extraordinary success in creating legislative change and public policy in health matters is respected and used today by national, state, and local governmental bodies.

New Models of Practice and Reimbursement

New practice models, and with them, new opportunities for advanced practice became apparent as nurse practitioners set up cooperative and independent practices. This type of nurse entrepreneurship began to push the frontiers of reimbursement policies. Their early business decisions reinforced the notion that advanced professional practice in the future would depend on the ability to produce income. Nurse practitioners were among the early nursing groups who focused on the need for reimbursable services in maintaining control and autonomy in practice.

Beginning of Service and Education Partnerships

Nurse practitioner education demanded closely supervised, mentored clinical practice. Because there were few field clinicians, faculty desired and were required to maintain individual practices. In negotiating academic appointments with practice components, the need for closer approximation of education and service arenas became apparent. Nurse practitioner faculty were among those for whom many types of appointment models were tested. Nurse practitioners established faculty practices and nursing centers. They helped to weave the early threads of clinical research into the cloth of the education, practice, and research fabric.

Nurse practitioners have moved through the last 20 years as effective providers of nursing services to an increasingly accepting public. Their continued value as primary providers has helped to define advanced nursing practice in the nonhospital setting. Even during the stressful times when the legitimacy of their practice in nursing, the quality of their care, competition with physicians, and the legality of practice came into question, nurse practitioners survived and have thrived. The mirror of the past reflects steps forward in tumultuous times and positive progress through controversial issues. The accomplishments were achieved through the strength of determined, disciplined, and competent productivity in the face of challenge. Nurses face similar circumstances today. The past gives us reason to believe that continued forward movement in nursing will occur.

A LANDSCAPE OF THE PRESENT

The present hallmarks of nurse practitioner practice today are signposts for future nursing practice: (a) direct patient care that is continuous and identifiable; (b) intradisciplinary and interdisciplinary principles and models of practice; and (c) accountability for outcomes that can be influenced, quantified, and evaluated. From the beginning, nurse practitioner practice was broadly conceptualized, with a focus on entry and access of populations into the health care system. Both results of national surveys and documentation of the recent history and experience of nurse practitioners have consistently provided evidence that the nurse practitioner has become an integral and viable component of the health care system (U.S. Congress, Office of Technical Assistance, 1986). Knowledge of the impact of varying models of health care based on research is increasing (Johnson & Freeborn, 1986; Siminoff, 1986). Few health care arenas and fewer patient populations have escaped the influence of nurse practitioner practice. Nurse practitioners are caring for the well, the worried well, the acutely ill person with minor illnesses, sicker groups of minorities, the poor, the elderly, and the chronically ill (American Nurses' Association, 1985; Fagin, 1987; Selby, 1985). They are broadly based in schools, clinics, and the workplace (ANA, 1985), shelters for the homeless, long-term care and life care facilities, home care, and acute care services in hospitals. It is this rich, ubiquitous quality of nurse practitioners to fit easily into multiple practice situations, and do well, that has resulted in some controversy. It is responsible for both the continued problems in education and practice surrounding nurse practitioners and for optimism about the continued success of nurse practitioners in the future.

Persistent Problems

In the 1980s, when nursing schools scurried to accommodate primary care programs into an essentially unchanged educational system (McGivern, 1986), several differences in perspective about the education and practice of nurse practitioners surfaced. Some persistent problems still plague nurse practitioners, such as (a) continued problems with titles and naming of these advanced practice nurses; (b) division and discord about what constitutes nurse practitioner education at the advanced practice level; and (c) divergence in developing educational programs with primary care principles.*

It is time that the first problem be negated. There simply is not sufficient time to resolve it permanently. A change in title is relatively unimportant considering the magnitude of the present problems in the health care system. More to the point, a change in title will cause major disruptions. Nurse practitioners are known by the public, other health care providers, legislators, and third-party payors by their present title. Energy should not be wasted in reconstructing programs or laws, or in the reeducating of the public that a change in title would demand. The high level of recognition obtained thus far should be built on. In so doing, the problem of titles will go away.

The second problem is fueled by attempts to classify both the product and the body of knowledge in master's programs within a single framework. Clinically oriented master's programs often label the product "clinical specialist" and the body of knowledge taught is directly related to the specialty area identified. Nurse practitioners, however, are generalists, and to some it may seem less clear what constitutes their educational program.

A no-nonsense approach to preparing nurses to provide direct care to consumers in unstructured sit-

---

*Mezey, M., & McGivern, D. (1986). *Nurses, nurse practitioners: The evolution of primary care*. Boston: Little, Brown. This study provides many, wide-ranging perspectives about issues in practice and education, controversies, health care systems, and other concerns related to primary care. It would be redundant to attempt to present the richness of the material contained. Thus the reader is urged to explore this book in detail for a review of the contemporary information presented in this chapter.

uations has often been seen as "skill training," rather than development of the complex elements required for the type of advanced practice provided by nurse practitioners. Because of the breadth of knowledge needed and the unpredictable nature of the practice arena, nurse practitioners must be taught reliable *processes* for finding and using information and resources.

A "generalist" nurse practitioner must have the expertise to apply a well-structured, but highly adaptable, process of assessment, decision making, and management to people in environments that change quickly and cannot be controlled by the nurse. Imaginative activation of patient and family initiative, making and accepting responsibility for independent decisions, working cooperatively in problem solving, developing an acute sense of timing and strategy, and perseverance in the face of unresolving problems are some of the behaviors and attributes developed. Graduates of nurse practitioner programs continue to practice in direct patient care services. They describe roles that require advanced practice skill and are satisfied with the graduate education they received (Jacobsen, 1987; Whitney & House, 1986). It is time to put to rest the differences in belief about what the content of nurse practitioner programs is. What is taught is apparently useful and effective.

Nurses and nursing need to focus on current problems facing all nursing educators: (a) determining who prospective students are and what they want to learn; (b) deciding what are the most useful concepts and content of advanced practice programs that should endure into the next century; (c) deciding how to cope with continued knowledge explosion; and (d) wrestling with the pragmatics of coalescing the needs of society, practicing nurses, and students within the realities of the educational process and its constraints. We need to use our collective wisdom to create curricular innovations that will provide *new* nursing models.

The third problem arises out of years of interchanging the words *primary care* with *nurse practitioner*. Mezey and McGivern (1986) suggest that we have reached the stage at which it is important to separate the words nurse practitioner and primary care:

The time is appropriate for the use of the term *primary care* to be differentiated from that of *nurse practitioner*. The continued disparity in the use of primary care among nurses, other professionals, and the public is detrimental to all concerned. It impedes communication and stunts the profession's efforts to positively exploit the experience gained from participation in primary care practice. The term *primary care* should be reserved to describe a mode of practice delivered in ambulatory settings; . . . the term *nurse practitioner* should be used to denote a nurse whose practice subsumes those components of care found in the original definition of primary care. . . . The *concept of primary care* and therefore the nurse practitioner role is transferable to broader population groups, such as those with chronic illness, and to other settings, including home, acute, and long-term care. (pp. 40–41)

This change in word use accommodates incorporation of the major principles of primary care into all appropriate levels of curriculum and nursing practice. It frees nurse practitioners to continue to define legitimately practice within developing health care arenas. Further it promotes intraprofessional understanding and cooperation about how to provide the elements of articulated care in a fragmented system, using the concept of primary care throughout.

CHANGES IN THE HEALTH CARE DELIVERY SYSTEM

The contextual relationships between nurses and the rest of the health care arena have always been important, but today they are vital to our understanding and planning in the future. A look at three major contextual variables, that is, health care providers, reimbursement issues, and societal needs, may give us some understanding of the complex environment within which we must plan the future for nursing.

Health Care Providers

Nurse practitioners were trained to practice in a climate of projected undersupply of primary care physicians, and were seen as the solution to the problem of providing primary care services to underserved populations. It is now projected that by 1990 there will be an oversupply of physicians, while nursing wrestles with what appears to be a severe and protracted undersupply of nurses. Data from the Cooperative Institutional Research Program in 1986 show that the number of freshmen women choosing medicine exceeded the number choosing nursing. It is estimated that by 1990, colleges will be graduating 16,000 MDs, while producing only 14,500 BSN nurses (Green, 1987).

There has been a consistent downward trend in physicians who declare primary care as their specialty (80% in 1931 to 15% in 1982) (Roemer, 1988). However, the number of physicians working in primary care facilities is increasing. With more female physicians seeking work, interest in part-time employment and in positions that provide more regularly scheduled working hours to accommodate families is sought. Salaries for these positions are competitive with nursing salaries. Physicians in specialty practice are also opting for some primary care positions to offset the decreasing need for specialty services. There has been speculation that these changes will toll the death knell for nurse practitioners. Yet most nurse practitioners have heard this tale before, and in the face of the present demographic and economic trends, they feel that the outlook for nurse practitioner practice is definitely positive.

There are increased numbers of health maintenance organizations (HMOs) and other prepaid practices, as well as community health centers in the last 10 years, all of which hire nurse practitioners in large numbers (Roemer, 1988). There is increased interest in preventive health maintenance among employers and the development of new fitness centers that employ nurse practitioners within industry. In hospitals, the percentage of nurses employed has increased, along with the higher ratio of staff nurse to patient (Aiken, 1987). Presently, house officers within hospitals are seeking fewer working hours through union activity. Because of their expertise in assessment and individual patient management, many nurse practitioners are being sought to follow patients in routine care within hospital walls, and to cover hours that house officers have traditionally

covered. Although this may appear to be a new form of physician substitution, it is an opportunity for nurse practitioners to change again the face of practice.

Reimbursement

Nursing has come a long way in its understanding of the role of economics and reimbursement in relationship to the future of nursing. Eli Ginzberg, at an invitational conference held at the University of Pennsylvania in 1987 to confront the nursing shortage issue, made a key observation: "The American public is friendly toward you, but the tough question is will they back that friendliness with more cash and other changes you seek?" (Ginzberg, 1987, p. 1600). Nurse practitioners are fully aware that they must be able to earn an income.

Prospective payment has affected the reorganization of services for hospitalized patients. Despite changes, much of the care delivered and paid for is still procedure-based. There are patients in need of prolonged and diverse types of nursing care who are excluded from payment. Home care, although widely touted, seldom reimburses appropriately, and families find themselves largely unsupported by both health care providers and payment mechanisms.

In caring for needy populations, many nurse practitioners in the past have been largely supported by salaries paid though public programs. The longevity of their practice somewhat depends on whether these programs are supported in the future. Even as prices continue to soar, there will be a concurrent loss in numbers of wage earners to support needy populations. Decisions regarding the percent of the GNP that the 20- to 45-year-old population is willing to spend for health care will influence what services are provided. As new forms of coverage for catastrophic care are designed and as new methods for dealing with high-cost tertiary care are devised, nurses must be willing to help determine the shape and focus of health care. The problems are complex, further confounded by the ever-increasing technological advances that would save and prolong life. Still if nurse practitioners want to be part of the future care of these populations, they have to be able to earn a living at it. Nursing will need to devote a great deal of energy to designing and lobbying for appropriate social programs that include nursing reimbursement if nursing services are to survive into the 21st century.

Health Needs of the Future

It is clear that there are changes in demographics that are helping to describe future health care systems. The "graying of America" is already a reality. There are growing numbers of homeless and over a million pregnant adolescents and their infants who still need care (Roemer, 1988). We live with the black box of acquired immunodeficiency syndrome (AIDS) statistics, which projects a death toll in 1991 of somewhere between 250,000 and 750,000, with no estimate of the number of people who will be ill with AIDS-related problems (Roemer, 1988). The cost of caring for these people will be substantial, and the bulk of the care will rest with nursing.

Substantial gains have been made in public health programs to decrease smoking and high blood pressure among the population. People now invest in fitness and health programs and eat healthier food. However, the numbers cannot be discounted that pertain to small infants with chronic, lifelong problems or to elderly with prolonged but not substantially improved lives—whose lives are being saved through better nursing care and advanced technology. These are the future patients, and decisions will have to be made on how best to care for them.

THE WINDOW OF THE FUTURE

Nurse practitioners looking through the window of the future should see a host of opportunities as direct health care providers in ambulatory, long-term, intermediate, and acute care settings. Nurse practitioners are already active in caring for the homeless, especially mothers and children, the chronically mentally ill, and the young, out-of-work man. Migrants, unemployed workers, the rural, and inner-city poor constitute a large portion of nurse practitioner practice. There is little doubt that nurse practitioners will continue to work with these under-served populations, but again nursing must be persistent in obtaining direct reimbursement for services.

There are also innovative roles for nurse practitioners in managed care and nursing centers, and as administrators of extended care services. Because nurses understand the system, they are able to act as liaisons and advocates for patients, and as risk managers and consultants in the insurance field. They understand what is written in the patient health record, and can translate for business organizations the meaning and importance of what is found in the health record. Nurses who know how to use resources efficiently will be hired as consultants to business and industry to help cut costs and halt the misuse of resources.

There are a number of roles that nurse practitioners can play in the future, but none is so important as the one that will shape a new type of practice for all of nursing, reach people who need nursing services, and act to unite nursing in an integrated nursing referral system.

A NURSING REFERRAL SYSTEM

Nurses need to redefine their major role as sources of referral within the health care system so that it includes nurses as a primary referral target. Nurses have to make new partnerships among themselves, redesign nursing positions to allow for fluidity between settings, and promote new alliances between practice, education, and research. It is imperative that nursing not only provide direct services, but also identify and operationalize a *nursing system* within which patients and nurses design patterns of care that best address known needs.

United efforts between schools of nursing and practice arenas will help create such a system. Once a nurse is involved deeply in both the provision of care *and* the generation of knowledge, she or he finds that it is impossible to draw boundaries around groups of patients or to ignore needed changes in either education or service that would strengthen both areas of nursing.

Nursing needs to think of a circle, a network wherein the acute care setting and all other practice settings are linked. Presently the interface between settings is ragged, barely integrated, and bereft of organization. Although 60% of nurses still work in hospitals (Aiken, 1987), they are simply not doing what they used to do. There are sicker patients in hospitals than in the past and more technical skills are needed. There is less time to prepare patients and their families for discharge. Patients are entering a community system unprepared for the degree of acuity and complexity of services needed. This higher level of illness has changed the practice of the community-based nurse, whether in home care or extended care facilities or in ambulatory settings. Faced with sicker patients and frightened families, nurse practitioners in the community setting spend a great number of hours merely finding out what was done for the patient in the acute care setting so that services provided will ensure a safe level of care. When patients must reenter the acute care setting, the reverse is true. The lack of coordination between practice settings causes the patient to suffer, the nurses involved to be frustrated, and worst of all, for costs to rise with no concurrent increase in quality of care. A truly integrated nurse referral system could eliminate most of these problems.

Nursing needs to build a network within which nurses who are based in different arenas can share in the care of patients. Nursing needs to find ways for nurses based in acute care settings to visit discharged patients in the community, and to help nurses there manage complex, continuing acute-care problems. Nursing needs to build a system that allows nurse practitioners to continue to care for patient's primary care needs when they are admitted to acute care settings. Nurse practitioners need to be able to refer directly to nurses in the acute care setting who are caring for the patient, and to have access to both the nurse and the patient to promote continuity of care on discharge. Nurse practitioners need consultant lists to be able to work in pairs with acute care clinical specialists when there is need for both acute and nonacute care nursing. Basically nurses need to work on the *interface* between groups of nurses, and to make contacts that truly refer patients from one nurse health care provider to an-

other. Nurse practitioners, and other nurses, do not need to form the circle to keep each other out, but to draw all nurses closer together and to link all of their talents and resources so that patients can truly benefit from them.

Nursing has again reached a turning point in the road followed by nurse practitioners. Their past is a true reflection of their abilities to be innovative and successful in practice. There is little chance that nurse practitioners will become extinct. Rather, they should be part of a closely knit network of nurses who share expertise, problems, and patients in an effort to create a system that makes sense in terms of human need, economics, and social good. Nurse practitioners have made remarkable gains, and it remains merely to link more colleagues together, and make the connections stronger. They can do it if they want to. In the process, they will gain title to the parts of health care that they want to call nursing.

REFERENCES

Aiken, L. (1978). Primary care: The challenge for nursing. In N. L. Chaska (Ed.), *The nursing profession: Views through the mist* (pp. 247–255). New York: McGraw-Hill.

Aiken, L. (1987). Breaking the shortage cycles (pp. 1616–1620). In Nurses for the future. *American Journal of Nursing*, 87 (12) (Suppl.), 1593–1648.

American Nurses' Association (ANA), Council of Primary Health Care Nurse Practitioners. (1985). *The scope of practice of the primary health care nurse practitioner*. Kansas City, MO: Author.

Fagin, C. (1987, April 1). *Nurses as one solution to the nation's health care problems*. Paper read at Presidential Forum with Ronald Reagan, College of Physicians of Philadelphia, Philadelphia, PA.

Ginzberg, E. (1987). Facing the facts and figures (pp. 1596–1600). In Nurses for the future. *American Journal of Nursing*, 87 (12) (Suppl.), 1593–1648.

Green, K. (1987). What freshman tell us (pp. 1610–1615). In Nurses for the future. *American Journal of Nursing*, 87, (12) (Suppl.), 1593–1648.

Jacobsen, B. (1987). *Survey of MSN Graduates*. Philadelphia: University of Pennsylvania, School of Nursing.

Johnson, R. E. & Freeborn, D. K. (1986, January). Comparing HMO physicians' attitudes toward nurse practitioners and physician's assistants. *Nurse Practitioner, 11* (1), 39–53.

McGivern, D. (1986). The unfullfulled promise in undergraduate education. In M. Mezey & D. McGivern (Eds.), *Nurses, nurse practitioner: The evolution of primary care* (pp. 86–100). Boston: Little, Brown.

Mezey, M., & McGivern, D. (1986). *Nurses, nurse practitioners: The evolution of primary care*. Boston: Little, Brown.

Roemer, R. (1988). The right to health care—gains and gaps. *American Journal of Public Health, 78,* 241–247.

Selby, T. (1985). Nurses meet challenges as cost cuts take toll. *American Nurse, 17* (10), 17.

Siminoff, L. (1986). Competition and primary care in the United States: Separating fact from fancy. *International Journal of Health Services, 16,* 57–69.

U.S. Congress, Office of Technical Assistance. (1986, December). *Nurse practitioners, physician's assistants and certified nurse-midwives: A policy analysis* (Health Technology Case Study 37, OTA-HCS-37). Washington, DC: U.S. Government Printing Office.

Whitney, R., & House, J. (1986). *Graduate survey 1983–1895, nurse practitioner program*. Philadelphia: University of Pennsylvania, School of Nursing.

✳ EDITOR'S QUESTIONS FOR DISCUSSION ✳

Discuss the public's perception of the nurse practitioner, what she or he does, how she or he does it, and where she or he does it. Do you agree with Whitney that the matter of title and the problems associated with titles for nurse practitioners, as well as differences in beliefs concerning what should be taught to nurse practitioners, are problems that should be ignored or forgotten? What is the basis for the misunderstandings and misconceptions about advanced nursing practice and specialty roles? What is the basis of the confusion regarding the content that is taught in nurse practitioner programs? How may the misunderstandings be corrected? If nurse practitioners are generalists, what is the difference between a nurse practitioner and a staff nurse?

What type of new nursing models could be suggested regarding curricular innovations for advanced nursing practice? Do Mezey and Mc-Givern differentiate specific definitions for the terms primary care and nurse practitioner? What assumptions are made about primary care and the nurse practitioner role? What should be the role of the nurse practitioner in providing care to specialized population groups such as AIDS patients, the underserved, and persons disenfranchised by the present health care system? What might be the differences between an integrated nursing referral system as advocated by Whitney and a nurse-operated corporation for nursing services? How specifically might one plan work to develop and operate an integrated nursing referral system?

44

An Impractical Dream or Possible Reality:

A faculty intramural private practice model

Brenda Lyon, D.N.S., R.N.

Nursing is a practice discipline; therefore, persons who teach nursing should practice. On the surface the statement sounds reasonable. In fact, it infers that practice should be a rule of conduct for academicians who teach nursing. Yet few faculty practice (Anderson & Pierson, 1983; Langfor, 1983). There are fundamental issues intrinsic to faculty practice that mitigate against it. These include insufficient time to devote to practice; lack of monetary, tenure, and promotion benefits of practice; and perception on the part of faculty that teaching students how to practice is equivalent to practice (Barger, 1986; Collison & Parsons, 1980; Holm, 1981; Jezek, 1980; Langfor, 1983; Millonig, 1986; Spero, 1980). A further concern is lack of comfort with the level of accountability that comes with charging directly for services rendered, as well as other "business" related matters. Developing workable solutions to these commonly cited issues will determine whether faculty practice is an impractical dream or a possible reality.

The purpose of this chapter is twofold: (a) to describe the faculty intramural private practice model developed at Indiana University School of Nursing, and (b) to discuss issues pertaining to the initiation and maintenance of faculty practice. Such issues include purpose, structure, faculty participation, fee structures, evaluation, and clinical scholarship. How the faculty and administration in a school deal with these common and difficult issues not only impact the success of the faculty intramural private practices, but also the future development of knowledge in nursing.

BACKGROUND

Indiana University School of Nursing sits in the center of a large medical center on the Indiana University/Purdue University Indianapolis (IUPUI) campus. The health professional schools on the campus include nursing and Indiana's only medical and dental schools. The degrees offered by the School of Nursing include ASN, BSN, MSN, and DNS. There were approximately 138 School of Nursing faculty on the Indianapolis campus and approximately 30 School of Nursing faculty located on five other Indiana University campuses throughout the state. Faculty in the schools of medicine and dentistry have faculty practice corporations. Therefore, faculty practice in the health sciences at the time we began work on the School of Nursing's faculty practice plan was not a new phenomenon to the University.

The author had a private practice in health and stress management for 7 years before requesting the Dean of the School of Nursing in 1983 to appoint a planning committee to develop and implement an intramural private practice model for faculty. The planning/development committee was appointed in late spring of that year and work on the faculty practice model began. During the initial phase of development the planning committee dealt with such central issues as purpose, whether or not to incorporate the faculty private practice, eligibility of faculty providers, liability, and incentives.

DEFINITION AND PURPOSE OF FACULTY PRACTICE

The question of purpose is of prime importance when formalizing a structure for faculty practice and is intertwined with the question, What is faculty practice? Members of the planning committee believed strongly that clinical scholarship must be a primary focus of faculty practice. Nursing's reason, unlike medicine's, to move away from apprentice-type hospital-based training to academia in the 1950s was to legitimatize the teaching and learning of the discipline, whereas medicine's move away from the apprentice system to an academic system was for the purpose of putting medicine in a place where it could "not only be taught but studied" (Stevens, 1971, p. 58).

There was considerable agreement on the planning committee that the purposes of the Office of Nursing Practice (ONP) should include the following: (a) the scientific study of phenomena of concern to nursing; (b) demonstration of nursing's autonomous scope of practice; and (c) the education of graduate students and practicing nurses. Scholarly practice, as conceived of by the planning committee, emphasizes the importance of utilization of research, generation of ideas, and generation of knowledge through practice-based research. In this scholarship model of practice the *faculty member is the primary provider of service* with education of students being a secondary purpose.

Nursing practice under the auspices of the ONP is limited to autonomous nursing activities. These are the diagnosis and treatment of *phenomena of concern to nursing* (Lyon, 1983; see also Chapter 34) Autonomous as used here means *self-directed* care, that is, the care is self-directed in that treatments do not legally require any type of delegation or authorization of a physician to be initiated (see box, Current and Desired Future Services for a listing of current services provided and future services proposed through ONP). In addition to practical reasons for the limitation to autonomous nursing activities, the planning committee strongly believed that the evolution of nursing science rests squarely with the study of what nursing uniquely contributes to a person's health. Such a limitation has not been without criticism, however, particularly from those who follow a nurse practitioner model of care. In a practical sense the limitation to autonomous or self-directed practice activities has been helpful because, as previously mentioned, the School of Nursing is located across the street from the state's only medical school. As can be readily appreciated, the discipline has not yet evolved to the point at which the practice of nurses providing substitute medical services is well received by the medical community. Some who have been doubtful about the limitation to autonomous nursing services have believed that the public would not desire or pay for the services. On the contrary, as demonstrated by my own practice in health and stress management, the public frequently not only needs but wants these services and is willing to pay for them. However, too often the public does not know that these services are available or that nurses can provide them. During the first year of operation, with minimal marketing effort, two faculty provided 69 professional service sessions to fee-paying clients.

STRUCTURE

Both business structure and internal structure within the administrative/faculty organization in the nursing school need to be dealt with when considering a faculty practice plan. An early question considered by our planning committee was whether or not to incorporate. The primary benefit of incorporating an academic practice unit at Indiana University

Current and desired future services

Current services

Professional Care Services:

Health and stress management self-care teaching/
counseling (care for adults who have physical
health problems/illness for which stress is the
primary or contributing etiology).

Sensory-motor facilitation of self-care (care for adolescents and adults who have experienced some
form of functional impairment caused by brain
damage).

Counseling/support services for families of persons
with Alzheimer's disease (includes evaluation of
home environment re: facilitation of functioning).

Self-care teaching/counseling to facilitate healthy
aging (includes health promotion and health deviation self-care).

Family/marriage counseling (focus is on improving
family/marital functioning).

Workshop/consultation areas:

Health and stress management self-care
Rehabilitation and rehabilitation nursing
Caring for an elderly family member
Developing a faculty practice
Autonomous nursing practice

Desired future services

Professional care services:

Diabetes education and self-care counseling (and
other chronic illnesses).

Facilitation of infant/child development.

Women's health (self-care counseling and teaching).

Parenting skills training.

is that faculty could accrue more than 20% over and above their academic salary. The start-up costs for establishing a corporation and the complexities of continuing its operation made the incorporation option unattractive for what faculty believed was a "trial" run.

The internal structure issue required more delib-eration to resolve than it took to articulate the pur-poses of faculty practice. The central question was, Should we organize the ONP under the auspices of faculty organization or under the auspices of the Dean's office? After considerable discussion the planning committee decided to organize the ONP under the auspices of the Dean's office. The benefits of such an organizational structure included (a) as-surance of a close administrative relationship be-tween the Dean and the director of the ONP; (b) sim-plification of decision making; (c) administrative support services for the collection and disbursement of fees; and (d) limitation of functional governance to only those faculty who provide services through the ONP.

Although the ONP is organized under the aus-pices of the Dean's office, it is governed by the fac-ulty providers in accordance with the ONP bylaws. The bylaws provide for a director; a five-member board, including the director, two ex-officio board members, the treasurer (appointed by the Dean), and the Dean. The board members, including the di-rector, are all faculty providers in the ONP. This type of structural relationship (Fig. 44-1) has facili-tated the operation of the ONP while maintaining pertinent faculty control over practices offered through the ONP.

FACULTY PARTICIPATION

To provide service through the ONP a faculty member must be approved for practice privileges. To be approved the faculty member submits the follow-ing to the ONP Credentials Committee chairperson: (a) a description/specification of the autonomous ser-vices to be provided; (b) documentation of educa-tional and practice-related experience that supports the competence of the faculty member in the auton-omous scope of practice described; (c) three letters of reference; (d) evidence of licensure; and (e) docu-mentation of professional liability insurance. Faculty approved for practice privileges in the ONP are re-viewed for reappointment every 2 years.

Several surmountable obstacles to faculty partici-pation in the ONP have been identified. The obsta-cles include insufficient time available to practice;

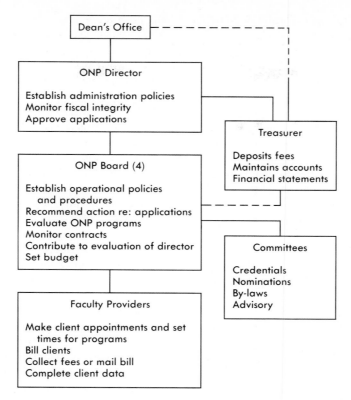

FIGURE 44-1

Structure and functional chart of the *Office of Nursing Practice* (ONP) at Indiana University School of Nursing.

lack of confidence and competence in delivering an autonomous service; lack of business knowledge; and the fact that practice per se is not a university mission, thus not contributive toward tenure promotion. In the following subsections each obstacle is discussed along with strategies that have been developed in an attempt to overcome the obstacle.

Strategies to Resolve Obstacles to Faculty Practice
Time commitment

A block to participation in faculty practice, commonly cited in the literature, is insufficient time (Barger & Bridges, 1987; Millonig, 1986). To help in overcoming this obstacle, the planning committee employed the following two strategies: (a) institution of an administrative approval process regarding amount of full-time-equivalent (FTE) time spent by a faculty member in the ONP, and (b) development of a fee-sharing reimbursement for ONP providers. When a faculty member applies to the ONP, the administrative person to whom the faculty member reports indicates the amount of the faculty member's FTE that may be allocated to ONP activities. Although a percentage of FTE time is administratively approved for each ONP provider, in actuality the time spent in providing services through the ONP is over and above the faculty member's full-time responsibilities. The reason for the overload is simply that there are no "extra" faculty, at this time, to offset the ONP FTE time spent by an ONP provider. Recognizing that distinct possibility, the planning committee believed that it was very important to provide faculty a monetary benefit (Smith, 1980) for participating in the ONP. The reimbursement plan is shown in Table 44-1.

The rationale for 45% of the "professional care service fee" going to the provider was based on profit-margin estimates for a faculty member in private practice. It was considered that, after paying for overhead, such a private practice would probably realize less than 45% of fees collected. In this case, the profit-margin estimate was influenced by data from medical practice plans, in addition to the personal experience of two faculty members who had supported private practices outside the School of Nursing. Although there is variability in the way medical schools distribute practice income, the average amount reimbursed to the faculty provider is 42% in salary compensation and 11% in fringe benefits (Curran & Riley, 1984). In Table 44-1 the percent reimbursement to faculty for workshops and consultation is substantially greater than that for professional care services. The reason for the difference is that the planning committee faculty would be encouraged to do practice-related workshops and consultations through the ONP. There is an Indiana University School of Nursing policy that a faculty member may not use School resources to develop and conduct workshops and/or consultations on a fee-for-service basis, unless the services are offered through the ONP.

The income generated by an ONP provider supplements the regular faculty salary. The funds generated for the ONP, at this time, provide a flexible

source of revenue to be used for research assistants, development, and travel money for ONP providers. The success of the ONP strategies in encouraging faculty participation is discussed later in the Evaluation and Summary sections.

Confidence and competence

Perhaps a more significant obstacle to participation in the ONP, and one that was not fully anticipated, is faculty confidence and competence or comfort in areas of autonomous nursing practice. Currently all six of the present ONP faculty providers are graduate faculty. Although undergraduate faculty have expressed interest in and excitement about the ONP, to date no undergraduate faculty have applied for practice privileges. On the surface the lack of undergraduate ONP providers could be attributed to differences in teaching loads; however, the graduate faculty practicing in the ONP have comparable teaching loads to undergraduate faculty. Additionally the graduate faculty have added responsibilities in research. After 2 years of talking with faculty about the ONP, I have found that, on the whole, faculty do not feel comfortable or confident in envisioning their participation in the activities of the ONP. It was not surprising that faculty would be somewhat uncomfortable, at least initially, with the high degree of visible accountability that accompanies the provision of a service for a direct fee. It was also not surprising that faculty would be uncomfortable initially with charging clients directly for their services, for example, questioning whether their services were worth a fee? It has been, however, somewhat surprising to discover the degree of lack of perceived competence in the provision of autonomous nursing services. In talking with many nurse academicians about nursing's autonomous scope of practice across the country, I am frequently asked, "If you don't do physical examinations to screen or treat medical problems, what do you do?" In fact, faculty at the School of Nursing often ask, "What could I do?" As these questions are contemplated, one is reminded of the extent that substantive content in nursing curricula is influenced by medical phenomena and medical knowledge, rather than knowledge about phenomena of unique concern to nursing. The

TABLE 44-1

Reimbursement plan: distribution by percent of fee charged

	PROFESSIONAL CARE SERVICES	WORKSHOP/ CONSULTATION SERVICES
ONP provider	45%	70%
ONP	45%	20%
School	10%	10%

Note: Fee charged to client is determined by the faculty providing the service.

fact that faculty are not comfortable in providing autonomous services on a fee-for-service basis does not mean that faculty are, in actuality, not competent in the provision of autonomous services. On the contrary, faculty in varying degrees teach students *nursing* care. The perceived lack of competence and resulting lack of confidence could be due to any or all of the following reasons: (a) faculty may have only a superficial knowledge of such phenomena as pain, grief, stress/coping, and other practice-based concerns, and do not have the depth of knowledge required to provide care on a direct fee-for-service basis; (b) faculty have not had sufficient opportunity to learn how to articulate their "know-how" in autonomous nursing practice; (c) faculty tend to magnify the "risks" of providing autonomous service and are so anxious about being accountable that they underestimate their knowledge and level of competence.

In response to the lack of confidence expressed by faculty, The author has met individually with faculty to help them identify and articulate areas of autonomous practice in which they have competence. Additionally ONP providers have offered to help faculty "articulate" their service areas. Perhaps a yet-untried strategy is to foster the development of a mentoring process. Just as faculty need mentoring in being a faculty member and conducting research, perhaps faculty who wish to participate in faculty private practice also need mentoring.

Business knowledge

Nurse academicians are typically not experienced in the "business" of practice. Although much of the business-related aspects of a faculty practice plan is handled at the administrative level, there is business knowledge that a provider needs, for example, setting fees and marketing. The ONP held sessions of 1 to 2 hours for small groups of faculty to discuss setting fees, billing, malpractice insurance, marketing assistance, and personal tax implications.

Faculty providers in the ONP typically offer services on a sliding scale. The vast majority of services are charged on an hourly basis and the highest hourly fee at present is $50. Third-party reimbursement has been obtained indirectly by some clients. That is, clients have received partial reimbursement for what was paid out-of-pocket by the client. Additionally hospital consultations have been reimbursed directly to the provider. The services provided through the ONP *are not substitutive medical services* and therefore third-party payors are not quick to pay. In Indiana, insurance companies may pay for health care services provided through the ONP. However, the services provided through the ONP are not technology-intensive, but rather typically are counseling/psychoeducational/teaching in nature and therefore are not costly. Since services are delivered on a learning model, clients are taught skills that would enable the client not to need the provider for a long period of time. The average number of sessions needed by a client is five. Third-party reimbursement is a target area that the ONP will be addressing systematically in the future.

Tenure and promotion

At Indiana University, tenure and promotion are based on research and publications, teaching, and service. Practice per see is not part of the university's mission. However, faculty practice provides rich opportunities for scholarship in nursing.

Of importance, ONP providers have discovered that doing research with clients for whom one is also the provider of care services raises important ethical dilemmas. The ethical issues are embedded in each phase of the encounter with the client and arise out of the conflicting goals or requirements of nursing care and nursing research (Table 44-2).

Although many methodologies could be used to study phenomena experienced by clients of a faculty practice, case study research is a particularly appropriate and useful methodology (Yin, 1984). However, when a client comes for a service, it is not only awkward but at times unethical to ask the client if data from sessions may be incorporated into a research project. It obviously would facilitate research endeavors to advertise for clients for funded research. Although advertising for clients helps eliminate some of the ethical dilemmas, it precludes the use of very rich data from clients who just come for a service. If meaningful research is to be generated through faculty practice during the 1990s, it is imperative that academicians who have a faculty prac-

TABLE 44-2
Ethical dilemmas of doing research in practice related to characteristics of nursing care and research

CHARACTERISTIC	NURSING CARE	RESEARCH
Initiation of encounter	Patient/client seeks care. (patient/client conveys need for assistance.)	Researcher seeks subjects. (Researcher conveys need for assistance.)
Purpose of contact	Professional to meet or assist patient/client in meeting need for care: serves the interests of the individual.	Generation of knowledge: serves the interest of society.
Informed consent	Informal	Formal
	Does not require approval from external body.	Requires approval from IRB.
	No regulations: professional acts in concert with Code of Ethics.	Regulations stipulating the components of consent.
	Consent occurs over time; at each session there is a little informing and consenting.	Consent typically occurs in one encounter.
Relationship between professional and patient/client (duty of care)	Extended	Brief
	Professional accepts patients who need care.	Protocol determines who are acceptable patients.
	Professional responsive to needs of individual/unique needs can be met.	Researcher responsive to the protocol/subjects are viewed normatively.
	Professional free to make decisions in conjunction with patient/client re: treatment.	Treatment is determined by the protocol.
Termination	When patient has achieved his or her goals.	When researcher has accomplished purpose.

tice deal effectively with the practice-research dilemmas, when the provider is also the researcher. In addition to the knowledge generation and theory testing opportunities through faculty practice, there are rich learning opportunities provided to graduate students. In the ONP the fee-for-service is waived or substantially reduced if the client agrees to see a graduate student under the supervision of a faculty provider. However, 90% to 95% of the ONP clients seek the services of a particular faculty provider who is known by reputation or by referral. It is common, therefore, for a client to decline the opportunity for fee waiver. Several clients, alternatively, have consented to work with a faculty provider in a demonstration room where a mirror is a one-way window with an observation classroom on the other side. A few clients, after achieving desired goals, have consented to participate in "grand-rounds" type of educational sessions, in which both students and faculty are invited to learn about the method and impact of services.

EVALUATION

Currently faculty participation in the ONP is low in terms of numbers of faculty approved to provide service (six faculty). It seems reasonable to project that a minimum of 20% of a school of nursing's teaching faculty would participate in faculty practice. At Indiana University this would mean approximately 25 to 30 faculty should be a target number over the next few years. Each of the obstacles to faculty practice discussed earlier in this chapter are surmountable but need continued attention to facilitate further faculty participation.

The ONP faculty providers have successfully met

revenue targets, even exceeding the goal of the second year. The first year of operation, the gross revenue goal was $4,000 and the ONP generated $3,818. For the second year, the gross revenue goal was $5,000 and the ONP realized $7,939.

The number of professional care services provided was 69 during the first year of operation, and 64 during the second year. In the first part of the third year, it is clear that the ONP will provide at least 80 professional care services by the end of the year. The average fee paid per service by clients is $28.00.

In addition to the professional care services, consultation and workshop services offered through the ONP have provided significant revenue. These services generated $1880 during the first year of operation, and $4390 in the second year. Projections for the third year of operation are that consultation and workshop services will generate $5000 and professional care services over $2000. Although there are six faculty approved to provide services, the figures reported above represent the efforts primarily of only two ONP providers. Currently for each faculty member who devotes *concerted* effort (15 to 20 hours per month over 10 months per year) to the ONP an average of almost $4000 of revenue is generated.

In addition to meeting financial goals at this point in our development, approximately 70% of the clients seen in the ONP are referred by previous clients. Such a large percentage of previous client referrals reflects a high degree of satisfaction with services; this is really our best marketing strategy. A follow-up evaluation of ONP services by clients, regarding the short- and long-term effects of the services received, is being developed by a doctoral student at the Indiana University School of Nursing in conjunction with an ONP faculty provider.

SUMMARY

Is a faculty intramural private practice model an impractical dream or a possible reality? The ONP has not fully overcome the obstacles to faculty participation; nonetheless, much has been learned during the first 2 years of operation that can be capital-
ized on in the future. Faculty participation can be facilitated if faculty are helped to identify, articulate, and develop competence in an autonomous area of nursing practice, through faculty development efforts and a mentoring process. As schools move to responsibility centers in the budgeting process, there will be greater incentive to structure faculty work loads in a manner that will encourage revenue-generating activities. Although not yet resolved, the identification of ethical issues inherent in being a practitioner-scholar will be helpful in evolving even greater opportunities for faculty scholarship. Capitalizing on the rich resource of scholarship provided through faculty practice will not only help practicing faculty meet tenure and promotion criteria, but will also generate important knowledge for the discipline.

It has been demonstrated through the ONP that an intramural private practice model is not only workable, but also has the potential to evolve into a significant source of revenue for a school of nursing. Although each school—depending on areas of faculty expertise, setting, and vision of nursing—will have differing models of faculty practice, a faculty intramural private practice is a possible reality!

REFERENCES

Anderson, E. R., and Pierson, P. (1983). An exploratory study of faculty practice: View of those faculty engaged in practice who teach in NLN-accredited baccalaureate program. *Western Journal of Nursing Research, 5,* 129–139.

Barger, S. (1986). Academic nursing centers: A demographic profile. *Journal of Professional Nursing, 2* (4), 246–251.

Barger, S. E., and Bridges, W. C. (1987). Nursing faculty practice: Institutional and individual facilitators and inhibitors. *Journal of Professional Nursing, 3* (6), 338–346.

Collison, C. R., and Parsons, M. A. (1980, November). Is practice a viable faculty role? *Nursing Outlook, 28,* 677–679.

Curran, C. R., and Riley, D. W. (1984, September/October). Faculty practice plans: Will they work for nurses? *Nursing Economics, 2,* 319–324.

Henderson, V. (1964). The nature of nursing. *Journal of Nursing, 64*(8), 62.

Holm, K. (1981). Faculty practice—noble intentions gone awry? *Nursing Outlook, 29*, 655–657.

Jezek, J. (1980). Economic realities of faculty practice. In National League for Nursing, *Cognitive dissonance: Interpreting and implementing faculty practice roles in nursing education* (pp. 37–41). New York: National League for Nursing.

Langfor, T. (1983). Faculty could practice if—and other myths. *Nursing Health Care, 4*, 515–517.

Lyon, B. (1983). *Nursing practice: An exemplication of the statutory definition*. Birmingham, AL: Pathway Press.

Millonig, V. (1986). Faculty practice: A view of its development, current benefits, and barriers. *Journal of Professional Nursing, 2*, 166–172.

Smith, G. R. (1980, November). Compensating faculty for their clinical practice. *Nursing Outlook*, 673–676.

Spero, J. (1980). Faculty practice as one component of the faculty role. In National League for Nursing, *Cognitive dissonance: Interpreting and implementing faculty practice roles in nursing education* (pp. 37–41). New York: National League for Nursing.

Stevens, R. (1971). *American medicine and the public interest*. New Haven: Yale University Press.

Yin, R. K. (1984). *Case study research: Design and methods*. Beverly Hills, CA: Sage Publications.

✳ EDITOR'S QUESTIONS FOR DISCUSSION ✳

Describe the various types of faculty nursing practice that have been developed and discuss the pros and cons of each model. Discuss the internal structure issues that need to be considered and resolved before the development of a faculty practice model. What criteria should be established regarding potential clients being faculty and students? What ethical issues must be resolved concerning potential clients? Should a faculty practice be considered a portion of the total work load of a faculty member?

What are the advantages and disadvantages in limiting a faculty practice to autonomous nursing activities? Can the phenomena of concern to nursing be studied and treated from an interdependent or collaborative practice mode? What ethical issues must be resolved regarding faculty practice and the development of research? How might a faculty nursing practice be developed in different types of settings such as acute care, outpatient clinics, home care, and community agencies?

Certification varies by specialty. ANA certifies adult, family, gerontological, pediatric, and school nurse practitioners. However, 80% of the pediatric nurse practitioners who are certified have achieved that status through the National Board of Pediatric Nurse Practitioners/Associates rather than through the ANA (Dickenson-Hazard, 1988). Obstetrical-gynecological nurse practitioners are certified by the Nurses' Association of the American College of Obstetricians and Gynecologists (NAACOG, 1984). Each of these certifying bodies requires registered nurse licensure, graduation from a recognized nurse practitioner program, and the successful completion of a certifying examination.

NURSE-MIDWIFERY

Traditionally, assisting with the birth process was considered a field for women and midwifery was a time-honored profession learned by apprenticeship (Leavitt, 1986). Obstetrics developed a medical specialty in the 19th century and other physicians added deliveries to their functions. Deliveries were moved from the home to the hospital, where analgesics and anesthesia were used, and promises of "painless childbirth" were made.

With the advent of the trained nurse most European countries developed nurse-midwifery as a specialty. Often a collaborative agreement was made, whereby nurse-midwives handled the normal deliveries and obstetricians took over for the problem cases. Nurse-midwifery was much slower to develop in the United States and the specialty has had to struggle for its existence (Litoff, 1978).

The first American nurse-midwifery training program was established in connection with the Maternity Center of New York City in 1932 (Tom, 1982). Unfortunately, many of the graduates of the program were prevented from practicing as midwives. They had to content themselves with serving as teachers or working in hospital maternity units. Nurse-midwives encountered the least opposition in the rural areas. Their best-known trailblazer was Mary Breckenridge of Kentucky. She established a service for mothers and children, which eventually came to be called the Frontier Nursing Service. Adopting the rule that if a husband could reach the nurse at the center, the nurse could make it back to the mother, nurses traveled on horseback and foot to the isolated hill residences (Breckenridge, 1952).

While the Frontier Nursing Service became a recognized outpost of expanded nursing function, nurse-midwives continued to be much less welcome in areas where there were more physicians. Such exclusion continued, despite the fact that research evidence indicated that lives could be saved by nurse-midwives. A landmark study carried out from 1960 to 1963 provided this evidence (Levy, Wilkinson, & Marine, 1971). The demonstration project employed two nurse-midwives to manage normal deliveries at the Madera County Hospital in rural California. They gave prenatal care, attended labor and delivery, and managed the care of the mothers and infants in the postpartum period. They were successful in breaking down cultural barriers between the patients and health care providers. The number of women seeking prenatal care and other preventive services increased significantly. Even more important was the fact that, during the span of the project, prematurity and neonatal mortality rates among the patient population fell significantly. Yet, when the project sponsors sought to institutionalize the practice and secure a change in the state law, which would have allowed nurse-midwives to continue practicing, they were unsuccessful because of opposition from the California Medical Association (CMA). When the CMA opposition forced the cancellation of the project, the neonatal mortality rate went from the project rate of 10.3 per 1000 live births to 32.1 per 1000 live births (Levy et al., 1971).

Because of the positive record of both nurse-midwives and nurse practitioners in caring for women from all social strata, including the socially and economically high-risk population, the Institute of Medicine recommended:

> More reliance should be placed on nurse-midwives and nurse practitioners to increase access to prenatal care for hard-to-reach, often high-risk groups. Maternity programs designed to serve socio-

National Federation of Specialty Nursing Organizations

American Association of Critical-Care Nurses (AACN)

American Association of Neuroscience Nurses (AANN)

American Association of Nurse Anesthetists (AANA)

American Association of Occupational Health Nurses (AAOHN)

American Association of Spinal Cord Injury Nurses (AASCIN)

American College of Nurse-Midwives (ACNM)

American Nephrology Nurses' Association (ANNA)

American Public Health Association (APHA) Nursing Section

American Society of Ophthalmic Registered Nurses, Inc. (ASORN)

American Society of Plastic and Reconstructive Surgical Nurses, Inc. (ASPRSN)

American Society of Post Anesthesia Nurses (ASPAN)

American Urological Association, Allied (AUAA)

Association for Practitioners in Infection Control (APIC)

Association of Pediatric Oncology Nurses (APON)

Association of Rehabilitation Nurses (ARN)

Emergency Nurses Association (ENA)

International Association for Enterostomal Therapy, Inc. (IAET)

Intravenous Nursing Society (INS)

National Association of Orthopaedic Nurses (NAON)

National Association of Pediatric Nurse Associates and Practitioners (NAPNAP)

National Association of School Nurses, Inc. (NASN)

National Flight Nurses Association (NFNA)

National Nurses Society on Addictions (NNSA)

Nurse Consultants Association, Inc. (NCA)

The Nurses' Association of the American College of Obstetricians and Gynecologists (NAACOG)

Oncology Nursing Society (ONS)

Society of Gastrointestinal Assistants, Inc. (SGA)

Society of Otolaryngology and Head-Neck Nurses, Inc. (SOHN)

From National Federation of Specialty Nursing Organizations. Member Organizations and Participants, July 21, 1987.

the health care team as divided into workers who focused on care, and those whose job it was to cure. Nursing was thought of as the caring profession. It followed that nurses should be interested primarily in the social and psychological problems that accompany illness, rather than in treating the actual illness. Nurses were described as maternal, expressive, supportive, and feminine while physicians were described as paternal, instrumental, masculine, and cure-oriented (ANA, 1965; Johnson, 1974; Kreuter, 1957; Rogers, 1964). The nurse practitioner role combined the care and cure elements, so it did not fit the format. Probably the most outspoken of the educators who did not favor nurse practitioners was Martha Rogers. She perceived the development of the nurse practitioner role as a ploy by physicians to lead nurses into "paying obeisance to an obsolete hierarchy" (Rogers, 1972, p. 42). She wanted nursing to be an independent profession and felt that the nurse practitioner movement was a step backward. She argued that those who became nurse practitioners left the nursing profession.

Educators who accepted this way of thinking were, naturally, unwilling to accept nurse practitioner programs in their schools. Consequently the lack of acceptance by educators was a powerful barrier to the early institutionalization of the educational programs within the mainstream of nursing education. Nevertheless, there were a few university nursing schools that were willing to set up nurse practitioner programs at the master's level. Gradually the fears and hostility lessened; the educational pattern was upgraded and switched from the certificate to the master's level. Women's health is now the only practitioner field left with any appreciable number of certificate programs. The master's degree programs are the norm in all other nurse practitioner specialties (Geolot, 1987; Sultz, Henry, Kinyon, Buck, & Bullough, 1983a, 1983b).

The nurse practitioner movement is now almost 25 years old and there are more than 15,000 nurse practitioners in practice. Six major nurse practitioner specialties have now emerged: pediatric, adult, geriatric, women's health care, and family health care nurse practitioners are the major specialties in the field. (U.S. Congress, 1986).

45

Advanced Specialty Practice:
Its development and legal authorization

Bonnie Bullough, Ph.D., R.N., F.A.A.N.

EARLY CLINICAL SPECIALIZATION

Clinical specialization in nursing is primarily a 20th century phenomenon. It started informally; nurses who wanted to know more about pediatrics or operating room technique would contract to work in the appropriate setting until they developed more expertise. Gradually hospital postgraduate courses were adopted. They formalized the educational process by adding lectures and demonstrations. Nevertheless, the emphasis was on experiential learning, which was regarded as the key to specialized knowledge and skills in the field. Isabel Stewart (1933) reported that there were six postgraduate courses already in existence in 1900, and the number grew rapidly after that time. The postgraduate nursing programs offered service to the hospital as well as an educational opportunity to the student.

Table 45-1 is adapted from a list of offerings published in the *American Journal of Nursing* in 1931 (Courses, 1931). It includes 242 separate offerings. Courses lasted from 1 week to 60 weeks with a median length between 12 and 14 weeks. Apparently, the most popular specialties were operating room technique and obstetrics. Certain specialties, such as laboratory, x-ray, dietetics, and physiotherapy, have since broken off from nursing to become separate occupations. The offerings summarized in the Table 45-1 were made by 127 hospitals with some

hospitals offering several types of courses. Some of the courses were offered with alternative time frames; for example, students could take a given course for 8 or 16 weeks.

The rapid growth of the hospital postgraduate courses as the focus of specialization and the reputed economic exploitation inherent in the pattern led the National League for Nursing Education (NLNE) to start considering the issue in 1933 (Stewart, 1933). This effort was not formalized until 1943, when the NLNE established a Committee on Postgraduate Clinical Nursing courses. The Committee (1944) found postgraduate courses of various levels. Some of the courses were offered to supplement basic programs that did not include a given specialty (i.e., psychiatric or orthopedic nursing), while others were aimed at keeping nurses up to date with new developments in the field. The majority, however, were aimed at producing advanced specialists. As a result of the study the Committee made recommendations for the education of advanced nursing specialists, and their ideas laid the groundwork for the reforms that occurred later in the century. The major recommendations were that postgraduate programs should be within the collegiate structure, and that they be credit bearing. This meant that most postgraduate courses should be at the baccalaureate level, since most registered nurses did not have that

TABLE 45-1

Hospital postgraduate nursing courses available in 1931

NURSING SPECIALTY	NUMBER	LENGTH IN WEEKS (RANGE)
General medical	7	8–24
Pediatric	19	8–24
Communicable disease	11	8–16
Tuberculosis	7	8–18
Psychiatric	11	8–26
General surgical	8	8–22
Gynecological	3	8–12
Obstetric	32	8–32
Operating room technique	37	8–32
Anesthesia	20	12–24
Out patient department	6*	4–24
Laboratory	22†	12–60
X-ray	14	8–60
Dietetics	12	4–24
Administration	9	4–24
Instruction	6	12–24
Supervision	5	16–35
Other	13‡	1–44

From Courses offered for graduate nurses. (1931). *American Journal of Nursing, 31,* 612–615.

*Included one offering in public health.

†Included a combined laboratory and x-ray course.

‡Included neurology, orthopedic, ophthalmic, ear, nose and throat, physiotherapy, receiving ward, doctor's office, private duty, field missionary, and hydrotherapy nursing.

degree. In addition, the Committee urged that the programs be based on terminal objectives, and that the fieldwork be well thought out and aimed at developing desired abilities, rather than furnishing service to the institution (Committee, 1944). Although times have changed, the basic goals of the Committee are still salient.

PUBLIC HEALTH NURSING

The first specialty to break away from the on-the-job-training model used by the early postgraduate courses was public health nursing. Using the model of the hospital postgraduate courses, several of the large urban visiting nurses' associations had started postgraduate courses in their agencies. However, in 1910 Lillian Wald changed the pattern by setting up a cooperative course that involved not just the Henry Street Settlement, but also Teachers College (Gold-

mark, 1923). When the 5-year collegiate programs started developing in 1916, most of them included an option for a specialty in public health nursing. The choices were ordinarily between a specialty in nursing education or public health with an occasional administrative focus. Thus public health nursing moved away from the other nursing specialties as its collegiate preparatory programs became more institutionalized with time.

However, in the post–World War II era the collegiate educational system was realigned. Specialization according to that system was dropped as educators started talking about the baccalaureate degree as a preparatory program for all professional nurses, rather than the specialists in public health, teaching, or administration. The Bridgman Report (1953) suggested this, and the Brown Report (1948) advocated two levels of nursing. Curricula were changed. Baccalaureate programs still included pub-

economically high-risk mothers should increase their use of such providers; and state laws should be supportive of nurse-midwifery practice and of collaborations between physicians and nurse-midwives/nurse practitioners. (1985, p. 161)

NURSE ANESTHESIA

The other nursing specialty that has been emerging as a master's degree level specialty is nurse anesthesia. Nurses started giving anesthesia as early as 1889, particularly in Catholic-affiliated hospitals (Clapesattle, 1943). Education for the role started in 1909 with the establishment of a course for nurse anesthetists in Portland, Oregon. Such courses quickly proliferated, with 20 such programs in operation in 1931 as shown in Table 45-1. The movement of nurses into anesthesia was possible partly because physicians had not seen it as an attractive field for specialization. Interns or colleagues of the surgeon were often pressed into service when an anesthetic was needed. The physicians who functioned in this role ordinarily did it without additional training (Thatcher, 1953).

However, eventually some physicians began to covet the territory of the nurse anesthetists and the role was challenged in the courts. In 1917, a Kentucky judge ruled in favor of nurse anesthesia and indicated that licensure laws are not written to benefit the professions. Furthermore, he ruled that they are written for the people and the people should not be deprived of the services of nurse anesthetists (*Frank v. South*, 1934). In 1937, a group of Los Angeles physicians sued a nurse anesthetist, Dagmar Nelson, arguing that she was illegally practicing medicine in violation of the California Medical Practice Act. Both the court decision and the appeal were in favor of Nelson on the technical grounds that the operating surgeon was in charge, and thus the nurse anesthetist was not practicing independently (Thatcher, 1953). This decision did much to lessen the negative pressure from physicians, but emphasized the subordinate role of the nurse.

The nurse anesthetists asked for a special section within the American Nurses' Association in 1930

(Gunn, 1984). The effort failed, so they organized the American Association of Nurse Anesthetists in 1931. The group established a certification program in 1945, and an accreditation program for nurse anesthesia programs in 1952. Recertification became mandatory in 1978 (Gunn, 1984). A baccalaureate degree was mandated for certification in 1987 and a master's degree in 1998.

NURSE PRACTICE ACTS

The development of the advanced nursing specialties has had a significant impact on nursing practice law. Nurse practice acts developed at the beginning of the 20th century to protect both nurses and the public (Bullough, 1980). These acts were necessarily state laws rather than federal statutes because the American Constitution included no mechanism for national licensure. The early nurse practice acts recognized nurses who had gone through a formal nursing educational program and differentiated them from untrained nurses. Starting in 1938 the laws were revised to divide the nursing role into a registered nurse and a practical nurse level (Bullough, 1976). During this same era nurses were seeking mandatory licensure to make it illegal for untrained persons to practice nursing. To achieve this goal it was necessary to spell out the nursing role. Thus, scope of function statements were written into the laws. In order to avoid controversy with medicine, nurses in many states suggested to legislators that a disclaimer be written into the nurse practice act indicating that nurses would not diagnose or treat patients (Bullough, 1984).

Consequently when the first nurse practitioner programs were started in 1965, the graduates were being prepared for a role that was outside the legal scope of practice in most states. Midwifery was recognized in New Mexico and New York City, although exemptions in some of the state laws written to cover lay midwives allowed nurse-midwives to practice. An important political task for nurses and their advocates has been to update the practice acts to accommodate the expanded nursing role.

The first state to change its practice act was

TABLE 45-3
State authorization of advanced nursing practice

STATES	CLINICAL NURSE SPECIALIST	RECOGNITION OF CERTIFICATION			PROTOCOLS	OTHER
		NURSE ANESTHETIST	NURSE PRACTITIONER	NURSE MIDWIFE		
Alabama		X	X	X	X	
Alaska		X				NM covered by NP statute
Arizona			X	X		
Arkansas	X	X	X	X		
California			X	X	X	
Colorado						NM under medical practice act
Connecticut			X	X	X	
Delaware	X			X	X	
Washington, D.C.					X	Hospital licensing act
Florida	X	X	X	X	X	
Georgia	X	X	X	X	X	
Hawaii		X	X	X		
Idaho		X	X	X		
Indiana						NM under medical practice act
Iowa		X	X	X		
Kansas		X	X	X		
Kentucky		X	X	X		NM covered by NP statute
Louisiana	X	X	X	X		
Maine		X	X	X		Physician delegated
Maryland		X	X	X		
Massachusetts	X	X	X	X		
Michigan		X	X	X		
Minnesota		X		X		
Mississippi		X	X	X	X	
Missouri					X	1983 Supreme Court decision
Montana				X		
Nebraska		X	X	X	X	

Idaho. In 1971, Idaho inserted the following clause after the prohibition against diagnosis and treatment:

> . . . except as may be authorized by rules and regulations jointly promulgated by the Idaho State Board of Medicine and the Idaho Board of Nursing which shall be implemented by the Idaho Board of Nursing. (Idaho Code, 1971, §54).

Following the passage of this amendment, the combined boards met and adopted regulations that called for agencies employing nurse practitioners to draw up policies and procedures to guide nursing practice. Thus the Idaho legislature and boards established two precedents: first, to utilize the power of the boards to draw up regulations to facilitate the expanded role; and, second, to use agency-generated protocols to guide the practice of the individual nurse.

Another necessary step to the accommodation of the nurse practitioner role was to expand the basic definition of the registered professional nurse. The definition was expanded by omitting or limiting the disclaimer against diagnosis and treatment by nurses, or by rewriting the definition of the regis-

TABLE 45-3

State authorization of advanced nursing practice—cont'd.

STATES	CLINICAL NURSE SPECIALIST	RECOGNITION OF CERTIFICATION			PROTOCOLS	OTHER
		NURSE ANESTHETIST	NURSE PRACTITIONER	NURSE MIDWIFE		
Nevada			X		X	NM covered by NP statute
New Hampshire		X	X	X	X	
New Jersey						NM regulated by Board of Examiners
New Mexico		X	X	X		
New York			X		X	
North Carolina			X	X		Regulations by Board of Nursing and Medicine
North Dakota	X	X	X	X		NM covered by NP statute
Ohio				X		NM under medical practice act
Oklahoma		X	X	X		
Oregon			X	X		
Pennsylvania		X	X	X	X	NM regulated by Board of Medicine
Rhode Island						NM regulated by Department of Health Rules
Tennessee			X	X		
Texas	X	X	X	X		
Utah	X	X	X	X	X	
Vermont	X		X	X	X	
Virgin Islands				X		
Virginia		X	X	X		
Washington	X	X	X	X	X	
West Virginia		X		X		
Wisconsin				X		
Wyoming	X	X	X	X		

NM, Nurse-Midwife; NP, Nurse Practitioner.

tered nurse using broader language. New York, in 1972, was the first state to carry this out (New York State Education Law, 1972). Most states have now expanded their basic definition of the functions of the registered nurse, removing the old prohibitions against nurses diagnosing. While this facilitates an expanded role for all registered nurses, it does not cover such nurse practitioner activities as writing prescriptions for medications or ordering laboratory tests. This creates a problem because most medical practice acts forbid these practices by anyone except physicians, dentists, osteopaths, and veterinarians.

Thus a statutory change is usually needed to allow nurses to carry these responsibilities.

Table 45-3 shows the two major approaches to this type of legal authorization. A system of state certification has evolved, allowing such activities for four types of advanced nursing specialties: nurse practitioners, nurse-midwives, nurse anesthetists, and clinical nurse specialists. A second approach to coverage are laws or regulations, which say that nurses can prescribe or carry out other medical functions when they are working under standing orders or protocols. The protocol approach has become more popular in recent years because of a 1983 Missouri Supreme Court decision supporting their use (Greenlaw, 1985). Missouri is one of the states that does not certify nurse practitioners or other specialists (Missouri Statutes, 1984). A case was brought by the Medical Board against five physicians, who were working with two nurse practitioners in a family planning clinic. The Board argued that the two nurse practitioners were functioning illegally. Their physician supervisors were charged with aiding and abetting the illegal practice of medicine. The Board won its case at the circuit court level, but the case was appealed to the Missouri State Supreme Court where the decision was reversed. The Court ruled that the practice of the two nurses was legal. Although the 1975 Missouri nurse practice act did not mention nurse practitioner activities, it was a broad general act, and the legitimization of the expanded nurse functions came from the use of standing orders and protocols (Greenlaw, 1984; Wolff, 1984).

The issue of which is the best approach to legal coverage is a controversial one among nurses. The American Nurses' Association (1981) supports the Missouri model of a broad-umbrella practice act, with no mention of the specialties in the nurse practice acts. Most nurse-midwives, nurse practitioners, and the legal advisors who support them would prefer certification by the states (Bullough, 1984; Greenlaw, 1984, 1985).

SUMMARY AND CONCLUSION

During the early part of the century, specialization in nursing was accomplished by self-identification and on-the-job learning. Hospital postgraduate courses furnished a framework for this type of education. Public health nursing was the first specialty to move its educational programs into the collegiate framework. In 1965, the federal government appropriated funds to upgrade nursing education and establish broad-scale graduate education in nursing. Federal funds facilitated the development of graduate-level specialties in nursing.

Certification of specialists, by a variety of specialty organizations, is a growing trend. Certification of one or more nursing specialties is now recognized in the statutes or regulations of most of the states. This state recognition is welcomed by the nurse practitioner specialties, nurse-midwifery, and nurse anesthetists. These groups need statutory authority to protect themselves from negative sanctions by medical societies and boards. State recognition is less of an issue among the clinical nurse specialists and other nursing specialties such as critical care nurses, operating room nurses, or emergency room nurses who face fewer boundary disputes with medicine.

The ANA has published two papers that are against state recognition of the specialties, so the issue is a controversial one. Probably, the ANA position is based on the nursing theoretical position, which divides caring and curing functions and considers curing a less wholesome enterprise for nurses. This objection to state recognition is probably a passing phase. In the future, the advanced specialties will be recognized as the professional level of nursing practice, and the profession will unite in seeking state recognition of certification.

REFERENCES

American Nurses' Association (ANA). (1965). *Educational preparation for nurse practitioners and assistants to nurses: A position paper*. [Pamphlet]. New York: Author.

American Nurses' Association (ANA). (1967). *Facts about nursing: A statistical summary*. New York: Author.

American Nurses' Association (ANA). (1981). *The nursing practice act: Suggested state legislation*. Kansas City, MO: Author.

American Nurses' Association (ANA). (1987). *The career credential, professional certification: 1987 certification catalog*. Kansas City, MO: Author.

The Boston Women's Health Book Collective. (1976). *Our bodies, ourselves: A book by and for women* (2nd ed.). New York: Simon & Schuster.

Breckenridge, M. (1952). *Wide neighborhood: A study of frontier nursing service*. New York: Harper.

Bridgman, M. (1953). *Collegiate education for nursing*. New York: Russell Sage Foundation.

Brown, E. L. (1948). *Nursing for the future: A report prepared for the National Nursing Council*. New York: Russell Sage Foundation.

Bullough, B. (1976). The law and the expanding nursing role. *American Journal of Public Health, 66,* 249–254.

Bullough, B. (1980). *The law and the expanding nursing role*. New York: Appleton-Century-Crofts.

Bullough, B. (1984). The current phase in the development of nurse practice acts. *Saint Louis University Law Journal, 28*, 365–395.

Clapesattle, H. (1943). *The doctors Mayo*. New York: Garden City Publishing Co.

Committee on Postgraduate Clinical Nursing Courses. (1944). Types of clinical courses for graduate nurses. *American Journal of Nursing, 44*, 1162–1165.

Courses offered for graduate nurses. (1931). *American Journal of Nursing, 31*, 612–615.

Dickenson-Hazard, N. (1988). News from the National Board: Pediatric nurse practitioners/associates certified by the National Board of Pediatric Practitioners/Associates. *Journal of Pediatric Health Care, 2*, 162–164.

Frank v. South, 194 S.W. 375, Kentucky (1934).

Geolot, D. (1987). Nurse practitioner education: Observations from a national perspective. *Nursing Outlook, 35*, 132–135.

Goldmark, J. (1923). The Committee for the Study of Nursing Education: *Nursing and nursing education in the United States*. New York: Macmillan.

Greenlaw, J. (1984). Sermchief v. Gonzales and the debate over advanced nursing practice legislation [Commentary]. *Law, Medicine and Health Care, 12*, 30–31.

Greenlaw, J. (1985). Definition and regulation of nursing practice: An historical survey. *Law, Medicine and Health Care, 13*, 117–121.

Gunn, I. (1984). Professional territoriality and the anesthesia experience. In B. Bullough, V. Bullough, & M. C. Soukup (Eds.), *Nursing issues and nursing strategies for the eighties*. New York: Springer Publishing.

Idaho Code, § 54-1413(e), 1971 revision.

Institute of Medicine, Committee to Study the Prevention of Low Birthweight, Division of Health Promotion and Disease Prevention. (1985). *Preventing low birthweight*. Washington, DC: National Academy Press.

Johnson, D. E. (1974). Development of a theory: A requisite for nursing as a primary health profession. *Nursing Research, 23*, 372–377.

Kalisch, P. A., & Kalisch, B. J. (1978). *The advance of American nursing*. Boston: Little, Brown.

Kreuter, F. R. (1957). What is good nursing care? *Nursing Outlook, 5*, 302–304.

Leavitt, J. W. (1986). *Brought to bed: Childbearing in America, 1750 to 1950*. New York: Oxford University Press.

Levy, B. S., Wilkinson, F. S., & Marine, W. M. (1971). Reducing neonatal mortality rate with nurse-midwives. *American Journal of Obstetrics and Gynecology, 109*, 50–58.

Litoff, B. (1978). *American midwives: 1860 to present*. Westport, CT: Greenwood Press.

Missouri Statutes, 335.016(8) (1984).

New York State Education Law, Op. Title 8, Article 130, §6901, 1972 revision.

The Nurses' Association of the American College of Obstetricians and Gynecologists and the American College of Obstetricians and Gynecologists (NAACOG). (1984). *The obstetric-gynecologic nurse practitioner*. Washington, DC: Author.

Rogers, M. E. (1964). *Reveille in nursing*. Philadelphia: F. A. Davis.

Rogers, M. E. (1972). Nursing: to be or not to be. *Nursing Outlook, 20*, 42–46.

Rosenfeld, P. (1985). *Nursing student census with policy implications, 1985* (Publication No. 19-2156). New York: National League for Nursing, Division of Policy and Research.

Silver, H. K., Ford, L. C., & Day, L. R. (1968). The pediatric nurse practitioner program. *Journal of the American Medical Association, 204*, 298–302.

Stewart, I. M. (1933). Post graduate education—old and new. *American Journal of Nursing, 33*, 361–369.

Sultz, H. A., Henry, O. M., Kinyon, L. J., Buck, G. M., & Bullough, B. (1983a). Part I. A decade of change for nurse practitioners. *Nursing Outlook, 31*, 138–141, 188.

Sultz, H. A., Henry, O. M., Kinyon, L. J., Buck, G. M., & Bullough, B. (1983b). Part II. Nurse practitioners: A decade of change. *Nursing Outlook, 31*, 216–219.

Thatcher, V. S. (1953). *A history of anesthesia: With emphasis on the nurse specialist*. Philadelphia: J. B. Lippincott.

Tom, S. (1982). Nurse midwifery: A developing profession. *Law, Medicine and Health care, 10*, 262–266.

U.S. Congress, Office of Technology Assessment. (1986, December). *Nurse practitioners, physician's assistants and certified nurse-midwives: A policy analysis* (Health Technology Case Study 37, OTA-HCS-37). Washington, DC: U.S. Government Printing Office.

Wolff, M. A. (1984). NLE rounds: Court upholds expanded practice role for nurses. *Law, Medicine & Health Care, 12*, 27–29.

✳ EDITOR'S QUESTIONS FOR DISCUSSION ✳

Explicate the issues and controversies that must be resolved within the profession regarding advanced specialty practice. What application does Bullough's chapter have for those written by Murphy (Chapter 5), Snyder (Chapter 15), Yasko and Dudjak (Chapter 41), Whitney (Chapter 43), and Lyon (Chapter 44)? Delineate the significance that the advanced nursing specialties have had on nursing practice law and acts. How justifiable and appropriate is it to have nurse practice acts changed for an expanded role? How possible may the omission or limitation of the disclaimer regarding diagnosis and treatment by nurses be a loophole mechanism for nurses to practice medicine under the aegis of a nurse practice law? Should nurses legally be able to make a medical diagnosis, write prescriptions, or order laboratory tests? How justifiable is it to expand nursing roles on the basis of the public's need for a particular type of care? Should it be law that determines what nursing practice is, or should nursing practice be determined by educational professional preparation and the profession of nursing? Which comes first—the need, role, and practice or the legal mandate? What is the process by which a practice act may be changed for nursing? What are the advantages and disadvantages of having a broadly stated nurse practice act for a state in relation to the development of nursing as a profession?

What is the difference between certification, licensure, credentialing, and accreditation? Give examples of each. Should nurse educators welcome the certification of specialists and the development of graduate programs for specialty areas in nursing that may or may not require additional statutory authority for practice? What are the advantages and disadvantages of certification of nurses? What are the implications of certificate programs for doctoral education? What issues may be of particular concern regarding nurse anesthesia programs that may not be as much of a concern to the profession as other nursing specialty programs? What relationships might be further established between perioperative nursing and nurse anesthesia programs?

planning will (a) be done on a timely basis, (b) identify patients who require posthospitalization planning, (c) document the plan, and (d) identify the available resources (JCAHO, 1988). Nursing responsibilities are delineated in the "Nursing Services" chapter of the manual and specific references relating to discharge planning have a broad scope. In addition to the standards that are applicable to all nursing care, the nurse in her or his discharge planning role, must provide instructions and individualized counseling to patients. Evidence of the instructions and that the patient or family understood the instructions must be documented in the patient's medical record. Nursing administration must have policies and procedures that relate to the role of the nursing staff in discharge planning.

Not all hospitals have sought JCAHO accreditation, nor do all hospitals participate in HCFA programs. Therefore to plan, implement, and monitor a comprehensive nursing discharge planning program, a nurse administrator must be knowledgeable about accrediting, licensing, and professional organizations' requirements. All these requirements must be met and synchronized to ensure an effective program.

JCAHO publishes its standards yearly in the *Accreditation Manual for Hospitals*. The HCFA Conditions for Participation in their entirety are in the *Federal Register* (1986, pp. 22010–22051).

Third-Party Payors

The more active role assumed by third-party payors, such as the health maintenance organizations (HMOs), in the use of health care resources is evidenced by the proliferation of restrictions and qualifiers on the use of resources. Some restrictions and qualifiers are:

1. Preadmission approvals
2. Restriction on weekend admissions
3. Second opinions
4. Medical record reviews
5. Preadmission testing
6. Deductibles and copayments
7. Approval for elective surgery

The public, for the most part, is not aware of behind-the-scenes restrictions placed on health care providers until they are personally affected by these restrictions. For example, Medicare has dictated admission criteria for the admission of its beneficiaries to a hospital. Medicare, after patient record review, will deny payment to the hospital if the criteria have not been met. The intensity of service criterion (one of the admission criteria) lists such requirements as (a) the patient requires intraveneous medications or fluid replacement; (b) the patient requires intensive care treatment; or (c) the patient requires vital sign monitoring every 2 hours or less. In essence, the admission criteria demand that the patient needs acute care provided by skilled health care providers. In addition to the government, other third-party payors are participating in the decisions involving the determinants of the quality of care.

In the past, quality of care was defined by the professionals in the field. With the escalation of health care costs, the emergence of consumer awareness, and a more active third-party payor, the definers of quality have shifted from professionals in the field to business and industry, government, and the consumer (Fair, 1987).

PROGRAM ELEMENTS

The requirements as listed by Medicare and the JCAHO should be augmented with the following suggested discharge planning program elements:

1. Statements on mission, philosophy, and purpose.
   1.1 Commitment by administration to the discharge planning program.
2. Goals and objectives.
3. Definition of discharge planning or continuum of care.
4. Identification of patient population to be served.
   4.1 Needs assessment
   4.2 High-risk groups
5. Organizational structure.
   5.1 Responsibility, accountability, power (designate *who* is in charge)
   5.2 Administrative control
   5.3 Program or department

5.4 Committees

    5.41 Planning

    5.42 Advisory

6. Job descriptions, performance criteria, performance appraisal.

    6.1 Measurable criteria

7. Standards of care.

    7.1 Individualized patient care plan

8. Regulations and accreditations.

    8.1 Government

    8.2 JCAHO

    8.3 Professional health care provider organizations

9. Policies and procedures.

10. Written agreements.

11. Interdisciplinary approach.

12. Education program.

    12.1 Staff—all disciplines

    12.2 Patient and family

    12.3 Community

13. Documentation and a shared data system.

    13.1 Forms

    13.2 Established communication network between members of the multidisciplinary team.

14. Referral—open, closed, automatic.

    14.1 Case finding

15. Resources.

    15.1 Internal

    15.2 Community

16. Quality assurance mechanisms.

    16.1 Outcomes

    16.2 Follow-up

    16.3 Data collection

    16.4 Annual review of program

17. Integration of finance.

PROGRAM ELEMENTS OF SPECIAL INTEREST TO NURSING

For the chief nurse executive, the program elements that require special planning and development are:

1. The need to assess all patients. The American Nurses' Association (ANA) states: "Not every patient/client will need a referral to another institution. But every patient/client should be assessed for continuing needs" (1975, p. 6).

2. The development of a tool to identify high-risk groups relevant to the individual agency (see box, High-Risk Categories for Discharge Planning).

3. The designation of a person who, in the final analysis, will be responsible and accountable for the individual patient discharge plan. The ANA states:

> The professional nurse is in a key position to serve as the coordinator for discharge planning; . . . although the responsibility for the coordination of this program should be delegated to one health professional, the responsibility for continuity of care planning cannot be delegated. (1975, pp. 5–6)

4. The development of quality assurance mechanisms that focus on patient care outcomes.

5. The definition of what discharge planning consists of in the individual agency.

UNRESOLVED ISSUES AND PROBLEMS

With the aforementioned basic requirements in mind, the final focus of this chapter can be addressed—unresolved problems and issues in the continuum of care. The first issues are, Who should be the discharge planner and what are the position requirements?

The discharge planner title has been used inappropriately across the country. In the interests of national clarity, the title should reflect the actual duties associated with the position or the title should be banned. In some hospitals, the individual so designated is actually responsible for the discharge planning for all or a designated group of patients; in other hospitals, the individual serves as a coordinator and staff advisor. Furthermore the title may be misleading to the nursing staff. If an agency has a discharge planner, the individual nurse planning care may think that she or he need not do discharge planning since this is "the job of the discharge planner." The ANA is very clear on this particular point and states: "Every professional nurse giving direct

High-risk categories for discharge planning

I. **Age**

1. Age 70 or older living alone or with a non-capable caregiver. (Age has consistently increased over the past decade from 62 to 65 to 70+ years.)
2. Minor.

II. **Residence**

1. Any person admitted to the hospital who does not reside in the area normally served by the hospital and who may need follow-up treatment and care.
2. Transfers from other facilities.
3. Unclear or no known place of residence ("street people," indigent, abandoned).

III. **Symptomatic and behavioral factors**

1. History of noncompliance to health care plan.
2. Readmissions within 30 days.
3. Attempted suicide or suicidal tendencies.
4. Possible or active substance abuse (alcohol, chemical).
5. Manipulative, aggressive, or other behavioral problems.

IV. **Social and familial**

1. No identification—John or Jane Doe.
2. No next of kin.
3. Family problems.
4. No known social support system.
5. Domestic violence.
6. Spiritual distress.
7. Financial problems.

V. **Medical** (Based on individual hospital's top 15 to 20 DRGs or other such data that reflect population being served.)

1. Multiple trauma.
2. Head and spinal cord injury.
3. Handicapped—visual, hearing, paralysis, and other progressive degenerative or debilitating conditions.
4. Chronic conditions—COPD, CHF, CVA, or any condition that may impair body function and growth.
5. Abuse—physical, psychological, failure to thrive.
6. Psychiatric patients.
7. History of multiple hospitalizations within a short period of time.
8. Joint replacement.
9. Terminal illness.
10. AIDS.
11. Patients taking multiple medications (OTC and prescription).
12. Obstetrics—high-risk or complicated pregnancy, single parent, minor, adoption.
13. Nutritional problems.

VI. **Nursing care and social service**

1. Patients in need of follow-up treatment, teaching, or referral to other agencies.
2. Patients with inadequate financial resources.
3. Patients currently being serviced by other agencies.
4. Patients who may require special equipment in the home.
5. Patients with changes in body image (stoma, plastic repair, burn).
6. Patients with cognitive deficiencies.
7. Patients requiring transportation, housekeeping, shopping, laundry, and other supportive services.

VII. **Activity limitations**

1. Visual, hearing deficit.
2. Unable to perform ADLs.

VIII. **Legal**

1. Guardianship.
2. Power of Attorney

Adapted with permission from criteria developed by Evelyn G. Hartigan in American Hospital Association. (1987). *Communicating quality care*. Chicago: Author.

care has a responsibility to plan for the continuity of care for the patient/client" (1975, p. 6).

A discharge planner, in a pure definition then, carries out the discharge plan for a group of patients. In contrast, a discharge planning coordinator (DPC) or director has a broader scope of function. The DPC coordinates the activities of the multidisciplinary team and serves as consultant and educator to these staff members. The DPC, in cooperation with the multidisciplinary team, is responsible for the planning, implementation, and evaluation of the discharge planning *program*. The DPC role has been assumed most often by a registered nurse or a social worker, although it is not limited to these professions.

The educational preparation of the DPC has not been defined, although nursing and social worker groups are studying this particular issue. Discussion centers on whether there should be an academic or professional degree required. If so, from what discipline or major? Is certification a more realistic answer? If so, what professional body shall define the criteria and guide the program? How often should the certification be renewed?

The second area of uncertainty is what are the basic elements of discharge planning and who defines them? When does discharge planning begin? When does it end? Who can assume responsibility for the efficient use of resources as the client moves back and forth on the wellness or illness spectrum? Who can assume the role of gatekeeper to the various care options? Who can assume responsibility for the efficient and effective use of resources over a client's lifetime? Many nurses see the nurse acting as a primary care provider and being the natural gatekeeper into the health care system.

A third issue to be resolved is the cost of discharge planning both in time, money, and personnel. Many agencies have added the responsibilities for discharge planning to already overburdened staff without adding the necessary budgets to support the discharge planning program. In addition, the need for clerical staff is seldom addressed. Record keeping, form completion, and follow-up telephone calls take up an enormous amount of time and effort. To use professional health care providers, nurses, and

social service workers for performing secretarial functions is a waste of professional time and reimbursement monies.

A fourth issue is the problem relating to the patient and family. Families have difficulty coping over time with ill family members requiring constant care in the home, such as the patient discharged on a ventilator. Some families are unwilling to, or cannot, provide the care required, or may refuse recommended nursing home or other care options. Support programs for the family taking care of an ill family member are scarce and are, more often than not, provided by voluntary agencies. Furthermore these agencies are overwhelmed by the needs created by deinstitutionalization, participative care, and ambulatory care options.

A fifth area of difficulty is the problem relating to physician cooperation and participation. Common complaints from nurses attempting to plan for discharge in a timely manner are that physicians order last-minute discharges, provide little or no preparation of family and patient for discharge, resist discharge planning, and do not participate in discharge planning conferences and rounds.

Finally, there are a myriad of problems connected with the lack of facilities, such as nursing home beds, support services, and so forth. There are also major issues that need to be addressed concerning delays in processing and approving care by government and other third-party payors, cumbersome paperwork, and the lack of computer systems for the processing of data. The greatest problem facing the health care industry is the decreasing numbers of health care workers, both professional and supportive. How excellence in care can continue to be provided, in an era of decreasing manpower and in an exploding technological era, is the challenge for health care providers as we move into the twenty-first century.

CONCLUSION

In conclusion, the nurse executive must be cognizant of the elements that currently constitute a continuum-of-care program, the requirements of the various government and professional groups, the issues and problems needing realistic and timely solutions, and the obligation to develop strategies to ensure that the needs of all concerned—patient, family, staff, reimbursers—are taken into account. In order to achieve the goal of a comprehensive discharge planning program, the nurse executive must meet external mandates and also assume a proactive role in affecting health legislation at local and national levels.

REFERENCES

American Hospital Association. (1987). *Communicating quality care*. Chicago: Author.

American Nurses' Association. (1975). *Continuity of care and discharge planning programs in institutions and community agencies*. Kansas City, MO: Author.

Evashwick, C. J., & Weiss, L. J. (1987). *Managing the Continuum of Care*. Rockville, MD: Aspen Publishers.

Fair, P. A. (1987). Taking a look at the forest: How the changes in the health care system are changing. *Journal of Quality Assurance, 9*(2), 18–21.

Hartigan, E. G., & Brown, D. J. (1985). Definitions, goals, benefits, principles. In E. G. Hartigan & D. J. Brown (Eds.), *Discharge planning for continuity of care* (p. 9). New York: National League for Nursing.

Health Care Financing Administration. (1986, June 17). Medicare/Medicaid: Conditions of participation for hospitals effective September 15, 1986. *Federal Register 51*(115), 22010–22051.

Joint Commission on Accreditation of Healthcare Organizations. (1988). *1989 Accreditation manual for hospitals*. Chicago: Author.

Omnibus Budget Reconciliation Act of 1986, Public Law 99-509.

✳ EDITOR'S QUESTIONS FOR DISCUSSION ✳

What specialized knowledge base is required for the position of discharge planning coordinator? Discuss methods and means of planning for discharge from the moment that a patient is admitted to an acute care institution. Provide examples of the various means and methods of carrying out discharge planning in institutions. What is the role of the staff nurse, primary care nurse, and case manager in discharge planning? How can discharge planning be monitored and evaluated in a health care setting? How can interfaces be developed between primary care nursing and case management in institutions for health care and in home health care agencies? How can continuity of care be ensured if there is not a specific coordinator for discharge planning?

47

Home Health Care:
Responding to need, growth, and cost containment

Violet H. Barkauskas, Ph.D., R.N., F.A.A.N.

Home care has been an organized system of care in the United States for approximately 100 years. Home care was developed in response to (a) the needs and preferences of families to care for ill and infirm members at home and (b) the limitations and costs of institutional care. Although institutional care has improved significantly in safety, quality, and scope during the past century, issues of preference, appropriateness, and cost remain; these latter factors are increasingly important in selection of a site for care when choice among alternate sites is logical and possible.

Nurses developed home care, integrated home nursing care into the overall health care system, and continue to be central and essential to home care. Nurses are the largest group of professional providers of home health care. Additionally nurses supervise much of the extensive personal care and support services provided in homes by paraprofessional personnel such as home health aides and homemakers, and nurses are the commonly designated coordinators of care in situations requiring multiple health care providers.

Two relatively recent, major events have served to catapult home care into an area of heightened interest and controversy. First, the Medicare legislation of the mid-1960s established national precedent for payment of home care through universally available, government health insurance; and second, the prospective payment legislation of the 1980s heightened interest in home care as a cost-effective alternative to hospitalization or continued hospitalization.

In the late 1980s home care is a large, growing, and complex segment of the health care industry. Contemporary circumstances in the field provide an environment for challenge, opportunity, and development for nursing.

Although all services provided to individuals in homes could be considered home care, the discussion in this chapter focuses on those programs minimally providing health care to individuals and families in their homes for purposes related to restoration of health and to long-term care. The following definition for home health care from Warhola (1980) provides context for the discussion:

> Home health care is that component of a continuum of comprehensive health care whereby health services are provided to individuals and families in their places of residence for the purpose of promoting, maintaining or restoring health, or of maximizing the level of independence, while minimizing the effects of disability and illness, including terminal

illness. Services appropriate to the needs of the individual patient and family are planned, coordinated, and made available by providers organized for the delivery of home health care through the use of employed staff, contractual arrangements, or a combination of the two patterns. Home health services are made available based upon patient care needs as determined by an objective patient assessment administered by a multidisciplinary team or a single health professional. Centralized professional coordination and care management are included. These services are provided under a plan of care that includes, but is not limited to, appropriate service components such as medical, dental, nursing, social work, pharmacy, laboratory, physical therapy, nutrition, homemaker—home health aide service, transportation, chore services, and provision of medical equipment and supplies. (1980, pp. 8–9).

HISTORICAL ROLE OF NURSING IN THE DEVELOPMENT OF HOME HEALTH CARE

During the late 1800s conditions in urban areas, created by the increasing numbers of immigrants living in overcrowded and otherwise unhealthy conditions and the subsequent epidemics, stimulated the development of programs of nursing service to the sick poor. The Henry Street Settlement in New York was probably the best known effort in the provision of home and community-based nursing and social services to this population, but this effort was not unique. During this time, home care became an accepted and relatively common service, as demonstrated by the establishment of 53 formal associations of visiting nurses across the country between 1885 and 1900 (Sullivan & Friedman, 1984).

Although the primary goal of the early visiting nurses was the care of the sick poor in their homes, visiting nurses soon discovered that prevention could make a major impact on illness and the need for restorative care. Therefore, the notion of patient and family teaching for purposes related to prevention was institutionalized early, as an essential component of practice. Other premises guiding these early services was that community-based nursing practice

required family and cultural focus and additional preparation beyond the basic, hospital-based nursing education of that day (Sullivan & Friedman, 1984.)

The successful practices of visiting nurses in the care of the sick, especially in prevention, were noted by other components of society. Shortly after home care nursing was established, the principles of community-based nursing practice were applied to other groups at risk of disease and in need of health promotion intervention. Thus home care nursing served as the base for the development of other community health nursing subspecialties, specifically industrial nursing, school nursing, and aggregate-focused public health nursing.

During the first half of the 20th century, the number of agencies providing care to the sick in homes also increased, with the growth occurring primarily in visiting nurse associations and health departments. In 1966, a total of 579 official health agencies, 506 visiting nurse associations, and 83 combined services of government and voluntary agencies provided home care and represented 92% of all home health care agencies (Spiegel, 1987).

The Medicare legislation of 1965 stimulated major growth in home health care agencies and changes in the agency sponsorship as demonstrated in Table 47-1. Additionally, professional nursing's centrality in home health care was institutionalized in the Medicare legislation, which required nursing participation in home health agency policy development and skilled nursing services as components of an agency's "Conditions of Participation" with the Medicare program (Medicare Home Health Agency Manual, 1968, Section B).

In the century since home care was formalized as a health service in the United States, home care has grown not only in size but also in the scope of services provided. Whereas nursing was the almost exclusive service provided by home care agencies until the Medicare legislation, many types of professional and paraprofessional health services are available through home care agencies today. Moreover, therapies thought experimental in hospitals only a decade ago are commonly provided in homes today. Given the contemporary emphases on cost containment,

TABLE 47-1

Medicare certified home care agencies: 1966–1985

	SPONSORSHIP												
	OFFICIAL HEALTH AGENCY		VISITING NURSE ASSOCIATION		COMBINED GOVERNMENT AND VOLUNTARY AGENCY		HOSPITAL		PROPRIETARY		OTHER		
YEAR	NO.	%	NO.	%	NO.	%	NO.	%	NO.	%	NO.	%	TOTAL
1966	579	45%	506	40%	83	7%	81	6%	0	0%	26	2%	1275
1975	1228	52%	525	22%	46	2%	287	12%	47	2%	212	9%	2345
1980	1253	41%	506	17%	59	2%	401	13%	230	8%	603	20%	3052
1985	1217	20%	519	9%	56	1%	1255	21%	1929	32%	986	17%	5962

Adapted from Spiegel, A. D., (1987). *Home health care* (2nd ed.). Owings Mills, MD: Rynd Publications. Copyright © 1987 by National Health Publishing. Used with permission of the publisher.

self-care, ambulatory care, and the large and growing number of elderly in communities, home care will continue to increase in prominence within the American health care system.

CURRENT ISSUES
The Financial Bases of Services

Currently home care is largely financed through third-party insurance, with the largest insurer being the federal and state governments through the Medicare, Medicaid, Title XX, and Older American Acts programs (Fisher, 1986). In addition, funding for home care is available through commercial health insurance companies and health maintenance organizations. Free home health care is irregularly available through philanthropic organizations and local governmental agencies. Because a large portion of home health care will be financed through public health insurance programs, home care will be in the public health policy domain for the foreseeable future (Grazier, 1986; Knollmueller, 1984).

In addition to displaying the overall growth of home care agencies, Table 47-1 also records the profound influence of funding availability on structure and sponsorship of home care agencies, which today reflect diverse sponsorship. The fastest growing types of home health agencies are those sponsored by hospitals and proprietary agencies.

Prospective payment, the health financing para-

digm of the 1980s, has had significant, both positive and negative, impact on home care. Prospective payment's incentive to reduce hospital costs through early discharge has resulted in increased home care need for patients who are being discharged quicker and sicker. However, the same cost-containment policy, which generated prospective payment for inpatient care, also has been directed to the home care field—the fastest growing sector of the health care system. Home care is experiencing unprecedented scrutiny of its agencies, practices, services, and utilization patterns (Bishop & Stassen, 1986; U.S. General Accounting Office, 1987).

Indication exists that prospective payment will be applied to home care (Van Gelder & Stassen, 1986). However, the notion of fixing a price for services in advance and by episode of care or for a specified time period is especially complicated when applied to home health care, for several reasons. First, the historical, retrospective payment mechanism in home care has been charge per visit for professional visits and charge per hour for paraprofessional services. Operationally, professional visits in home care have varied greatly in length of direct care time and are subject to additional variation in indirect care time, for example, because of travel and coordination activities and services. Second, a standardized resource allocation index for an episode of care, such as days of hospital length of stay, does not currently exist for home care.

Quality of Care

Given the remote and isolated context in which home care services are delivered, the assessment and maintenance of quality care in the field is a major concern. Home care is generally provided in patients' homes and unobserved by others except patients and family members. Additionally, the individuals providing care to the same patient usually do not encounter each other either in the patient's home or elsewhere. Therefore, the quality of care is largely indirectly monitored, primarily through the documentation in patients' records. The covertness of practice and the associated issues of quality have been designated a "black box" by the American Bar Association (1986) in recent testimony to Congress.

A large portion of the home care is provided (a) by home health aides, who are legally accountable to nursing for delegated nursing functions, and (b) by homemakers, who may be supervised by a variety of health care professionals. The quality and safety of the care of home health aides and homemakers have recently received significant public attention; paraprofessionals in home care have been indicted for various crimes against their patients, including theft and murder. Incumbents in these roles tend to have low educational levels and to come from low-income and other disadvantaged groups. The frustrations and temptations inherent in isolated care situations are major risk management issues for home care nursing.

Although nurses are involved in the training and supervision of paraprofessionals in home care, organized nursing has done little to develop and assure standards for their training and supervision. Given the increasing dependence of the elderly and handicapped on paraprofessional home care providers, the need for safeguards is urgent. Because the care provided by paraprofessional health care providers is largely delegated nursing function, the involvement of organized nursing in policies and issues related to their practice is relevant, responsible, and overdue.

Prediction of Utilization

Various researchers and policy analysts have considered methods to apply the major health care fi-nancing paradigm of the 1980s—prospective payment according to some patient classification system—to home care. The diagnosis related group (DRG) system for classifying patients for hospital services is considered inadequate for home care because it does not take into account the nursing problems and needs of patients, the resources available within homes, nor environmental factors affecting patients and their care. Moreover, although length of stay is an adequate financial index for hospitalized patients, the concept has little meaning for home care; patients with identical lengths of stay consume varying amounts of resources across agencies and geographical regions, measured by numbers of encounters or hours of direct and indirect service (Ballard & McNamara, 1983; Benjamin, 1985; Berk & Bernstein, 1985). In home care, some index of resources used—rather than length of stay—will have more meaning because of the largely part-time and intermittent nature of most home care service programs.

Various factors have impact on the establishment of a prospective payment system for home care. Such influences include lack of an adequate, historical data base for documenting amount of service provided across categories of patients; lack of a standardized data base for describing patients; lack of criteria for assessing outcomes of services; lack of standardized criteria for determining needs and allocating resources; and lack of a formula to measure resource deficits, given the abilities of the patient and informal caregiver contribution.

Because it is likely that some type of prospective payment or capitation system for home care will be established for home care in the near future, a patient classification system for resource allocation is essential. A number of nursing, practice-based tools for classification are in development. These include the following:

1. A five-group classification system was developed by the Visiting Nurse Association of New Haven to measure rehabilitation potential of patients (Daubert, 1979). This system has been used in quality assurance programs and as a basis for care plan development. However, categories are probably too general to

measure potential resource needs with any precision.

2. The Visiting Nurse Association of Omaha (Martin, Scheet, Crews, & Simmons, 1986; Simmons, 1980), developed and validated a classification scheme for nursing diagnoses managed in community health programs. The scheme includes 40 health problems in environmental, psychosocial, physiological, and health-related behaviors areas. Although the problems inventoried in the system have utility for planning and communication, their relationship to resource utilization is unknown.

3. A caseload or work load analysis tool developed by Allen, Easley, and Storfjell (1986) classifies patients according to difficulty based on clinical judgment of assessed teaching, physical care, and psychosocial needs. The validity, reliability, and predictive ability of this tool have not been evaluated.

4. The Visiting Nurse Association of Los Angeles (Churness, Kleffel, Jacobson, & Onodera, 1986) developed a home health service patient classification system reflecting the amount of skilled nursing care required by patients with specific treatment needs. These investigators noted significant variability in nursing visit time for similar treatment needs and identified some of the factors affecting length of nursing visit.

Other attempts to identify and measure the effects of nursing and other provided home care services on home care patients have been published (Hardy, 1984; Harris, Santoferraro, & Silva, 1985; Larson & Cerniglia-Lowensen, 1987; Roeder, 1984). Generally these studies have demonstrated broad variability in resource use among patients, as measured by total number of visits, scope of services provided by health professional and ancillary personnel within visits, amount of time allocated to visits, and total cost for an episode of care. However, most of the measurement efforts have been limited by (a) tools whose validity and reliability have not been established, (b) small sample sizes, and (c) data collection limited to a few agencies or only one agency.

Productivity

Productivity, a major issue in all health care systems, is especially complicated in home care. Some of the major, time-related factors are out of the control of agencies—specifically travel time, amounts of resources available in homes, obstacles to care in homes and communities, unpredictable situations in homes, and amounts of indirect services (usually not reimbursable) needed by some clients, for example, report of new symptoms to a physician, arranging transportation to a clinic, or the amount of documentation required by third-party payors.

The current fee-per-visit fee structure for home care reimbursement serves as an *incentive* for numerous, short, focused, treatment-oriented visits by health care providers and, in contrast, such a structure serves as a *disincentive* for family-focused, comprehensive care with thorough follow-up and coordination. A prospective payment or a capitation system of reimbursement for home care could allow for flexibility and experimentation in site, length, and content of encounters based on needs and problems. However—given the goal of cost containment in any system—data, monitoring, and discipline are needed to assure that fixed resources are appropriately shared across an aggregate of clients.

NURSING ISSUES
Control of Nursing Practice Within Home Health Care

The Medicare health insurance program is only one of the mechanisms by which nurses are reimbursed for home care services. However, the role of nursing in home health care warrants analysis from the perspective of the Medicare program operations because it is the major funding source for home care services and serves as a model for other government and private insurance benefits. Two anomalies in the Medicare program have had substantive effect on nursing practice; these are (a) the focus on acute care benefits when the major health problems of the elderly are either chronic illnesses or are affected by the presence of chronic illnesses, and (b) the major deference to physician control of reimbursable services.

Although physicians have not been a major group of home health care providers, physicians are required to authorize all home care services in the Medicare program. Operationally, although physicians are involved in decisions for and authorize referrals to home care, plans of treatment for home care are usually completed either by discharge planners in hospitals or by nurses in home care agencies after the first assessment visit. In the case of hospital-initiated referrals, the plans of treatment often require alteration because of unique circumstances of particular home situations. Although physicians are the undisputed experts in delegated medical functions, physicians are the gatekeepers of care for all other home care professionals. In a recent article, Reinhard (1986) discusses the limitations of the medical model in directing public policy in health care reimbursement for the elderly, whose health needs are more oriented to nursing services than medical services.

Although Medicare regulations acknowledge the competencies of registered nurses in health teaching, coordination, and similar activities, reimbursement is allowed only for skilled, intermittent nursing services to homebound patients. To meet the requirement of skilled nursing, the patient must need services either because a technical procedure is required or because the patient's condition is so unstable that a less technical procedure would be unsafe unless performed by a registered nurse (*Medicare Home Health Agency Manual*, 1968).

Largely in response to patient needs, evidence exists that nurses have been negligent in adhering to Medicare funding regulations and have requested and received Medicare reimbursement for services other than those specified in the Medicare legislation and regulations. Various studies have documented nurses' predilection toward overprovision of services and reluctance to discharge patients when the justification for reimbursable services has ceased (Mundinger, 1983; U.S. General Accounting Office, 1979, 1981). The patient advocacy demonstrated in the evidence is laudable, but over time, "backdoor" approaches to funding services have created an aura of fiscal irresponsibility around the profession that invites scrutiny. If patients are not receiving needed services and are being harmed by denial or inaccessibility, documentation and lobbying advocacy approaches are more appropriate than manipulation of documentation.

Care of the Caregivers

Community-based nursing practice has a strong history of philosophical orientation toward family-centered care, in which family is viewed as client, resource, and environment. Current home care issues impacting nurses' interactions and interventions with caregivers include the following: (a) the demand for more "in-kind" contribution from the family in the home care of its members; (b) the growing complexity of the care needs of home care clients; and (c) increasing numbers of very sick clients being maintained in their homes. Logically nurses should be paying increasing attention to the learning, counseling, and support needs of informal health care providers. The paradox here is that, while third-party agencies presume family care to be necessary to support patient care, nursing care to families in behalf of their own or the client's health is an inconsistently reimbursable service in most funding programs and rarely deemed a sufficient, exclusive reason for reimbursement of services.

In addition to general family needs in the cases of acute illness and altering responses to chronic illnesses, respite care is increasingly being recognized as useful in an effective home care system. Respite care provides various types of concrete intermittent relief to the caregiver and enables the caregiver to remain in the role (Hooyman, Gonyea, & Montgomery, 1985). Examples include "time off" for families who are involved with 24-hour care of chronically ill persons, often children who are homebound and dependent on technological life support systems. Often home care agencies participate in the identification of families needing respite care and coordinate such services using paid professional or paraprofessional workers or volunteers.

Caregivers reflect varying competencies, commitments, and needs. Caregiver status must be assessed to determine services needed, to assess safety of home care, and to determine the extent to which the caregiver can participate in care. A special and increasingly prevalent problem in home care for the elderly is that the caregivers of many elderly patients are themselves elderly, and they have low physical tolerance for intensive caregiving over extended periods of time. Nurses have identified the at-risk status of caregivers and are experimenting with group-based interventions with them (Pesznecker & Zahlis, 1986). However, much more study is needed to determine the needs of caregivers and to design relevant, efficient interventions.

The development of valid and reliable tools for the assessment of caregiver competencies, such as the cost of care index (Kosberg & Cairl, 1986), are imperative for nursing practice. Use of such tools could not only justify the need for professional nursing interventions with caregivers, but also evaluate the efficacy of such interventions.

Measurement of Nursing Practice and Its Effectiveness

The unit of service in home health care, both for statistical as well as reporting purposes, has been the home visit. This unit of service measurement is too global to describe adequately or evaluate nursing practice. Funding agencies have required some specification of provided services as components of the documentation required for reimbursement; nonetheless, the usual listing of reimbursed services consists primarily of physical treatments and services. Such listing tends to omit many of the other domains of nursing practice, for example, counseling, work with caregivers, referral, and coordination services.

The development of a taxonomy of nursing services is a priority for all the specialties in nursing. Given the "covertness" of home care nursing, the need for a standardized, valid, and reliable taxonomy is perhaps even more critical to that field. Several researchers have completed preliminary work toward the development of taxonomies of services (Barkauskas, 1987; Martin et al., 1986). Striking agreement exists among the preliminary taxonomies developed through various methods in different agencies. Therefore, the establishment of a taxonomy for the field is close, but additional research is required.

The concern about cost has heightened the urgency for nursing to continue the exploration of the effectiveness of its services. Demonstration of the effectiveness of nursing is complicated by a number of situational factors. These include the relatively short total amount of time in nurse-patient encounters, especially in home care; the multidisciplinary context of health care; and nursing's focus on preventive and supportive care.

An outcome scheme for home care has been developed by Martin et al. (1986). Using both medical and nursing diagnoses as the bases, each health problem is ordinarily scored—at admission and after a period of intervention—according to change in the following areas: knowledge, behavior, and status. The scheme has not yet been tested for reliability and validity, but it holds promise in pilot testing.

Coordination with Remote Health Care Providers

Nurses, through assignment or default, often assume the role of patient care coordinators. Reasons for this include: (a) nurses are the most ubiquitous home care providers; (b) they often develop the plan of care; and (c) they are responsible for the referrals to other home health care providers. In contrast to the situation in other health care systems, the members of the "team" providing care to a given home care patient are unlikely to be working for the same agency, unlikely to have met each other before, and unlikely to meet in the course of care for a given patient. Therefore, it becomes a burden of the patient, the caregivers, and the nurses to maintain a sense of organization and evaluation in particular cases.

Although nurses are logical case managers for patients needing complex care arrangements or long-term, community-based care, a number of current organizational arrangements relating to nursing in home care agencies mitigates against nursing's systematic development of this role. Specifically, one such factor is the encouragement of nurses and other staff to work from their homes (rather than offices), because of the costs of travel and office time.

Another deterrent is the hiring of a significant and growing number of contract or per diem nurses, which increases the documentation and coordination load on the full-time and supervisory staff within agencies. Given these conditions, nurses' abilities to be case managers in many patient situations may be limited by and may vary according to agency structure and operations.

Education of Nursing Practitioners

Although all baccalaureate students receive experience in community health nursing and many baccalaureate nursing students receive some experience in home care, preparation in home care is not required within undergraduate nursing education programs. Nor is preparation in community health nursing required in associate degree or diploma programs in nursing. Therefore, no basic nursing program predictably prepares staff nurses for the home care field; the orientation to the field and the continuing education within it is largely a function of the service sector.

One of the reasons for inconsistency in preparation for home care is that home care experiences for the basic student are difficult to organize and execute. The largely independent nature of practice creates difficulties with student supervision, which largely must be done vicariously through conferences and recording. Complexity of documentation, and related reimbursement regulations, compounded by concerns about payment denials, cause home care administrators concern about intermittent, novice practitioners. The part-time and structured nature of the scheduling of student experiences creates conflicts with patients' potential needs for follow-up, continuity, and coordination. Because of legal and reimbursement issues, agencies are sometimes reluctant to provide experiences, except to only the most advanced of undergraduate students.

Given the growth in the field and the growing need for staff nurses in home care, it is imperative that nursing students receive minimally adequate preparation for generalist roles in home care. The notion of minimal adequacy for home care has yet to be discussed formally by the nursing profession, but

it would seem to be an important agenda item. Community and family care are well emphasized in a recent publication, *Essentials of College and University Education for Professional Nursing* by the American Association of Colleges of Nursing (1986), which could serve as a base for the discussion.

Graduate preparation for home care roles is a recent innovation in nursing. The first program to be funded by the Advanced Nurse Training Grant Program of the Division of Nursing (U.S. Department of Health and Human Services) was conceptualized as a subspecialty within community health nursing (Barkauskas, Clemen-Stone, Blaha, & Smith, 1984). This program was initiated in 1984. Strong, documented interest in home care by graduate program leadership suggests that a substantive number of graduate programs will include home care educational options within the next decade (Barkauskas, Blaha, & Ging, 1986).

Maintenance of clinical competence is a major issue for home care nurses and employing agencies, especially those based solely in the community. Contributing factors are the isolation of home care practice; the infrequency of contact with colleagues; and the rapidity with which therapies, initially designed for institutional application, are being developed and integrated into the home. Evidence exists that learned skills atrophy over time in home care practice without learning reinforcement (Clarke, Goggin, Webber-Jones, Vacek, & Aderholdt, 1986). Nursing staff within hospital-based home care agencies potentially have access to colleagues, consultants, and other resources within the same institution (Lerman, 1987).

FUTURE POTENTIAL FOR HOME CARE NURSING

There is strong evidence that the trend from institutional care to community-based and home care will continue (Somers, 1986). Evidence is found in demographic trends, cost-containment initiatives, and client's preferences.

The projected, dramatic increases in the numbers of elderly in the population and the associated proportion represented by them in the population, as well as increased longevity, have strong implications for the growth of community-based health services. The elderly's need for and increasing use of home care services is well documented (Hogstel, 1985; Stone, 1986; U.S. General Accounting Office, 1977, 1986).

It is likely that all health insurance will be organized around some type of prospective payment or capitation arrangement, in which the responsibility of the health care agency will be to provide adequate care for fixed, predictable costs (Van Gelder & Stassen, 1986). In this system, the health care agency will have significant flexibility regarding the services provided within general guidelines of the funding agency. This situation could stimulate responsible, individualized allocation of resources to patients according to needs and circumstances, or it could generate a "stinginess" or restriction of access that might be harmful to patients (Newman & Autio, 1986).

Various studies have indicated that home health care is a cost-effective alternative for institutional care for patients needing short-term services related to acute illnesses, in which the institutional alternative is usually extended acute hospitalization and the cost per day is hundreds of dollars. However, the findings are inconsistent among studies of long-term home care services, in which the alternative is nursing home care and the cost per day is usually under $100 per day (Capitman, 1986; Capitman, Haskins, & Bernstein, 1986; Gaumer et al., 1986; Hughes, 1985; Hughes, Corday, & Spiker, 1984; Palmer, 1982).

Clients are becoming increasingly vocal about their preferences for home and community-based care, and they are seeking assistance for self-care (Friedman, 1986). This trend is appropriate because partnership between consumers and providers holds promise for achievement of the primary governmental goal of cost containment.

The strong institutionalization and need for community-based and home care services in the United States will continue to provide a structure for the development of home care nursing for some time to come. Nurses are notable among health care providers as having aptness for determining the needs of

populations and matching resources with needs. They continue to be acceptable health care providers with broad-based, generalist skills and a knowledge base sufficient for the provision of a variety of commonly needed health care services.

Areas of particular importance to nursing care in the home relate to (a) the establishment of the nurse as a formal case manager in appropriate situations, (b) the continued integration of technology into the home, and (c) the use of computers in home care. Contemporary demographics and the changing picture of contemporary families will create case management needs for large numbers of elderly living alone. Whereas nurses have been informal case managers for many years, availability of reimbursement has produced competition and confusion among health professionals for the provision of formal, case management services (Levine & Fleming, 1986). Although many types of health professionals can be appropriate case managers, it is important that nurses continue to articulate abilities and develop strengths in this area of practice.

Hospital-based technology will continue to be integrated into the home. As this occurs, both hospital-based and community-based nurses need to provide leadership in evaluating the safety of home management and the mechanisms by which patients and caregivers can most effectively manage therapies and their associated sequelae.

Computer technology holds major promise for participating in the resolution of many problematic aspects of home care. Computers can facilitate communication among patients and health care providers, communication among health care providers, documentation, coordination of care, and patient education. Therefore, it would be logical for nurses to (a) conceptualize application of computer technology, (b) establish linkages with technological disciplines leading the development of computer applications, and (c) experiment with applications.

Nurses need to research and develop their roles in home care, as well as the home care field itself. The material presented in this chapter has indicated major knowledge deficits regarding the clients of nursing services, the services provided, and the effects of services. Therefore, nurses have little other than anecdotal material and humanistic values to contribute to the ongoing debates on public policies that will strongly influence the design of home care delivery. Tensions among need, cost, and quality will continue into the future, and nurses will need to understand the related issues and debates and to participate in the development and evaluation of resolutions (Hogstel, 1985; Mundinger, 1983; Stuart-Siddall, 1986).

REFERENCES

Allen, C. E., Easley, C., & Storfjell, J. I. (1986). Cost management through caseload/workload analysis. In F. A. Shaffer (Ed.), *Patients and purse strings: Patient classification and cost management* (pp. 331–346). New York: National League for Nursing.

American Association of Colleges of Nursing. (1986). *Essentials of college and university education for professional nursing*. Washington, DC: Author.

American Bar Association. (1986). *The black box of home care quality: A report presented by the chairman of the Select Committee on Aging, House of Representatives*. Washington, DC: U.S. Government Printing Office.

Ballard, S., & McNamara, R. (1983). Quantifying nursing needs in home health care. *Nursing Research, 32,* 236–241.

Barkauskas, V. H. (1987). *Taxonomy for nursing home care services*. Unpublished manuscript, Visiting Nurse Service of New York.

Barkauskas, V. H., Blaha, A. J., & Ging, T. (1986, September). *Current status of graduate nursing education in home health care*. Paper presented at the Annual Meeting of the American Public Health Association, Las Vegas, NV.

Barkauskas, V. H., Clemen-Stone, S., Blaha, A. J., & Smith, A. S. (1984, November). *Essential graduate curriculum content for the preparation of nurse managers for home health care*. Paper presented at the Annual Meeting of the American Public Health Association, Anaheim, CA.

Benjamin, A. E. (1985). Determinants of state variations in home health utilization and expenditures under Medicare. *Medical Care, 24,* 535–547.

Berk, M. L., & Bernstein, A. (1985). Use of home health services: Some findings from the National Medical Care Expenditure Survey. *Home Health Care Services Quarterly, 6*(1), 13–23.

Bishop, C. E., & Stassen, M. (1986). Prospective reimbursement for home health care: Context for an evolving policy. *Pride Institute Journal of Long Term Health Care, 5*(1), 17–26.

Capitman, J. A. (1986). Community-based long-term care models, target groups, and impacts on service. *Gerontologist, 26,* 389–397.

Capitman, J. A., Haskins, B., & Bernstein, J. (1986). Case management approaches in coordinated community-oriented long-term care demonstrations. *Gerontologist, 26,* 398–404.

Churness, V. H., Kleffel, D., Jacobson, J., & Onodera, M. (1986). Development of a patient classification system for home health nursing. In F. A. Shaffer (Ed.), *Patients and purse strings: Patient classification and cost management* (pp. 319–330). New York: National League for Nursing.

Clarke, J. H., Goggin, J. E., Webber-Jones, J. E., Vacek, P. M., & Aderholdt, S. (1986). Educating rural home health care nurses in respiratory assessment: An evaluation study. *Public Health Nursing, 3,* 101–110.

Daubert, E. A. (1979). A patient classification system and outcome criteria. *Nursing Outlook, 6,* 450–454.

Fisher, R. (1986). *Review of home health care payor practices and related literature*. Unpublished paper, Center for Health Policy Studies, Columbia, MD.

Friedman, J. (1986). *Home health care: A complete guide for patients and their families*. New York: W. W. Norton.

Gaumer, G. L., Birnbaum, H., Pratter, F., Burke, R., Franklin, S., & Ellingson-Otto, K. (1986). Impact of the New York long-term home health care program. *Medical Care, 24,* 641–653.

Grazier, K. L. (1986). The impact of reimbursement policy on home health care. *Pride Institute Journal of Long Term Health Care, 5*(1), 12–16.

Hardy, J. A. (1984). A patient classification system for home health patients. *Caring, 3*(9), 26–27.

Harris, M. D., Santoferraro, C., & Silva, S. (1985). A patient classification system in home health care. *Nursing Economics, 3,* 278–282.

Hogstel, M. O. (1985). *Home nursing care for the elderly*. Bowie, MD: Brady Communications Co.

Hooyman, N., Gonyea, J., & Montgomery, R. (1985). The impact of in-home services termination on care givers. *Gerontologist, 25,* 141–145.

Hughes, S. L. (1985). Apples and oranges? A review of evaluations of community-based long-term care. *Health Services Research, 20,* 461–488.

Hughes, S. L., Corday, D. S., & Spiker, V. A. (1984). Evaluation of a long-term home care program. *Medical Care, 22,* 460–476.

Knollmueller, R. N. (1984). Funding home care in a climate of cost containment. *Public Health Nursing, 1*(1), 16–22.

Kosberg, J. I., & Cairl, R. E. (1986). The cost of care index: A case management tool for screening informal care providers. *Gerontologist, 3*, 273–278.

Larson, E., & Cerniglia-Lowensen, J. (1987). State case mix systems for reimbursing long-term care for the elderly. *Nursing Economics, 5*(2), 77–81.

Lerman, D. (Ed.). (1987). *Home care: Positioning the hospital for the future*. Chicago: American Hospital Publishing, Inc.

Levine, I. S., & Fleming, M. (1986). *Human resource development: Issues in case management*. Rockville, MD: National Institute of Mental Health.

Martin, K. S., Scheet, N. J., Crews, C. C., & Simmons, D. A. (1986). *Client management information system for community health nursing agencies,* (NTIS Accession No. HRP-0907023). Washington, DC: Division of Nursing, USDHHS.

Medicare Home Health Agency Manual (Publication No. 11). (1968). Washington, DC: U.S. Department of Health and Human Services, Health Care Financing Administration.

Mundinger, M. O. (1983). *Home care controversy: Too little, too late, too costly*. Rockville, MD: Aspen Systems Corporation.

Newman, M., & Autio, S. (1986). *Nursing in a prospective payment system health care environment*. Minneapolis: University of Minnesota.

Palmer, H. (1982). Home care. In R. J. Vogel & H. C. Palmer (Eds.), *Long-term care: Perspectives from research and demonstrations* (pp. 337–390). Washington, DC: U.S. Department of Health and Human Services, Health Care Financing Administration.

Pesznecker, B. L., & Zahlis, E. (1986). Establishing mutual-help groups for family-member care givers: A new role for community health nurses. *Public Health Nursing, 3*(1), 29–37.

Reinhard, S. (1986). Financing long-term health care of the elderly: Dismantling the medical model. *Public Health Nursing, 3*(1), 3–22.

Roeder, B. (1984). Diagnosis-specific home care: A model for the future. *Caring, 2*(12), 39–42.

Simmons, D. (1980). *A classification scheme for client problems in community health nursing* (DHHS Publication No. HRA 80-16 HRP-0501501). Washington, DC: U.S. Department of Health and Human Services.

Somers, A. R. (1986). The changing demand for health services: A historical perspective and some thoughts for the future. *Inquiry, 23*, 395–402.

Spiegel, A. D. (1987). *Home Health Care* (2nd ed.). Owings Mills, MD: Rynd Publications.

Stuart-Siddall, S. (1986). *Home health care nursing: Administrative and clinical perspectives*. Rockville, MD: Aspen Systems Corporation.

Stone, R. (1986). Aging in the eighties, age 65 years and over-use of community services (DHHS Publication No. PHS 86-1250). *NCHS Advance Data from Vital and Health Statistics*. Hyattsville, MD: Public Health Service, National Center for Health Statistics.

Sullivan, J. A., & Friedman, M. M. (1984). History of nursing in the community: From the beginning. In J. A. Sullivan (Ed), *Directions in community health nursing* (pp. 3–43). Boston: Blackwell Scientific Publications.

U.S. General Accounting Office. (1977). *Home health— The need for a national policy to better provide for the elderly*. (Report No./GAO/HRD 78-19). Washington, DC: Author.

U.S. General Accounting Office. (1979). *Home health care services—Tighter controls needed* (Report No./GAO/HRD-79-17). Washington, DC: Author.

U.S. General Accounting Office. (1981). *Medicare home health services: A difficult program to control* (Report No./GAO/HRD-81-155). Washington, DC: Author.

U.S. General Accounting Office. (1986). *Elderly needs and costs* (Report No./GAO/HRD-86-135). Washington, DC: Author.

U.S. General Accounting Office. (1987). *Medicare: Need to strengthen home health care payment controls and address unmet needs* (Report No. GAO/HRD-87-9). Washington, DC: Author.

Van Gelder, S., & Stassen, M. (1986). Home health care in the era of hospital prospective payment: Evidence and thoughts about the future. *Pride Institute Journal of Long Term Health Care, 5*(1), 3–11.

Warhola, C. R. (1980). *Planning for home health services: A resource handbook* (DHHS Publication No. HRA 80-14017). Washington, DC: U.S. Department of Health and Human Services.

✳   **EDITOR'S QUESTIONS FOR DISCUSSION**   ✳

How has prospective payment impacted home care? Discuss how the factors can be resolved that have impacted the establishment of a prospective payment system for home care. What is the likelihood that all health insurance will be organized around some type of prospective payment or capitation arrangement in the future? What variables need to be considered regarding a prospective payment or capitation system of reimbursement for home care? What political strategies, mechanisms, and processes should be considered and implemented to change the Medicare program requirements to make it possible for nurses to authorize and be reimbursed for home care services? What might be the role of discharge planners in acute care, long-term care, extended care, or intermediate care facilities for authorizing home care, health care visits, and reimbursement for nurses? What provisions need to be considered for reimbursement of services to caregivers in a home care situation?

What is the status of developing a patient classification system and taxonomy of nursing services in home care? What issues are involved in terms of measuring, monitoring, and evaluating the quality of care in home care situations? How might clinical competence be assured and maintained for home care nurses and employing agencies? What should be the preparation necessary for nurses providing professional home health care services? How might the role of case manager be defined in home care? How might home care experiences best be designed for the generic nursing student? What alternative models might be used for nursing students for learning experience in home care? What are the possible applications of computer technology in home care?

48

A World View of Nursing Practice:
An international perspective

Barbara J. Brown, Ed.D., R.N., F.A.A.N.

No matter where the nurse is educated or in what society she or he is practicing, international nursing has a common base of knowledge, skills, and competencies. The founder of modern nursing, Florence Nightingale, has probably had a greater influence on the care of the sick than any other single individual (Kelly, 1985). The image of Florence Nightingale as the "gentle, caring Lady of the Lamp, caring, full of compassion for the soldiers of the Crimean" (Pavey, cited in Kelly, 1985, p.34) is an accurate one, but no more so than that of the strong-willed administrator who used her considerable knowledge of sanitation, nutrition, logistics, statistics, and politics to develop a new system of nursing education, practice, and overall health care.

The nursing profession has expanded vastly since the days of Florence Nightingale. However, throughout the world not all of the criteria of professionalism are yet met. Nursing remains the only health profession in which most of its practitioners are educated at less than baccalaureate level. Furthermore many nurses lack commitment to the profession. The very society in which they live frequently makes it difficult for women to have such a commitment for a career or lifework. Contemporary Western world nursing has struggled through the admonitions of Florence Nightingale in "qualifying ourselves—as a man does for his work" (Kelly, 1985, p.34). Miss Nightin-

gale saw nursing as a professive art, in which to stand still was to go backward. She advocated continuing education and professional development, saying:

A woman who thinks of herself, now I am a full nurse, a skillful nurse, I have learned all there is to be learned. Take my word for it, she does not know what nursing is and she will never know. She has gone back already. (Pavey, cited in Kelly, 1985, p. 34).

International nursing practice requires the utmost in adaptation, flexibility, innovation, and creativity in addition to, above all, upholding the basis and foundation of nursing practice. Adaptation to nursing practice internationally is based on variations in organizational cultures—those deep sets of beliefs about the way work should be organized and the manner in which authority should be exercised. For example, reward and control of organizational members usually is different in an international organizational culture. Moreover, time perspective and planning vary, and the degree of conformity and initiative of subordinates that is considered desirable is usually significantly less than in the Western world. Other potential differences are the individual and collective decision-making and control processes that operate. The key to adaptation to organizational culture is recognition and acceptance of the kinds of people that the organization employs. Factors involved are the nature of career aspirations of the employees, their social status, their occupational mobility, and their prior education.

ADJUSTMENT TO LIVING AND WORKING IN A NEW CULTURE

An international nurse must adjust to the work environment and living conditions in a new culture. Each location of practice has its endemic socioeconomic and educational requirements and a known concept of community living from birth to death. There must be constant interaction between the nurse and nurses of other nationalities, including but not limited to those of the country in which the nurse is practicing; furthermore work and social life must be integrated. Language represents a crucial factor in international nursing practice. In such an environment, the necessity for working in a language that is completely strange and of working through interpreters is a struggle. The difficulty is compounded when there are nurses from many different nationalities working in a foreign country, each of whom has a different foundation in a common language. The problem is even further exacerbated when none of these nurses are able to speak the language of the people being served. Identifying common nursing terminology and methods of practice and developing an international nursing model become a great challenge in such a setting.

To adjust to living and working in a new culture, it is important that the nurse relaxes and enjoys easy communication with people from the nurse's own social contacts. Nursing practice is influenced almost imperceptibly by the international nurse's attitude toward local people and especially toward national counterparts, colleagues, and administrators with whom the nurse has contact.

The nurse's attitude toward the culture of the people will either ease adjustment to a new cultural situation or make it more difficult. Making the individual adjustment in personal life and contacts is crucial for adjustment in an international setting. Each person working internationally starts with certain personal motives for entering international nursing

service. These reasons may include increased financial reward, enjoyment of travel, interest in other ways of living, humanistic service to an underserved people, or a liking for meeting new people.

International nursing practice requires sudden adaptation when it is realized that the initial impetus to practice in a foreign culture does not always continue the way the nurse anticipated. Motives for practice should be clear to the nurse, when trying to work out adjustments in new situations. Often, international nurses experience a change in their philosophy of life and work. Suddenly isolated from familiar cultural routes, the nurse will wonder from time to time about what constituted the most influential factor in her or his professional development— whether it was the teaching in the basic school of nursing, what the nurse has worked out in practice, the influence of the new culture, or still other factors that had the greatest influence on the individual's thinking. It is desirable for the international nurse to have a philosophy of nursing practice in the new practice environment; otherwise understanding the views of all involved in the specific international setting will be impossible.

Another adjustment factor is the progressive discovery of the need for flexibility in planning, teaching, and practicing nursing techniques. A strong foundation in nursing practice standards that has been developed by the nurse and inherited in that nurse's cultural tradition often are ignored or bypassed in the international work in which she or he is engaged. Time management is a typical example. Lack of punctuality, waste of time, postponement of action, and major adjustments to time requirements often frustrate the nurse; eventually the nurse may even adjust more to time wastage factors than to time utilization factors.

The independent aspect of nursing practice is not found internationally. It is rare to find nursing students who study by themselves; a Western nurse in an international environment may expect to teach everything, and what the nurse teaches will then be the main source of the student's knowledge. Bedside nursing practice in hospitals and clinics is a constant source of surprise in international nursing and calls for drastic rethinking of standards.

Adaptation to a new culture in a strange and far-away land requires the same skills as adaptation to a different community in one's homeland. There is rarely a homogeneous culture, either economically or ethnically. The predominant culture will be influenced by forms of urban and rural life and the degree of education or lack of it that people have; these factors may influence greatly the way in which a nurse practices internationally. Recollection of illiterate and uneducated members of one's own nation will help the nurse to accept and work through traditional cultural patterns in another nation.

Understanding the main variations of culture in an international setting greatly enhances the nurse's ability to practice. An example is the predominantly male-dominated society of Saudi Arabia. In both hospitals and clinics, men and women are treated separately and quite differently; thus both settings may have two separate areas for handling men and women patients. Furthermore in Saudi Arabia respect for the custom of women to remain veiled and covered creates unique challenges, particularly in taking a nursing history or doing a nursing assessment.

Although a nurse in international nursing practice may have some idea of the customs in a certain country, the value that the people place on the practice of their culture is frequently not fully comprehended by the nurse. Customs may be identified as certain strange or striking facets of people's patterns of living, and these patterns make a coherent whole. These facets may relate to basic ideas people have about health and disease, ideas that they have acquired over generations and subsequently handed down. They may arise because certain members of families have authority in matters of health and are anxious both to preserve their authority and maintain certain ways of behavior. For example, it is not uncommon to have a Saudi Arabian patient present with scars covering certain parts of the patient's body, caused by burning or cauterization received from their traditional medicine healers to ward off evil spirits. China, Japan, and other Asian countries have traditional healers as well as Western healers.

If an international nurse refers to such behavior as superstitious, this will interfere with her or his acceptance and with the opportunity for leading the patient to more modern or scientific methods of treatment. Unscientific, irrational ideas embedded in traditional religion are part of a person's ancient beliefs; using these beliefs constructively is one way in which people are indoctrinated to practice health. If an attitude sets up a gulf between the people who are trying to give care and the individuals who are seeking care, many barriers can be created. Of attitudes involved, change on the part of the international nurse is highly important, in approaching people to break through their traditional methods and substitute basic modern health patterns as a new value for them. Customs, which may be strange and unfamiliar to one not of that country, should be integrated into the health care system and become part of a continuous caring process in helping people adapt to better hygiene and new ways. The challenge then for international nursing practice is to find out what will enable different communities to accept new ideas in managing their own health.

ASSISTING COMMUNITIES TO ADAPT

In Saudi Arabia, the first contact with the health care system is the physician or clinic. There are many primary care dispensaries in each region of the Kingdom. Many hospitals support community outreach clinics staffed with nurses, physicians, and pharmacists, generally from Third World countries. The secondary level of care is obtained from proprietary or government-financed hospitals, which are general or less technical in nature. Hospitals associated with the university medical schools conform to this category, in contrast to such hospitals found in the Western world. Tertiary care subdivides into two groups of hospitals. One group of hospitals focuses on specific diseases or medical areas; these are psychiatric hospitals, fever hospitals, and maternity and children's hospitals. The second type of hospitals offers sophisticated diagnostic testing and technically advanced treatment—examples are the King Khaled Eye Specialist Hospital and King Faisal Specialist Hospital and Research Center in Riyadh. Both are referral facilities serving the entire Kingdom and the

Middle East countries. Until recently, patients were sent abroad at government expense for specialized treatment. This practice has been curtailed as access to health care has improved within the Kingdom (Mills, 1986).

INTERPERSONAL RELATIONS PROBLEMS OF THE MULTINATIONAL NURSE

Understanding the health plan of the country in which the nurse works and adapting to the varied ways of implementing this plan as well as to the attitudes of the local people is crucial to success. It is important to realize that the plans and schemes all exist within the total cultural context of the country, that is, not merely in an education program or in a central health administration such as the country's ministry of health.

In a complex research and referral center, where nursing and medical staff are often drawn from more than 25 countries, the multinational aspect of nursing practice is compounded within a cross-cultural context. The international expatriate work force includes citizens of countries such as Afghanistan, Australia, Austria, Bangladesh, Belgium, Britain, Canada, China, Denmark, Egypt, Eritrea, Ethiopia, France, Germany, Holland, India, Indonesia, Iraq, Ireland, Italy, Japan, Jordan, Kenya, Korea, Lebanon, Malaysia, New Zealand, Pakistan, Palestine, Philippines, Singapore, Sri Lanka, Sudan, Syria, Taiwan, Thailand, Turkey, the United States, West India, Yemen, and other countries, including other Middle Eastern countries. The result is that patient populations as well as workers exhibit a wide diversity in language, ethnicity, culture, and national and international mix. This presents an opportunity for development of cultural synergy in a multinational, international setting.

Multinational is defined as "of, relating to, or involving more than two nations" (Webster's, 1983, p. 779). Relating as colleagues to more than two nationalities not only affords diversity among the nursing and medical staff, but also introduces the nurse to unusual points of view. The resultant increased stress and conflict require utmost delicate political leadership to attain consensus on philosophy and mission in order to provide cohesive patient care in such an international practice setting.

International is defined as "of, relating to, or affecting two or more nations; . . . of relating to, or constituting a group or association having members of two or more nations; . . . active, known, or reaching beyond national boundaries" (Webster's, 1983, p. 632). Table 48-1 categorizes the nationality of the nursing services staff in an international practice environment in Saudi Arabia. It is obvious that nursing services in this Saudi Arabian medical facility truly represent an international mix.

Cultural synergy refers to a dynamic process whereby persons with two often-opposing views interact, requiring both empathy and sensitivity to interpret signals by others in adapting and learning. It is combined action in working together. The total effect of the joint action is greater than the sum of the effects of independent action. Cultural synergy does not signify compromise, yet in true synergy nothing is given up or lost. In explaining cultural synergy, Moran and Harris (1982) provide examples from Saudi Arabia. While facilities and resources may be comparable to the Western world, many patients and workers in the Saudi Arabian environment are clearly Third World nationals.

TABLE 48-1

Nationality mix of nursing services staff at King Faisal Specialist Hospital and Research Centre, Saudi Arabia

CATEGORY	NUMBER	PERCENTAGE
United States	332	33
Philippines	157	16
Canada	127	12
United Kingdom*	116	11
Egypt	86	8
Scandinavia	43	4
Lebanon	40	4
Other†	120	12
TOTAL	1021	100

*United Kingdom includes Australia and New Zealand.
†Other includes Ethiopia, Somalia, Jordan, Yemen, Pakistan, India, Malaysia, and Singapore.

Diseases in Saudi Arabia are quite different from those found in the Western world. Traffic fatalities are the leading causes of death, and infant mortality (118 per 1000) is among the highest in the world. Life expectancy is 56.4 years. Major health problems are trauma, cancer, and a wide range of viral, bacterial, and parasitic infections. Congenital diseases caused by consanguineous marriages create a unique challenge in the care of infants and children. The spectrum of stress-related diseases is increasing as the international setting modernizes (Mills, 1986). For example, placing premature infants with multiple defects in a neonatal intensive care unit—when there is only one respirator for two or three infants—results in death from infectious disease within the first 6 months of life. In such cases, it is questionable whether life should have been prolonged in the first place.

Many of the problems of interpersonal relationships in this complex multinational setting relate to the image of the nurse. Involved are questions of status—how the nursing profession ranks in the country of practice, how this may differ from that in the various multinational countries represented by these nurses, and how nursing is viewed in relation to auxiliary nursing ranks in each of these settings. A hierarchical system is universal in the medical and nursing world, but the forms of hierarchy and the relationships of different groups in the hierarchy vary greatly from one country to another. Questions of status may concern relations between the administrator, doctor, nurse, and other professionals, but questions also may be closely connected to the education of the nurse or how the nurse is regarded in the nurse's own country. "Autonomy, accountability, responsibility for one's actions, legal accountability—all these have not yet become part of every nurse's mental outlook but progress is being made" (Holleran, 1988, p. 73).

Attempting to unify nursing in an international setting presents an unprecedented opportunity for the nurse administrator. The status of nursing needs to be viewed in relation to status patterns of the culture as a whole. In a culture in which women are less valued and physical contact with others is perceived as demeaning, nursing as a profession certainly has less than a professional image. In such an environment, autonomy is considered impossible or unacceptable by nurses themselves as well as by other professionals.

Moreover, determination of the economic worth of nurses, as reflected in salaries, results in inadequate pay to nurses for practice in many countries in the international setting and also in differential pay to multinational nurses. This creates alienation among nurses, since a nurse from one country may be paid more than a nurse from another country, depending on the status of nursing in one's home country. The nurse wants to improve nursing services; however, the resistance that is met because of questions of equity in salary and status, differentiating nurses from one country to another, has to be accepted as part of the cultural context in which the nurse is practicing.

In a country that is Muslim based, the seclusion of women does not allow for women to be out alone or to undertake public work unless protected and supervised. Therefore public health nursing is more difficult to accomplish, depending on progressive change in the people's thinking and attitude toward nurses that would allow community nursing to occur.

PROBLEMS IN NURSE RELATIONSHIPS WITH PATIENTS AND WITH PHYSICIANS

Patients' reactions to hospitalization, doctor and patient relationships, and nurse and patient relationships are frequently under study by social scientists. International nursing blends patients into a modern hospital community, with services, treatment, and relationships quite different from their native settings. For example, a Bedouin child, accustomed to living a nomadic existence in the desert in tents, when hospitalized over a prolonged period of time, adopts the culture of the people caring for him or her more than the culture of the society from which the child came. The sharp contrast and conflict that exist between the hospital's routine and treatment and that which is available in the Bedouin tents creates incongruences that can lead to alienation of the parents. A case in point is a boy who was hospitalized for up to 4 years, who spoke English better than Arabic, and who adopted Western behaviors to the point that his family no longer wanted him to live with them.

Nurses practicing in such a setting need to pay attention to deep-rooted cultural traditions and integrate them into the caring process. In many areas of the developing world, physicians outnumber professional nurses. Physicians have primary responsibility for determining and teaching the theoretical content of the nursing curriculum, while the nursing instructors monitor the students in their clinical work on the hospital wards. Too frequently, because nursing faculty are few in number, no effort is made to correlate theory with practice (Ohlson & Franklin, 1985).

Because physicians become the primary teachers of nurses in developing countries, a multinational work force of nursing varies from "handmaids" of the physician to the independent, articulate, clinical decision makers representative of the Western world. If the work force of nursing has practiced primarily in the dependent role of the nurse following physician's orders, the expectation to practice as independent clinical decision makers requires a substantial educational support system; this must be provided to enable nurses from differing countries and educational backgrounds to develop the competencies and skills essential to the nursing process. Both stronger collaborative practice, with effective nurse and physician relationships, and clinical competency partnered with leadership skills enable nursing to move forward; these factors enhance the potential for changing nursing practice from a traditional to a more comprehensive professional decision-making practice.

AN INTERNATIONAL NURSING PRACTICE MODEL

Clearly, the basic adjustment issues and problems of practicing nursing in the international setting exemplify problems that have been faced throughout the international nurse's career. Major issues relate to the universal need for available, accessible, respectable health care. Key recommendations include (a) changes in the health care system; (b) greater utilization of nursing personnel in health care planning; and (c) reforms in basic and postbasic nursing education to enable nurses to provide care in community settings rather than only or primarily in tertiary care centers (Ohlson & Franklin, 1985). In assuming leadership and creating a professional practice environment, the nursing leader should have identified the issues confronting nursing in the respective country and have articulated its vision for the future of nursing as a profession in that country. This leadership involves collaboration with other health care personnel or persons responsible for making decisions about health care planning and implementation. An international nursing care model is shown in Figure 48-1.

The definition of nursing practice, through a common philosophy of nursing expressed in the international nursing care model in Figure 48-1, focuses on the patient and the family. This includes defining their needs; allowing them to keep control of their lives throughout the health care system; making them viable members of the health care team, which requires a tremendous amount of teaching and, perhaps necessarily, a language translator; providing for support at home, in whatever environment or circumstances that occur; and enabling the family unit to participate in the care.

In order to help the patient and the family, it is essential that the international nurse be capable of all of the following: (a) comprehensive assessment; (b) planning of care; (c) teaching; (d) coordinating and evaluating for discharge planning, and collaborating with the doctor and community resources. The latter is particularly necessary to follow through on the required interventions, which are based on the medical diagnosis and the medical treatment plan for continuous interface with health promotion and maintenance.

If the nurse is to be able to apply this conceptual model of nursing, then the primary professional roles of nursing practice, teaching, consultation, research, and administration are essential. Each nurse must have a strong, competency-based, clinical practice identity, familiarity, and comfort level in order to practice internationally. Whether the nurse is teaching or practicing nursing, the ability to teach both patients and nurses is a key requirement in the

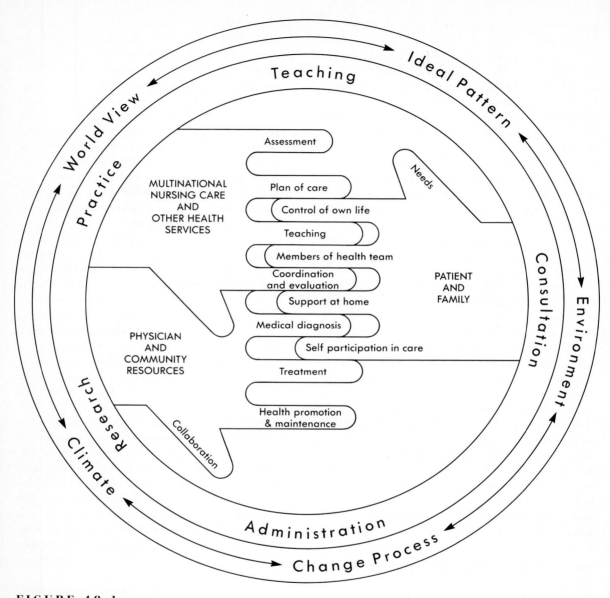

FIGURE 48-1

International nursing care model.

role of a professional nurse. The consultation role requires unique communication skills, facing language and cultural difficulties encountered in coping in an environment that is foreign. The ability to communicate in the local language not only facili-

tates communication, but also provides greater opportunity for mutual understanding and goodwill (Ohlson & Franklin, 1985).

A nursing consultant in an international setting will find a wealth of opportunity for international mutual exchange. Of foremost importance is recognizing that the American system is not necessarily applicable in all environments; many adaptations are essential if one is to be a credible consultant in the international setting. Professionally we have to give as well as receive, and while many think that this means going abroad as an expert, it also means giving to foreign nurses in one's own country (Holleran, 1988).

The development of nursing depends on research conducted by those who know and practice nursing. With few exceptions, such research has been minimal in developing areas of the world and in some developed countries as well. Primary health care offers abundant opportunity to study systematically problems relevant to nursing practice, nursing administration, and nursing education.

In developing nursing research, nurses with advanced preparation are essential to articulate clinically competent research design and adapt to the culture and community in which the research is conducted. A nurse researcher at King Faisal Specialist Hospital in Saudi Arabia has just completed a longitudinal study of child growth and development, using the Brazelton assessment, that has resulted in changing practice both in medicine and nursing. A videotape is one of the outcomes that will help doctors and nurses to evaluate the coping mechanisms and strategies of infants in their early developmental stages. This research required the nurse investigator to move into the community and to visit patients and families in their homes. The side effect of "beginning to intrude" into the cultural community leads the way for creation of a home care and community health based nursing system as part of the total health care system at King Faisal Specialty Hospital and Research Centre. The outcome of such research therefore far exceeds the intent for which the study was designed.

Administration in the international practice setting requires the utmost in adaptation skills, patience, flexibility, understanding, and willingness to learn and grow—especially in developing collegial relationships at the administrative level with doctors and administrators who are not accustomed to women at such high-level status. The integration of nursing as a partner in planning and decision making is dependent on the status of nursing in the country's health care system and the status of women in their culture. A strong foundation in administrative science assists the nurse leader in adapting the administrative process to the international setting. Initially a clear assessment must be made of what exists and what represents a world view of nursing within the specific practice setting and its relationship to the health care system as a whole.

Establishing an ideal pattern of goals in a long-range planning process is essential to move the organization from what exists to what ought to be. The environment, including financial and physical resources, provides constraints in enabling the change process to occur. Of priority is the creation of a climate that enables the strength of all nurses within the practice setting to develop a comprehensive unified approach that is consistent in demonstrating competency in nursing practice and administration. A climate that is open and allows each nurse from each country represented to participate equally is essential to enable a change process in developing an international practice environment. Such participation should include the creation of a nursing model and the development of unified nursing practice.

American nurses might well be reminded of the historical development of the profession in the United States when considering the problems faced by nurses today in less developed countries. They too had the problems of inadequate numbers of nurses, the need for leadership development, and low status as a profession. However, as one reflects on the evolution of nursing and the constant conflict and discourse regarding professionalization and requirement of a baccalaureate degree for entry into practice, the gaps between nursing evolution in the United States and the international setting become wider. The challenge to overcome these gaps, however, are mutual concerns internationally. A common base for nursing practice and concerns for social justice, in the face of sobering facts about unequal goods and service for health care in the world, motivate each nurse internationally to provide the strength and leadership to create the change that is essential. Such change includes the action needed to support the beliefs that all peoples of the world should be able to meet their basic health needs, such as access to the means for maintaining healthy and hygienic living conditions and the opportunity to receive help for at least the most common illnesses.

CONCLUSION

A recent consultation visit to a rural area of Saudi Arabia created increased awareness of the need for well-qualified, clinically capable nurses to become more involved in assisting people of the world to meet their basic health needs. Visitation to a chest and fever hospital, reminiscent of the tuberculosis hospital still in existence in America in the 1950s, revealed patients young and old in desperate situations. Frady (1970) has said there is

> no way actually to make a true deep passage through the fierce experience of another people, another place, without being seriously touched yourself; possibly even damaged: real understanding probably had to be personally expensive in some important way, had to issue finally out of one's own involvement and trauma. (p. 57)

International nursing practice enables a greater awareness of one's own cultural and ethical values; it is a rewarding and growing experience. The international nurse learns to accept other ways of life as they exist and attempts to influence health care with available, accessible, and economical resources. Simple hygiene measures of water, electricity, and basic technology become significant priorities in adaptation to a basic standard of nursing practice. The world's health care depends on nurses' ability to move forward in comprehensive professional practice and achieve equality in the relationship that nurses must maintain with patients and other providers of health care.

REFERENCES

Frady, M. (1970). An American innocent in the Middle East. *Harper's Magazine, 241* (1445), 55–80.

Holleran, C. (1988). Nursing beyond national boundaries: The 21st century. *Nursing Outlook, 36* (2), 72–75.

Kelly, L. Y. (1985). *Dimensions of professional nursing* (5th ed.). New York: Macmillan.

Mills, A. C. (1986). Saudi Arabia: An overview of nursing and health. *Focus on Critical Care, 13* (1), 50–56.

Moran, R. T., & Harris, P. R. (1982). *Managing cultural synergy (International management productivity series, Vol. 2)*. Houston: Gulf Publishing.

Ohlson, V., & Franklin, M. (1985). An international perspective on nursing practice. *Monographs Series Heading: Issues in Professional Nursing Practice, 6* (N P - 68 F - 2 M)

Webster's ninth new collegiate dictionary. (1983). Springfield, MA: Merriam-Webster, Inc.

✳   **EDITOR'S QUESTIONS FOR DISCUSSION**   ✳

What are the primary adjustments that must be made personally and professionally in international nursing practice in various cultures? What types of adaptation are essential for a nurse who aspires to practice international nursing? Discuss some strategies by which nurses can best prepare themselves for international nursing practice. What are the implications of Brown's chapter for those written by Jensen and Lindeman (Chapter 18), and Rosenblum (Chapter 19) for preparing persons educationally for international nursing practice? How might a nurse assess her or his ability to be an effective international nurse? How do cultural differences impact nursing practice in a country? How might values and attitudes differ among nurses in different cultures who practice as international nurses?

How might decision making, control, and accountability differ in the practice of nursing in various countries?

Discuss the strategies by which nursing as a profession might be unified in an international setting. What may be a common base of knowledge, skills, and competencies in international nursing? How might the development of a common philosophy of nursing be possible on an international basis when it has been extremely difficult to establish on a national basis? What might be the predominant role of a nurse in international nursing practice? What are the primary issues of concern in the development of nursing education programs and professional nursing practice on an international basis?

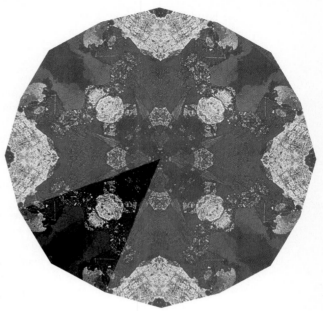

PART VI

NURSING ADMINISTRATION—SERVICE

Kaleidoscopes that reflect administration in service and academe are designed by nurse administrators. The two images—service and academia—are molded by similar elements and substances, called management functions and processes, into forms that represent management roles. There are sufficient differences between the two images as specialty areas and each is addressed as a separate part of this volume.

The focal point in the kaleidoscope of the service world in nursing is the patient. The nursing service administrator is charged with creating a total environment conducive to the provision of high-quality care. The following chapters unveil portions of blueprints formed by administrators for directing and guiding the nursing world of service.

Gail Wolf in Chapter 49 illustrates the challenges that must be met in designing an environment that contributes to quality, cost-effective care. She targets the essential elements in all service settings, including nursing services.

Anne Lynn Porter in Chapter 50 explains further the need to maximize human resources. She elucidates the clinical advancement system, its structural components, and processes for offering a professional practice of nursing and rewards to staff nurses.

The adhesive that holds the elements together in the kaleidoscope of nursing service is that of nursing governance. In Chapter 51 Tim Porter-O'Grady reflects on management structures and models for nursing administration in which the practicing nurse is at the hub.

Factors that exacerbate the nursing shortage and present an unattractive image of nursing to nurses must be minimized. Nancy Graham and Christine Sheppard in Chapter 52 build on the view previously introduced. They promote shared value systems and nursing role clarification in recruiting and retaining the staff nurse for satisfying nursing practice.

Diana Weaver in Chapter 53 enlarges the scope of nursing administration. She envisions nursing care activities based on cost-effective models for using resources.

There is another aspect of environment that increasingly has been coming to the fore, that is, collective bargaining. Marian Martin Pettengill in Chapter 54 looks at the legal and economic environment of collective bargaining in nursing. Pettengill discusses some resolutions for resolving the conflict between nursing management and labor.

The dilemma of organizational and professional conflict can be resolved through strategic planning. Marjorie Beyers in Chapter 55 shows how strategic planning is the key to numerous corporate structure results.

Educational preparation for nurse managers and executives is an imperative need that many nurses are realizing. The scope of administrative practice requires leadership and management designers and integrators who are exceptionally equipped. Marian Sides in Chapter 56 offers data for preparation of these roles as perceived from the practice arena. In Chapter 57 Norma L. Chaska and Judith W. Alexander further enlarge the data base regarding educational preparation needs.

It is clear that administrators are the prime facilitators for the service environment. They direct and coordinate numerous patient care and management activities. In so doing, they thrive on meeting many challenges to create appropriate designs for superior patient care.

utilizing our resources wisely. We need to determine not only if we are doing the job correctly, but also if we are doing the correct job to get the desired outcome.

A first step in this process is examining what is fact and what is folklore concerning nursing practice. I believe there are several myths under which we practice that fail to maximize our resources and detract from the quality of care that nurses are capable of providing.

Myth 1 — Nurses Practice Nursing

Nurses do an excellent job implementing the medical regimen prescribed for patients. Tasks such as medication administration, intravenous administration, cardiac monitoring, and the like constitute the dependent role of nursing, and represent nursing's response in implementing the medical regimen. Although nursing's medical scope of practice is important, there is also an independent or autonomous scope of nursing practice. This aspect of the role involves assisting patients in their responses to health conditions and includes such activities as skin care, mouth care, and teaching, to name a few. The dependent aspect of nursing practice is implemented far more frequently than the autonomous aspect for a variety of reasons. It is more widely taught in schools of nursing, it is task-oriented, valued by organizations, and more widely understood. However, nurses who have implemented the autonomous aspects of their role have achieved some very impressive patient outcomes. We need to quantify these outcomes, and help nurses understand how to better implement this aspect of their role.

Nurses may also fail to practice nursing because they are too busy performing nonnursing work. It is an obvious misuse of valuable nursing resources to have nurses function as dietary aides, housekeepers, and messenger-escorts, to name only a few of the frequently encountered roles. This work can be delegated to less skilled personnel. On the other hand, there are aspects of patient care such as basic respiratory therapy or physical therapy that could potentially be more cost-effectively integrated into daily patient care by nursing.

Finally, nurses fail to practice nursing as efficiently as they could, largely because of system deficiencies. For example, much of the nursing documentation required by hospitals is repetitive, nonessential, and expensive. Change of shift reports can consume numerous nursing man-hours. Hospitals need to examine these issues and become as nursing-supportive as they are physician-supportive through use of dictaphones, computerization, bedside terminals, and similar means to free nurses for nursing practice.

Myth 2 — Good Nurses Meet Patients' Health Care Needs

Nurses have incredible expectations about what they "should" accomplish for patients, and consistently feel as though they have failed when there is not enough time to do everything. In truth, many patients have extensive needs that can never be satisfied. We need to become more realistic, and spend quality time focused on achieving the most critical patient outcomes.

Myth 3 — The Way We've Always Done It Is the Best Way to Do It

A great deal of nursing practice is based on ritual. It is so ingrained into our thinking, that we never even question the wisdom of our actions. For example, in most hospitals patients get bathed every day (and on day shift) whether they need or want it. Beds are changed religiously, even if they are clean. Vital signs are taken, even when there is no reason to suspect any physiological change. We waste time on inconsequential tasks and are frustrated because there is no time for health care teaching or psychological support of a patient.

We must change our thinking. In order for hospitals to survive, every aspect of care must contribute to a positive patient care outcome. We can no longer afford meaningless rituals. We must systematically and scientifically challenge the folklores of nursing practice and determine which aspects are based on fact and which are based on fiction.

In conclusion, the crisis we are facing in health

care presents a significant challenge in finding new ways of balancing both the quality and cost of care. Nursing has the answer to many of the questions for accomplishing this. We are being given the opportunity to influence how health care will be provided in the future through the creation of new and better approaches to care. The danger is that we will lose our courage, our vision, and fail to ask "what if . . ." We cannot afford to allow this to happen, but must surge forward into our new frontier.

REFERENCES

Donabedian, A. (1987). Five essential questions from the management of quality in health care. *Health Management Quarterly, 9*(1), 6.

Ehrat, K. S. (1987). The cost-quality balance: An analysis of quality, effectiveness, efficiency, and cost. *Journal of Nursing Administration, 17*(5), 6–13.

Fralic, M. F. (1988). Tracking cost while keeping quality alive (and well). *Journal of Nursing Administration, 18*(4), 7–8.

How consumers perceive health care quality. (1988). *Hospitals, 62*(7), 84.

Pincus, J. D. (1986). Communication: key contributor to effectiveness—the research. *Journal of Nursing Administration, 16*(9), 19–25.

Quality, not ads, increase physician loyalty. (1987). *Hospitals, 61*(12), 56.

Wolf, G. A. (1986). Communication: key contributor to effectiveness—a nurse executive responds. *Journal of Nursing Administration, 16*(9), 26–28.

✳ EDITOR'S QUESTIONS FOR DISCUSSION ✳

What conflicts in professional nursing practice are caused by differences between professional and organizational value systems? How can the two value systems be reconciled for the benefit of patient care? What are the characteristics of an excellent environment for professional practice? What specific strategies might a nurse executive use for developing a positive environment? How might nurses attain control over factors that influence their practice that they have not previously been able to influence?

What are the critical factors in team building? Propose a process by which a strong team can be built for nursing administration. What are the critical issues involved concerning measuring the quality of care and cost? Present various methodologies for measuring the quality of care and determining the relationship between quality, effectiveness, efficiency, and cost. How do the suggestions in Chapter 52, by Graham and Sheppard and Chapter 53, by Weaver relate to the values discussed in this chapter?

50

Clinical Advancement Systems

Anne Lynn Porter, Ph.D., R.N.

Clinical advancement systems, often referred to as clinical ladders, were first widely introduced into nursing service departments during the nursing shortage of the late 1970s. At that time nurse "burnout" was a much-discussed phenomenon as staff nurses expressed dissatisfaction with their roles and the hospital system in which they functioned. Hospital and nursing administrators responded to the crisis by introducing a variety of incentives, including salary increases, flexible staffing methods, bonuses, and others. In an effort to link rewards to professional performance many hospitals initiated clinical advancement systems. Based on a conceptual model described by Zimmer (1972) clinical advancement systems specified levels of performance behaviors that guided the professional development of the staff nurse and were accompanied by incremental rewards, most often salary increases. Although the structure and mechanisms of these promotional systems varied from institution to institution, their goals were to develop and reward clinical competence and expertise in staff nurses. The nursing literature has reported the success of these programs in narrative accounts, but formal research data related to the programs are limited.

ISSUES

The current critical nursing shortage finds many nurse executives reevaluating clinical advancement systems. Once again there is a need to increase rewards for the staff nurse in order to retain these nurses at the bedside. There is a continuing need for professional development and evaluation systems. Clinical competence in nursing must be described, recognized, and rewarded to maintain delivery of quality patient care. Development of clinical advancement systems where none exist and the redesign of early advancement systems are appropriate responses to the situation. Today, however, more questions are being asked regarding these systems:

Will clinical advancement systems enhance recruitment during a shortage?

Will these systems have a long-term effect on nurse retention?

How do these systems enhance career development?

Do the levels of performance imply levels of productivity?

Does the cost of program implementation and maintenance justify the outcomes?

Little research data have been reported to answer objectively these questions, but experiences from institutions that have had clinical advancement systems in place over several years can provide some knowledge of the issues involved.

Effect on Recruitment and Retention

The presence of a clinical advancement system influences nurses' decisions when seeking a nursing position and nurses' tenure in a position. For nurses who are deciding where they will work, the presence of a clinical advancement system is a "marker" for a professional department of nursing. The Magnet Hospital study reported that "staff nurses consider a career ladder to be an essential component of professional development. They perceive it from two major perspectives: (a) as a personnel benefit, and (b) as an educational program for professional growth and career development" (American Academy of Nursing, 1983, p. 36). When a nurse executive analyzes whether a clinical advancement system is appropriate for a given setting as a recruitment measure, the local market must be considered. In some locations, most area hospitals have a clinical advancement system, and they are a component of a professional nursing model that is expected by nurses seeking positions. In other settings where the systems are not common, an advancement system might give a hospital the competitive edge in recruiting nurses.

Clinical advancement systems are reported to positively affect nurse retention. Several hospitals have reported decreased staff turnover that was attributed to the initiation of a clinical advancement system. However, nurse supply in the area, availability of positions, salary rates, and other factors may have been intervening variables (Alt & Houston, 1986; Ulsafer-Van Lanin, 1981; Wine & Mapstone 1981).

Effect on Career Development

The unique features of the nursing career must be acknowledged when programs, such as clinical advancement systems, are designed for nursing career development. Lortie (1975) described characteristics of teaching that apply to nursing as well. Most people enter a profession at a level where they are involved in some of the least valued activities and work toward more important tasks. In most cases, junior members of an organization must take on the "dirty work" (Schein, 1978). For teaching, however, the most valued activity—student-teacher interac-

tion—occurs immediately in the career. The nurse, like the teacher, is immediately performing the activity that is most important in the career. The nursing career is built around a body of knowledge that relates to the care of the patient, and the philosophy of nursing places the highest value on interactions with patients (Styles, 1982). Patient contact can be the most rewarding aspect of nursing. The nurse in entering the career at the staff nurse level has, in a sense, the most "valued" position in nursing. The staff nurse views promotions only as moving away from the important activity of patient care.

The entry pattern into nursing contributes to the lack of staging in the profession. The work to be accomplished by a staff nurse must be suitable to relative neophytes and is described in terms of minimum expected behaviors in job descriptions. Care at the bedside is differentiated by the expertise of the individual nurse, but this often relates more directly to the intelligence, motivation, and energy of the nurse at any career point rather than to a planned career development stage. The development stages of a nursing career are compressed in comparison with other professions. Staff nurses arrive at full levels of responsibility early in their careers. They are also required to have an immediate grasp of the knowledge needed to practice. Nurses are delivering patient care to patients with complex care problems within the first year after graduation.

Financial reward for the staff nurse follows predictable patterns dependent on length of service or a merit system, or both. There is a reasonable salary structure for the beginning staff nurse, but nurses who have lengthy experience as staff nurses are seldom compensated a great deal more. There is often less than a $5,000 difference between the annual salary of a new graduate and a nurse with 20 years' experience. This structure is similar to that of teachers, which Lortie (1975) describes as being predictable and relatively unstaged. He uses the term "front-loaded" to describe the rewards that are placed early in the career. This results in the problem of motivation in a profession in which the future does not hold the promise of advancement and appropriate financial reward. For nurses in staff positions there are few opportunities open and salaries are compressed when an advancement system is not in place.

Clinical advancement systems offer the opportunity for lateral movement and career growth in clinical nursing practice. Lateral movement within a career is a positive force for individual motivation and for long-term development. When economic constraints occur, opportunities for lateral growth can also enhance job interest despite minimal financial rewards (Smith, 1982). Care must be taken, however, not to substitute diversity for fiscal reward.

Clinical advancement systems:

Recognize patient care as the most valued nursing activity

Describe advanced practice behaviors

Reduce salary compression

Promote lateral growth

Thus clinical advancement systems restructure the staff nurse career to eliminate negative structural elements including limits on growth potential, recognition, and compensation.

Effect on Productivity

Quantitative data demonstrating the effect of clinical advancement systems on productivity of staff nurses have not been reported. Use of patient classification data to compare caseloads of nurses in various levels of an advancement system would yield a beginning comparative data base. Nurse executives who have had experience with advancement systems believe that there is an increase in productivity that includes the ability to care for more complex patients and to handle a larger caseload. The nurses in advanced levels demonstrate the ability to address flexibly a wide variety of clinical problems. Expertise and flexibility in patient care situations result in cost efficiencies.

As nurse executives seek to restructure the work of nurses to meet the demands of a shrinking pool of nurses, the performance criteria of a clinical advancement system spell out the professional functions of the nurse. Other activities, which nurses may currently perform, can be delegated to assisting or support service personnel. Thus nursing productivity for critical nursing tasks can be increased.

Quality of patient care also benefits from nurses who are participants in an advancement system. Nurses in advanced levels practice in a more collaborative manner with physicians and other health care professionals, introduce innovation into their own practice, and individualize patient care. As resources to other staff members these nurses affect the quality of care for patients beyond their own assignment or caseload. Those activities that affect patient care indirectly, such as policy formation, setting standards for care, and monitoring activities required by the Joint Commission on the Accreditation of Healthcare Organizations (JCAHO) are also important to recognize as contributing to the quality of patient care.

COST OF THE SYSTEM

The costs involved in establishing and maintaining a clinical advancement system include (a) the development costs for the program; (b) the costs involved in creating a salary structure with several levels of pay; and (c) the ongoing costs of incentive pay for performance. Initial costs for program design and implementation vary widely depending on whether external consultation is used, the degree of participation by nursing staff and administrators, and the length of time it takes to implement the program. Development of the advancement system must involve staff nurse representation from a wide variety of service areas, key nursing management, and human resources staff. Even when external consultants lead the design process, the staff involvement is essential for assuring compatibility of the system with institutional goals and ownership of the program by the nursing staff. While it is difficult to manage with staffing shortages, it is advisable to design and implement the program in a relatively short period of time, for example, 6 months. The process of implementing these programs involves widespread change. Anxiety accompanies the change process. Therefore, from a cost and climate perspective it is wise to accelerate the process.

The salary structure for clinical advancement systems involves the development of pay grades and ranges for each level of the system. These pay ranges overlap, but must have a significant spread between range midpoints. Increases from level to level vary, and generally they range from 2.5% to 10%. The development of the several pay grades allows for greater spread among staff nurse salaries. In hospitals without clinical advancement systems staff nurses' salaries increase only 27% from the minimum average salary to the maximum, whereas the increases in systems with several levels for staff nurses are reported to be as high as 51% (Beyers, Mullner, Byre, & Whitehead, 1983). These increases, of course, increase costs, which must be evaluated in respect to expenses that are reduced by the presence of an advancement system. Recruitment expenses, inefficiencies created by staff turnover, and missed profit caused by staffing shortages may decrease in the presence of an advancement system that helps to fill the nursing positions. Harder to evaluate are the cost savings involved when the nursing staff is more experienced, efficient, and therefore more cost-effective in delivering care.

CLINICAL ADVANCEMENT SYSTEM COMPONENTS

Establishment of a clinical advancement system in nursing involves the design of the structural components of the system including:

Organizational framework
Performance criteria
Rules and processes
Performance evaluation system
Reward structure

Each of these components contains elements that are critical to the system. For example, the reward structure includes the compensation related to advancement and the recognition mechanisms for participating nurses.

Organizational Framework

Clinical advancement systems in nursing should reflect by structure and design the philosophy, mission, and conceptual framework of the hospital and its department of nursing. Goals of clinical advancement programs most frequently mentioned include (a) to improve the quality of patient care by increasing the clinical competence of nursing staff; (b) to provide a professional career development system; (c) to reward nurses who have demonstrated clinical competence; (d) to establish an evaluation system for nurses; and (e) to recruit and retain nurses for bedside nursing positions. The selection of goals for the program communicates the priority of the department of nursing. The behavioral criteria for each level of practice in the system are organized by a professional nursing practice framework. Common organizing elements are nursing process, leadership or management, education, research, and quality assurance. The selection of the organizers conveys those elements of professional practice that will be projected to the nursing staff and should reflect the belief system of the organization. Elements, such as patient education, collaborative practice, interpersonal communication, or community service, can be used as organizers if emphasis in these areas is desired. The organizing elements selected become the framework for the behavioral criteria.

Determination of the number of levels in a clinical advancement system can draw on the experience of successful systems in other settings, but it must be accompanied by an analysis of environmental factors, demographic data, and established goals. The majority of clinical advancement systems have from four to six levels. Some of these programs include the clinical nurse specialist role as the upper level. Analysis of staff nurse turnover and length of employment will indicate whether an advancement system should be designed to provide career growth over a relatively short 4- to 5-year tenure or a longer period of time. Research by Benner (1984) identified five levels of expertise in nursing from novice to expert. Study of Benner's work, which includes rich descriptions of the varying levels of clinical expertise, is helpful in determining the number of levels for a program. Sanford (1987) believes that all clinical advancement programs should be based on Benner's development model for clinical excellence.

Performance Criteria

The development of performance criteria is the single most critical element that affects the success of the clinical advancement system. Criteria need to reflect those elements of professional nursing practice that can be observed or measured. Sufficient distinction must be indicated between levels to allow for accurate evaluation. Variations in performance occur on a continuum for any given behavior, but a statement must be written to describe a point on the continuum for each level of performance. Stem statements with items indicating quality, quantity, or complexity are written for each important aspect of behavior (Sierra-Franco, 1984). Most behavioral statements include a level-specific statement for each of the levels. There are a few areas in which a behavior may not be expected to occur until an advanced level is attained. Some other behaviors may be fully developed during the first or second level of the system. For example, attainment of clinical skills may be completed during the second or third level, while participation in community health initiatives may begin at these levels. Behaviors are written in a sequential manner so that growth from level to level is evident.

Rules and Processes

The process by which staff nurses will relate to the system and the rules that will govern that process, are specified in detail as a component of the advancement system. Eligibility for participation in the program specifies whether part-time nurses, float pool nurses, and nurses in such roles as intravenous therapy team, or infection control, as well as others will be included in the program. These decisions are based on analysis of these functions to determine if the full range of professional nursing can be practiced in the roles and if adequate continuity of evaluation of performance is possible. The placement of nursing staff in a newly developed clinical advancement system can be accomplished in several different ways.

Nurses may be placed in the lower levels of the system based on years of nursing experience and al-lowed the option of seeking movement to a higher level after demonstrating that current performance exceeds the level of initial placement. This is the most efficient method of initial placement. Its disadvantage is that it does not immediately acknowledge individual differences in performance. Another method of placement is to allow nurses to apply for a position in the level that best reflects their current performance. Involving peers in initial placement decisions can provide individualized feedback to nurses and result in more accurate placement. Newly hired nurses can enter clinical advancement systems at the initial or an advanced level depending on experience and salary requirements.

Performance Evaluation System

Evaluation of individual nurse performance occurs on an annual basis and when a nurse has qualified for advancement in the system. Some systems use identical processes for these evaluations, while others use a more comprehensive process for advancement decisions. The annual evaluation process should be congruent with the performance appraisal system in place within the institution. The timing of the performance appraisal, the reporting of the evaluation results, and the annual pay increase recommendation should follow the hospital's established practice. The annual evaluation in a clinical advancement system will require additional documentation for the professional practice behaviors and may include such components as peer review. Clinical advancement structures can be used within hospitals with performance appraisal systems that reward staff for longevity in a system, but they are most appropriate conceptually in pay-for-performance systems. The process of advancement from one level to the next involves an evaluation of performance that is usually more extensive than the annual evaluation. Decisions related to movement from one level to the next are frequently made by a unit nurse manager in the beginning levels of the system. These decisions are sometimes made in conjunction with peer evaluation. Many advancement systems have a review committee to determine placement in the higher levels of the system. These committees consist primarily of nurses who have achieved advanced placement in the system, in addition to management or education staff as resources.

A variety of tools can be used for evaluation, such as simple checklists to record performance of the behaviors, anecdotal notes, critical incident technique tools, and others. Many systems rely on a portfolio system that requires nurses to assemble documentation of their performance with charting and care-plan samples, continuing education certificates, and similar documents. Care must be taken to reduce the paperwork involved in the evaluation process as much as possible. With current staffing constraints there is little time available for staff to collect evidence of performance. The danger also exists that staff will interpret a heavy emphasis on documentation as a message that the ability to assemble a portfolio is more important than the ability to deliver patient care. One way to reduce some of the paperwork is to emphasize a peer review format of evaluation. These systems can be designed to emphasize a peer observation of performance that reduces the need for written samples of performance. Peer review systems also help to emphasize the professional responsibility of nurses to monitor the clinical practice on their units.

In an attempt to develop evaluation systems that are completely objective, some clinical advancement systems rely on point systems for placement within the system. Point systems are appropriately used to determine performance-based merit increases, but they are seldom effective if used alone to determine advancement in the system. With a point system, advancement decisions appear to be arbitrary, since a few points on the scale may separate a level-two from a level-three nurse. A holistic view of the nurse's performance measured against the behaviors of a given level is more effective. Just as a nursing director is expected to meet all of the position expectations of the director position, the nurse in a level-three position, for example, is expected to meet all of the expectations of the level-three position, not to select and have acquired points from a menu of expectations.

Policies for the clinical advancement system must include specific information regarding transfers from one nursing unit to another, resolving situations in which nurses fail to maintain their level of behaviors, and the appeal process. These policies are developed by the committee designing the clinical advancement system and are approved through nursing administration and human resources.

Reward Structure

Most clinical advancement systems include financial incentives as a critical element in the program. To be successful the fiscal reward attached to advancement must be a significant dollar figure, but the dollar figure varies greatly among the various local markets for nurses. In addition to financial rewards, recognition in the form of new titles for each level of staff nurse, ceremonies to celebrate advancement, mention in in-house publications, and opportunities for participation in organizational decision making should be emphasized. Other rewards that may be built into the advancement system are tuition or continuing education reimbursement, certification program expenses, paid time off, and scheduling preferences.

SUMMARY

Clinical advancement systems offer one approach to the development of a satisfying and productive role for the staff nurse. Development of a clinical advancement system offers nurses the opportunity to define nursing practice in a concrete terms, to examine the functions of the staff nurses in relation to professional practice, and to build rewards for professional behavior into the staff nurse role.

REFERENCES

Alt, J. M., & Houston, G. (1986). *Nursing career ladders: A practical manual*. Rockville, MD: Aspen Systems Corporation.

American Academy of Nursing. (1983). *Magnet hospitals: Attraction and retention of professional nurses*. Kansas City, MO: American Nurses' Association.

Benner, P. (1984). *From novice to expert*. Menlo Park, CA: Addison-Wesley.

Beyers, M., Mullner, R., Byre, C. S., & Whitehead, S. F. (1983). Results of the Nursing Personnel Survey, Part 1: RN recruitment and orientation. *Journal of Nursing Administration*, *13*, (4), 34–37.

Lortie, D. (1975). *Schoolteacher*. Chicago: University of Chicago Press.

Sanford, R. (1987). Clinical ladders: Do they serve their purpose? *Journal of Nursing Administration*, *17*, 34–37.

Schein, E. (1978). *Career dynamics*. Reading, MA: Addison-Wesley.

Sierra-Franco, M. (Ed.). (1984). *Staff nurse performance criteria and appraisal system* (Stanford Nursing Monograph Series No. 2). Stanford, CA: Stanford University Medical Center, Nursing Services.

Smith, D. (1982). Creating opportunity for clinical nursing advancement. In J. Wood & G. Zilm (Eds.), *Energizing the work place* (pp. 60–70). Vancouver, British Columbia, Canada: Canadian College of Health Service Executives.

Styles, M. M. (1982). *On nursing*. St. Louis: C. V. Mosby.

Ulsafer-Van Lanin, J. (1981). Lateral promotion keeps skilled nurses in direct patient care. *Hospitals*, *55* (5), 87–90.

Wine, J., & Mapstone, S. (1981). Clinical advancement. *Nursing Administration Quarterly*, *6* (1), 65–68.

Zimmer, M. J. (1972). Rationale for a ladder for clinical advancement. *Journal of Nursing Administration*, *1* (11), 18–24.

✳ EDITOR'S QUESTIONS FOR DISCUSSION ✳

How may clinical advancement systems be used as an effective recruitment and retention tool? Construct a clinical ladder system for an institution based on three levels of clinical practice. What should be the predominant criteria for each level? How can salaries and merit increases be connected to the various levels of a clinical ladder? Should there be ratios established for the number of personnel that can be allocated in one level? What options might there be for the person who has reached the highest level of a clinical ladder in terms of rewards and salary increases?

What is the difference between performance appraisal systems and advancement systems or structures? Discuss the pros and cons of various tools and designs of performance appraisal systems and advancement tools or structures. Who should develop the policies and procedure related to the development of advancement systems? What should the composition of a review committee be for an advancement system? Construct a possible management ladder system for institutions. What criteria for management ladder levels might be included for a management ladder? At what point should a staff nurse be provided the option to retain a clinical advancement track or pursue a management advancement track?

51

Nursing Governance in a Transitional Era

Tim Porter-O'Grady, Ed. D., R.N., C.N.A.A.

It certainly would not be extreme to state that the nursing profession is in the midst of an era of major social change. We are moving from industrial models of production, organizational design, and human relations management to a highly integrated technological model influencing the management of the future workplaces of America (Naisbitt, 1984). This technological transformation is working a change on society not previously experienced in any other social transition in history. The advent of the information age, the radical acceleration of the applications of technology, the communication networks established throughout the world, and the ability to make decisions with a great deal of data in split-second time are all having a major impact. The effect is on how work gets done and the way work relates to people and to the world (Toffler, 1980).

IMPACT ON THE NURSE

Clearly there is no arena that has felt any greater impact of technology than has health care. At the heart of the health care delivery system is the nursing professional struggling to deal with the meaning of the technological change. The professional is simultaneously trying to meet the demands in utilizing and applying technology to facilitate and enhance patient care.

This individual is often responsible for integrating, facilitating, and coordinating the application of technology in the delivery of health care services. Consequently it is the nurse who feels the greatest impact of the demands of this transition. However, it is also the nurse who feels the greatest inertness of the management structure that governs these activities. The nurse is capable of making high-level decisions, utilizing technology, and undertaking major strategies leading to healing, wellness, or improved patient circumstances. Many times, however, the organizational constructs within which she or he must operate do not clearly facilitate the nurse in the exercise of a demanding role.

CAREER CHOICES FOR WOMEN

Complicating the issue today is the fact that there are many other career choices available to women in the current marketplace. Traditionally women were relegated to positions in teaching or nursing or other "feminine" jobs and roles. Now they have a whole host of available choices different from and perhaps more rewarding, at first glance, than either nursing or teaching. Women are choosing to go into the major professions of law, medicine, engineering, architecture, science, and many other careers. As a result, there is a net decline in both the interest and enrollments in nursing schools. This occurs at a time when the need for nursing skills and the demands on the nursing professional are growing at an accelerating rate. Further complicating the issue are the concerns and feelings of nurses related to the organizations of which they are a part. Nurses today deal with the struggles and issues of their own value, role, and contribution to health care. Nurses have, in many ways, concluded that the workplace is not sensitive or structured in a way that facilitates parallel and equilateral roles with other health care professionals—notably physicians—in the health care workplace. The common complaints of lack of respect, no opportunity to grow, lack of influence on decision making, no control over one's own practice or circumstances, limited time with patients, too much paperwork, and not enough pay are all indicative of the internal struggles between the professional nurse and the workplace (National Commission on Nursing Implementation Project, 1986, 1987).

All too often the nurse's complaints are legitimate. The organizational structure that governs most hospital organizations is archaic at best. It represents highly segmented hierarchical industrial models that are rigidly defined, clearly enumerated, and carefully structured. Within this context the delineation of professional roles for the nurse falls within the control of the institution. As a result, the nurse's role becomes precisely what the institution defines for it regardless of the values, beliefs, and understandings of that role by the nursing profession and the individual professional. Most nursing administrators who manage nursing organizations tend to maintain decentralized, but essentially authority-based, structures within the professional practice of nursing. The management role becomes central to the exercise of control and authority in the organization. Concentration on the development of managers, the careful definition of their roles, and the education of the manager in human relations skills all reaffirm the hierarchical nature of most nursing organizations.

What is not clearly articulated is whether health care organizations believe that nurses are professional. The issue is that if the nurse is a professional there are environmental, relational, social, and structural elements that best represent the governance and management of professionals.

These are different from the traditional industrial models. Professional management systems demand a different kind of approach. Without addressing this fundamental reality the work of the nurse will always remain subject to discord, conflict, and question.

ORGANIZATIONAL STRUCTURE

The basic question becomes, What is the best structure, organizational framework, and relational system for management of the professional worker? What are the characteristics of the professional that require an approach that reflects these unique characteristics, and how should the organization be structured in order to address them? Finally what are the changing demands of the health care system that indicate a specific and concerted need to address the issue of management, organization, and structuring for the professional worker? In responding to these needs, appropriate and significant changes must occur in the organizational system in order to effect a positive outcome for the nursing profession, and for those who are recipients of nursing services.

The first issue relates to the need to delineate clearly that nursing is a profession, meets the characteristics of professional definition, and acts and behaves within a professional context. The change agent, therefore, must "buy into" at least the following vital elements:

- A professional has a social mandate to utilize and exercise judgment on behalf of the client in a way in which the client could not do so for himself or herself.
- The professional nurse's role is such that no other person without the professional preparation for the role could adequately and appropriately undertake it to the degree essential to fulfill the social mandate.
- The nurse seeks and maintains equity with other professionals. Therefore, the nurse has

the attendant authority and role in decisions that affect her or his practice, in conjunction with decisions that affect the health care practices of all involved disciplines. The professional nurse has the opportunity to participate fully as an interdependent member of the health care team. The nurse must clearly be parallel in status, equal in function, and respected for the nurse's unique contribution in the delivery of health care.

If these applied professional characteristics of the nurse are to be clearly articulated with the delivery of patient care services, the organizational design within which the nurse must work to accomplish these ends must be different from that generally experienced. The archaic management and administrative structure of most health care organizations do not adequately address this reality. In most management structures it is the manager and not the practicing nurse who is accountable for the output and outcomes of the delivery system (Callahan & Wall, 1987). For accountability to operate, the accountable individual must have the authority, autonomy, and control over his or her actions to the degree that this person can directly influence outcomes. Generally the nursing manager is responsible for assuring outcomes, instead of the practicing nurse, through the authority and control given by the institution to the nurse manager. No one should be surprised if ownership and accountability stop there and do not successfully transfer to staff nurses.

In a professionally delineated organization, standards of practice, process, outcomes, quality, and evaluation are determined directly by the practitioners, articulated by them, and defined by them in terms of both their structure and operation. This is clearly a different process from the traditional industrial model approaches. In professional governance models the management team is empowered by the professional organization to ensure that the practitioner-defined frameworks operate within the context defined by the peer process, and unfold consistent with the mandates of the professional organization. The belief here is that the professional determines the standards and frameworks in which professional practice unfolds. From this determination the me-

chanics for assuring that practice unfolds as defined, are derived, developed, and structured by the corporate nursing staff. It is assured that each professional meets the obligation she or he has agreed to undertake. The obligation exists within the context of the values provided for the nurse's role by the profession and the corporate nursing organization. The manager therefore becomes a moderator of the process, assuming that the mechanisms of the operating system are designed to support this professional framework (Naisbitt & Aburdene, 1985).

STRUCTURE AND GOVERNANCE

Professional staff governance demands a different focus on the structuring of the organization. Moving away from the traditional hierarchy, professionals need a more incorporative, integrative organizational framework that simply defines where accountability exists—and provides within the structure a way to express accountability. It is important that structures

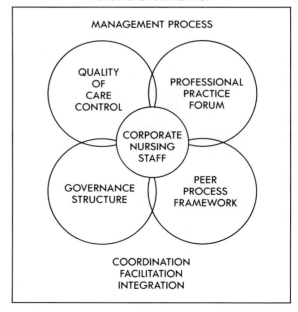

FIGURE 51-1

Professional governance model for nursing.

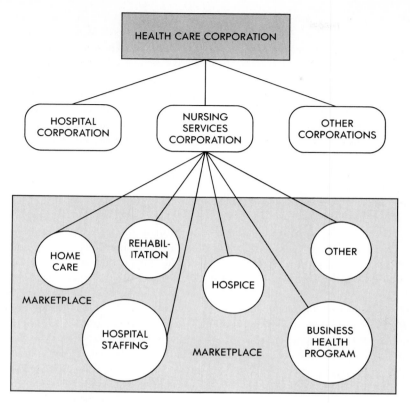

FIGURE 51-2

The nursing service corporation in the health care delivery
system of the 21st century.

be evolved that allow the professional to experience
truly the obligation of practicing within a professional context. Structures need to incorporate the
demands and roles of professional nursing into practice behaviors regardless of the setting (Fig. 51-1).

In the coming age, settings reflecting a wide array
of health care systems will continue to expand. The
role of the nursing professional will reflect an increasing call for nurses to practice in smaller work
units and to assume more responsibility for individual practice behaviors (Fig. 51-2).

To ensure that the individual professional is capable of working in this kind of setting, the overall
organizational structure must provide a market-
based "bottom-to-top" approach. In a professional

organization the expectations and the demands of the
structure should clearly indicate to the professional
nurse that accountability originates with her or him,
and is not shifted away nor is the nurse insulated
from the realities of that accountability. The framework that holds the nurse to accountability in the
future will be functionally and clinically described
and will be structured and articulated within the
context of a peer-defined and peer-operated framework.

RULES OF ORGANIZATION

The new organizational structure of the future will
have to provide an opportunity for the professional

nurse to incorporate the following roles in her nursing practice:

- Obtain privileges for membership on the nursing staff. Utilizing a privileging framework, the nurse presents evidence of the individual credentials, experience, capabilities, and leadership in the area for which she or he is seeking the privilege to practice nursing.
- Participate in a peer-based evaluation system, which looks specifically at the nurse's ability to practice, to integrate well with the organizational system, and to contribute to the defined goals and objectives of the delivery system of which the nurse is a part.
- Provide leadership in the organizational and practice decision-making arenas, not just advice and service. This occurs in the context of accountability and authority for those decisions.
- Share in the evaluation of the effectiveness of the delivery of nursing care services, within both a business and a practice context. The nurse should have an eye to the clear economic and clinical value of the services provided.

CHANGING SERVICE STRUCTURE

The arena for nursing practice is becoming broader in scope yet narrower in function. As previously indicated, smaller and smaller units of clinical activity will undertake a broader range of health care services because corporate structures will continually decentralize based on specified market demands (Waterman, 1987). Each of these unique entities that are offering clinical services will have to stand alone. The nurse practicing in this frameworks will have a broader role than has been traditionally expected in the more centralized, defined unit of service.

The hospital traditionally was organized to provide a multitude of care services within one context in one setting. In the decentralized health care delivery systems, the settings and context for the delivery of services will be wide and variable. From businesses to communities, to homes, to service institutions, homeless shelters, community programs, and

a whole host of other service frameworks not yet conceived, nurses will have to practice in flexible arrangements. These flexible arrangements cannot always be prospectively defined. Each service provider will have to represent closely the specific arena of service that is being offered within the context of the market out of which it is derived. Because of market variability, flexibility in both structure and design will be central to the success of the individual health care services.

No longer will institutions be designing service structures merely to accommodate the organizational and structural needs of the institution. Because the market now determines the health care delivery system, it will be essential that each of the service-providing organizations be structured and designed within the context of the market it serves. The needs framework of the market will clearly describe the functional service framework of those who will provide the service. This is different from the traditional framework for organizations. Usually the hospital structured services to represent both its needs and the needs of its clients. To maintain appropriate systems management and control, often the service structures represented more of the institutional values than it did consumers' values. However, in today's marketplace, to be successful the service provider must design structures that are convenient and serviceable to the consumer. This provides the flexibility necessary to meet the consumers' needs and to ensure financial viability both in the short term and in meeting the institution's long-term objectives.

BROADENING THE NURSE'S SKILLS

In the future, nurses will have to look at incorporating broader-based skills for the management of these clinical health service providers as a part of their clinical practice. The traditional supervisory, policy-based control mechanisms found in the management structures of large institutions will no longer be viable models for the management and operations of these smaller units of service. Because of this, nurses will need to be able to exercise more independent roles in the functioning and the delivery of the clinical health care services they are providing. Also the nurse must be able to incorporate into the practice roles management skills such as budgeting, resource control, personnel skills, business planning, consumer relations, and the like. In other words, the nurse must be able to develop more clearly her or his understanding of the service and economic products of nursing practice.

This is certainly a new role for the practicing nurse as she or he prepares for newer delivery models. However, these new roles are not optional. Mechanisms must therefore be developed in academic centers, as well as in continuing educational development processes within service institutions.

The nurse of today is not prepared to deal with the service, productivity, and economic realities associated with nursing practice and decentralized units of service. Therefore in order to be able to incorporate these roles and skills into the clinical service framework, the nurse will have to undertake further development in primary practice systems. The expectation is that nurses are moving to service frameworks where they have a broader role to play in governance, management, economics, and the delivery of the service itself. The nurse has a broader role to play in practicing nursing within a larger health care context. A fuller professional practice of nursing will be defined within this broad framework and will be described within a clinical and business context.

THE REQUIREMENTS OF NEW MODELS

Governance and structural models will therefore have to incorporate a broader range of roles in the control and governance systems within newer organizational models. Basic expectations of nurses' roles indicate a broader familiarity with the implications of practice as well as the process of practice. Practicing nurses in these newer settings will have to integrate more clearly the relationship between their service, the value of that service, and the outcomes they achieve. The organizational and governance frameworks must therefore reflect the role of the practicing nurse in both defining and carrying out these activities. Hence governance models will have to be more incorporative of clinical processes, val-

ues, and practices than they have in the past and reflect less industrial-based management strategies, treating them as remnants from the past.

NEWER EXECUTIVE PROCESSES

These newer models create a whole new set of variables to be concerned with as nurses work to unfold a much more integrative and highly complex health care delivery system. Since nurses will continue to play increasingly central roles in the delivery of services, being positioned and prepared for these services become vital to the success of the profession's response to new market demands. To ensure that this happens, the following processes will have to be a part of the transitional program of nursing services as they confront the newer designs for organizing nursing services and respond to the clinical demands of these newer models:

1. The nurse executive will have to reexamine the role of leader in the organization. This leader must assess the way in which organizational relationships are described. The organization will need to be restructured from the market and practice framework outward, rather than from the organizational and management hierarchy downward.

2. Practicing nurses will have to develop a broader concept of their role. They will need (a) a clearer understanding of the meaning of accountability, and (b) mechanisms for establishing the authority, autonomy, and control over decentralized services, which are necessary to maintain the services' integrity and response to the market.

3. Unique and creative strategies for integrating multidimensional and multilateral services being provided by nurses will have to be incorporated into the organizational design. Nursing services of the future may share only one common denominator, the fact that nurses offer these services. The wide range of services, which keep them distinct from each other, will have to be carefully managed. Consistent and coordinative mechanisms will need to be designed to maintain nursing corporate integra-

tion at the governance level of the nursing organization.

4. Changes in the role of the nurse—from a primarily dependent provider to a primarily interdependent provider of services—with all of the attendant changes in role, behavior, character, and practice will have to be incorporated into the ongoing career development of practicing nurses. It is at this point that issues related to the appropriate preparation and education of the nurse for these roles take on operational significance. Discussions regarding the educational preparation of the clinical health care provider for these roles must clearly center on the demands of the roles, the expectations for performance, and the outcomes desired. Utilizing this context, differentiated practice models in nursing will have to be carefully defined and implemented.

5. The relationship of the corporate nursing organization to the health service corporation of which it is a part will have to be assessed. Changes in the relationship of nursing to other major categories of the health care corporation must be clarified. This is important particularly in the way in which nursing relates, decides policy, implements response to economic demands, and fulfills the mission of the organization. Therefore, leadership in nursing must play a significant role at the corporate policy and mission level. Roles and relationships related to governance at the board level will be critical. Relationships at the highest executive levels of the corporate health care structure will be central to the success of the nursing corporate effort in delivering nursing services in a multilateral service structure.

It is in the quality of the response to the previously mentioned issues that the nursing organization will position itself to be successful in a market-based economy. Health care systems will continue to evolve. Much change will be experienced in the transition to newer practice models over the next two decades. Financial, service, and market characteristics will continue to be in a state of flux. What is necessary in nursing is the development of newer organizational systems and structures. These are needed to respond strongly to the changes in the marketplace in sufficiently brief time to define and meet the needs of that market as it develops further permutations. The corporate nursing organization and the profession, of which it is a constituent, can no longer wait for other forums of the health care delivery system to identify their appropriate role in responding to the marketplace.

As the National Commission on Nursing Implementation Project (1987) has made clear, nurses are professionals who provide health care services. If this is true, then nurses position themselves to be available to those services as they become a valued and important part of the health care delivery system. Economic, social, and market positioning is central to the success of the delivery of nursing services as we move toward the 21st century.

The ability of the nursing organization to structure itself utilizing professional practice models—rather than hierarchial or industrial models—will be key to the nursing organization's ability to respond to these market demands, and to provide leadership for the health care delivery system. To the extent that nursing leaders can respond incisively to these important governance and operational issues, nursing's position, role, and leadership in the health care delivery system will either be diminished or enhanced. As to which it will be, as always, the choice is ours.

REFERENCES

Callahan, C. B., & Wall, L. L. (1987). Participative management: A contingiency approach. *Journal of Nursing Administration, 17* (9), 9–15.

Naisbitt J., & Aburdene P. (1985). *Reinventing the corporation*. New York: Warner Books.

Naisbitt, J. (1984). *Megatrends*. New York: Warner Books.

National Commission on Nursing Implementation Project. (1986). *Report of the First Invitational Conference*. Milwaukee: Author.

National Commission on Nursing Implementation Project.

(1987). *Report of the Second Invitational Conference*. San Diego: Author.

Toffler, A. (1980). *The third wave*. New York: William Morrow & Co.

Waterman, R. H. (1987). *The renewal factor: How the best get and keep the competitive edge*. New York: Bantam Books.

✳ EDITOR'S QUESTIONS FOR DISCUSSION ✳

What are the implications and relationships in this chapter for those written by Lyon (Chapter 34), Wolf (Chapter 49), Graham and Sheppard (Chapter 52), and Weaver (Chapter 53)? What is the best structure, organizational framework, and relational system for management of the professional worker and why? Design possible structures that would capitalize on the professional aspects of nursing practice. What specific type of decision making requires autonomous nursing practice for professional nurses? What specific inputs, outputs, and outcomes are to be accountable by professional nurses in practice? How is this type of accountability different for the nurse manager than the staff nurse?

How can standards for nursing practice be interdependent with standards held by and for structures in organizations? What method and process is most effective in developing and implementing a peer-based evaluation system? What factors inhibit the successful utilization of a peer evaluation system? What interventions can be made to correct problems in a peer evaluation system? What type of skills will be needed in the management of clinical service providers of the future? What type of transitional programs for nursing service should be developed in either academic settings, continuing education programs, or staff development programs to prepare professional staff nurses for new models of providing clinical care and professional care?

Realities in Retention and Recruitment

Nancy O. Graham, Dr. P.H., R.N.
Christine Sheppard, R.N.

Nurses provide 95% of the care a patient receives while hospitalized

> (American Academy of Nursing, 1983, p. 1)

Nurses' central dilemma is:

The order to care in a society that refuses to value caring.

> (Reverby, 1987, p. 5)

Both the institutional image and the personal image presented by the nurse greatly affect customer satisfaction with hospital service.

> (Curran, 1987, p. 1)

Too many service companies have concentrated on cost cutting efficiencies they can quantify, rather than adding to their product's value by listening carefully and . . . providing the service their customers want.

> (Peters, 1987, p. 6)

These quotes are indicative of the organizational, social, and economic milieu of today's health care environment. The nation's hospitals are struggling with a new environment of prospective payment, increased regulation, reduced demand for inpatient services, increased competition from physicians in ambulatory settings—and now—the national nursing shortage. Some administrators have said that the nursing shortage is a national health care crisis.

This shortage is the result of many factors, for example, a precipitous decline in nursing school enrollment, a decline in the size of the cohort of 18-year-olds, an increase in career options for women, poor working conditions (weekend work, shift rotation, overtime), and a lack of a strong public image of the nurse's role as a professional. Addressing the retention and the recruitment of nurses in this changing environment requires great flexibility on both the macro and micro levels. For example, on the macro level, while the burden of solving much of the current nursing shortage falls on the providers of health service, this responsibility is shared by government, by the education sector, and by professional associations. State and federal governments provide a substantial amount of funds that support the health care industry, the education sector prepares those who enter the health care industry, and the professional associations ensure that professional standards and issues are addressed. Solutions to the recruitment and retention dilemma require extensive cooperation and coordination of these groups. Explanation and development of other issues relating to recruitment and retention that need to be dealt with on the macro level include portable pensions, retraining classes, scholarships, loan forgiveness, and education and marketing.

At the micro, or hospital level, greater attention must be given to retaining the current work force. Job satisfaction is critical to any strategy that strives to ensure an adequate supply of nurses. Management must be bold in discarding much of its inheritance; what works today may not work 6 months from now.

There are many variables in a sound hospital retention program. Leadership is a key factor. Positive attitudes of management and staff are fundamental. Intense communication is required to foster involvement of the nurses. It is imperative to listen constantly and share information and ideas. To make it work you must believe there is much worth listening to. Flexibility, feedback, and action are essential. Wholesale participation of the nurses is a must. And then recognize, recognize, the nurse. (Peters, 1987).

PRELIMINARY GROUNDWORK

The focus of this chapter is retention of nurses: the realities for individual hospitals. Before getting into the specifics, certain groundwork must be laid. First, in a viable retention program there must be a *value* system that is shared by all participants from members of the board to every employee. This may be one of the most crucial requirements for sound management in the changing health care organization of the future (American Academy of Nursing, 1983). Everyone must buy into a core philosophy of how the organization works. Individual and organizational values must be congruent, must be clear, and must be exciting. The hospital and the nursing department must have a sound set of beliefs on which they base all action. The basic philosophy, spirit, and drive have far more to do with retention than organizational structure, technological resources, or economic resources. There must a belief in being the best, a belief in the importance of people, a belief in giving superior care, and these beliefs must permeate all other departments (Kramer & Schmalenberg, 1988b).

Second, the *roles* of both nursing management and staff nurses must be clarified. These roles in recent years have become more collegial and collaborative. The congruency of role expectation between nursing administration and staff nurses appears to be a strong retention factor (American Academy of Nursing, 1983). Role clarification between staff nurses and physicians is necessary. For instance, despite the fact that hospital patients today are more acutely ill and require constant monitoring and intervention, there has been little formal recognition of the impact of the nurse's role in clinical decision-making. The shift in medicine from general to specialty practice has resulted in multiple physician specialists caring for a single patient. The nurse needs to synthesize continually and coordinate the care of the many physicians. Despite these factors, there has been little recognition of the expanded role of the nurse (Aiken, 1982).

In addition, the nurse must synthesize and coordinate the care of the patient rendered by other disciplines. The nurse is the only primary caregiver who is with the patient 24 hours a day and assumes the responsibilities of physical therapist, respiratory therapist, social worker, and nutritionist. Furthermore the nurse often assumes tasks that normally fall to other departments such as housekeeping, transport, and messengers. Such situations create role ambiguity that must be clarified. The nurse must be recognized as the facilitator of all direct patient care, and she or he must have the authority to control the support services and other resources that indirectly affect patient care (Aiken, 1982).

RECRUITMENT

Job fairs, career days, and advertising are all part of recruitment. However, one of the most important ingredients in recruitment starts with the interview. Managers need to elicit commitment from the onset. The interviewer needs to address the realities of modern nursing—hard work, responsibility, accountability, ongoing educational demands, technological know-how, and the ability to care compassionately in a society that may not place a value on caring (Reverby, 1987).

The recruiting process should be intense and straightforward. The interviewer should concentrate on traits that many would consider soft. Nursing management must become adept at assessing teamwork, flexibility, courtesy, and a commitment to patient care. An impressive resume is no guarantee of success (Peters, 1987). It is important to hire people who have a value system in agreement with the one you are trying to promote (Kramer & Schmalenberg, 1988b).

RETENTION—THE REALITIES FOR INDIVIDUAL HOSPITALS

The goals of a retention program are to allow nurses to practice nursing and to make the hospital the place where the nurse wants to work. They are not mutually exclusive.

Nurses at the Bedside

The first goal of the retention program is to bring the nurse back to the bedside of the patient. Nurses want to practice nursing. This simply means bringing the art, science, and spirit of nursing that is taught in the schools to the patient's bedside—in order to deliver the care that meets the needs of each individual patient. Unfortunately, in today's health care milieu, nurses feel that they cannot practice nursing, that the obstacles between them and their patients are often insurmountable. These obstacles have not appeared overnight as part of a deliberate or systematic plan to obstruct the delivery of patient care by nurses ("Consider This," 1988). They are, in fact, related to multiple factors in society, in government, and in health care institutions that have converged at this point in time. These factors, as demonstrated in Figure 52-1 have had the greatest impact on the people who are directly involved in providing patient care, the nurses.

The institution of prospective reimbursement and diagnosis related groups (DRGs) has resulted in an increase in patient acuity and a shorter length of stay. Patients have a greater need than ever before for nursing time, self-care education, emotional and social support, and discharge planning. The demands of treating a more acutely ill patient population in a shortened period of time has resulted in inadequate nursing time available for patients. Thus nurses feel guilty, frustrated, and unfulfilled.

To correct this, hospitals must recognize the economic relationship between the nurse and the services rendered. However, the reimbursement environment has led hospitals to consider shrinking financial resources and the "bottom line." It is clear that a financial commitment to qualified nurses is a worthwhile investment and the risk of making that investment now versus deferring it is a cost opportunity lost. The health care industry must change the message to nurses from "do more with less" to "more nurses mean quality patient care."

Another economic solution for hospitals is to recognize nursing units as profit or revenue centers rather than as cost centers. Nursing managers should control operations not just from the expense side of the budget but from the revenue side as well. The time has come for costing out of nursing services. These solutions involve the nurse in a partic-

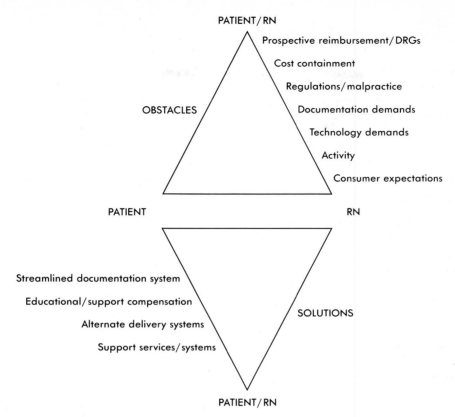

PATIENT/RN

Prospective reimbursement/DRGs

Cost containment

Regulations/malpractice

OBSTACLES   Documentation demands

Technology demands

Activity

Consumer expectations

PATIENT   RN

Streamlined documentation system

Educational/support compensation

Alternate delivery systems   SOLUTIONS

Support services/systems

PATIENT/RN

FIGURE 52-1

Obstacles and solutions in patient-nurse relations.

ipatory and responsible way in the survival of the institution (Buerhaus, 1987).

Increasing governmental, outside agency, and third-party regulation, combined with rising malpractice threats, have mandated voluminous documentation by the nurse as a primary caregiver. Valuable time that should be spent on patient comfort and well-being is being spent on paperwork. Documentation and charting systems must be evaluated and streamlined to facilitate this important process of translating care to records. Staff nurses must actively participate in this change if it is to be effective.

Technological advances from computerized monitoring systems to complex diagnostic testing demand sophisticated knowledge and ability of the nurse, but also require time-consuming attention to "hardware details." Nurses must "monitor the monitors" as well as the patients. Faced with increased patient care demands and the demands of high technology, it is the caring details of nursing that suffer. Once again, nurses are in a situation that frustrates their efforts in delivering bedside care. Not only do nurses have to spend more time with high-tech equipment, but they have to spend more time learning about and keeping up with technology without commensurate compensation for their knowledge and skills.

Hospitals need to demonstrate a commitment to continuing education for nurses. Time must be allocated for continuing education, time that nurses perceive as education time and not time away from patient care. Tuition reimbursement, conference time, salary education differential, recognition for specialty certification, and career ladders that support ongoing education are necessary.

The shift in demographics and in attitudes of patients as consumers has been translated into higher expectations for the nurse who is working with fewer and fewer resources. The patient population is elderly, is sicker, has a high proportion of patients with AIDS or chronic multisystem diseases, resulting in a dramatic increase in the need for nursing care. Educated consumers believe that good care is their right and they have high expectations about the care that they receive. The consumer believes "more is better" and the nurses are faced with "doing more with less." This results in frustrated consumers and nurses. Solutions include evaluation of alternate care delivery systems, such as faculty practice and case management. Staff nurse participation is vital to the success of these programs. Adequate support services must be provided to address nonnursing tasks and functions, for example, transport, messengers, housekeeping, and dietary aides. An interdepartmental espirit de corps is imperative. A commitment to flexibility and change by hospitals must be translated into action.

The dramatic changes that have created today's health care milieu have not changed the basic premise of health care: patients want to be nursed back to health and nurses want to practice nursing. A sound hospital retention program will ensure that the patient and the nurse are brought together in an environment that meets both of these needs.

The Hospital as a Place of Work

The second goal of a nurse retention program is to make the hospital an attractive place to work. To implement a retention program the issues listed in Figure 52-2 must be addressed. The retention program must be dynamic; what works today may not work tomorrow.

The factors reflecting dissatisfaction with hospital employment can be grouped into the following categories (Prescott, 1987):

1. Salary and benefits.

2. Control over basic working conditions, for example, hours, shifts.
3. Professional issues, including autonomy, respect, and promotional opportunity.

While the economic and benefit packages are important and need to be addressed, they are not the only concern. Flexible scheduling and control over hours are important. Nurses want to participate in clinical and managerial decisions that affect their practice. Collaboration with other team members is essential for the quality of patient care and for the satisfaction of the nurse. Participation in decisions and self-governance empower the nurse. Opportunities must be given for growth and advancement by use of education programs, clinical career ladders, and recognition programs. Making the hospital an attractive place to work (i.e., improving basic working conditions, paying competitive wages and benefits, providing opportunities for growth and advancement, allowing authority over practice, and truly valuing the nurses' contribution to patient care) is a cornerstone in a retention program (Prescott, 1987).

Administration must *believe* that the staff nurse is the one essential, irreplaceable link in the delivery of patient care (Kramer & Schmalenberg, 1988a). The nurse must be well educated, must be included in policy and practice decisions, and must feel appreciated and valued as an integral member of the hospital's health team. The core philosophy of the hospital and the nurse must be in harmony.

Leaders need to develop a culture in which people work hard and enjoy coming to work. An effective leader has a vision of the future and works with everyone to buy into such a vision. The climate must be positive with a sincere caring for each person. Staff recognition must be wholehearted and plentiful. The expectations must be clear, exciting, and pervasive. A sense of commitment fosters retention. When there is a clear mission and a purpose, productivity increases and commitment solidifies.

Visible management is a requisite for today's hospital. Management must be ever-present to encourage the nurses to be comfortable with change, innovation, and risk taking. People should be encouraged to learn from their mistakes and to try again.

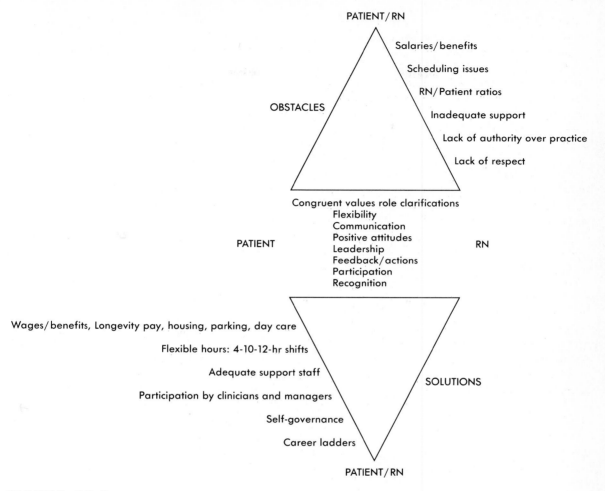

FIGURE 52-2

Obstacles and solutions in the hospital environment.

Today's effective leader must listen, take action, give feedback, teach, cajole, care, and comfort. To listen, per se, is the single best tool for empowering large numbers of people. This also helps to create an energetic esprit de corps. On a unit with excellent retention, the staff have high energy and a sense that nothing can stop them. This spirit is electric, contagious, and encompassed in the culture of the organization (Kerfoot, 1988).

There is no one solution to rectify the problems of getting the nurse back to the bedside and in making the hospital an attractive place to work. While issues must be addressed by the federal and state governments, by the education sector, and through professional associations, the focus of this chapter has been the realities for the individual hospital. The current reality as demonstrated in Figure 52-3 includes issues that impact on the nurse and on the hospital.

The result of ignoring these issues will affect both

RN

Salaries
Lack of control over lives/scheduling
RN-patient ratios
Inadequate support services
Lack of authority over practice
Lack of recognition/respect
Limited promotional opportunities

HOSPITAL

DRGs
Cost containment
Regulations, legal issues, documentation demands
Technological demands
Patient acuity, elderly, AIDS
Consumer expectations

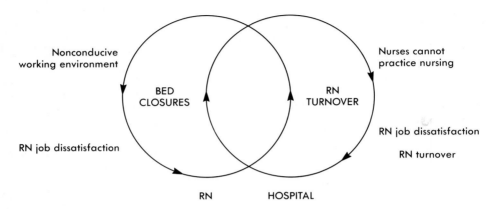

FIGURE 52-3

Current realities: impact on nurses and hospitals.

RN

Professional recognition
Autonomy in practice
Improved scheduling/self-governance
Improved salary/benefits
Sense of value/recognition

HOSPITAL

Participative fiscal control
Costing nursing services
Streamlined documentation
Educational support/compensation
Alternate delivery systems
Support services/systems

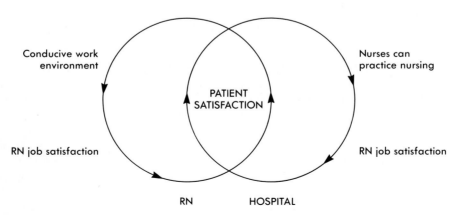

FIGURE 52-4

Future realities: impact on nurses and hospitals.

cal) that define the parameters for collective bargaining. These regulate such functions as the recognition, certification, negotiation, and implementation of collective bargaining outcomes—both labor contract content and implementation. The major legislation to minimize disruption to the economy from nurse labor-management disputes is the 1974 Amendment to the National Labor Relations Act (NLRA) governing nurses employed in the private sector (Flanagan, 1986; Stevens, 1980; Werther & Lockhart, 1976). The NLRA sets restrictions on actions by employers and unions in the private sector to prevent disruption of the health care industry and to ensure previously denied worker rights to health care employees.

State labor laws, such as right-to-work and right to organize and bargain legislation, further define the parameters of union and employer activities in relation to public sector employees. Other ancillary legislation affecting worker rights are: (a) federal legislation on safe working conditions by the Occupational Safety and Health Act of 1970 (OSHA), employment discrimination by the Civil Rights Act of 1964, and wages by the Fair Labor Standards Act of 1938; and (b) state insurance health rate regulations. Right-to-work legislation is perceived as decreasing union's chances of winning elections, decreasing the level of union activity, and supporting management's resistance to unionization (Becker, 1983; Juris & Maxey, 1981; Kochan & Wheeler, 1975). In contrast, right to organize and bargain legislation facilitates unions organizing workers. Becker (1983) and Tanner, Weinstein, and Ahomuty (1979) reported that unions in states with laws facilitating collective bargaining in nonprofit hospitals before the passage of the 1974 NLRA amendment had higher union election and victory rates than those unions in states without such legislation.

State insurance regulations affect the resources that hospital management has available to meet union demands, particularly wage-related issues (Becker, 1983; Becker, Sloan, & Steinwald, 1982). Legislated mandatory continuing education may be considered a "mandatory" bargaining issue, thus requiring employers and labor to codify educational provisions. Worker rights are covered by OSHA.

Civil rights legislation and amendments to the Social Security Act at times supercede areas covered under NLRA and state and local labor laws.

The National Labor Relations Board has a central and a regional director whose interpretations and administrative rulings on the NLRA and court decisions on such issues as bargaining unit composition, management domination, and "fire at will" doctrine further direct the actions of management and labor participants. For example, the Supreme Court's five-to-three decision in the *Communications Workers of America v. Beck* case protects employees who choose not to join a union, even though their institution is represented by a collective bargaining unit, by allowing them to regain any portion of their dues spent on activities related to collective bargaining ("Little Effect," 1988). Federal and state appointments to these administrative and judicial bodies further mold the labor relations legal environment. The myriad of legislation, administrative rulings and interpretations, and court decisions affects both directly and indirectly the bargaining process, its participants, and bargaining outcomes.

Economic Environment

The economic environment refers to those labor-monetary factors such as labor supply and demand, prevailing income, wage rates, and urbanization that, in part, determine the marketplace in which unionization and collective bargaining take place. These factors are the resources needed to support or to deter unionization. Of specific importance are the wealth of and number of health care personnel within a specific geographical area. According to Fennell (1982) and Becker (1983), the higher the levels of each of these indicators, the richer the area is in needed resources. Becker contended that in high per capita income areas, there are more resources to resist unionization than in low per capita areas; areas with high levels of per capita income were not traditionally strong areas of union support.

Common economic variables used in labor research are per capita income for a defined geographical area; ratio of registered nurses (RNs) to total population in an area; total population per defined geographical area, and type of geographical location, that is, urban, rural, or suburban. In research by Juris and Maxey (1981) and Pettengill (1988), these economic variables were found not to be significant in unionization of professionals and specifically nurses. However, Pettengill reported the following trends. State nurses' associations (SNAs) negotiated contracts more frequently than trade and service unions (TSUs) in not-for-profit hospitals located in areas with high per capita income, high RN ratios, and high total population. TSUs organized nurses more frequently than state nurses' associations in metropolitan areas where union chances of success are generally higher (Becker, 1983; Juris & Maxey, 1981). Thus both SNAs and TSUs competed for nurses in economic environments rich in resources. However, SNAs also organized nurses located in rural areas, thus demonstrating their commitment to all nurses regardless of geographical location.

Further discussion of the potential labor supply as an economic factor includes the percent of full-time and part-time employees. Within hospital nursing, there is a large supply of part-time employees, who may or may not be covered by contracts. The extent to which the nursing shortage of the 1980s influences these percentages needs to be researched. However, if the present trend in facility unionization spreads over into health labor relations, there could be additional efforts to organize more fully the part-time work segment (Blum, 1988).

Another economic environmental factor considered to influence union activity is the emergence of prospective payment systems and state cost review boards. Schramm (1977) stated that systems designed to control or both control and regulate health care costs determined the available supply of dollars budgeted for labor costs; therefore monetary amounts were guaranteed before actual negotiations. However, Abramson (1978) contended that management within this economic environment may go above its "ceiling" and try to maneuver unions into negotiating with these fiscal parties for additional dollars.

Emergence of these regulatory groups intent on controlling hospital cost has altered the character of health care labor relations. Multilateral collective bargaining has replaced the traditional bipartite labor-management process (Pettengill, 1985). Multiple actors influence negotiations directly and indirectly. Within this environment, labor and management relinquish some of their decision-making authority to other parties in order to resolve conflict.

When considering the economic environment, no discussion is complete without reference to labor costs and the concept of monopsony—the dominance of one employer controlling the worker market. Monopsony has been applied to nursing by Link and Landon (1975), and supported by the common knowledge that over 60% of the possible nurse labor supply works in hospitals. Link and Landon contended that monopsony restricts wages and consequently affects union demands for wage compensation. Two major trends are found within this complex economic environment. First, there has been reported a positive collective bargaining effect on wages and fringe benefits by Becker et al. (1982). They reported, based on their summary of available literature, that unions have had a smaller effect on professional nurses' and other professionals' wages than on those of nonprofessional occupations. Their contention is substantiated by the work of economists like Sloan and Elnicki (1978), Link and Landon (1976), and Feldman and Scheffler (1982), who reported varying increases in nursing salaries with an average increase of about 6%.

The second trend is that collective bargaining affects a hospital employee's pay even when he or she is not a union member. Feldman and Scheffler (1982) and Becker (1979) reported that internal spillover effects raise compensation from 1% to 8%. Measures of external spillover, in which wage activity of one unionized hospital affects pay levels in a neighboring nonunionized hospital, are imprecise, but generally are considered to occur (Becker et al., 1982).

The final economic environmental factor for consideration is the impact of unionization on hospital costs. When the impact of strike activity is excluded from analysis, Becker et al. (1982), in their review of existing literature, reported that a conservative estimate of the full union effect on real hospital expenditures is about 10%. Becker et al. (1982) stated: "This estimate implies that hospital union growth raised real spending on hospital care by about 5 percent during the 1970's as compared to the 67 percent increase actually observed" (p. 11).

MANAGEMENT, UNION, AND WORKER CHARACTERISTICS
Management Characteristics

The management (organization) demographic characteristics applied to health care labor relations are often used in research on nursing labor relations. The primary management variables include hospital (agency) ownership and bed size, and management rights. The former variables have been examined by Alexander and Bloom (1987), Juris (1977), Juris and Maxey (1981), and Pettengill (1988), who provided data on overall hospital complexity, labor pool available for unionization, and differences in propensity for unionization by different union types.

Regarding hospital bed size, the larger the hospital's bed capacity, the more resources and bureaucracy exist to deal with unions; thus, larger hospitals are less resistant to unionization than smaller hospitals (Becker, 1983). From the union's perspective, larger hospitals offer greater return on the union's investment. Also greater worker-employee distance found in larger institutions makes worker dissatisfaction more likely, and therefore unionization more appealing. While Juris (1977) and Becker (1983) reported that the most unionized hospitals were those in bed-size categories of 300 and above, Pettengill (1988) in her study of unionized hospital nurses reported that a majority of the 95 hospitals studied were under 300 beds regardless of SNA or TSU representation. The American Hospital Association's 1987 Nursing Personnel Survey (AHA, 1987) supported Pettengill's findings, and further reported that hospitals between 200 and 299 beds and very large institutions (500 or more beds) were unionized at 1.5 times the national rate.

Hospital ownership has been identified as a factor in propensity for unionization. Juris and Maxey (1981) stated that union influence

would be generally greeted in the private sector since the public sector hospital bargaining often occurs within the context of city- or state-wide collective bargaining processes which may impose structural constraints on the size or scope of the settlement unions can obtain. (p. 28)

Becker (1983) stated that from the union's perspective, employee loyalty to religious hospitals made them difficult to organize, whereas profit-making hospitals had financial resources for wage and fringe benefit issues. In contrast, management in for-profit hospitals perceived themselves as having greater administrative prerogatives, and being more resistant to unionization than administrators of voluntary and religious hospitals (Becker, 1983). The findings of Wakim (1976), Pettengill (1988), and those from the AHA 1987 Nursing Personnel Survey (AHA, 1987) supported the contention that not-for-profit hospitals were more likely to have unionized nurses than investor-owned institutions.

Management rights is considered another characteristic and prerogative of management. The employer has the right to direct the work of employees; to maintain efficiency of agency operation; to fire, suspend, and retain employees; and to promote, demote, transfer, and assign employees. Within health care labor relations, these rights are deemed necessary for there to exist the staffing needed for quality care (Metzger, 1979). Somers (1975) and Zimmerman (1975) cautioned against union intrusion into those management rights that included formulation of macroeconomic policy. Metzger further contended: "When a union extracts a concession to limit sub-contracting, it is in effect controlling the hospital's ability to deliver patient care at a level which may be less costly and more efficient (not always, but the possibility exists)" (p. 29).

However, research by Juris and Maxey (1981) and Pettengill (1987, 1988) showed a growing trend toward encroachment by the unions on management's right to determine staffing utilization. Specifically Pettengill reported that TSUs were more likely to negotiate contract language affecting staffing determinations of subcontracting than were SNAs. In addition, the nursing shortage of the 1980s may result in labor challenging management's prerogatives to use float pools, nurse registries, and subcontracted nursing personnel and in management insisting on utilizing these resources.

Union Characteristics

Within nursing there exists union dualism. Union dualism should not be confused with coalition bargaining, which is defined as two or more unions bargaining jointly for a common master contract for all employees within a single institution. Union dualism refers to the presence of dual union actors, that is, a state nurses' association and a conventional trade or service union, who compete for the right to represent professional employees (Walker & Lawler, 1979). Walker and Lawler's conceptualization of union dualism distinguishes between aggressive unions, which place priority on the distribution of management power among employees, and protective unions, in which the priority is employee dissatisfaction with the responsiveness of the incumbent management. Within this framework, Walker and Lawler identified the American Nurses' Association and its constituent states as a "protective" union since it was concerned with protecting or restoring an environment of professionalism and collegiality, generally by nonmilitant strategies.

Trade and service unions, such as the American Federation of Teachers (AFT) and the National Union of Hospital Care Employees (1199), were categorized as "aggressive" unions that sought to improve salaries and working conditions, which sometimes had liberal or populist views on social issues, and which were willing to strike to achieve their objectives. Authors such as Colangelo (1980), Donaldson and Warner (1974), Seldon (1972), and Pettengill (1988) agreed that the opposing ideological postures of different union types affected the negotiating process and dictated, in part, the bargaining outcomes. Furthermore research by Juris and Maxey (1981), Pettengill, (1987, 1988), and Wakim (1976) on specific contract outcomes for unionized professional and nonprofessional employees and nurses by different union types substantiated these differences. Pettengill's research further documented differences by SNAs and TSUs for negotiated contract provisions on staffing determinations, education, and decision-making provisions.

In addition, union dualism exists in primarily highly urbanized areas where there are more available hospitals from which to compete (Pettengill,

1988). The AHA 1987 Nursing Personnel Survey reported that SNAs were the collective bargaining agents in 60% of organized hospitals; TSUs were a distant second with 26.7% (AHA, 1987). TSUs and SNAs are similar in their propensity to organize not-for-profit rather than profit, investor-owned hospitals (Pettengill, 1988). TSUs are more likely to cross state boundaries, whereas SNAs' contracts are generally restricted to one state.

SNAs are more likely to have homogeneous or all–Registered Nurse (all-RN) bargaining units than are TSUs. This characteristic may not prevail in the future because of recent challenges to the "community of interest doctrine" and movement toward a "disparity of interest test" for determining bargaining unit composition (Flanagan, 1988). Rather than the National Labor Relations Board accepting prima facie all-RN bargaining units, petitioning RN employees, SNAs, and TSUs have had to establish sharper than usual differences in wages, hours, and working conditions from those of other professionals and nonprofessionals. This evolving need, coupled with NLRB surveillance of supervisor dominance within SNAs' governing boards, has led some SNAs to insulate their union activities from other association activities ("Major Bylaws," 1986).

Worker Characteristics

Characteristics of nurses seeking union representation and attitudes of nurses toward collective bargaining have been frequent areas for nursing research. Researchers have focused on the perceptions and attitudes of staff nurses and nursing administrators toward professionalism and unionism (Beletz, 1980; Levi, 1980; Pettengill, 1983; Sargis, 1978). Denton (1976) examined the relationships between job satisfaction and contract clause provisions. Hunter, Bamberg, Castiglia, and McCausland (1986) studied job satisfaction and propensity for unionization. They maintained that although not statistically significant, the data seemed to indicate that (a) collective bargaining cannot help improve a job; and (b) a trend toward nurses who are not represented by collective bargaining being more dissatisfied with their jobs than those who are represented.

The work of Kleingartner (1973), Levi (1980), Pettengill (1983), and Ponak (1981) examined the influence of nursing as a profession or a semiprofession or occupation on bargaining outcomes. Kleingartner (whose results were validated by Ponak) maintained that if nurses perceived their work as an occupation or semiprofession, they were more likely to be interested in short-run job and work rewards (Level I goals), rather than longer-run career and professional goals and objectives generally associated with a profession (Level II goals). In contrast, if the nurses viewed nursing as a profession, then there would be more activity to negotiate contract provisions that encompassed concepts of autonomy, occupational integrity and identification, individual satisfaction and career development, and economic security and enhancement. Pettengill's research (1983) on attitudes of unionized nurses toward professionalism showed that autonomy was perceived by the sample studied as antithetical to unionization. These findings suggest that the desired outcomes by nurses seeking representation require assessment by labor, management, and the employees involved before selection of a bargaining agent and contract negotiations.

The final characteristic of the work force is the presence of functional redundancy, that is, others can be substituted for nurses' work. Nursing's inability to define legally and control its practice domain has been a factor in strike activity (Levi, 1980), contract resolution (Levi, 1980), layoffs, and, most likely, in the current movement by the American Medical Association for "registered care technologists" (RCTs) (Page, 1988).

BARGAINING ISSUES AND OUTCOMES
Bargaining Unit Composition

As previously mentioned, bargaining unit composition is a central issue in nursing collective bargaining. In the past, the community of interest doctrine was applied to all-RN bargaining units. This doctrine refers to grouping together only employees with substantial mutual interests in wages, hours, and working conditions of employment (Pointer &

Metzger, 1975). However, the community of interest doctrine has been repeatedly challenged by the disparity of interest test, that is, grouping of different employees who have similar job functions and responsibilities. As the National Labor Relations Board examined this issue, labor and management continued to assert their respective viewpoints. For management, units with all professionals may (a) be easier to defeat, (b) more accurately reflect the homogeneity of the professional worker, and (c) more appropriately reflect the multidisciplinary teams in which the various professionals regularly interact. Management has also argued that separate professional units are not cost-effective, hinder efficient utilization of staff, and lead to multiple strikes or strike threats (Flanagan, 1988). For labor, the posture taken on this issue may well depend on union type. State nurses' associations maintain that their exists a strong community of interest that is not shared by other professionals, because of nurses' 24-hour responsibility for patient care, intermittent communication with other professionals, and distinct wage market for nurses (Flanagan, 1988). The TSUs stance on the disparity of interest test is dependent on their past practices of including nonnurses in RN bargaining units, their assessment of the economic ramifications of bargaining unit expansion, their acknowledged different ideology, and their assertion that they negotiated professional issues (Pettengill, 1988). The National Labor Relations Board, responding to the testimony by management and labor, on September 1, 1988 ruled on the 1982 St. Francis case. They sanctioned eight bargaining units, one of which is an all-RN bargaining unit. Thus they reaffirmed the community of interest doctrine (Bureau of National Affairs, 1988). How this decision will affect those SNAs who have insulated their collective bargaining components will require careful watching. What will be the reaction by TSUs who are more likely to include RNs with other professional and nonprofessional groups? What will be the response by nurses who favor expanding the American Nurses' Association (ANA) membership structure? What will be management's next move? All of these questions are unanswerable at this time.

Delineation of Professional Issues for Negotiation

In general, economic gains as advocated by Cleland (1978), Jacox (1980), and Zimmerman (1981) were a paramount issue in the collective bargaining outcomes for nursing. Additionally the ANA has proclaimed an indivisibility of patient care policies, working conditions, and economic benefits (Gideon, 1979). These authors concurred that the ambiguity of the phrase, "and other working conditions of employment," gives license to negotiations that directly affect such professional issues as autonomy, determination of staffing ratios, and control over quality of care.

Jacox (1980) has contended that the general consensus of the nursing profession on the definition of the working conditions phrase distinguishes nursing collective bargaining from traditional bargaining models in which the primary focus is salaries and fringe benefits. She maintained that professional concerns were mandatory bargaining issues. Other authors, such as Castrey and Castrey (1980) and Flanagan (1986), have also identified professional issues that should be subsumed under working conditions. These include (a) release time for continuing education, program fees, and expenses for workshops; (b) participation on committees, for example, patient care, employment condition, and joint practice committees; (c) involvement in staffing determinations, that is, setting staffing ratios and patterns for general and specialty units, and assessing use of float pools, temporary assignments, and subcontracting; (d) establishment of clinical career ladders; and (e) inclusion of a code of ethics, standards of practice, and state practice acts.

However, the actual inclusion of these professional provisions varies over time and by union type. Wakim (1976) in her comparison of 50 SNA and 50 TSU contracts reported that (a) SNAs significantly differed from TSUs on inclusion of professional standards committees; (b) TSUs were more oriented toward economic issues; (c) SNA contracts were more inclusive of both professional and economic issues; and (d) inclusion of both economic and professional concerns was determined by the number of years over which collective bargaining was practiced in a hospital. In 1977 Miller, Becker, and Krinsky reported that nursing hospital contracts in a tristate region were silent on patient care issues of staffing, job assignments, and working conditions. While some contracts included a joint study committee, the authority and scope were unclear. Juris (1977) included nursing contracts with the general category of health care contracts and found some provision for "decision making" input on professional issues through use of joint study committees. Educational leave was mentioned in almost one half of the sampled contracts. Juris assumed that SNAs were the dominant negotiator of nursing contracts.

The 1988 ANA analysis of 190 SNA contracts documented that they contained provisions that addressed practice concerns not shared by other professions (Flanagan, 1988). Flanagan stated: "Agreements, for example, commonly established nursing practice committees to address such issues as standards of nursing care, means of alleviating the nursing shortage, the use of temporary nurses hired through outside agencies, and other staffing concerns" (p. 26). Pettengill's research (1987, 1988) on contract inclusion of professional issues showed that SNAs were more likely to include provisions on decision making and education, whereas TSUs were more likely to include provisions on staffing determinations.

The above research supports the contention that working condition clauses indeed reflect professional concerns, but also that there is variability in their negotiation by union type. Although the contract sets guidelines for management, labor, and employee on these matters, questions remain concerning what extent negotiated professional provisions alter the work environment sufficiently to affect worker satisfaction, commitment, retention, turnover, absenteeism, and quality of patient care, as well as from whose perspective these effects are perceived to occur?

FUTURE DIRECTIONS

Legal and economic climate, management, union and employee characteristics, and bargaining issues and outcomes interrelate to create a system of collective bargaining aimed at resolving management-labor conflict. The viability of the collective bargaining system, not only within nursing but in general, has been questioned. There has been a decline and then an increase in the unionized hospital nurse population. The 1980 AHA Special Survey on Selected Topics estimated that 18.5% of the 7000 hospitals in the survey had nurse contracts (Pettengill, 1988); the AHA 1985 survey reported 12.9%, and the 1987 survey, 14.8% (AHA, 1987).

Some explanations for the variability include inaccurate reporting, confusion in coding categories, and reluctance to share data. The distribution of unions continues with over 60% of the contracts negotiated by SNAs and 26% negotiated by TSUs (AHA, 1987; Pettengill, 1988). As the SNAs expand their union representation and TSUs continue their activities to include other professionals and nonprofessionals in RN bargaining units, there is potential for union growth. Management's response to nurse dissatisfaction and to pressure to resolve the perceived nursing shortage of the late 1980s will be crucial in determining whether union activity surges and what issues will be negotiated. Collective bargaining endeavors are affected by the nursing wage compression. Will the unions (and management) be able to take a proactive response to this problem, or continue their reactive short-term approach to wages? Will there be changes in bargaining table priorities, that is, wages traded off for control over practice and staffing; hours traded for expanded benefit packages; educational reimbursement traded for job security?

Union survival may well, in part, depend on the resolution of the entry-into-practice issue. Hunter et al. (1986) found that associate degree nurses (ADN) were more likely to favor unionization than baccalaureate (BSN) nurses. Even with the overall decrease in nurse supply, more ADN than BSN nurses are prepared for the profession.

Hospital acquisitions and establishment of multihospital facility systems further affect the future of nursing labor relations. The NLRB examines whether the "single employer" theory applies, that is, if separate and independent entities exist or if shared or common management, ownership, operations, and actual control over labor relations exist (Brent, 1987). If the single employer theory is applied, then questions arise on whether or not the bargaining unit should be multifacility. Furthermore if a unionized facility acquires a nonunionized facility, employees may be "accreted" or added to an existing unit, thus extending the collective bargaining contract to newly acquired nurse employees whose community of interest with existing bargaining units requires assessment.

Again, the issue of bargaining unit composition is raised. It is doubtful that the NLRB's September 1988 ruling puts the issue to rest. The dynamic nature of nursing, unions' need to survive economically, and management's assessment of what nursing care it needs to provide, are only three variables constantly playing on this doctrine.

Research on factors affecting unionization of nurses is crucial. Little is known on how unionization affects recruitment and retention or how it affects patient outcomes. While research documents different contract content by union type, further research is needed to determine if these differences reflect the professional or occupational orientation of the affected nurses, management, or union. Contract implementation remains another area for study, with such questions as, Are their differences in contract implementation by union type? What level of conflict must exist during contract implementation for successful renegotiation?

The collective bargaining of nurses is a complex system within a complex practice market. Understanding of one system requires knowledge of the other. Ultimately the goal of both is harmony in order to provide what the consumer demands—quality patient care.

REFERENCES

Abramson, A. (1978). Collective bargaining in the health care industry. In J. D. Jacobson (Ed.), *Labor relations in the health care industry* (pp. 69–80). New York: Practicing Law Institute.

Alexander, J. A., & Bloom, J. R. (1987). Collective bargaining in hospitals: An organizational and environmental analysis. *Journal of Health and Social Behavior, 28,* 60–73.

American Hospital Association (AHA). (1987). *Report of*

the 1987 Hospital Nursing Personnel Survey. Chicago: Author.

Becker, E. R. (1979). Union impact on wages and fringe benefits of hospital non-professionals. *Quarterly Review of Economics and Business, 19*(4), 27–44.

Becker, E. R. (1983). Structural determinants of union activity in hospitals. *Journal of Health, Politics, Policy and Law, 7,* 889–910.

Becker, E. R., Sloan, F. A., & Steinwald, B. (1982). Union activity in hospitals: Past, present and future. *Health Care Financing Review, 3*(4), 1–13.

Beletz, E. E. (1980). Organized nurses view their collective bargaining. *Supervisor Nurse, 11*(9), 39–46.

Blum, D. A. (1988, May 11). New bargaining units in 1987 comprised only part-time professors and assistants. *Chronicle of Higher Education,* p. A18.

Brent, N. (1987). Mergers and venture, implications and options: Legal and ethical. In M. M. Pettengill & L. A. Young (Eds.), *Mergers and ventures: Creative responses to shifting resources, Midwest Alliance in Nursing Eighth Annual Fall Workshop* (pp. 37–48). Indianapolis: Midwest Alliance in Nursing.

Bureau of National Affairs. (1988, September 1). *Daily Labor Report,* p. 60.

Castrey, B., & Castrey, R. (1980). Mediation—What it is, what it does. *The Journal of Nursing Administration, 10*(9), 18–21.

Cleland, V. (1978). Shared governance in a professional bargaining model. *Journal of Nursing Administration, 8*(5), 39–43.

Colangelo, M. (1980). The professional association and collective bargaining. *Supervisor Nurse, 11*(9), 27–32.

Denton, J. (1976). Attitudes toward alternative methods of unions and professional associations. *Nursing Research, 25,* 178–180.

Donaldson, L., & Warner, M. (1974). Structure of organizations in occupational association. *Nursing Research, 27,* 721–738.

Feldman, R. D., & Scheffler, R. M. (1982). The effects of labor unions on hospital employee wages. *Industrial and Labor Relations Review, 35*(2), 196–206.

Fennell, M. L. (1982). Hospital clusters. *Journal of Health and Social Behavior, 23* (3), 65–84.

Flanagan, L. (1986). *Braving new frontiers.* Kansas City, MO: American Nurses' Association.

Flanagan, L. (1988, March). All-RN rule to have major impact. *American Nurse,* p. 26.

Gideon, J. (1979). The American Nurses' Association: A professional model for collective bargaining. *Journal of Health and Human Resources Administration, 2,* 13–27.

Hechenberger, N. B. (1988). The future of nursing education administration. *Journal of Professional Nursing, 4,* 279–284.

Hunter, J. K., Bamberg, D., Castiglia, P. T., & McCausland, L. L. (1986). Job satisfaction: Is collective bargaining the answer? *Nursing Management, 17*(3), 56–60.

Jacox, A. (1980). Collective action: The basis for professionalism. *Supervisor Nurse, 11*(9), 22–24.

Juris, H. A. (1977). Labor agreements in the hospital industry: A study of collective bargaining outputs. *Labor Law Journal, 28,* 504–511.

Juris, H. A., & Maxey, C. (1981). *The impact of hospital unionism* (DHHS Publication No. HSO1557). Washington, DC: National Center for Health Sciences Research, U.S. Department of Health and Human Services.

Kleingartner, A. (1973). Collective bargaining between salaried professionals and public sector management. *Public Administration Review, 33,* 165–173.

Kochan, T. A., & Wheeler, H. (1975). Municipal collective bargaining: A model and analysis of bargaining outcomes. *Industrial and Labor Relations Review, 29*(3), 46–66.

Levi, M. (1980). Functional redundancy and the process of professionalism: The case of registered nurses in the U.S. *Journal of Health, Politics, Policy and Law, 5,* 333–353.

Link, C. R., & Landon, J. H. (1975). Monopsony and union power in the market for nurses. *Southern Economic Journal, 41,* 649–659.

Link, C. R., & Landon, J. H. (1976). Market structure, nonpecuniary factors, and professional salaries: Registered nurses. *Journal of Economics and Business, 28*(2), 151–155.

Little effect on faculty unions seen in court ruling. (1988, July 13). *Chronicle of Higher Education,* p. A16.

Major bylaws changes proposed. (1986). *Michigan Nurse, 59*(7), 15.

Metzger, N. (1979). Unions impact on hospital management. *Journal of Health and Human Resources, 2*(1), 28–39.

Miller, R. U., Becker, B., & Krinsky, E. (1977). Union effects on hospital administration: Preliminary results from a three-state study. *Labor Law Journal, 28,* 512–518.

Page, L. (1988, August 26). AMA, nursing groups still split on RCT proposal. *American Medical News,* pp. 1, 19.

Pettengill, M. M. (1983). Psychometric re-assessment of

the Hall Professional Inventory. *Western Journal of Nursing Research, 5*(3), 65.

Pettengill, M. M. (1985). Multilateral collective bargaining and the health care industry: Implications for nursing. *Journal of Professional Nursing, 1,* 275–282.

Pettengill, M. M. (1987). The relationship between union labor environmental characteristics, union dualism, and negotiated labor contracts. *Proceedings of the Winter Meeting of the Industrial Relations Research Association.* Madison, WI: Industrial Relations Research Association.

Pettengill, M. M. (1988). Economic and general welfare. In M. K. Stull & S. Pinkerton (Eds.), *Current strategies for nurse administrators* (pp. 255–272). Rockville, MD: Aspen Publishing Corporation.

Pointer, D. D., & Metzger, N. (1975). *The National Labor Relations Act.* New York: Spectrum Publications.

Ponak, A. M. (1981). Registered nurses and collective bargaining: An analysis of job related goals. *Industrial and Labor Relations Review, 34,* 396–407.

Sargis, N. (1978). Will nursing director's attitudes affect future collective bargaining? *Journal of Nursing Administration, 8*(6), 21–26.

Schramm, C. (1977). The role of hospital cost regulatory agencies in collective bargaining. *Proceedings of the Spring Meeting of the Industrial Relations Research Association.* Madison, WI: Industrial Relations Research Association.

Seldon, W. (1972). Professional associations—Their primary functions. *Journal of Allied Health, 11,* 25–28, 1972.

Sloan, F. A., & Elnicki, R. (1978). Professional nurse wage-setting in hospitals. In R. Scheffler (Ed.), *Research in Health Economics* (pp. 217–254). Greenwich, CT: JAI Press.

Somers, G. G. (1975). Collective bargaining and the social economic contract. *Proceedings of the 28th Annual Meeting of the Industrial Relations Research Association* (pp. 1–7). Madison, WI: Industrial Relations Research Association.

Stevens, B. (1980). *The Nurse as Executive* (2nd ed.). Wakefield, MA: Nursing Resources.

Tanner, L. D., Weinstein, H. G., & Ahomuty, A.L. (1979). *Impact of the 1974 Health Care Amendment to the NLRA on Collective Bargaining in the Health Care Industry.* Washington, DC: Department of Labor, Federal Mediation and Conciliation Service.

Wakim, J. (1976). *A comparison of collective bargaining agreements negotiated by registered nurses by different bargaining agents.* Unpublished doctoral dissertation, School of Education, Indiana University, Bloomington, IN.

Walker, J., & Lawler, J. J. (1979). Dual unions and political processes in organizations. *Industrial Relations, 18*(1), 32–43.

Werther, W., & Lockhart, C. (1976). *Labor relations in the health professions.* Boston, MA: Little, Brown.

Zimmerman, A. (1975). The industrial model. *American Journal of Nursing, 75,* 284–286.

Zimmerman, A. (1981). Collective bargaining in the hospital: The nurse's right, the professional association's responsibility. In J. C. McCloskey & H. Grace (Eds.), *Current issues in nursing* (pp. 423–430). Boston, MA: Blackwell Scientific Publications.

✳ EDITOR'S QUESTIONS FOR DISCUSSION ✳

What is the difference between state nurses' associations being able to negotiate contracts, and that done by trade and service unions? In multilateral collective bargaining, how do the multiple actors influence negotiations? Why would unions have a smaller effect on professional nurses and other professionals' wages than for nonprofessional occupations? How and why would collective bargaining affect a hospital employee's pay even when he or she is not a union member? What are the variables in relation to the size of a hospital that influence the tendency for a nursing staff to become unionized? Why should not-for-profit hospitals be more likely to have unionized nurses than investor-owned institutions? What would be the difference between an investor-owned institution and one owned by a voluntary or religious order?

To what extent do Pettengill's findings pertain to the degree of professionalism that a nurse may or may not have? Discuss whether nursing's inability to define legally and control its practice domain is the key factor in the movement by the AMA for RCTs. What is the community of interest doctrine and the disparity of interest test, and what implications do these have on threaten ing the sanctioning of all-RN bargaining units? What variables are related to the composition of the bargaining unit issue? What advantages or disadvantages are there for the profession of nursing to have all-RN bargaining units? To what extent do you believe that the ANA represents a trade association rather than a professional association? Discuss whether or not you believe that the "working conditions" clause should include a reference to professional issues such as autonomy, staffing ratios, and quality of care as bargaining issues. Are there relationships between the quality of care that a patient receives and whether or not an institution has unionized nurses? What structures can be developed within a department of nursing to ensure professional practice, professional rights being advocated, realistic and equitable salaries, and fringe benefits being maintained without a union or collective bargaining? What are implications for unionization in the profession in relation to the entry level of professional nursing practice? To what extent does the professional or occupational orientation of nurses affect the negotiated content of a contract, as well as the difference in contracts according to the type of union?

55

Strategic Planning for Nursing Service:

Finances and resources

Marjorie Beyers, Ph.D., R.N., F.A.A.N.

Strategic planning is a vehicle for responding to and shaping change. Changes in health care delivery and in nursing service have not only been well documented but they have also been experienced by nurses in all types of health care agencies. Resources for delivering quality nursing care, which have never been plentiful, are now even more constrained. Continued ability to provide quality nursing care now requires prospective planning and negotiation to ensure adequate resources. Strategic planning provides the methodology for these processes.

THE STRATEGIC PLANNING APPROACH

Strategic thinking is becoming integrated into daily living. Developing strategies to realize goals is part of everyday communication at work, at home, and at play. Strategizing is a way of managing control in a time of rapid change. It has become an accepted way to cope with uncertainty, ambiguity, and complexity. Effective strategic planning is now a necessary component of pathways to achievement. Formerly considered an executive management and governance function, strategic planning is an integral part of management at every level. Nursing ser-

vice executives in today's world participate in strategic planning for overall organizational plans as well as for specific plans for nursing service. Strategic planning is a process in which decisions are made about how to design and deliver services, the resources needed for effective services, and the organizational structure to enable service delivery. The strategic plan is negotiated and developed through review and comment processes. Once approved, the strategic plan becomes a blueprint that provides direction for operational decision making. Perhaps the most important change is that strategic planning has fostered strategic thinking that, in turn, influences organizational behaviors. Nurses must now use the processes of strategic planning to maintain and improve the quality of nursing services. They must think strategically in all decisions.

How does strategic planning influence organizational behaviors? What leadership factors are important in strategic planning and implementation of strategic planning processes?

Strategic planning in nursing services incorporates both the planning processes and implementation. Decision making is the critical aspect of strategic planning in every phase. The basic concept underlying strategic planning is that organizational actions must be thoughtfully and purposefully developed prospectively.

Studies have shown that effective organizations have executive management teams that make decisions for the long and short term. This high-level, participative decision-making influences present and future success. Executive management teams engage in strategic planning to allocate organizational and financial resources. Members of the executive management team provide a spectrum of varied expertise and also influence their respective constituencies to achieve cooperation and understanding of the strategic plans. The result is shared organizational goals. In addition, each constituency develops its own strategic plan as a subset of the organization-wide strategic plan. These subset strategic plans ensure that the diverse work of each part of the organization contributes to the whole. Consequently decision making throughout every level of the organization is focused on a common purpose designed to carry the organization from the present to the future. All decisions, including day-to-day and long-term, are influenced by this focus.

Strategic planning in most nursing services has focused on planning for staffing. Development of business approaches to service delivery, such as product or service line management, has broadened this focus to include total resources needed to provide services. Planning to meet future service demand for effective, profitable, services is now essential. Nursing service executives are decision makers, the authors and implementers of the strategic plans. Successful strategic planning is now possible because data are more readily available about current experience in service delivery. Key factors that will influence services, such as demographic changes, technology development, and others, can also be projected.

PURPOSES OF STRATEGIC PLANNING

Strategic planning serves to position effectively the organization for success. Clear identification of mission and values is basic to strategic planning processes. The strategic questions are, Where is the organization now? Where should it be in 2, 5, or 10 years? How do we get there? Goals are set forth and progressive activities are delineated to achieve goals. Steps are taken to acquire or allocate resources accordingly. Contemporary strategic planning does not occur at the expense of short-term planning. Organizations need to balance short-term with long-term actions to maintain and develop their purposes. Formerly, strategic planning was often an exercise in projecting the future by envisioning the future and what the organization would look like in that future. Strategic planning now encompasses the set of activities that begins now and moves in progressive steps into the future. Provision for periodic evaluation, and refining or revision of programs and services at critical points in the strategic planning process ensure flexibility and adaptability. Hrebiniak and Joyce (1986) present a useful approach to strategic planning that encourages short-term thinking with appropriate strategic controls to meet strategic needs. In their view, strategic plans should be reduced in scope to manageable and logical short-term activities characterized by interdependence and diversity within organizations.

The purposes of strategic planning from Hrebiniak and Joyce's perspective (1986) include developing the structure to support the accomplishment of strategic plans, defining actions and time frames for accomplishment, establishing performance standards, agreeing on short-term operational implementation, and facilitating decision making. A logical consistency in short-term and long-term activities and goals is achieved through strategic planning in a manner that absorbs uncertainty and deals effectively with relationships between and among events. "The need is to derive and employ short term measures of performance that relate logically to long term plans and objectives" (Hrebiniak & Joyce, 1986, p. 7). These authors consider the need for subsets within the organization to deal effectively with their specific areas of function while contributing to organizational goals. They also suggest that the organizational business unit, or program, or product life cycles need to be identified to integrate short- and long-term goals. Strategic controls that involve evaluating predetermined performance measures with the appropriate analysis and action allow for ongoing achievement of strategic goals.

Strategic planning for nursing service thus involves evaluation of short-term performance in relation to long-term strategic goals. Nursing service, whether organized as a department, a division, or in a matrix, is one of the hospital's core businesses. Nursing services are part of almost every "product line." Nursing service can be a separate product line as in home care or skilled nursing care. Nursing service management requires the same types of information that businesses use in their strategic planning processes. Nursing service must define a useful approach to strategic planning appropriate to its business.

One example of an approach to strategic planning presented by Olivia, Day, and DeSarbo (1987) is the use of a Strategy Map. Unique characteristics of the business, performance of the competitors, and appropriate organizational performance standards are identified in this mapping. For example, target strategies may include product quality, employee productivity, customer types, and research and development. Strategic performance targets may include market share, return on investment, cash flow, and growth. If the strategic plan calls for development in a defined service, progress toward achievement is monitored through evaluation of how well the strategic activities are meeting the goals, and how actual performance measures up to the targeted levels designated in the strategic plan.

Strategic planning processes, like organizations, are undergoing transition. Hayes (1985) depicts the differences between traditional and contemporary strategic planning. Traditional approaches involve the definition of objectives and outlining actions and resources needed to accomplish objectives. Today's strategic planning involves a means-end approach, in which organizations choose the ends and develop ways to get to desired outcomes. This ends-ways-means sequencing in strategic planning allows focus on far vision, while developing the small steps or strategic leaps toward the ends. This approach is based on assumptions that the organization's mission and values remain stable, and also requires evaluation of the competition and environment. Means allows developing of the organization's capabilities. Strategic planning benefits the organization by providing a sense of organizational unity and cohesiveness in action. Organizational integration occurs through a shared set of goals and a common vision, which also serve to keep the organization moving ahead.

Strategic planning, to be effective, must take place at different levels in the organization to further strategic accomplishments. Hospitalwide strategic plans need nursing service subset plans. Strategic planning throughout the organization is a relatively new approach. The new integrated strategic planning applies the same concepts and processes at different levels throughout the organization.

Viewing strategic planning as an integrated set of processes provides for adaptability within the organization's subsets. Involvement of people in clarifying objectives, responding to market changes, and enacting organizational goals is more likely to occur when the organization moves as an integrated force. Thus nursing service moves within and with the hospital to achieve overall plans, leading to success in overall performance and to all who participate. The nurse executive and nurse managers throughout the organization are leaders in processes of strategic planning. Developing leadership for strategic planning is particularly necessary during the time when the organization is shifting from bureaucratic, traditional organizational behaviors to participative management.

LEADERSHIP IN STRATEGIC PLANNING

Leadership qualities and styles are important ingredients of strategic planning and implementation processes (Isenberg, 1987). Health professionals, such as nurses, have formal education and experience in the work of the profession. Integrated strategic planning, as described in the previous section, requires that professionals become involved in strategic planning to make the organization dynamic.

In health care, clinical professionals are acknowledging the importance of their involvement in planning. This acknowledgement is characterized by role ambiguity for some. Traditional strategic planning involved top administration and governance, and focused on financial performance. Today's strategic planning is increasingly integrated in the organization. Clinical professionals in the traditional approach concentrated on clinical practice appropriate for their respective disciplines. The integrated approach forces participants to learn organizational strategic planning processes, and to translate clinical practice outcomes to organizational strategies, which lead to overall financial performance strategies. Separation of the domains of clinical practice and business strategies were respected as essential to ethical, quality practice. Now the two domains are expected to be integrated.

Lorsch and Mathias (1987) provide insights into the potential dilemmas faced by the clinical professionals. The clinical professional domain and the business domain were distinguished as follows: clinicians provided the service and consequently were in the "operations" component of the organization; business experts dealt with organizational strategy and management. Lorsch and Mathias identify the producing managers as responsible for both management and provision of the services. These producing managers can guide their colleagues to balance the fine lines between professional autonomy and organizational commitment. Respect, collaboration, flattened organizational structures, webs of complex communication networks in all directions within the organization, and streamlined measurement systems support the producing managers. Rewarding performance helps to balance the producing manager's functions. Not every clinician can be or wants to be a manager. Those who effectively manage, in these authors' view, must be perceived as being people of integrity, dependability, and trust. They must understand and meet the needs of their professional constituents, and must be able to enhance each professional's ability to make decisions in an environment characterized by complexity and uncertainty.

Another dimension of the potential conflict for professionals is engaging in competitive strategy. Clinical values and outcomes are based on universal standards of performance rather than corporate competition. In today's world of health care, appropriate sharing of clinical values and appropriate develop-

ment of clinical corporate performance to meet corporate goals are necessary. Involvement of professionals in competitive corporate strategy depends on developing a strong commitment to it. Porter (1987) offers an agenda to develop this commitment. First, processes must be defined for purposes of adding value through shared expertise or services. Second, core businesses essential to corporate strategy should be identified and stabilized. Third, horizontal relationships among core businesses should be developed to capture the potential for new businesses that could develop from them. Fourth, the potential for sharing should be developed from the strengths of the core business units. In this approach, different organizational units are more likely to collaborate in development of new programs with the fewest integration problems. Fifth, opportunities for this sharing, for transferring different skills to develop new products, should be supported. Sixth, restructuring should occur as appropriate to build the new group of businesses; and seventh, the diversification should pay dividends to shareholders. In a nonprofit organization, profitability would be used instead of dividends. All of these steps require building a strong corporate identity. Implemented with respect to ethical values of professionals, these steps can be effectively applied in the strategic planning processes for production of health care services.

Hamermesh's description (1986) of types of strategic planning illustrates one way to develop multiple strategic plans in an organization that allows integration of corporate and professional specific plans. The three types he described are business strategy, corporate strategy, and institutional strategy. Business strategy is unique to the unit of business, whereas corporate strategy refers to the overall organization's decisions about what businesses to develop, and what resources to allocate to corporate strategies. Institutional strategy refers to mission, values, and commitment to them through a sense of purpose shared by employees. This approach expands the focus of strategic planning on performance measures to include traditionally used ones such as financial targets and market share, with the addition of the overall purpose and mission of the organization in relation to outcomes.

Strategic planning for health care services can be developed in multiple sets for the corporate level, which involves the top administration and governance; for the institutional level when the hospital is part of a multiinstitutional system; and for the business level. Hospital departments or functional units, as a product or service line, can be compared to business units. In all cases, how nursing is placed organizationally in the corporation, institution, and business determines how nursing services participate in planning, and how strategic plans for nursing are developed. In all cases, management styles that produce the best strategic results can be developed to improve integration between the corporate and business units.

Corporate strategic plans are increasingly being used to develop strategic business unit plans that are highly integrated across units. The business unit strategies are derived from the corporate strategic plans to achieve good integration toward overall goals. While this approach can lead to some loss of business unit autonomy and diminished flexibility, there is increased involvement in review and approval processes. Strategic controls in this approach are balanced between the business and the corporate goals. Financial control is based on the business unit financial planning targets as approved by corporate staff. Planning success is thus evaluated by the implementation results compared with targets.

Strategic planning effectiveness depends as much on management of implementation as on the design of the strategic planning process. Gray (1986) reported a study of strategic planning in which the most common problems found were preimplementation problems. Six problems identified were (a) poor line manager preparation; (b) faulty business unit definition; (c) vague goals; (d) inadequate base of information for action plans; (e) poorly handled review of business unit plans; and (f) inadequate links between strategic planning and organizational control systems. Integration of strategic planning in the organization appears to be important to successful implementation. The results of this study reinforce the positive aspects of balanced, integrated strategic planning for organizations.

SUPPORT SYSTEMS FOR STRATEGIC PLANNING

Resources for strategic planning must be identified in planning the actions to implement the plans. Contemporary strategic planning depends on quality information about the services, production parameters, market share, and financial outcomes. Fredericks and Venkatraman (1988) developed an approach to strategic planning support based on the belief that effective strategy for today's environment requires analysis of multidimensional inputs. Implementation likewise requires lining strategic plans with organizational controls such as budget, productivity, and others. In their multidimensional framework, key strategy issues are organized in five dimensions. The first is described as the value chain, which incorporates inputs of market share, cash flow, size, pricing, and cost of capital, as well as internal performance targets for productivity and quality. The second dimension is analysis of product line performance, including relationships between product lines. The third dimension is market segmentation involving analysis of customer demographics and selection of products. Competitor analysis constitutes the fourth dimension. The fifth dimension involves forecasting and developing scenarios of market evolution.

Forecasting and scenario development were vanguards of strategic planning in the 1960s and 1970s. Rapid changes in recent times made these trend-based incremental methods less effective because environmental factors have interrupted the trends. The evolving strategic planning processes require quality data about appropriate inputs selected for strategic analysis. Computer systems now allow more complex analysis than previously possible.

Nursing service must have adequate information for strategic planning. The focus of information systems in nursing has been on planning for staffing using patient classification systems. In some settings, costs and prices have been assigned to nursing service. In other settings, nursing orders are being used to determine both resource needs and financial performance. The field of information systems for nursing service calls for immediate development to ensure that nurses can effectively develop strategic plans, because decisions in today's environment depend on adequate data.

DESIGN OF STRATEGIC PLANNING PROCESSES

There are several different ways to design strategic planning processes in organizations. In some instances, organizational learning about strategic planning is promoted through use of a packaged approach. Some organizations relegate strategic planning to the corporate office, and they develop business plans for setting performance targets for organizational units. In other organizations, each business unit may develop a strategic plan that complements the overall organizational strategic plan. As previously mentioned, varying interpretations of what a strategic plan is can be found in actual practice. Strategy more often has been interpreted as the long-term visionary plan, and business planning as the short-term department, project, or program level approach to performance targets and outcome goals. Now the strategic plan is becoming a sequenced set of activities that lead to long-term results.

Some authors (Slavin & Pinto, 1987) have renewed discussion of the differences between strategy and tactics to explain the differences between the overall plan for goal achievement and the more immediate, circumscribed operational tasks. The important aspect of strategic planning from the practitioner's view is to understand the organization's approach to strategic planning. The quality of participation in strategic planning depends on common understanding among those who provide input and are involved in decision making.

Elements of strategic planning tend to be similar in most approaches. Description of the current status is the first step. Data about key organizational factors are collected to describe current status. The quality of the strategic plan depends on selection of meaningful factors. Description of services, for example, should include scope of services, market share, customer response, cost, revenue, return on investment, capital outlay, and the competition. An environmental assessment is another key element in strategic planning. This assessment includes information such as demographic trends, market segments, customer selection profiles, and technological changes that are either in progress or anticipated. Economic, societal, and political trends that may impact customer utilization, market share or financial performance, or anticipated changes in resource availability and cost are also assessed. Evaluation of the current staff, qualifications needed to accomplish plans, and the potential for recruiting new employees may involve both internal and external environmental assessment. Finally reimbursement trends, regulatory changes, and sources of financing (e.g., philanthropy) are included in this assessment.

Analysis of all data inputs then provides the basis for developing strategies. Strengthening services, revising or deleting those estimated to show reduced profitability, or developing services to gain a market share are some examples. Decisions are made about the relative importance of retaining unprofitable services. In some strategic planning designs, scenarios are developed to depict what might occur given stated assumptions about future customers, competitors, changes in service technology, and other factors. The strategic plan is then developed from the organizational mission and value statements.

Strategies may include actions, such as developing a new image; stabilizing core services; instituting new ventures; changing work force composition and distribution; implementing new productivity measures; forming new organizational relationships, including affiliations, acquisitions, mergers or divestiture of existing resources; making changes in the organizational structure; or engaging in leadership or skill development or training. Strategic planning at this stage incorporates timing for activities that must be accomplished as progressive actions that lead to long-term goals. Life cycles of products or services are projected to schedule evaluation at critical times in the life cycle. Performance targets for every aspect of the plan are determined. Financial performance targets represent the quantitative type of performance goals. Customer survey responses to evaluate effects of change is an example of a qualitative measure translated to quantitative targets for performance.

The combination of overall strategic planning with business unit planning complements the overall plan that is used. This approach distinguishes between the more short-term business actions and long-term plans needed to attain corporate goals. Business planning focuses on the operational aspects of the organization and emphasizes the short-term components of the strategic plan. Market share, competition, production targets, organizational resources, and internal and external inputs needed, including human resources are examples. Business plans include financial data such as (a) costs of providing services or producing products; (b) projected revenues; (c) market share targets; and (d) financing sources, pricing trends, volumes, and regulatory and reimbursement variables. Business plans include a narrative description of each component along with financial information. A number of business planning guidebooks, software programs, pro forms, and other tools are now available to guide the process for those seeking help.

STRATEGIC PLANNING FOR NURSING SERVICES

Preserving the caring value of nursing is critical to the present and future success of nursing service. Nursing service is one of health care's core "businesses," critical to the future success of health care delivery organizations. The essence of nursing is the caring and nurturing of individuals. An environmental assessment pertinent to strategic planning in nursing contains a number of consequential issues and problems. First and most serious is the availability of qualified nurses to meet societal demands for caring nursing service (Fry, 1988). Second in importance is the mixed public image of nursing reflected in varied expectations of nurses by nursing's many publics: purchasers of nursing services; recipients of the service; practitioners; physicians; administrators; and other health professionals. Third in order of consequence is the resulting lack of an agreed-upon economic base for nursing service. Some might rightfully argue that the economic base is the most critical for strategic planning. Fourth is how nursing fits into newly developing health care delivery system modes. For example, how do nurses fit into the scheme of managed care? Do nurses have a major role in health promotion? Will nursing capture its role in the care of the chronically ill and elderly? Will nursing be the health profession cohort that moves to care for the indigent, the health care poor, and those with needs that have yet to be legitimized in reimbursement policies and regulations? These questions are basic to defining the best approach for nursing service in the overall strategic planning processes in organizations. Nursing service is integral to every level of strategic planning in health care organizations. The organizationwide involvement in strategic planning for nursing service carries with it the imperative to move beyond traditional views of nursing. Service organizations are developing a "new worldview" of nursing service and increasingly varied ways of organizing health care services. A new vision is needed to define clearly how nursing contributes to the whole, and in this new vision the value of caring must be preserved.

A pragmatic organizational view of strategic planning in nursing service must acknowledge that nursing care is now delivered in different types of organizations: hospitals, long-term care, skilled nursing care, occupational health in industry and businesses, school health programs, ambulatory care, and home care. These services may be provided by one corporation, or in combinations of separate corporations. Increasingly the affiliations, agreements, and contracts for care delivery cut across previously well-defined sectors within health care. Consequently the mission and values of the respective organizations reflect many different views of the populations served, the demand for services, and other strategic planning inputs. Nursing must now have a common value system that incorporates the service ethic with caring practice competence. The legal sanction and implications for nursing practice are similar across settings at the nursing practice level. The differentiation of nursing service according to settings is more attuned to the delivery aspects of care than the actual care rendered for different patients. Decreased length of hospital stay, combined with increased use of ambulatory and home care, and increased self-care by patients and families, have all contributed to diminishing the differences in nursing practice according to settings.

The continued differentiation among types of nurses and nursing care specialization, according to settings rather than patient care, may be a barrier to effective strategic planning, particularly in organizations with many services provided across settings. The traditional view, of patterning nursing service according to the organizational needs, is appropriate for organizational components of planning. These organizational differences, however, need to be conceptualized with attention to nursing's universal practice standards. Growth of nursing service in an increasingly, insurance-based health care market depends on clarity in nursing practice across settings. Cost and price, now guided by reimbursement schedules, need to be studied according to universality in practice outcomes, in addition to differences in delivering the care in different settings.

The stage for strategic planning in nursing service must be set with nursing practice standards as a given and with organizational mission and values being the basis of how this nursing practice is delivered, in what settings for targeted populations, and as a component of the broader health care delivery plan. Truly effective strategic planning opens new vistas for exploration so that the planners deal with what ought to be or could be rather than perpetuating what is.

Moving from current practices to future potential is more easily discussed than activated, however. The first step is to create a mind-set for change. Strategic planning for nursing service in an organization must fit the way nursing fits into the organizational structure. Nursing may be considered as a component in the overall institutional plan. In this scheme, development of the nursing resource, recruitment and retention of nurses, standards of practice, productivity, and cost price parameters are the major inputs to strategic planning. If nursing is a separate department or division, a type of business strategic planning can be effectively accomplished. When nursing is a component of a service or product line, strategic planning for nursing inputs is integrated with other essential inputs for the service-line strategic planning. The internal organizational context for strategic planning should be understood before selecting a design for the processes.

Strategic planning for nursing service in long-term, skilled nursing care or in home care organizations is becoming as complex as planning in hospital nursing service. In some cases, one nurse executive is accountable for nursing service as a core service used in several different business lines, including nursing in the different settings of hospital and home care. Because nursing services are human resource intensive, the major resource for nursing service delivery is the nursing staff. Thus, qualified nursing staff is the major strategic resource in all types of planning. Another major resource is the material component, the disposable equipment and supplies needed to provide the care. To support nurses in their function, a third resource is needed: information systems for planning, scheduling, cost accounting, and productivity data basic to decision making. Strategic plans for nursing service must begin with the current status and build toward the strategic goals. For example, if qualified nurses are not currently in place, the strategic plan must include ways to recruit and retain them. Optimum utilization of qualified nursing staff should be strategized. Nurses must be involved in determining the resources needed to deliver care, as well as in determining the care standards. Strategic planning thus incorporates developing or acquiring resources not currently available. The strategic plan may include development of information systems to provide cost, productivity, and quality data needed to evaluate performance outcomes. These data are essential to nursing service planning in all settings. Finally the framework used to deliver nursing service must be strategized. A new image of nursing requires new organizations that enable rather than dictate nursing practice.

REFERENCES

Fredericks, P., & Venkatraman, N. (1988). The rise of strategy support systems. *Sloan Management Review, 29* (3), 47–54.

Fry, S. T. (1988). The ethic of caring: Can it survive in nursing? *Nursing Outlook, 36,* 46.

Gray, D. H. (1986). Uses and misuses of strategic planning. *Harvard Business Review, 86*, (1) 89–96.

Hamermesh, R. G. (1986). Making plans strategic. *Harvard Business Review, 86* (4), 115–120.

Hayes, R. (1985). Strategic planning: Forward in reverse? *Harvard Business Review, 85* (6), 111–119.

Hrebiniak, L. G., & Joyce, W. E. (1986). The strategic importance of managing myopia. *Sloan Management Review, 28* (1), 6–14.

Isenberg, D. J. (1987). The tactic of strategic opportunism. *Harvard Business Review, 87* (2), 92–97.

Lorsch, J. W., & Mathias, P. M. (1987). When professionals have to manage. *Harvard Business Review, 87* (4), 78–83.

Olivia, T. A., Day, D. L., & DeSarbo, W. S. (1987). Selecting competitive tactics: Try a strategy map. *Sloan Management Review, 28* (3), 5–15.

Porter, M. E. (1987). From competitive advantage to corporate strategy. *Harvard Business Review, 87* (3), 43–59.

Slavin, D. P., & Pinto, J. K. (1987). Balancing strategy and tactics in project implementation. *Sloan Management Review, 29*, 33–41.

✳ EDITOR'S QUESTIONS FOR DISCUSSION ✳

What is the difference between strategic planning and other types of planning? Who should be involved in strategic planning for departments of nursing? What approaches to strategic planning are most effective for nursing service? At what "levels" within nursing service might strategic planning occur and how might the levels be interfaced? What leadership qualities and processes are most conducive to effective strategic planning and implementation? What dilemmas must be resolved in strategic planning and how? How might strategic planning most effectively be integrated throughout an organization that has departments?

What resources are essential for effective strategic planning? Design two strategic planning processes that might be used in nursing service. How might the strategic planning processes be evaluated for nursing service? What might be the key differences in developing strategic planning in and for nursing service departments and academic departments of a university? What specific applications from business should be made for effective strategic planning in both service and academic organizations?

56

Preparing the Corporate Nurse Executive and Nurse Manager:
Perspectives from the practice arena

Marian B. Sides, Ph.D., R.N.

Health care in America is undergoing rapid change as advances in medicine, science, and technology expand the horizons of industry. Futurists predict that health care will soon be the largest single industry in the United States, both in absolute size and rate of growth.

Organizations as vehicles for health care delivery can no longer be taken for granted as unchanging eternal monuments of the past. They are rapidly becoming high-energy systems in complex corporations. Their survival will depend largely on the ability of their leaders to meet effectively the growing demands of today's society (Kaiser, 1986).

These radical changes in the health care arena are reshaping the roles of nurse executives. The management of nursing services, once couched in a stable and predictable environment, now faces dramatic and unprecedented challenge in a new corporate world, characterized by uncertainty and chaos. Nurse executives must be educationally prepared not only to survive these unsettling years but also to provide effective leadership in the restructuring and delivery of health care for a better future.

The nursing literature since 1980 has begun to address with increasing regularity common themes in executive nurse preparation for the new corporate culture in health care. This chapter presents the key concepts that shape the executive manager role as viewed from the practice arena. A curricular framework that would adequately prepare a nurse executive for the corporate world of work is suggested.

According to *Webster's Ninth New Collegiate Dictionary* (Mish, 1988), *executive* means any person whose function is to administer or manage affairs. An executive may be similarly defined as a person or group having administrative or managerial authority in an organization (Sovie, 1987). For purposes of this chapter, the word *executive* will be used to symbolize the nurse who holds the top management position within a nursing organization.

Administrative hierarchies within nursing vary considerably from one organization to another. In this chapter the administrative core is considered as stratified into three levels: the senior nurse manager who is commonly titled a Vice-President for Nursing; the middle manager, frequently called a Clinical Director, Supervisor, or Director; and the first-line manager, commonly termed a Clinical Manager, Unit Manager, or Head Nurse.

Participants in this study were asked to identify at least five job skills that they perceived as essen-

TABLE 56-1

Skills identified by first-line managers as important for effective job performance

SKILL AREAS	FREQUENCY OF PERCEIVED IMPORTANCE ($N = 40$)
Financial management	36
Communication	34
Personal management	30
Decision making	28
Information systems	26
Motivation	26
Marketing	25
Planning	22
Organizational behavior	19
Managing change	19
Clinical concepts	18
Stress management	12
Time management	12
Assertiveness	9
Conflict resolution	8
Labor relations	8
Performance evaluation	6
Research	6
Negotiating	3
Leadership	3

tial to effective job performance (Table 56-1). The key skills that were identified are discussed in the chapter. Specific views of participants are occasionally augmented by selected perspectives from the literature.

FIRST-LINE MANAGER

The discussion of role preparation for the first-line manager is based on interviews and survey responses of 40 nurses who currently function as first-line managers. All participants work in tertiary care settings of 300 beds or more and have been employed in their current positions for a minimum of 2 years. Their educational backgrounds vary from diploma-educated nurses working on the BSN degree to master's prepared nurses working on doctoral degrees.

Financial Management and Budgeting

Concepts in financial management and budget preparation were believed to be the most needed area of growth for the first-line manager. The development, management, and evaluation of a budget are key responsibilities of the unit-based manager today.

Traditionally nurses in the first-line management role were only passively involved in the budgeting process. The advent of diagnosis related groups (DRGs), increasing emphasis on controlling costs, and changes in reimbursement systems escalated the need for greater precision in planning, monitoring, and controlling the operating budget. These demands led to a decentralization of the budgeting process and greater accountability for the first-line manager.

Volume and acuity changes dictate the need for precision and control in the budget process. Today only the sickest phase of a patient's illness is spent in a hospital. Patients are discharged far before recovery is complete and they achieve varying levels of wellness. As patient volume and acuity fluctuate, dollars must be allocated and distributed accordingly to meet patient care demands.

Communication

Most managers view effective communication as the foundation of the manager's role. Communication has many dimensions in the emerging corporate mileau and holds unique challenges for the first-line manager.

The need to understand the organization's channels of communication, and knowing when and where information is shared, is vital to the manager's survival, success, and job satisfaction. Effective listening is viewed as an important skill that will enhance communication with subordinates and foster a trust relationship. Managers express the need to develop sophistication in communicating difficult and unpopular decisions to subordinates in ways that will achieve understanding and acceptance. For example, in one institution, the Director of Nursing decided to cut caregivers in a particular cost center. The unit manager had to communicate to the staff the rationale for this decision and seek their support and help in identifying appropriate and creative measures to assure quality care with fewer resources.

The first-line manager represents the clinical unit in the broader organization. This role requires skill in communicating effectively with groups of people from many disciplines who have different objectives, interests, and values even though they are all working toward common organizational goals. The competition and pressures of organizational politics call for sophistication in negotiating skills, compromising, conflict resolution, and persuasion in order to achieve the goals of a complex organization.

Personnel Management

The importance of personnel management is described in many ways by first-line managers. A key interest is invested in the ability to recruit and retain nurses.

Interest in personnel management spans the scope of interviewing, educating, performance appraisal, and controlling absenteeism and turnover. The ability to support, guide, coach, and discipline effectively is frequently expressed.

One nurse manager described her interest in learning how to triage management issues. Everything does not have the same index of importance and learning how to juggle and balance clinical issues with personnel issues was a skill she needed to master.

Decision Making

The management of change requires skill in decision making and effective problem solving. First-line managers believe that theoretical as well as clinical experience is necessary for refinement of decision-making skills. Scenarios drawn from actual clinical situations can be used to exercise decisions analysis and to evaluate the effectiveness of decisions.

Respondents felt that it was important to share decision making by including staff nurses in the process. One example of shared decision making described by a clinical manager was the placement of clinical problems in a unit newsletter, seeking staff

nurse response and increasing awareness of the issues. The use of staff meetings and clinical roundtables are mechanisms for group decision-making.

A critical decision path taken every day is staffing for patient care requirements. The first-line manager faces this issue on a 24-hour basis. She or he must determine the delicate balance between the number and mix of staff to meet care requirements while remaining within the unit's budget.

Information Systems

A newfound respect for the management of information is emerging as computer technology expands and electronic communication begins to play a greater role in health care. Unit-based managers value automated systems as an immediate and powerful technology for managing patient care and improving the quality of work life for nurses.

First-line managers are rapidly adopting a new corporate mind-set with cost savings and productivity as an important bottom line. They believe that reliable automation can reduce costs now created by manual systems. Automated order entry and results reporting can enhance communication with ancillary and support services. Automation can save hours of time spent by nurses in using manual systems and can expedite the delivery of care.

Motivation

A valued skill of the nurse manager is the ability to motivate employees to higher levels of productivity and job satisfaction. One of the most important management tools is the skill to increase the motivation of subordinates and achieve a strong sense of pride and commitment to the goals of the organization. Respondents believe that they could motivate staff by increasing opportunities for professional growth, recognition, and autonomy in the work environment.

Marketing

Interest in marketing is sharply focused on promoting the profession, in an effort to attract and retain good nurses. The current nursing shortage has prompted institutions to give high priority to internal and external marketing efforts.

Managers believe that they must take an active role in promoting the services and opportunities of their units to nurses in the marketplace. What does this hospital offer that's different from any other? Why should a nurse want to work here?

This same marketing framework must be applied to the consumer of services. The first-line manager must be sensitive to patient satisfaction in providing care (product), in creating an environment that is conducive to convalescence and wellness (place), in offering a variety of patient amenities (promotion), at a cost-effective but reasonable expense to the patient (price) (Strasen 1987).

Planning

Health care delivery today is characterized by change and complexity. The first-line manager is often faced with situations in which many activities are occurring at once. Effective planning lends control over a complex and changing environment.

Planning at the unit level may be short term, such as getting through the shift, or long term, for example, opening up a new unit. Both require systematic thinking in advance as a basis for doing. First-line managers perceive planning for change as a critical skill for effective job performance.

Organizational Behavior

Effective job performance for the first-line manager requires a general understanding of how organizations work. A knowledge of the infrastructure and the functional dynamics of an organization enable the nurse manager to establish meaningful role relationships and thus make more effective decisions.

Organizational effectiveness is dependent on the degree to which its participants know and contribute to organizational goals. For example, if the institution plans to increase the patient satisfaction index by 20%, the unit-based manager must establish an action plan to contribute to that end. If the strategic planning team of an organization decides to expand bone marrow transplant cases on the adult hematology service, the unit-based manager must calculate the impact of this plan on patient acuity, staffing patterns, supply budget, and perhaps volume. Goal achievement is a team effort. While each manager contributes her or his particular skill and knowledge, the team as a whole is responsible for the outcome.

The first-line manager fills one of the most critical administrative roles in the hospital. Positioned at the juncture between the Division's Director of Nursing and staff nurse, the unit-based manager has the unique responsibility of conveying the goals of the organization to staff nurses and interpreting its strategic direction in a manner that is meaningful and useful to them.

Managing Change

First-line managers view the management of change as a critical skill for job success at all levels. Change requires ongoing communication and effective strategies to motivate staff to understand, accept, and support changes. Especially in environments where change is rapid, the manager has little time to execute the change process. A plan to open six additional beds by the weekend, for example, leaves little time to devise appropriate staffing and secure needed supplies. The announcement of the expansion of the unit secretary's job responsibilities to improve unit efficiency leaves little time to train, prepare, and test personnel skills. Program developments, downsizing, expansion, consolidation, decentralization, and redesigning are examples of change activities that continue to flavor the milieu and challenge the nurse manager.

Clinical Concepts

Respondents pointed out that the first-line manager must have a thorough knowledge of relevant clinical concepts and be clinically competent to practice nursing. A broad theoretical base in the science of nursing is necessary to evaluate patient care needs as well as the quality of patient care provided. Other situations that require a strong clinical knowledge base include identification of opportunities for research, recognizing need for staff or patient education, and knowing how and when to get involved in clinical problem-solving.

The effective clinician displays a sense of confidence in the ability to lead and guide the staff in clinical decision-making and problem-solving. The first-line manager is a highly visible role model for nurses on the unit. The ability to roll up one's sleeves and help when times get tough earns credibility and respect from subordinates and others.

MIDDLE MANAGER

The role of the middle manager, especially in large institutions, provides a critical interface between the chief nurse executive and the first-line managers. The middle manager provides the juncture for the conversion of strategic goals of the institution into operational goals at divisional and unit levels.

The fundamental principles and skills that essentially prepare the first-line manager are likewise necessary for effective preparation of the middle manager. These skills have unique implications for the middle manager and are discussed within the context as perceived by managers functioning in the role. A survey was conducted and interviews held with 20 nurses in middle management roles in institutions varying in size from 300 to 850 beds. The middle manager role varies among institutions, depending on the Chief Executive Nurse's distribution of staff support functions and specialty assignments.

Communication

Communication skills are vital to effective performance of the middle manager. The communication pattern of a middle manager shows a network that is broader in scope than the first-line manager with horizontal integration across the divisions to ensure continuity in departmental operations. Effective communication is viewed as a tool to establish a cohesive and desirable infrastructure within the division.

The middle manager forms the connecting bridge between senior management and first-line management and is the vital link for transmission of strategic goals to the division and for the relaying of progress toward achieving goals from the division back to senior management.

Strategic Planning

The middle management level in an organization is strategically positioned to present the organization's mission to first-line managers and to provide the direction and momentum for appropriate divisional participation. The middle manager must have a strategic planning mentality, that is, the ability to conceptualize the divisional role within the context of the entire institution. Middle managers believe that they must be prepared and educated to develop goals that will coincide with the broad organizational goals and to develop a plan that will ensure a productive management effort toward these goals. One of the critical skill needs expressed by middle managers was knowing how to allocate limited resources to projects and programs in a timely manner and to maximize efficiency and effectiveness in achieving goals.

Organizational Skills

The scope of responsibility of the middle manager spans multiple units within a division, as well as groups and individuals in the broader organization. The ability to set priorities and to organize work effectively is a skill perceived as critical to successful performance of the middle manager. Organizational skill development depends on one's ability to focus on the preestablished goals of the department and to allocate time and resources primarily to those activities that will contribute most significantly to achieving the goals. The ability to delegate effectively is also viewed as a critical skill for the middle manager that will enhance the effectiveness of organizational skills.

Personnel Management

The management of personnel is one of the most critical challenges faced by the middle manager. Participants identified four areas of particular concern in the management of work performance of subordinates. They include the ability to (a) motivate employees; (b) promote a positive attitude; (c) develop creative thinking; and (d) promote critical thinking and problem solving.

Motivation refers to the acquisition of goal-directed behavior as it relates to the work situation; it involves encouraging individuals to contribute productively to the organization while achieving personal job satisfaction. The management of employee attitudes is a particular concern, especially in work environments characterized by constant change, uncertainty, and chaos. The ability to promote positive attitudes in employees who feel threatened and insecure in an environment that is unpredictable is a continuous challenge.

Responses from middle managers point out the importance of developing creative and critical thinking in themselves as well as subordinates. The familiar cliché, "Work smarter not harder," must be applied in order to survive the turbulent health care industry today.

Clinical Skills

In-depth clinical skills are not viewed as essential for middle managers. Middle managers believe that they must be knowledgeable enough about the nursing discipline to make intelligent judgments and decisions for the division, and to analyze critically and evaluate the effectiveness of clinical operations and the quality of patient care.

SENIOR NURSE MANAGER

The senior nurse manager is the chief nurse executive (CNE) who holds the top administrative position in the nursing hierarchy. The CNE is frequently a member of the institution's senior management team.

The skill profile for a CNE is drawn from qualitative interviews with 20 chief executives from corporate health care institutions, varying in size from 350 to 850 beds. Skills in business administration and the nursing discipline were viewed as basic necessities or "givens" in the executive role and therefore were not explored or examined in the interview process. The executive skills identified by CNEs as essential for effective job performance establish a unique corporate profile that sets them apart from their subordinates in the management hierarchy. These skills are displayed in Table 56-2 and are briefly discussed in the narrative to follow.

TABLE 56-2
Executive skills perceived as important for the chief nurse executive role

SKILL AREAS	FREQUENCY OF PERCEIVED IMPORTANCE ($N = 20$)
Leadership	18
Strategic planning	18
Self-confidence	12
Political savvy	12
Creativity	11
Critical thinking	6
Humor	4
Flexibility	3
Risk taking	3

Leadership

Effective leadership was identified as one of the most essential skills of the CNE. Some see the leader as a visionary who forecasts the future and inspires followers to chart its course. The effective nurse executive sets the tone for the nursing organization. This person establishes standards and expectations for the department and models behavior that will effectively achieve its goals. The effective leader accepts responsibility for success and failure within the department. As Harry Truman once said, "The buck stops here." If you don't get to the bottom line you haven't done the job.

The trends in institutional downsizing and retrenchment in middle management place additional responsibilities on the CNE as leader. For example, reduction in positions, terminations, and layoffs must be handled diplomatically. A good leader is honest, direct, and decisive in these actions, thus showing respect and support for the affected individuals. Here is where the CNE gains respect, credibility, and trust in the organization.

Strategic Planning

The chief nurse executive must not only know where the organization is headed, but must play an active role in charting the course. The CNE participates in establishing the institution's strategic initiatives and then shapes nursing's program accordingly. For example, if the institution decides to expand its primary care base, the CNE must create a plan for increasing nursing's role in primary care.

Respondents believed that a key strategic initiative for the CNE is to effect greater integration of nursing into the broader institution. The CNE participates in analyzing regional and national health care trends and their impact on the institution. For example, how does the shift of payor mix from private pay to Medicaid and the shift from commercial reimbursement to managed care impact our financial systems? How do we plan care for a changing population? The CNE must be sufficiently freed from clinical operations to keep abreast of current health care events and forecasted trends so that nursing can be proactive in the marketplace.

Self-Confidence

Effective executives have self-confidence. They operate from a position of strength because they know themselves and believe in themselves. They have an excellent command of the job and know where they are going.

Some respondents believed that effectiveness is a blend between personality and knowledge. Sometimes success is less knowledge and more personality, the ability to project oneself in a confident manner. If you can make people think you know what you are doing, that is more than half the battle.

Self-confident executives are able to attract the support and cooperation of others. Employees are usually willing to invest their time and efforts to follow leaders who project themselves in a self-assuring, optimistic, and decisive manner.

Confidence is built through experience. Effective executives are more confident if they have "been there before" and did it right. They can perform with certainty and can predict outcomes more accurately.

Political Savvy

The chief nurse executive must establish political savvy in the organization. Participants identified

several key attributes that would enhance one's effectiveness in the political arena.

An effective executive uses a direct style of communication. It is important to be clear about the rules of the department and what is expected of employees. One must be honest and up front to avoid misunderstanding and confusion. The effective executive has strong interpersonal and networking skills. Executives believe that it is important to be highly visible with the right people, at the right time, in the right way.

The effective executive knows how to use power to get things done. This political skill is not a single force but is a culmination of clarity in purpose, commitment, persistence, ability to persuade, and decisiveness. Political astuteness can be learned. Political behavior and institutional politics are based on fundamental principles that can be taught; however, direct observation of the political arena and personal involvement in its process will enhance skill acquisition.

Creative and Critical Skills

Increasing competition among health care institutions has challenged executives to find creative, unique, and different approaches to health care delivery. We must experiment in ways that will simultaneously cut costs, improve services, satisfy customers, and provide job satisfaction for employees. At the same time, we must strengthen critical thinking skills, the ability to solve problems quickly in a cost-effective way.

Humor

Participants viewed the ability to maintain a sense of humor as an important skill for anyone in a high-stress environment. One must not become engulfed by the problems and chaos of the organization. You must be able to move away from a tense situation, find appropriate releases for stress, and find occasion to laugh and humor the events. This approach often reduces job stress and enhances effective thinking and decision making.

The effective CNE knows how to build tactfully

humor into presentations, committee meetings, and casual conversations. People enjoy being around individuals who are interesting and at the same time have something worthwhile to say.

Flexibility

The ability to survive and be productive in an environment that is constantly changing requires a flexible mind-set and a positive attitude. The effective CNE establishes, plans, and plays out the consequences of probable outcomes. Contingency plans should be created in anticipation of unexpected circumstances. The CNE who looks ahead and is ready to move in different directions maintains control and is able to make the systems run in a disciplined way.

Risk Taking

Risk taking is essential to getting ahead. The executive who remains within the certainty zone and chooses only what can be clearly seen will never move forward. Respondents believed that the effective risk taker makes mistakes. If you do not make mistakes, you are not taking risks. Mistakes expand with more responsibility. Therefore, strategy and outcome probabilities must be carefully calculated to minimize risks and reduce error.

ANALYSIS

The skill profile described for three levels of nurse managers shows some unique distinctions among levels, while at the same time clearly portraying a common skill base. Several particular skill patterns evolved that have implications for educational preparation of the executive and manager. The CNE is viewed as a hospital administrator whose role responsibilities are closely integrated with organizational goals. Business skills play an integral role in the manager's job performance at all three levels. Corporate responsibilities are increasingly important as one progresses up the administrative hierarchy. Professional activities related to nursing practices and clinical operations decrease as one moves higher in administration (Fig. 56-1).

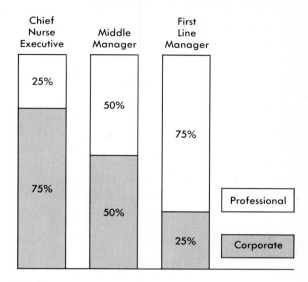

FIGURE 56-1

Profile of role preparation in professional and corporate skills for the three levels of nursing management.

Affective or interpersonal skills are perceived as essential to job success. Effective learning requires direct involvement in its process. These skills cannot be fully developed and refined through formal academic preparation nor can the complexity of the practice arena be fully appreciated without participating in it.

Curriculum Profile

The educational preparation of the nurse executive and managers at all levels in the nursing hierarchy should include a combination of formal education and experiential learning. A core curriculum in three key areas frames this course of study. The first area is basic business administration concepts including budgeting, marketing, personnel management, strategic planning, quantitative methods, organizational design, politics, and information management. The second area of content is advanced concepts in nursing and health care including theories, research, and forecasting trends. The third is experiential learning such as corporate fellowships or administrative practicums. This core curriculum is created from views and perceptions of the nurse manager in practicing roles. It coincides closely with concepts proposed in a recent study to determine essential preparation of nurse executives (Fralic, 1987).

The first-line manager, middle manager, and CNE should be prepared with a basic nursing degree. They should have a graduate degree that will provide a solid foundation in the nursing discipline, health care administration, and basic business principles.

The CNE should have 3 to 5 years experience in a line management position to master the skills described in this chapter. A postgraduate component would enhance skill development and adjustment to the corporate role.

Doctoral education is desirable for the CNE role in many major medical centers. It adds prestige to the nursing discipline. The effective doctorally prepared nurse usually has skills in research, writing for publication, public speaking, or some specialized area that add clout and credibility within nursing and among disciplines.

SUMMARY

This chapter provides a synthesis of ideas for the educational preparation of nurse executives and managers practicing in tertiary health care settings. The management of nursing services in health care today requires increasing sensitivity to the business and corporate nature of its operations while simultaneously developing the discipline of nursing.

As health care in American undergoes rapid change, nurse executives and managers at all levels of the hierarchy are encouraged to continue to exert their influence in effectively managing the delivery of health care services for a better tomorrow.

REFERENCES

Fralic, M. F. (1987). Pattern of preparation: The nurse executive. *Journal of Nursing Administration*, *17*, 35–38.

Kaiser, L. (1986, November). *Organizations as energy systems*. Paper presented at the 93rd Annual Meeting of the Association of Military Surgeons of the United States, San Antonio, TX.

Mish, F. (Ed.). (1988). *Webster's ninth new collegiate dictionary*. Springfield, MA: Merriam-Webster.

Sovie, M. D. (1987). Exceptional executive leadership shapes nursing's future. *Nursing Economics*, *5*, 13–20.

Strasen, L. (1987). *Key business skills for nurse managers*. Philadelphia: J. B. Lippincott, pp. 162–163.

✳ EDITOR'S QUESTIONS FOR DISCUSSION ✳

Critique Sides's study in terms of design, methodology, sampling, data analysis, and interpretation. Discuss the common themes that are being emphasized in the preparation of the nurse executive and executive manager. What are the similarities and differences in findings between this study and that conducted by Chaska and Alexander (Chapter 57)? How do the studies and findings by Sides and by Chaska and Alexander complement each other? What other issues need to be addressed regarding the preparation of nurse executives?

57

Academic Preparation of Nurse Managers and Nurse Executives

Norma L. Chaska, Ph.D., R.N., F.A.A.N.
Judith W. Alexander, Ph.D., R.N.

Nationally, little consensus exists as to the appropriate academic program for preparation of nurse managers and executives, and there is even less consensus regarding program content for varying levels of practice (McCloskey, Gardner, Johnson, & Maas, 1988; Wagner, Henry, Giovinco, & Blanks, 1988). Heretofore, most graduate programs for nursing administration have been developed along a generic, traditional approach by offering content in organizational theory, organization behavior, management of human resources, financial management, and a role practicum. Some programs have also included a varying degree of advanced clinical nursing content.

PURPOSE OF THE STUDY

A survey was conducted to obtain an inventory of needs and content areas for the academic preparation of nurses as nurse managers and nurse executives. Nurse executives were queried concerning the content deemed essential for the practice of nursing administration and how students could more effectively be prepared for management and administration.

Assessment of needs is essential for program evaluation and future planning of nursing adminis-

tration programs. The changing practice scene demands that programs offer content that is critical to the effectiveness and success at various levels in nursing administration. Nurse managers and executives are thrust into the midst of settings in which advanced knowledge is essential from personnel, organization, and business management perspectives, as well as from the perspectives of clinical nursing practice and patient management. Business orientation and patient care need to be more effectively synthesized for high-quality care and effective management.

In the practice setting, increased emphasis has been placed on cost-effectiveness in utilization of human resources, the environment of corporate structures, sophisticated technology, product line management, and strategic financial planning. Furthermore, concentrated efforts to increase high-quality care have focused on such means as primary nursing or case management. In sum, there is great demand to balance quality care and costs.

The effect of these factors is that nursing administration is increasingly being viewed as the management of nursing systems. The previous dichotomous perspective of nursing administration as the management of either patients or personnel (nurses) is obsolete. It is currently acknowledged that nursing administration must include both patient care and resource management. In a true nursing system the patient is the central focus and concern. One can visualize the patient as the hub in the huge wheel of a nursing system. The wheel has numerous layers of nursing management levels. All levels must revolve around and for the patient. The closer and more direct an inner layer of a system interfaces with the patient, the more particular the clinical knowledge base and patient care management that is utilized. The further removed from direct patient care that a system level is, the more specific the operations knowledge base and business management that is applied.

All nurse administrators in a nursing system need both clinical nursing knowledge and management knowledge. Given the various levels in a nursing system, the questions are: What is the most appropriate and effective *mix* of clinical nursing and management knowledge for each level within a nursing system? What should that knowledge consist of and how best might persons obtain the knowledge? A nursing system may be defined as having at least three levels of management: beginning or entry level, primarily the providers of direct patient care; intermediate or mid-level, such as unit managers; and advanced or executive level, such as directors or vice-presidents of nursing.

Conflict and confusion exist among management practitioners and educators on what the academic preparation should be for nursing administration. Graduate programs for nursing administration are obligated to provide the best academic preparation possible in line with needs of the practice of nursing administration. To function successfully in a health care delivery system that is continuously undergoing major transitions requires strategic preparation.

CONCEPTUAL FRAMEWORK

The conceptual framework that directed the questions for the survey in this study was based on role and adult learning theories. Information about these theories and how they were used to develop the survey questions is presented below.

Role theory is a set of interrelated concepts and

hypothetical formulations that predict how persons will perform in a given role (Biddle, 1979; Conway, 1988). One perspective in role theory has evolved as a result of focusing on social systems that are pre-planned, task-oriented, and hierarchical. This perspective is that roles in organizations are assumed to be associated with identified social positions and generated by normative expectations (Biddle, 1986; Biddle & Thomas, 1979). However, norms may vary and reflect the official demands of organizations, as well as the pressures of formal and informal groups. Norms are also the result of education, socialization, and experiences. Such may be the case for expectations in relation to the various levels of management roles in the social system of nursing. The American Nurses' Association (ANA, 1978) recognized three levels of management in nursing: first-line (entry), mid-level, and executive. Thus the management roles for these levels were the foci for the study reported here. Although ANA (1988) has recently revised its documents pertaining to standards and roles, the designation of three levels of management is appropriate for this study, given its use and present status in many nursing administration programs.

Knowles (1980) developed a model of adult learning based on andragogy theory. According to Knowles's model, self-direction is essential to the self-concept of the adult; thus the learning climate must be conducive to allowing learners to have significant input into the diagnosis of learning needs and the development of programs. Knowles taught that programs should be built as a result of a positive learning climate. Action-learning techniques should be used that emphasize practical application and allow adults to free themselves from preconceptions and learn from experience. Adults tend to have a problem-centered orientation to learning. Often adults come to the learning activity because of some inadequacy in coping with current problems. Knowles (1980) further advised that adult learning experiences need to coincide with the learner's developmental tasks.

A framework adapted from Knowles's theory was the foundation for the survey questions pertaining to preparation of nurses for management positions and questions on the management content of programs. Nursing administration is an integrated discipline in which content must be drawn from both clinical nursing and management; therefore the framework further provided the basis for queries on the teaching and learning methodologies used in integrating and synthesizing management and nursing content in graduate programs for nurse administrators. Given that nurse managers are first professional nurses and then managers, questions were developed to elicit the need for clinical content, academic preparation, and experience essential for each of the three levels in nursing administration. Finally questions were phrased to ascertain the types of degree programs needed to prepare nurses for management roles.

BACKGROUND FOR THE STUDY AND REVIEW OF THE LITERATURE

The background information for this study was obtained through extensive telephone conversations with 18 nurse executives who were members of the American Organization of Nurse Executives (AONE) and a review of the literature. Consensus emerged that a crisis is evolving in the preparation of nurses for management and executive positions. The crisis has further been pointed out in the literature (Henry, 1989). Academic preparation for nursing administration has been a continuing and increasingly more significant issue in the health care scene. According to the interviews of nurse executives and the literature, three issues continue to be unresolved: (a) the amount of clinical content that should be included in nursing administration programs; (b) identification of and consensus on the critical content to be included in programs; and (c) opinion on whether programs should be differentiated for distinct role levels in administration.

Clinical Content

Poulin (1979) and Rotkovitch (1979) have argued the need for a clinical component in management preparation. Both support a base of clinical skills and information about clinical phenomena for the nurse administrator, but believe that clinical experi-

ence should be obtained and clinical skills developed before entering a graduate program. Subsequently other authors have advised specific content in the preparation of nurse administrators. Advocated is leadership content with skill development that would enable provision and supervision of quality nursing care. Blair (1976), at the University of Colorado, and McCloskey, Kerfoot, Molen, and Mathis (1986), at the University of Iowa, have described their nursing administration graduate programs. Both programs place varying emphasis on clinical nursing, nursing theory, administration, and research. However, both programs encountered difficulties in resolving curricula issues surrounding (a) the interpretation of both clinical nursing and management; (b) the length of the programs; and (c) the expertise of the faculty.

Overall Content

Duffy and Gold (1980) studied nurses prepared in nursing and nonnursing graduate programs. These investigators concluded that nurses prepared in nursing programs believed that they were "best prepared" to handle clinical problems, whereas those persons prepared in nonnursing programs had more confidence in their financial and leadership skills. Since both clinical and management skills are essential to the successful implementation of the roles in nursing administration, synthesis of the two disciplines for content as one program is essential (Fralic, 1987; Stevens, 1982). Both Fralic and Stevens propose that such synthesis should be in a graduate nursing program.

Wagner et al. (1988) completed a literature review that addressed the curriculum content and evolution in the education of nurse administrators. They found a broadening of the curricula emphasis in recent years to (a) general economic concerns (in addition to budgeting); (b) focus on total organizations and political environments; (c) concern for the array of issues related to human resource management, productivity, and design of new nursing roles; and (d) emphasis on total health care systems, new structures in those systems, and new technology such as computerized information systems.

Preparation for Various Management Levels

The final issue raised in the literature is whether there should be different types of programs that clearly focus on different levels of management—the entry, mid-level, and executive. Cleland (1984) described a conceptual educational model that reflects the need for management content to be provided and augmented at every curricular level. For example, entry level nurse managers should be prepared in master's of nursing (MSN) programs providing a clinical major with a management minor; and executive level management preparation should be the focus of the postgraduate (certificate) program. Doctoral programs in nursing that offer an area of concentration in administration should provide an environment for student research and development in managerial sciences.

McCloskey, Gardner, Johnson, and Mass (1988) suggested that the master's program in nursing be designed to provide a broad-based introduction to leadership and management and to the role of the nurse administrator, in preparation for the role at the level of head nurse or director of a small agency. A doctoral program that offers a concentration in nursing administration should emphasize research, statistics, and additional content needed at the level of nurse executive in a tertiary care facility. Damewood (1988) interviewed 11 clinical directors in middle management positions concerning their thoughts about the preparation of middle managers. The results indicated that educators with the help of practicing nurse managers must (a) specify the critical skills and competencies for the middle management level; (b) identify learning activities that promote these skills and competencies; and (c) utilize qualified, experienced nurse middle-managers to precept students during the practice experience within the educational program. Various authors (McCloskey et al., 1988; Damewood, 1988) have also expressed concern regarding the balance between research and role preparation of nurse managers at the mid and executive levels. Christman (1987) offered possible solutions for resolving some of the concerns expressed, such as the development of more doctoral programs for professional role preparation.

DEFINITION OF TERMS

The following definitions were used for this study:

Entry management level is the lowest level management position in a nursing organization, whereby assigned titles are equivalent to such traditional designations as shift charge nurse, assistant head nurse, or head nurse.

Mid-management level refers to any management position between the lowest and highest levels of nursing administration, whereby assigned titles are equivalent to such traditional designations as supervisor, coordinator, or assistant director.

Executive management level is the highest level management position in a nursing organization, whereby assigned titles are equivalent to such traditional designations as director of nursing, vice-president of nursing, or assistant (hospital) administrator.

METHODOLOGY
Sample

Initially the presidents of the 61 chapters of the American Organization of Nurse Executives (AONE) were contacted by letter. They were informed of the purpose of the study, the nature of potential involvement being solicited, and the provision for protection of subjects and responses. The content of this letter was approved by the university institutional review board. Those who agreed to participate in the primary sample for this study then returned an addressed, stamped postcard. In addition to their agreement, they were asked to indicate the names and phone numbers of two nurse executives from their state who, by virtue of their expertise and qualifications, would also be eligible to participate in this study. One follow-up letter was sent to those presidents who did not respond to the original letter. Letters then were sent to the peer referral group, that is, those nurse executives named by the respondent presidents. These letters advised these individuals that they were recommended for participation in the study and also provided the information initially given to the primary sample. Telephone calls were made to the referral group to ascertain their willingness to participate. As a final result of these mailings and telephone calls, 43 AONE chapter presidents and 43 referred nurse executives participated in the study. Further, 15 nurses, renowned in the profession as executives, were recruited by the investigators for participation in this study. Thus a total of 101 nurse executives made up the sample in this study.

Interview Consistency

Data were collected by means of telephone interviews conducted by the investigators. A semistructured questionnaire, consisting of 10 broad open-ended questions, was used to direct the interview. The investigators were concerned that the items addressed in the questionnaire were asked the same way and that the participants interpreted the questions in the same manner. Thus, extensive notes of interviews with 10 subjects were compared between the coinvestigators. The investigators indeed used the same approach and the participants were consistent in their interpretation of the questions. However, it was noted that the technique utilized differed slightly for two of the questions. The data for those questions were coded differently, separately, and analyzed independently from the main study data.

Data Collection

Telephone calls were made to each participant to establish an interview appointment. The telephone interview varied from 20 minutes to 1 hour. Variations occurred owing to participants' desires to explain further, discuss, or expand their responses. Numerous participants explored additional aspects of the broadly based, open-ended questions. For example, in citing a need for increasing the management content taught in baccalaureate programs, some participants offered additional suggestions regarding curricula differentiation between associate degree and baccalaureate programs.

Ten basic open-ended questions were phrased to ascertain the respondents' attitudes toward (a) academic preparation and content for the three levels of nursing; (b) advanced clinical content essential for the three levels; (c) focus of doctoral programs in nursing administration; and (d) methods for synthesizing management and nursing content. Demographic data on the participants were also obtained regarding age, sex, years in position, years in nursing administration, level of academic preparation, size and nature of the employing agency, position titles for the various levels of nursing in the employing agency, state of employment, and membership in AONE.

FINDINGS
Demographic Data

The sample consisted of 95 women and 6 men. The average age of the participants was 45.9 years with, a range from 31 to 63 years.

The majority (73) of the participants in this study had earned a master's degree, with 55 of the degrees earned in nursing and 18 in nonnursing programs. Twelve respondents indicated that they held a doctoral degree, but only three were earned in nursing. Nine participants held a baccalaureate, 5 a diploma, and 1 indicated an associate as their highest degree.

The basic education for these nurse executives ranged from practical nurse programs to baccalaureate degree programs in nursing. From the basic programs, 42 participants had baccalaureate degrees, 47 had diplomas, 10 had associate degrees, and 2 were graduates of licensed practical nurse programs.

The average length of time that participants were in their present position was 6.3 years, ranging from 1 to 23 years. The average number of total years that participants held a position was 15.8 years, with a range from 4 to 30 years. All but nine of these nurse executives were members of AONE.

The hospitals in which these nurse executives were employed ranged in size from 39 to 1000 beds and represented all geographical regions of the United States including Hawaii. Thirty-four states were represented. Three participants were not employed by hospitals. A variety of titles existed for positions of nurse executives, ranging from the traditional titles of director of nursing or chief nurse, to corporate titles such as vice-president, chairman, administrator, and associate executive director. Great variation also was reflected in the number of management levels for nursing administration existing within a given institution. The number of these levels reported varied from two to six. Again, titles for management positions below the nurse executive level reflected both traditional titles such as assistant director of nursing, supervisors, and head nurse as well as the more recent titles of clinical coordinator, clinical manager, and clinical director.

Academic preparation

Participants were asked what they believe should be the academic preparation for nursing administration at the three different management position levels. As shown in Table 57-1 the majority of the participants believed that the academic preparation for the entry level management position should be the baccalaureate degree in nursing. For the mid-level manager, 50 respondents stated that the academic preparation should be the master's degree in nursing, while 34 persons recommended experience, and 4 respondents believed that a nonnursing master's degree was appropriate. Some respondents did not specify the major area in the nursing master's program for the mid-level position, while 23 suggested nursing administration for the major and 13 advised clinical nursing as the major in a master's program.

In responding to the "best preparation" for the position of nurse executive, 65 respondents recommended a master's degree in nursing. That number was followed by 22 respondents who indicated a nonnursing master's degree, and 11 participants who believed that the "best preparation" was a doctoral degree. Three respondents either did not make a recommendation or recommended a baccalaureate in health administration. As shown in Table 57-1 most respondents suggested for the nurse executive position a master's degree in nursing with a major area of concentration in nursing administration, or a dual degree in business or health administration, while only one participant believed a master's degree in nursing with a clinical major was needed.

TABLE 57-1

Academic preparation for three management levels in nursing administration

		RESPONDENTS*
Entry level		
Less than baccalaureate		2
Experience		4
Nursing baccalaureate		77
Master's degree in nursing		18
Mid-level		
Experience		34
Master's degree in nursing		50
Nursing administration	23	
Nursing clinical	13	
Not specified	14	
Nonnursing master's degree		4
No response		13
Executive level		
None		0
Baccalaureate in health administration		3
Master's degree in nursing		65
Nursing administration	31	
Nursing clinical	1	
Dual degree or at least nonnursing courses	29	
Program unspecified	4	
Nonnursing master's degree		22
MBA	13	
MPH, MHA, other	9	
Doctorate		11
Nursing doctorate	9	

*($N = 101$).
MPH, Master of Public Health; MHA, Master of Health Administration.

Content areas

Open-ended questions were used to elicit what the nurse executives believed the content should be in the academic preparation for nurse administrators. The data in Table 57-2 illustrate that there should be a difference in the content and depth in the preparation for the various levels. For the entry level management position, the content areas men-

TABLE 57-2

Percent responding to each content area and rank order of content for preparation at three management levels

	PERCENT AND (RANK) FOR EACH LEVEL		
	ENTRY	MID LEVEL	EXECUTIVE
Finance—Budget—Costs—Accounting	71(1)	86(1)	64(1)
Communication—Interpersonal Skill—Human Relations—Group Dynamics	69(2)	64(3)	55(4)
Leadership—Delegation—Motivation	62(3)	NA	NA
Clinical competencies	62(3)	55(4)	NA
Problem Solving— Decision Making—Clinical Thinking	54(5)	15(19)	34(16)
Planning—Short-term Priority Setting—Time Management	53(6)	NA	NA
Personnel Management— Labor Relations—Counseling	44(7)	65(2)	38(12)
Management Philosophies—Theory	43(8)	NA	NA
Politics—Conflict—Organizational Politics—Conflict—Organizational Mechanisms	33(9)	40(8)	49(7)
Staff Patterns—Scheduling	23(10)	NA	NA
Other Areas	15(11)	NA	NA
Legal-Ethical	14(12)	19(16)	38(13)
Statistics—Data Analysis—Research Skills	13(13)	19(16)	32(17)
Computers—Information Systems	11(14)	19(16)	40(11)
Broad Basis in Liberal Arts	8(15)	NA	NA
Planning—Mission—Corporate Strategic Planning—Forecasting	NA	45(5)	55(4)
Public Relations	NA	44(6)	41(10)
Evaluation—Develop Standards—Quality Assurance	NA	41(7)	22(19)
Resource Allocation— Productivity Staffing	NA	39(9)	44(8)
Broad Health Care Orientation	NA	37(10)	61(2)
Marketing	NA	34(11)	38(13)
Change	NA	32(12)	35(15)
Labor Relations—Collective Bargaining—Negotiation	NA	24(13)	25(18)
Health Economics	NA	22(14)	57(3)
Law—Regulation—Reimbursement	NA	21(15)	54(6)
Product Line Management	NA	7(20)	16(20)
Health Policy	NA	NA	44(8)

NA, Not applicable.

tioned by more than 50% of the respondents were (a) finance, (b) communication, (c) leadership, (d) clinical competencies, (e) problem solving, and (f) short-term planning. Only four content areas—finance, personnel management, communication, clinical competencies—were mentioned by 50% of the executives for mid-level positions. Notably, although prominently mentioned for the entry level management position, content areas of leadership,

short-term planning, and problem solving were either not mentioned at all or mentioned less frequently as content for the mid-level position. Finance was mentioned by 86% of the respondents for the mid-level position, as compared with 71% who suggested finance for the entry level position.

For the executive level, substantial differences were noted in the content recommended for this level of preparation in comparison with the entry level and mid-level positions. Finance continued to be ranked first, being mentioned by 64% of the participants, and communication content also ranked high. The planning focus for the executive level was on strategic planning, whereas at the entry level the focus was toward planning time and short-term goals. The content areas of broad health care orientation, health economics, and legal regulation were other suggested areas for the executive level, indicated by more than 50% of the respondents. Following closely was politics as a critical content area for executives.

The findings concerning the need for a broad liberal arts base in management should be noted. Minimal need of liberal arts content was indicated for the entry level management position. No acknowledgement of liberal arts was identified in the preparation for mid-level and executive level management.

Advanced clinical content

The participants were asked what kind and amount of advanced clinical content were essential for each level of nursing management. Advanced clinical content was defined in the telephone interview as clinical content beyond that provided in the basic nursing program.

It is demonstrated in Table 57-3 that the nurse executives participating in this study believe that the type and amount of advanced clinical content needed is dependent on the nurse manager's situation (area of assignment or supervision) and the level of management. For the entry level management position, most of the participants indicated that advanced clinical content was not needed, or if needed, it depended on the clinical area assigned to the entry level manager. In contrast, many more respondents stated that for the mid-level position, either advanced clinical experience or some type of advanced clinical content was needed. However, at the executive level the majority believed that advanced clinical content was not needed.

Teaching and Learning Methodologies

Agreement was not significant among the respondents as to teaching and learning methodologies rec-

TABLE 57-3

Advanced clinical content for three management levels in nursing administration

	RESPONDENTS*
Entry level	
None	42
Depends on situation	21
Experience	8
CE−certification	12
Master's content	18
Mid-level	
None	28
Depends on situation	19
Experience	33
CE−certification	14
Master's content	23
Executive level	
None	53
Depends on situation	0
Experience	33
CE−certification	9
Master's content	14
Doctoral content	4

*Respondents gave a combination of answers.

ommended to synthesize and integrate the management and nursing content in graduate programs. Each of the following methodologies—program flexibility, practicum experience, and personalized advisement—were suggested but by less than a third of the respondents.

Relationships between demographic variables and responses

To test whether or not the results previously discussed were related to any of the demographic characteristics of the sample, chi-square analysis was employed. In general, few demographic variables were significantly related to participants' responses concerning the academic preparation of nurse managers and executives. The criterion for statistical significance was set at $p < 0.05$.

There was no relationship between demographic variables and responses concerning preparation of nurse managers for the entry level management position. The only demographic characteristic significantly related to preparation for a mid-level position was number of years that the respondent was in a current position. The fewer the years in a current position, the more likely a master's degree in nursing was recommended as the appropriate preparation for a mid-level management position. Respondents who were in their current position from 7 to 15 years were more likely to believe that experience was the most important qualifier to prepare for an intermediate level management position.

Several demographic variables were significantly related to responses concerning the preparation for the nurse executive position. Both the highest level of education attained by the respondent and the teaching status of their hospital were related to that dependent variable. In general, respondents were most likely to suggest that the "best preparation" for the executive position should be the level of education that they had received themselves: those with doctorates recommended a doctoral degree, those with nonnursing master's degrees suggested nonnursing master's degrees, and those with a master's degree in nursing believed that a master's degree in nursing or dual degree was best. The exception to this trend was indicated by those who held a diploma or an undergraduate degree. Respondents who held a baccalaureate degree advised a master's degree in nursing for the "best preparation." Participants with a diploma or an associate degree stated that the nonnursing master's degree provided the "best preparation." Respondents employed by teaching institutions were more likely to select the "best" academic preparation for the nurse executive to be the master's degree in nursing or a dual degree. Whereas those employed by other types of facilities were divided as to the best preparation, indicating responses that were distributed equally among numerous types of graduate program to prepare nurse executives.

Three demographic variables were significantly related to type and amount of advanced clinical content indicated as being essential for the nursing ad-

ministration positions. One variable was related to the entry level and two were related to the executive level. Bed size of the employing organization was significantly related to advanced clinical content needed for the entry level position, whereas the age of the respondents and their highest education level were related to advanced clinical content for the nurse executive. Nurse executives employed in smaller hospitals were significantly more likely to state that advanced clinical content is not needed for the entry level position. Respondents from small hospitals who indicated that it was necessary believed that advanced clinical content should be obtained through certification. Respondents from hospitals with over 600 beds were significantly more likely to state that the nurse executive should have advanced clinical knowledge and that clinical experience should be the primary method for obtaining the content.

The most frequent response by all age-groups was that no advanced clinical content was needed for the nurse executive. However, respondents from age 45 to 49 were more likely to indicate certification, and subjects over the age of 50 were more likely to suggest doctoral education as means to attain advanced clinical content. Those respondents with associate, baccalaureate, or master's degrees were significantly more likely to indicate that no advanced academic clinical content was needed for the nurse executive, whereas subjects with a doctoral degree were more likely to state that the nurse executive needed significant clinical experience or doctoral level clinical content for an advanced clinical knowledge base.

DISCUSSION

The results of this study offer direction for nurse educators to refine and develop further programs in nursing administration. Role theory suggests that expectations for various aspects of the management role differ with different levels in nursing administration (Biddle, 1986). The needs for academic preparation vary just as roles differ. Respondents in this study believe the appropriate preparation for an entry level management position is the baccalaureate degree in nursing. At the mid-level positions, the master's degree in nursing degree was recommended as the type of program that best prepared nurses for the management role.

The discipline of nursing administration was suggested more often as a major area for concentration than the clinical area. However, this finding must be placed in the context of this study. Nurse executives with less than 7 years in their current position advised that approach, while nurse executives with 7 to 15 years experience in their current position were convinced that experience was more important than academic preparation. The seasoned nurse executives' responses may reflect significant understanding and appreciation for role operationalization and the difficulty that some master's-prepared nurses have in assuming and establishing a management role. Overall these results are consistent with the model proposed by Cleland (1984).

For the nurse executive most of the respondents posited that the best academic preparation was the master's degree in nursing with a major in nursing administration. This finding must be interpreted with caution, as both the education of the respondents and the size of their employing institution were related to their response. However, the differences in their recommendations were related to the type of master's program rather than differences concerning the need for a master's program.

The findings regarding the best preparation are contrary to what is currently being considered by educators and practitioners. The current emphasis is that education for nursing administration should include a significant amount of content in business administration (Henry, 1989). In spite of the excessive credit requirements, dual master's degrees—nursing and business administration—increasingly are being considered for nurse executives. It would appear that the critical content and program most frequently advocated by the nurse executives in this study, that is, master's programs in nursing with a major area in nursing administration, may effectively meet needs. The design and resources for such programs remain critical variables.

The findings concerning academic preparation suggest a great need for inclusion of management content in baccalaureate programs for nurses, to pre-pare them for entry level management positions. Clearly completion of a master's program in nursing is the appropriate academic preparation for a mid-level or executive management level position. Generally those programs should have a major focus in nursing administration; however, the data do not clearly indicate this. For the mid-level manager, a clinical master's degree is very acceptable.

The differentiation of management content for the various positions suggests that there are discrete management roles in nursing administration. It appears that preparation for entry level management requires broad-based management knowledge. Decision making concerning budgets and personnel may be a prime facet of the mid-level management role. Significant authority and responsibility are inherent in the mid-level managerial role for many organizations. The need was realistically identified for substantive content in the areas of finance and personnel management. However, the respondents' total lack of mentioning leadership knowledge and short-term planning ability, and minimal responses for problem-solving and decision-making abilities for the mid-level management role should be of great concern. It is unlikely that mid-level managers would obtain sufficient knowledge in those areas from broad-based content in a program to prepare entry level managers. Mid-level managers must fulfill major leadership roles. Frequently they are the primary synthesizers or integrators of clinical and management content. Furthermore they are the "blenders" among staff nurses, entry level management, and executive management in the corporate structure. Exceptional academic preparation for the role is vital.

The role of the nurse executive is very different from other management roles in nursing administration. The role focus is specialized at the executive level. Extensive knowledge is required in content areas that nurses seldom have had the opportunity to access or acquire. Therein frequently lies the argument that nurses may be best prepared for that role totally in programs aside from the discipline of nursing. However, the data from this study do not support that belief. Indeed the findings suggest that the most effective nurse executive may be one who appropriately integrates advanced nursing and management content within the confines of a nursing graduate program. The liaison and unification of nursing and management appear to be in demand and essential for optimum provision of quality care and success for departments of nursing administration.

The findings concerning a liberal arts base were very unexpected. These findings are contrary to what is increasingly and commonly being advocated for baccalaureate nursing programs by educators. It is further disconcerting that the nurse executives in this study cited no need of a liberal arts background for mid-level and executive management. It appears that these nurse executives place little value on a liberal arts education and they appear to place a higher value as indicated by the data on tasks and technical competence (see Table 57-2). Given nursing's humanistic orientation, this finding is puzzling. The question should be addressed as to how nurse executives conceptualize or understand the benefits of a liberal arts education.

The nurse executives in this study did not perceive advanced clinical content an essential for persons in entry level management positions. Because of increasing acuity of patients and complexity in needs for care, this finding also was unexpected. However, professional nurses who are in entry level management positions may be viewed as having extensive current clinical knowledge, either by virtue of being recent graduates from basic programs or because of ongoing experience in providing direct patient care. Experience is a variable that was highly valued by the respondents. It also is a variable that should have significant implications for and within graduate programs.

IMPLICATIONS

The type of management content to include in graduate programs for nursing administration has been a continuing concern to nurse educators. The findings of this study concerning the identification of critical content were similar to the results of other studies (Duffy & Gold, 1980; Wagner et al., 1988). A relevant aspect of this study was that not only were content areas identified, but a ranking of their importance for different nursing management levels was obtained.

The findings do not support the idea that specific management content, such as leadership indicated for one management level, is not used at or needed for higher levels of management. Rather, it is assumed that programs should build on content for higher position levels that were first identified for a lower level management position. Furthermore the point is that each management level requires specific substantive knowledge to be focused on as content in an academic program. The content primarily addressed should be that deemed most critical and essential to a particular position. Consequently graduate programs for nursing administration wisely may elect to develop content focused for a specific management role in nursing administration.

In summary, finance and communication should be emphasized for all management levels, but in different depth. Clinical competencies are particularly important for the entry and the mid-management levels, while content that addresses leadership, problem solving, and short-term planning are important *primarily* for the entry level position. Personnel management and public relations knowledge and skill are needed predominantly at the mid-level position. Long-range planning skills are critical for both mid-level and executive level management positions. Finally a broad health care perspective and significant knowledge about health economics, regulation and reimbursement, and political acumen are highly desired for the nurse executive.

The type and degree of advanced clinical content should vary according to the management position. For both the entry and executive levels the norm may be that clinical content beyond the basic nursing education is not needed. However, that norm should be adjusted for entry level management in certain clinical areas such as intensive care. Advanced experience, master's degree content, or certification for clinical practice are recommended for the mid-management level. As for the other recommendations concerning academic preparation, the findings pertaining to advanced clinical content for the nurse executive must be considered with caution. There were intervening variables that could not be controlled in this study.

The preceding findings and discussion provide salient information about the content for nursing administration programs. However, the education process still needs to be further explored and developed. Adult learning theory (Knowles, 1980) postulates ideas concerning teaching and learning methodologies that may be applicable for graduate programs to prepare nurse managers and executives. This study did not generate a clear direction regarding processes for synthesizing nursing and management content. The suggestions of program flexibility, extensive practicum experiences, and personalized advisement are consistent with Knowles's theory. Given the differences in academic and clinical content recommended by the nurse executives, preparation for the various nursing positions in nursing administration and proper counsel, based on individual career goals and experience, would seem to be essential. Further study is warranted regarding the issues. Strategic assessment, planning, implementation, and evaluation concerning content critical in the practice of nursing administration and for programs educating nurse administrators must be an ongoing process. The challenge remains constant to explicate the academic clinical nursing and management knowledge and practice experience needed to prepare an effective nurse administrator.

REFERENCES

American Nurses' Association (ANA). (1978). *Roles, responsibilities, and qualifications for nurse administrators*. Kansas City, MO: Author.

American Nurses' Association (ANA). (1988). *Standards for organized nursing services and responsibilities of nurse administrators across all settings*. Kansas City, MO: Author.

Biddle, B. J. (1979). *Role theory: Expectations, identities, and behaviors*. New York: Academic Press.

Biddle, B. J. (1986). Recent developments in role theory. In R. H. Turner & J. F. Short, Jr. (Eds.). *Annual Review of Sociology, Vol. 12* (pp. 67–92). Palo Alto, CA: Annual Reviews Inc.

Biddle, B. J., & Thomas, E. J. (Eds.). (1979). *Role theory: Concepts and research*. Huntington, NY: Robert E. Krieger Publishing Co.

Blair, E. (1976). Needed: Nursing administration leaders. *Nursing Outlook, 24,* 550–554.

Christman, L. (1987). A view of the future. *Nursing Outlook, 35,* 216–218.

Cleland, V. (1984). An articulated model for preparing nursing administrators. *Journal of Nursing Administration, 14* (10), 23–31.

Conway, M. E. (1988). Theoretical approaches to the study of roles (2nd ed.). In M. Hardy & M. E. Conway (Eds.). *Role theory: Perspectives for health professionals* (pp. 63–72). St. Louis: Appleton-Lange.

Damewood, D. M. (1988). Targeting student learning at the critical skills of the middle manager. *Journal of Nursing Administration, 18*(3), 6, 38.

Duffy, M. E., & Gold, N. E. (1980). Education for nursing administration: What investment yields highest returns? *Journal of Nursing Administration, 10*(9), 31–38.

Fralic, M. F. (1987). Patterns of preparation: The nurse executive. *Journal of Nursing Administration, 17*(7,8), 35–38.

Henry, B. (1989). The crisis in nursing administration education [Department column education for administration]. *The Journal of Nursing Administration, 19*(3),6,7,28.

Knowles, M. S. (1980). *The modern practice of adult education: From pedagogy to andragogy*. New York: Association Press.

McCloskey, J. C., Gardner, D., Johnson, M., & Maas, M. (1988). What is the study of nursing service administration? *Journal of Professional Nursing, 4*(2), 92–98.

McCloskey, J. C., Kerfoot, K., Molen, M., & Mathis, S. (1986). Educating nursing administrators: One program's answer. *Nursing and Health Care, 7,* 505–508.

Poulin, M. A. (1979). Education for nursing administrators: An epilogue. *Nursing Administration Quarterly, 14*(3), 37–41.

Rotkovitch, R. (1979). A clinical component in education for nursing administration? *Nursing Outlook, 24,* 668–671.

Stevens, B. (1982). The role of today's nurse executive: Implications for education. *Developing a curriculum for the nursing service administrator role* (Publication No. 15-1902, pp. 29–36). New York: National League for Nursing.

Wagner, L., Henry, B., Giovinco, G., & Blanks, C. (1988). Suggestions for graduate education in nursing service administration. *Journal of Nursing Education, 27,* 210–218.

✳ EDITOR'S QUESTIONS FOR DISCUSSION ✳

Critique the study design, methodology, data analysis, and interpretation of the findings. How valid and reliable are the findings? What alternative explanations could be offered for the findings? What are the strengths and limitations of the study? What are critical issues that need to be addressed in conducting studies where telephone interviews are the means of collecting data?

What relationship exists between content suggested in this study and the preparation of nurses for the new manager and clinical roles in future delivery models as proposed by Porter-O'Grady (Chapter 51)? Design a curriculum for the preparation of nurse managers and executives based on findings of the Chaska and Alexander' study in this chapter and that conducted by Sides (Chapter 56). What strategies might be used to synthesize effectively nursing and management content in one curriculum for nurse administrators? Discuss the pros and cons of offering different levels of nursing management as major areas of preparation in the same or different programs for nursing administration. How might resources for nursing administration programs be more effectively used or shared between universities?

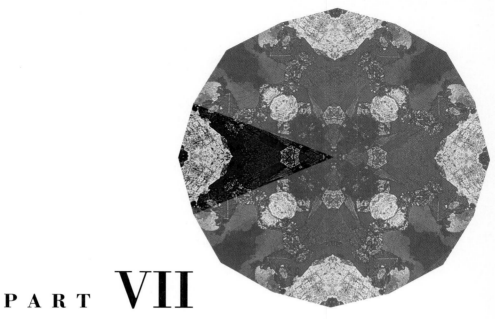

PART VII

NURSING ADMINISTRATION— ACADEMIC

The center of attraction in the kaleidoscope of academic administration is the student. The designer (academic administrator) must be somewhat magically creative in forming, developing, and evaluating new models for providing education. Faculty resources and support services are the elements that are highlighted in this section.

The chapters show how structure, process, and personnel may most effectively be developed and used to result in relevant learning and high-quality outcomes. Sue Hegyvary in Chapter 58 initiates the design of this structure by a discussion of the variables that influence the shape of governance, administration, and organization of schools. Multiple dimensions and views of organizational assessment are addressed.

Joan Farrell in Chapter 59 suggests that vision in academic administration include critical concepts from the business enterprise. She shows how the image and effectiveness of professional nursing schools can be enhanced by using business strategies and marketing techniques.

In Chapter 60 Constance M. Baker portrays how old structure and images can be transformed into new models and modes of operation for success in facing the challenges of academic administration. She focuses on the need for consistent innovation in higher education. Five critical dimensions of change are discussed as an exemplary model.

Geraldene Felton in Chapter 61 addresses the heart and hub of academic administration: academic nursing's covenant with quality. Felton brings into view serious challenges and reveals nursing's most important asset for ultimately producing and determining nursing's contribution to society.

Rosalee Yeaworth in Chapter 62 exposes the influence of politics and economics on nursing and nursing education. She advocates the need for nursing schools and organizations to negotiate superordinate goals and form alliances. Quality nursing service and education cannot be provided without such unification.

How can institutions and organizations select effective administrators and leaders? Norma L. Chaska in Chapter 63 provides direction and counsel regarding this significant issue. She advocates the use of professional search and screen committees. Values, as they relate to inherent ethical practices and effective functioning of a search committee, are explored in depth. Stages in the search and selection process are shown in a detailed flowchart. Troublesome areas are addressed and recommendations are offered for a successful search and screen committee.

It can be seen that there are many leadership patterns and styles for the kaleidoscope of academic administration. Regardless of the style that is marketed or advocated there is one function that remains supreme. The academic administrator remains the designer for facilitating professional directions and models in practice, research, and education. How to provide most effectively the adhesive that best holds the pieces together within a kaleidoscope for a consistent, constant view remains the management challenge.

58

Organizational Structures for Administration and Governance

Sue T. Hegyvary, Ph.D., R.N., F.A.A.N.

Both the popular and the scientific literature on excellence in organizations place a high value on participative management and sense of organizational mission. Some organizations have given concentrated and deliberate attention to an increasingly egalitarian style of conducting their business. Others give lip service to employee participation programs and persist with a highly centralized bureaucratic form of organization. Several of these variables may remain ill-defined in a scientific sense, but they refuse to be ignored in analyses of structure, organizational behavior, and productivity.

Schools of nursing as organizational entities cover the range of possibilities in organizational style. Some are hard-line bureaucracies; others more collegial. At the same time they contain a complex set of variables that influence and shape the governance, administration, and organization of schools.

This chapter addresses the concepts of governance, administration, and organization as they pertain to schools of nursing and explores both pressures and counterpressures in our shifting organizational environments. The importance of organizational structure is addressed in relation to multiple

dimensions of organizational assessment. This analysis attempts to portray a set of variables that as a composite will assist faculties and administrators in exploring alternative structures for governance and administration.

TRADITIONS IN ACADEMIA

There is considerable spoken and written opinion that universities are a unique type of organization. Although an organized community of scholars differs in many ways from some other types of organizations, the view of universities as unique is contested. The traditions of academia help to explain why the university has been perceived as a unique type of organization.

For centuries academia has enjoyed being set apart from the routine problems and processes of society. Academics have long been designated as the intellectual elite of society. In return, their job has been the transmission of knowledge from one generation to another and the generation of new knowledge for the benefit, enjoyment, improvement, or simply for the cerebral activity of future generations. The medieval robes, the ivy-covered walls, and professors meditating on grand thoughts have perpetuated the image of otherworldliness.

A driving force within the university environment

The author is grateful to Kathryn Barnard, Ph.D., F.A.A.N., and Pamela H. Mitchell, M.S.N., F.A.A.N., for their comments on this paper.

is the tradition of academia as a community of scholars. The norm of this community of scholars is that each person pursues standards of excellence and goals centered on knowledge. The explicit belief is that only in an environment with freedom of inquiry and freedom of expression will the quest for knowledge thrive.

These traditions of academia arose at a time when the general population was mostly illiterate or at least was very limited in formal schooling. The educated few enjoyed great respect and privilege because they possessed the power and uniqueness of expert knowledge. Indeed societies that have not protected and promoted the freedom of expression of their intelligentsia have paid dearly in subsequent generations.

While we retain and wish to retain many of the traditions of the academic community, the external environment has changed dramatically. No longer is it true that those protected within the halls of ivy are society's only brain trust. As the level of education and other means for developing and disseminating knowledge have increased in the population at large, those outside the university have placed greater demands on academia to make sense. This gradual and irreversible shift in the societal environment has created many pressures and counterpressures both within and external to the university.

Organizational structures in academia also are steeped in tradition. As academic institutions grew in size and number, there was a need for some form of organization. Lawrence and Lorsch (1967) observed that as organizations increase in size they tend to differentiate into subunits, such as schools or departments. With increased differentiation there also is an increased need for integrating mechanisms among the subunits. At the same time, because the differentiated subunits tend to be areas of specialized knowledge, there also is increasing interdependence among them.

Predictably, the necessities of organization have presented some unwelcome interference and threat to the purity of unlimited academic freedom. Organizations have determined the space, the salaries, the need for materials to pursue and disseminate knowledge, and other essentials of work. The administra-

tive component has been seen at best as a necessary evil.

The classic and most persistent form of organization is the Weberian bureaucracy. Scholars in academia abhor the bureaucratic model. The university most vividly illustrates the inherent conflict between bureaucratic and collegial models. Boulding (1975) noted that American universities tend to be organized as corporate structures with a typically bureaucratic type of hierarchy, but at the same time continue to hold on to the values of the medieval collegial university, that is, a community of scholars. Academics often assume that the university is unique in this internal conflict. In fact, it also exists in other types of settings in modern society.

The "professional-bureaucratic dilemma" has been described for decades in industrial organizations. Although the "professional" represents a particular type of academic with some intensified pressures and counterpressures, as is discussed later, scholars in nonacademic organizations report the same conflicts. As Scott (1982) described:

> Professionals see themselves as moral, autonomous actors, responsible and accountable for their own decisions, hence, needing to resist all efforts to regulate their actions. (p. 229)

The scholar, scientist, or professional holds to certain standards and traditions that focus specifically on knowledge—its generation, dissemination, or utilization. Expert knowledge and judgment are the primary driving forces in the mentality and work style of these individuals. The values and worldview of the professional may result in conflicts in a bureaucratic organizational context. Scott (1982) further noted that professionals

> are likely to resist external control arrangements on principle, believing that even if a particular rule may not be objectionable, the idea of administrative rules and the precedent for them must be resisted. (p. 229)

In contrast, the corporate organization has its own mission and goals. It must rely heavily on expert knowledge and judgment for the achievement of organizational goals. If the scholar and professional have the same goals as corporate managers, there may be little conflict. Even when they share the same general goals, however, such as quality care for all patients, scholars and professionals may find themselves at odds with managers of operations. Whether the conflicts relate to the O-rings on a spaceship or visiting rights of a hospitalized person, the potential for conflict of purposes and decisions is great. Each decision is a test of one's loyalty to the goals of academia and professional practice versus the need for control of chaos or meeting the business purposes of the organization.

Cohen and March (1974) described the university as organized anarchy. Scientists in industry are assumed to have subscribed to the goals of an industry by choosing to work there. Although academics in the university may subscribe to the overall goals of the university, they are generally less willing than industrial employees to tolerate the imposition of bureaucratic procedures and expectations. This difference is the source of debates and conflicts about governance and administration in universities.

GOVERNANCE AND ADMINISTRATION

Faculty governance or shared governance has become a rallying cry in recent years. Rarely are the words spoken without emotional overtones. Given the traditions of the academic community, as well as the shifting organizational environment and the pressure it creates, the question of governance is legitimate and predictable. If faculty are a community of scholars charged with the responsibility of assuring the appropriate knowledge base for future generations, the imposition of a purely bureaucratic style of administration is inappropriate.

An assumption in a hard-line bureaucracy is that administrative officers are best equipped to make decisions; workers should comply with those decisions in accordance with the division of labor, their task assignments, and the hierarchy of authority within the organization. These assumptions and premises are the antithesis of the norms of a community of scholars.

A central difficulty in discussions of governance and administration is the frequent equating of ad-

ministration with bureaucracy. To many people, bureaucracy denotes "red tape," impersonality, and rigid, thoughtless adherence to designated procedures. Although this function (and dysfunction) of bureaucracy is not inherent in its formal definition, everyone's personal experience with "the bureaucracy" sets up negative expectations of other administrators and structures. Since administrators have the job of making the organization work to meet its goals, this negative view of administration, while frustrating, is also predictable.

The basic questions regarding governance and administration, then, center on the rational and efficient balance of powers among faculty and administrative personnel. Styles (1983) defined administration as "the total structure and set of operations by which the organization is led" and governance as "the decision-making apparatus in which various members and constituencies participate with administration to guide the organization along its way, especially at key junctures" (p. 283). Governance is the joint determination of policy, while administration is the management and implementation of policy (Styles, 1983).

Styles (1983) outlined complementary faculty and administrative domains and roles in academic governance. This model also clearly indicates that some individuals fill dual roles as both administrators and faculty. Activities and issues in the domain of faculty governance include policy determination related to curriculum and instruction, educational policy, research, and faculty status. In the complementary administrative domain is policy determination regarding resource acquisition, resource allocation, and nonacademic services.

Even greater in number, however, are the joint faculty and administrative roles and tasks regarding administrative policies, consultative participation in matters of mutual concern, approaches in implementing various faculty policies, and joint participation in the decision-making process. Stating this separation and sharing of powers conceptually sounds easy; defining a structure for it is not so simple.

In her superb exploration of faculty governance, Styles (1983) identified some variables that help to define acceptable structures for governance and administration. Among the questions she raised are the following:

1. What are the levels of decision making within the organization?
2. What is the nature of participation within the various levels and the phases in the decision-making process?
3. To what extent is the organization centralized or decentralized among its decision-making units and what is the relative degree of autonomy?
4. What is the clarity of all participants' perceptions of the decision-making process?
5. Who has the legitimate formal power and authority to command resources necessary to implement decisions?

Responses to these questions require assessment of many variables in an organization. Since norms, values, and expectations differ across organizations, it follows that structures and functions also may differ.

PROFESSIONAL TRADITIONS

Just as the faculty of a university hold the community of scholars as their most sacred norm, professionals revere the "community of practitioners." The two are parallel in many ways. As illustrated for centuries in the craft guilds, the community of practitioners sets and maintains its own standards of excellence and evaluates its practitioners as peers. The profession bases its existence on a unique body of knowledge that guides the practice of its members. The traditional definition of a profession also has included variables such as a code of ethics, specified training required for practice, and autonomy and self-governance of the community of practitioners.

External pressures on a community of practitioners have increased with a more educated population, parallel to the shifting environment of academia. Because of the need of professionals to interact more closely and positively with their external environments, recent organizational analyses have referred to professions not just as a community of

practitioners in an area of knowledge and skill, but as political entities (Hall, 1983).

The community of scholars and the community of practitioners share the dilemmas of changing norms and expectations in a shifting organizational environment. This fact was described by Baldridge (1971) as follows:

> On the modern campus today we see neither the rigid formal aspects of bureaucracy nor the calm, consensus-directed elements of an academic collegium. On the contrary student riots cripple the campus, professors form unions and strike, administrators defend their traditional positions, and external interest groups and irate governors invade the academic halls. . . . These groups articulate their interests in many different ways, bringing pressure to bear on the decision making process on any number of angles, and using power and force wherever it is available and necessary. Once articulated, power and influence go through a complex process until policies are shaped, re-shaped and forged from the competing claims of multiple groups. All this is a dynamic process, a process clearly indicating that the university is best understood as a "politicized" institution. (pp. 8–9)

Every part of a university is a point of pressure and counterpressure between traditions, ideals, realities, and relevance. Professional schools, such as schools and colleges of nursing, share the assets and liabilities of both the community of scholars in the university and the community of practitioners in the profession. Sorting out the multiple effects on governance, administration, and organization of schools of nursing necessitates recognition of this position of the "double whammy."

THE ENVIRONMENTS OF SCHOOLS OF NURSING

Schools of nursing in universities are a part of the traditional academic community with its rights and privileges, as well as its high expectations. At the same time, faculty of the school of nursing are part of the community of practitioners in the profession, if not by current involvement, at least by professional identity.

Faculty of schools of nursing differ even within schools in their identity with the traditions of these two communities. Faculty who identify far more closely with the community of scholars may express more resistance toward administrative decisions as well as greater variance with the expectations from the professional community outside the university. For others, closer identity with the current realities and difficulties of nursing practitioners guides their behaviors toward the professional community. Herein lies a source of considerable conflict within faculties of schools of nursing.

Although the traditions of professions as discussed above center on the unique body of knowledge, autonomy in practice, peer determination, and enforcement of standards of practice, and so on, nursing has not fully met these standards in its practice. Nurses have little voice in hospital organizations. Furthermore the organization of the work of nursing continues to follow a strongly bureaucratic tradition. Hospitals and most health care agencies emphasize division of labor, task specialization, reporting relationships, domains of authority, maintenance of records—the traditional definition of a bureaucratic organization. Hospitals remain particularly entrenched in that tradition.

Nursing faculty who have been quite accustomed to working in this heavily bureaucratic environment may be slower to question the rights and responsibilities of faculty for self-governance. In many schools of nursing, the dean remains the center of power and authority with no complementary organization or expectation for power and authority among nonadministrative faculty. Furthermore, unless several other faculty, including administrative faculty, are professionally and academically mature, the dean also may shoulder the responsibility for faculty development, as well as decisions of academic policy. The dean may be the central authority for all matters by tradition, by preference, or by default. Failure to move to a more collegial model as faculty become more professionally and organizationally mature sets the stage for increasing strain within the school.

The most severe earthquakes occur when the tectonic plates are locked, with both sides unmovable and subjected to increasing pressures. This analogy portrays the intensity of conflict in many schools over the issues of governance and administration. If the administrative style has persisted with strongly bureaucratic traditions over many decades, despite counterpressures toward a more collegial model, the quake lines are drawn. Schools of nursing are not unique in this potential or actual conflict. As nurses who are university faculty members continue to develop in their maturity toward participation as a true community of scholars, the discomfort with a bureaucratic administration increases accordingly.

At the same time, faculty in schools of nursing have increasing pressures to organize themselves to be more responsive to the practice community. What then are the goals and missions of the school? More clearly stated, what business are we in? Clearly our business is that of knowledge, but what aspect of knowledge? In our role as scholars, is our business specific to the generation and dissemination of knowledge, that is, research and teaching? Or, because we are also are a part of a community of practitioners, is part of our business also involvement in some way in the utilization of knowledge?

Again, more philosophical issues in the academic community must be brought to the surface in these arguments. At the heart of the issue is the faculty's interpretation of the social contract. As faculty we insist and must insist, within reason, on the freedom of inquiry and freedom of expression of ideas. We vigorously guard the essential neutrality of the university. In many institutions, particularly public universities, there are safeguards against university competition with the local business community. Yet American society increasingly regards higher education as both a right and a service to society. There are growing expectations of relevance and response to societal needs. A highly visible example is the pressure on schools of nursing in universities to respond to the nursing shortage.

Who then owns the university and its schools? At least, who owns the soul of the university? Who shapes its goals and missions and determines the scope of its business enterprises? What happens to the local economy if the university drags its feet in the production of engineers and business administrators? What happens in health care if the university fails to increase the preparation of nurses for care of the local citizenry? Are these issues of governance or administration? Are they to be determined within or external to the university?

It is illogical and inappropriate to assume that a faculty is simply a self-governing community of scholars, isolated from their constituents and protected from all interference in the pursuit of knowledge. It also would be inappropriate to define administration as the locus of all decision making or the only linking pins to the external environment. What emerges is a picture of growing complexity of decisions, processes, procedures, practices, and organizational styles that evades simple prescription and final conclusion. There are no simple prescriptions for governance, administration, or organization in schools of nursing.

THE EMERGENCE OF THE ENTREPRENEURIAL MODEL

Nursing faculty in universities have matured dramatically in their ability to participate in the academic community and to meet its standards. In addition to the pressures and counterpressures in the academic-collegial and bureaucratic models, a third dimension—the entrepreneurial model, has emerged in recent decades. Many faculty see the entrepreneurial model as a welcome change from the restricted resources of universities, particularly the funding for research. Other faculty, however, see the entrepreneurial model as a threat to academic standards and an excessive response to pressures external to the university.

There are two major types of entrepreneurial activity in schools of nursing. Both have numerous implications for governance, administration, and organization. The first is the conduct of research. In schools where research programs are more established, programs often have grown like topsy on the basis of funding. The allocation of personnel and space, and indeed a growing imbalance of powers often have derived from the availability of funds for research. These imbalances are not limited to professional schools, but have been particularly evident there because of the expectation of these schools to

respond to societal needs. In some schools of nursing, more than half the school's budget comes from external "soft" funding.

A second type of entrepreneurial activity is pursuit of faculty practice either on an individual or a group basis. Faculty practice in universities is fraught with controversy. Is the legitimate role of faculty to utilize knowledge? Or is it to generate and disseminate knowledge? Or is it all three? Perhaps *even more at issue is who shall decide*. If a faculty leans very heavily toward the entrepreneurial mode in its arrangements for practice, does it then lose some of the essential qualities of academia as the community of scholars? These debates are rampant in schools of nursing and certainly have no final conclusions. (In fact, are not any "final conclusions" the antithesis of academia?)

These questions exemplify the role of nursing faculty as participants in the community of scholars and the community of practitioners. A basic tenant of the social contract is the continued examination of the nature of our responsibilities in our society. The mechanisms for pursuing these decisions and implementing our actions are embodied in the debates about governance, administration, and organization.

THE EMERGENCE OF COLLEGIAL MODELS

The literature about excellence in numerous types of organizations repeatedly emphasizes the dynamic nature of decision-making processes. Furthermore the emerging structures for decision making emphasize participation at multiple levels of organization and decreasing the various "levels" of hierarchy. The National Aeronautics and Space Administration (NASA) invented matrix organization to stimulate creativity and productivity (Baber, 1983). Would a bureaucratic organization in NASA find us still never having set foot on the moon?

Excellence does not depend on any prescribed organizational structure. Yet some structure is necessary for a large group of people to pursue their activities in harmony and clarity. The NASA precedent, the emergence of models of shared governance, and the increasing numbers of educated people in the work force require new approaches to old dilemmas.

While collegial models may be a breath of fresh air, they also have some pitfalls. Just as administration is often equated with bureaucratic style, faculty governance and collegiality often are equated with decision consensus. Arrival at total agreement in any group is difficult. If the expectation is discussion of every item to the point of consensus, indeed there is a greatly diminished probability of any change. Collegiality denotes that the prevailing norm in decision making is discussion among colleagues and participative management. In no way does it require a vote or consensus on every decision.

This reality and the dual existence of administration and governance require clarity in the structure about major topics of decision. Areas of particular controversy include decisions about appointments, promotions, and tenure, salaries, and allocation of other resources such as space and personnel. In a collegial model, the purely "administrative" nature of these decisions is challenged.

Bolman and Deal (1984) gave new insights to meet these challenges in their approach to understanding and managing organizations. They defined organizations along four dimensions that they refer to as frames. The structural frame often receives primary emphasis, although it may be of secondary importance in some organizations. The structural frame includes the goal direction, organizational units, and mechanisms of operation of the organization. The human resource frame refers to the effective response to human needs, both within and external to the organization, and the appropriate use of human resources toward the achievement of goals. The third frame, the political frame, refers to the coalitions, conflicts, and problems of resource allocation. The symbolic frame embodies the shared values, traditions, symbols, and cohesion of all persons in the organization.

Using these four frames in their analysis of many organizations, Bolman and Deal (1984) concluded with this assessment:

> The environment of most organizations will continue to change rapidly in the coming years. Such changes inevitably create possibilities for misalign-

ment of the domains represented by the four frames. Individual resistance to both change and organizational inertia can be powerful forces leading to rigidity and defensiveness in the face of new conditions. . . . In the face of bewildering changes some institutions are standing pat and running the risk of extinction. Others are moving aggressively to realign their goals, human resources, political dynamics, and culture. Those that succeed will be the successful of the future. (p. 291)

Analysis of the three concepts of governance, administration, and structures; the findings of studies reported in the organizational literature; and personal experiences repeatedly indicate the complexity and ambiguity of the environments of schools of nursing. Nursing's leap to define a formal organizational structure represents a grasp for certainty in our roles and behaviors, in the face of an uncertain and turbulent environment. This chapter does not present proposed structures for schools of nursing to prescribe their mechanisms or definitions of governance and administration. Structures are enabling mechanisms to achieve goals. As goals and environments change, structures may have to be changed accordingly.

In a mature organization, the central questions relate more to mission than to structure. Mission is our substance; structure is merely the form for the present. Collegiality in governance and administration helps us to retain that essential focus.

SUMMARY

Universities and their component schools often view themselves as a unique type of organization. Indeed there are some traditions that are specific to academia. However, universities are increasingly akin to some other organizations, and face many of the dilemmas confronted in business and industrial organizations.

As society has growing expectations for relevance in academic work, the university mission and goals will need continuous examination and probable change over time. These issues are particularly evident in professional schools, such as schools of nursing.

Professional schools in universities face a continuing and increasing set of pressures and counterpressures. These forces are most visibly represented in two traditions: the community of scholars and the community of practitioners. As organizations with a mixed agenda in their mission statements, nursing schools are attempting to respond to a variety of demands from within the community of scholars as well as within the community of practitioners of nursing.

As has been demonstrated in other types of organizations, appropriate responses will change over time. Structures for managing these changes similarly will be dynamic. The concepts, definitions, and structures for governance and administration will require continued analysis and change if we are to meet our obligations to society.

REFERENCES

Baber, W. F. (1983). *Organizing the future: Matrix models for the postindustrial polity*. Birmingham: University of Alabama Press.

Baldridge, J. V. (1971). *Power and conflict in the university*. New York: John Wiley & Sons.

Bolman, L. G., & Deal, T. E. (1984). *Modern approaches to understanding and managing organizations*. San Francisco, Jossey-Bass.

Boulding, K. (1975). Quality versus equality: The dilemma of the university. *Daedalus, 2*, 298–303.

Cohen, M., & March, J. (1974). *Leadership and ambiguity*. New York: McGraw-Hill.

Hall, R. H. (1983). *The professions, employed professionals and the professional organization*. Paper presented at Midwest Sociological Society, Kansas City, MO.

Lawrence, P. R., & Lorsch, J. W. (1967). *Organization and environment: Managing differentiation and integration*. Boston: Harvard University.

Scott W. R. (1982). Managing professional work: Three models of control for health organizations. Health Services Research, *17* (3),213–240.

Styles, M. M. (1983). Faculty governance. In M. E. Conway & O. Andruski (Eds.): *Administrative theory and practice: Issues in higher education in nursing* (pp. 283–302). Norwalk, CT: Appleton-Century-Crofts.

✳   **EDITOR'S QUESTIONS FOR DISCUSSION**   ✳

How can faculty as a community of scholars legitimately govern themselves to prevent the traditional, inherent conflicts between academics and professionalism in bureaucracies? How can power be balanced between faculty and administrators? What types of checks and balances can be initiated or included in a system? What conflicts may or may not exist in the model outlined by Hegyvary in which a person holds a dual role as an administrator and faculty member? What activities are clearly in the domain of faculty governance? What type of "gray areas" exist between administrative and faculty decision making and roles? Are decisions regarding what types of nurses should be prepared decisions that should be issues of governance or administration? What criteria should be used to determine decisions or roles in the gray areas? What similarities do or do not exist between the community of practitioners and the community of scholars? What is the sources or sources of conflict within faculties of schools of nursing? How might conflict most effectively be addressed in schools of nursing? How can working relationships be facilitated and increased in schools of nursing? Should faculty organize themselves professionally?

What are the key variables that need to be addressed in providing structure prescriptions for governance, administration, and organization in schools of nursing? What structure options or models will encourage faculty development and growth? What qualities and qualifications need to exist in an organization in order to have a matrix-type organization be effective for the institution? Propose various structures for schools of nursing in light of specific types of goals and different missions and goals that schools of nursing may have. What are the assumptions, rationale, advantages, and disadvantages for each of the proposed structures? Apply the four frames for analyzing organizations in introducing change into a school of nursing. Define first a major change you would wish to introduce, and follow through with an indication of specific processes to bring about such change.

CHAPTER 59

Academia as Big Business

Joan Farrell, Ph.D., R.N.

For decades colleges and universities have tended to operate under the assumption that they were exempt from problems of big business even though their budgets, their staffs, and their physical plants clearly put them in a position not unlike business and industry. Most have had difficulty viewing education as a product and therefore have been slow to recognize the value of business concepts in managing the academic environment. The historical view of scholars sitting around pontificating about the fate of the world is no longer a valued concept that will serve academia for the next decade, nor help institutions of higher education learn to plan for and manage in the next century.

Universities make up one of the largest industries in the nation but, according to some experts, are the least businesslike and in many instances are mismanaged. They are threatened by decline and bankruptcy with a prediction that 10% to 30% of America's 3100 colleges and universities will close their doors or merge by 1995 (Keller, 1983). Some institutions are more vulnerable than others, but these predictions apply to institutions of all sizes, public and private alike.

SERVICE INSTITUTIONS

Colleges and universities are categorized as service institutions along with hospitals, churches, social agencies, and government authorities. Service institutions are in some respects different from other businesses and industries, but not different enough to ignore business aspects of management. Critics of academia as big business are quick to point out the constraints to using sound business practices and claim that the differences are profound enough to justify the old ways of operation. The argument is that the educational product is an intangible item and therefore cannot be bought and sold like other products. Others contend that the self-governing nature of faculties make the idea of a business operation impossible in higher education. Some claim that service institutions suffer from a lack of good men and women, and that institutions do not perform well because of weak leadership, not because of traditional management techniques. Faculties are cited for being less proficient than their counterparts in industry. It is pointed out that low salaries encourage the best and the brightest to reject academic positions.

Drucker (1974) believes that these attitudes are only excuses for ignoring the value of business practices in academia. He, however, presents the notion that there is one very real difference in service institutions. The real difference has to do with money and, more specifically, with the budget process. Businesses are paid for goods and products, for satisfying customers. Customer satisfaction is known to be a way of assuring long-term success. Academic agencies, on the other hand, are by and large paid by budget allocation, a predetermined sum usually

The style and features of a program refer to how it looks to the public and include where and how the offering is presented. Style should be designed for a specific consumer group and it is best never to impose a style without good reason. Style deals with image, and a positive image is the first step to successful programming. Features refer more to specifics of the program or service and include the time, the cost, the number of hours per week, and the instructional setting.

Quality is a well-known term to educators and is an accepted concept in academia as well as in business. Quality of education has been measured and remeasured. It has been assessed correctly and incorrectly. Quality is acknowledged as one of the most important aspects of an academic offering, yet it is difficult to achieve agreement of the indicators of quality. Sometimes the determinant quality is subjective, since it represents a level of performance of the provider. Many educators depend on quality alone to sell their programs and tend to minimize the importance of style and features. It is not unusual for consumers to pay for a program of only reasonable quality, if all other variables are satisfactory. Successful institutions strive for perfection in all market elements: style, features, quality, packaging, and branding. Packaging and branding are the most difficult considerations for academicians to accept as they attempt to apply business concepts to education.

Packaging and branding of courses takes place by colleges and universities, but in most cases these elements of marketing are not carried out systematically and their value is usually underestimated. Generally it is understood that a product in industry must be wrapped in an attractive, colorful package that stimulates buyer interest. The college campus, its buildings and general environment, is considered to be the package in which educational products are delivered to the public. However, excuses are made for dreary classrooms that are inadequate to accommodate class size, and special features, such as access for the handicapped, are rarely considered. More times than not, academia assumes that words of wisdom from learned professors alone will attract students. Even when budgets are tight, attention to minor cosmetic improvements of the environment attract consumers, particularly in times of high competition. Some consumers enroll in colleges and universities close to home for economic and family reasons no matter what the environment offers. However, those who are paying high tuition give increasing thought on how and where they spend their money on education. In these situations, attention to packaging can be a powerful recruitment tool.

The last of the product characteristics is branding, by and large, a foreign word to academia. Educators are in the habit of labeling courses, programs, and services with mundane names like Health Science I or Nursing II. These labels are usually unexciting and tell the consumer very little about content. It is not uncommon to talk about courses by numbers: NUR601, PIO346. This approach leaves much to be desired and certainly does not encourage the inquisitive student. The excuse usually given is that most of the courses are required, and therefore labeling and branding of courses in an interesting way is unnecessary. It is forgotten that some students do not come to college only for the requirement, but to enrich their lives and maximize their educational opportunity. Special students who have flexibility will be attracted to interesting courses. Branding of an educational offering may be a new concept, but there is no good reason not to try new labels.

PRICING AND DISTRIBUTION

Pricing education has gotten out of hand and has come to mean one thing in America. Setting the price for education has meant raising tuition every year since the early 1970s. The public complains about high tuition but has come to expect regular price increases for higher education. Students and their families look for increased opportunities for scholarships, loans, and government aid. In the aggregate, this behavior leads to unprecedented cost increases no matter who pays the bills.

Growing criticism has generated a multitude of explanations for the tuition increases. The nation's colleges and universities, our defenders claim, are

✳ EDITOR'S QUESTIONS FOR DISCUSSION ✳

How might an accurate assessment of the stage or cycle that an academic institution is in affect a leader's plan for change? What endogenous factors as indicated by Farrell were present in the setting illustrated by Baker (Chapter 60)? What type of leader and leadership for an academic institution may be appropriate for each stage of the four stages in an institution's life cycle? What strategies can be proposed both for an accurate assessment of the stage as well as for intervening or reversing negative events within the life cycle. What are the methods and processes by which a leader and manager may move an institution to a desired position on the life-cycle curve? What programs currently exist in many schools of nursing that have a limited life cycle?

How can a dean best assess his or her academic institution for the appropriate product-mix of education programs and related services offered to students? What are the pros and cons for deans in schools of nursing sharing resources and defining target populations for students? What factors contribute to decreasing enrollments of students and utilization of various programs in nursing? What strategies can be used by deans of nursing to reverse the decline in enrollments and attract potential students? What marketing strategies might be more appropriate than others to attract potential nursing students

into programs? Indicate various means by which the packaging of programs can be made attractive for the potential student. What should the label of a course convey to students? How might branding be applied to the titling of courses? What are criteria for the measurement of quality in education programs? How can consensus best be obtained for indicators of quality in programs? How can a nursing dean best determine what programs are most needed in the geographical area, and the potential for attracting students, qualified faculty, and resources?

Why is the actual cost of higher education greater than the direct cost to the student? Propose strategies for potential students being able to pay for the more accurate cost of education. What are the advantages and disadvantages regarding the price strategy of usage maximization? What implications are there for quality in programs emphasizing usage maximization? What risks are involved in keeping low caps on tuition costs? What is the impact of pricing methods on the potential quality of education programs? What strategies can be suggested for the effective use of various pricing methods for programs? What are examples of unit pricing, two-part pricing, and term pricing that might exist in a university and in schools of nursing?

60

College Transformation:
Changing to compete

Constance M. Baker, Ed. D., R.N.

Change is the hallmark of survival. Most chief executives know that consistent innovation aimed at producing a quality, cost-effective product ensures longevity. The challenge is to orchestrate systematically institutional change.

A verified theory of how change occurs in colleges and universities does not exist. Usually change in institutions of higher education is based on theoretical models of the change process and practical experience in overcoming resistance. The major change models associated with colleges and universities are (a) the rational planning approach found in research, development, and diffusion; (b) action research using problem solving and organizational development; (c) social interaction aimed at persuading opinion leaders; (d) the political conflict model used by special interest groups; and (e) adaptive development with systems theory and contingency theory (Nordvall, 1982). Essentially, these models are based on various conceptions of the decision-making process and include collegial, bureaucratic, and political approaches (Baldridge & Deal, 1975). The practical advice in the literature describes actual change projects and enlightening experiences in relation to coping with resistance.

This chapter presents a case study that describes how a large, locally oriented nursing school with a credible performance record was transformed into an internationally focused, competitive institution. Neither the dean nor the school where the transformation occurred are identified in the case study. Attention is given to first, a description of the setting and situation; second, the vision developed and held by the dean, the chief executive of the school of nursing; third, a five-dimensional model for the change effort; and fourth, reflections on the future of the school.

FORMING A VISION

In 1981 the College of Nursing in the case study presented here was 23 years old, housed in a modern spacious facility on the main campus and guided by its seventh dean, an acting dean. It had (a) just undergone a critical external review of the master's degree program by the Commission on Higher Education; (b) offered a large generic baccalaureate program that dominated the college; and (c) was anticipating a revisit by the National League for Nursing concerning the associate degree program, which had been placed on warning. The majority of the faculty held a master's degree received from one university, and none of the 10 doctorally prepared faculty held nursing doctorates. Considerable covert turmoil existed among the faculty, and the external community was openly critical. The university administration was (a) young and energetic, (b) committed to moving the university into the forefront of higher education, (c) frustrated with nursing and nurses, and (d) determined to resolve the College of Nursing's problems.

The new dean, an experienced academic administrator, believed that (a) nursing is a credible academic discipline, with an evolving science base; (b) the values of science should undergird academic behavior; and (c) leadership is critical for nursing to assume its place in the university (Morris, 1981). The university administration made a commitment to these ideals and to the College of Nursing during the dean's preemployment interviews, but it needed to be nurtured and the university administration needed facts about academic nursing.

Assuming the deanship of a large college of nursing is accompanied by wishes, hopes, fears, and—ideally—a strong compelling vision. Bennis and Nanus (1985) consider a vision as a mental picture of a desired future state. A vision is a pragmatic dream that can serve to inspire action. A vision pulls people together around some future state that is important, but nearly impossible to realize; thus there is an element of risk, excitement, and intrigue. They suggest that all of us are visionaries, but we are not encouraged to express our vision or we are too afraid to take risks. A vision serves many purposes; it (a) inspires individual behavior; (b) provides a common bond among group members; (c) dictates goals; (d) influences organizational structure; and (e) offers guidelines for work appraisal. The process of developing a vision requires time to reflect on the past, the present, and the future. It is necessary to review past successes and shortcomings, present conditions and resources, and future trends and needs. Such a review is the first step in developing a vision.

An assessment of the College of Nursing was deliberately conducted by the new dean with assistance from knowledgeable persons inside and outside the college. The next step in forming a vision was to consider the needs of the state and the external environment and to match the philosophy of the university with the characteristics of the college and the dean's beliefs (Keller, 1983). The dean's overar-

ching vision was to use academic nursing to transform significantly the nursing profession in the state in 5 years. This vision required an academic organization with a diverse faculty and student body that would produce excellent graduates, clinically relevant research, and visible professional leadership. Considerable change was required to achieve this vision, and the change needed to be carefully orchestrated to maximize the use of resources.

A MODEL FOR CHANGE

In the case study, attention was focused on five dimensions of organizational change: the college culture, management skills, college reorganization, participants, and the rewards (Kilmann, 1984). Each of these dimensions was studied to identify specific problem areas and to select techniques for implementing change. Each dimension was then systematically introduced in an integrated fashion, based on the capacity for change of the majority of the faculty and the organization. Efforts were made to set priorities by determining which changes would be easiest and most needed and which changes could be postponed.

College Culture

The culture of a college includes the shared beliefs, attitudes, norms, values, and rituals that are learned and provide the force behind formal written policies. Any efforts aimed at permanent change must focus on managing the cultural system by identifying the actual culture, articulating what is needed to achieve the vision, and dealing with culture gaps. For example, in this case study many dimensions of the culture of the College of Nursing were revealed in the nursing commencement. The event was called the "pinning ceremony." Students wore their nurse uniforms; faculty wore street clothes; master's graduates were not included; the speakers were favorite teachers who described anecdotes; class awards were given to the secretary and student counselor who contributed to student "survival"; and as the students received their pins, the majority embraced the faculty. This ritual had considerable potential to communicate the values of professional nursing and to teach and reinforce the academic model, but it needed to be altered drastically. First, the name was changed to "nursing convocation." Faculty were expected to wear academic regalia; master's students were invited to receive academic hoods; within a year, all students were required to wear academic regalia; awards were given for excellence in education, research, and service; and congratulations were offered with handshakes. Thus ceremonies and rituals were used to close the gap between the college culture and the vision for the future, in which rituals serve to renew values and commitment.

Since culture is an intangible and pervasive aspect of an organization, any effort at implementing change requires the culture to be deliberately managed. In the case study, the 25th anniversary of the baccalaureate program was an opportunity to review history, project future trends, and elicit alumni's support. All the former nursing deans and acting deans were invited to the campus to present a short overview of their tenure as dean, followed by the current dean's vision of the future. An alumni association was launched, officers were elected, and efforts at fund raising were begun. This celebration (a) communicated a respect for the past and the necessity to go forward; (b) invited the participation of all parties in shaping the future; and (c) set the course for the changes necessary to achieve the vision.

Management Skill

The second dimension of college change is the dean's repertoire of skills brought to the position. In this case study, one of the early questions posed was what dean behaviors will challenge the old culture and reinforce efforts at implementing the vision. In response, it was concluded important that the dean act openly and consistently with the expectations of the vision, while maintaining high optimism and positive attitudes toward the effort.

All new administrators have a "honeymoon" when considerable change can be introduced, if the risk is taken. During this time the dean launched several new "traditions." For example, on the first day of the

school year a general faculty meeting was held. At this time the dean (a) made a formal presentation on the state of the College of Nursing, (b) interpreted the budget and annual salary adjustments, and (c) introduced new faculty. Additionally the assistant deans and committee chairs set the stage for the coming year by reporting accomplishments and outlining annual goals. This effort was aimed at communicating the vision and enlisting everyone's participation. An example of another new activity was a "TGIF coffee hour" with the dean on Friday mornings, to further the dean's accessibility to the faculty. Attendance at this function varied depending on the time of the year, but it proved to be of value for informal communication.

Within a month after the new dean arrived, the recently retired provost telephoned the dean to discuss nursing's outdated promotion and tenure criteria and to offer his assistance to the tenured faculty to revise the criteria. This telephone call gave the dean additional legitimacy to call for an examination and revision of the criteria. A second immediate issue involved faculty requests for part-time employment to pursue doctoral study, in the absence of any approved guidelines to respond effectively. The dean charged the tenured faculty with using the American Association of University Professors work load statement to draft a comparable work load statement for the College of Nursing (AAUP, 1969), the process of which produced meaningful discussions regarding the missions of the university and college. The one-page document went through nine drafts over 1½ years before faculty consensus was reached. Faculty discussions during this process revealed such outdated college values as rigid work hours and provided an opportunity to establish new values such as the legitimacy of faculty scholarship. All of these activities are critical to achieving the vision of a credible academic discipline. Criteria for appointment, promotion, and tenure must be in accord with other disciplines; time must be protected to ensure faculty scholarship; and faculty must know the expectations of the dean and the university administrators.

Relationships with the community were in need of immediate attention. Strategies included making presentations to the medical associations, meeting

adequate to reinforce performance that contributed to achieving the vision. The overall conditions were such that the intrinsic rewards derived from the nature of the work would be maximum.

Outcomes

In summary, a powerful vision spawned a multidimensional approach to implementing change. This approach integrated five dimensions of organizational life and suggested that each dimension had to be carefully sequenced to maximize efforts toward achieving the vision. Such an approach required time, energy, and commitment but the outcomes were very apparent. Faculty and student morale was high. Nursing took its place in the university and the community: a nurse became the highest funded researcher in the university; nurses chaired two university committees; and nurses led professional organizations, consulted in practice settings, and served on government committees. It was extremely rewarding to watch faculty and student behavior become more in line with the vision of academic nursing.

FUTURE PROJECTIONS

Setting an agenda for the future requires consideration of the organization and its mission within the environmental context. Organizations have a life cycle and evolve from one stage of development to the next in the process of maturation. Baker (1981) has documented differences between nursing departments along the organizational life cycle and differences in management style as departments mature.

Organizational and personal vitality require regular reexamination of goals in relation to environmental challenges and organizational accomplishments. New technology in health care, shifts in population and demographics, scarcities in human and capital resources, and growing emphasis on quality influence revision of college goals. With the number of doctorally prepared faculty over 50% in the College of Nursing, the need for administrative guidance was diminished enough that the size of the administrative structure could be decreased. Strategic planning, data-based decision making, and an ongoing program of institutional evaluation will ensure that future changes are made for the advantage of the student, the consumer.

In summary, major changes were implemented in a college of nursing during the recent past through the use of a multidimensional model. Efforts were made to challenge deliberately and shape the college culture, exercise maximum control over administrative management style, and reorganize in a manner that facilitated the professional success of all involved. These efforts served to advance the success of this college of nursing, recruit and socialize the faculty, and reward all who contributed to achieving the vision. Changes through the use of a multidimensional model must be ongoing to ensure the future preparation of academic nursing that will meet the challenges of the 21st century.

REFERENCES

American Association of University Professors (AAUP). (1969). *Academic freedom and tenure: A handbook*. Washington, DC: Author.

Baker, CM (1981). The development of academic departments and governance in colleges of nursing. In JC McCloskey & HK Grace (Eds.), *Current issues in nursing* (pp. 451–459). Boston: Blackwell Scientific Publications.

Baldridge, JV, & Deal, TE (Eds.). (1975). *Managing change in educational organizations*. Berkeley: McCutchen.

Bennis, W, & Nanus, B (1985). *Leaders*. New York: Harper & Row.

Brody, J (1985, March 26). Laying on of hands gains new respect. *New York Times*, p. 17.

Kanter, RM (1983). *The change masters*. New York: Simon & Schuster.

Keller, G (1983). *Academic strategy*. Baltimore: Johns Hopkins University Press.

Kilmann, RH (1984). *Beyond the quick fix*. San Francisco: Jossey-Bass.

Morris, VC (1981). *Deaning: Middle management in academe*. Urbana: University of Illinois Press.

Nordvall, RC (1982). *The process of change in higher education institutions* (AAHE-ERIC/Higher Education Research Report No. 7). Washington, DC: American Association for Higher Education.

✳ EDITOR'S QUESTIONS FOR DISCUSSION ✳

What are the possible methods by which an assessment of a school or college of nursing might be done? How can one be assured that the data obtained in the assessment are valid and reliable? How does a vision of a dean influence the dynamics and organizational culture? What is the process by which rituals, behaviors, and values may be altered most effectively? What are the methods and processes by which systematic change can be orchestrated? What are the stages and steps within the change process? To what extent must each step and stage be planned before implementation of the change? How does one establish priorities in introducing, planning, implementing, and evaluating change? How are timing and pacing critical factors in the change process? Identify the restraining forces and the driving forces concerning change in the case study detailed in this chapter. How can one determine when an institution is ready to move from one step or stage in the change process to another? How can a dean increase the driving forces for change and decrease the restraining or resisting forces against change? How can a dean bring into play residual forces to increase, inhibit, or prevent further change? How might chaos be used as a medium for introducing and implementing change? What are the advantages and disadvantages of constant, continuous change within an organization? Should or how can a change or changes be stabilized or maintained as a steady state?

What factors are critical for the acceptance and implementation of major decisions in change? How can an academic administrator best determine when additional information or input regarding a possible decision should be obtained versus when to move ahead in change? What type of communication is most effective in promoting and implementing change? How can and do administrators and faculty discern a difference between what is stated in a communication versus what is actually meant? How can diversity promote conflict rather than unity within an organization regarding purpose, goals, objectives, and values? In bringing new staff and personnel into an organization, how can a shared unity of purpose be developed? What are criteria that might be used for evaluating the success of the change process? What implications does Chapter 58, by Hegyvary have for the process of change as outlined by Baker? What are the assumptions, advantages, and disadvantages of matrix-type structure or designs? What is the difference between decentralized decision making and decentralized functions, and how might these differences be shown in an organization's design? What are other frameworks for introducing, planning, implementing, and evaluating change?

61

Nursing and the Academic Enterprise:
A covenant with quality

Geraldene Felton, Ed.D., R.N., F.A.A.N.

A university is its people, individually and collectively. Nurse faculty in universities sense how much nursing owes to the process that identifies and nurtures devoted scholars and teachers and their commitment to reaffirm a covenant with quality. The covenant with quality helps us make the case that education is about life, and not just work, and that nursing is a good way to live a life.

The covenant with quality is directly attributable to many ongoing changes in schools of nursing. We are caught up in the buoyant force of intellectual curiosity. There is an increase in the number of doctorally prepared faculty. Some schools are moving toward the concept of one faculty—away from separate undergraduate faculty and graduate faculty (Forni & Welch, 1987). In many schools, appointment to the rank of assistant professor requires the doctorate as it does in other academic disciplines. In some schools, faculty role is conceptualized in the collegiate sense—one role that embraces three complementary and overarching responsibilities: teaching, public service, and research to improve professional practice and to demonstrate its effect on health.

Major publications painstakingly document that

through all this change nursing has remained steadfast in its commitment to excellence in educating women and men for lives of leadership in their communities, their state, their nation, and the world; for contribution to the profession; and for lives of personal satisfaction and individual fulfillment. In answer to the question, "Why go to nursing school?", a nursing graduate could truthfully answer, "To get a skill that allows one to do things that are really useful to people."

There are still major issues to be addressed to make the covenant with quality more coherent. These include the leadership challenge, the trend in strengthening educational standards, racial diversity in higher education, and the roles of the nurse in academia.

LEADERSHIP AS THE ART OF THE POSSIBLE

In noting the increased incidence of universities looking to lawyers for leadership as presidents, Thomas Ehrlich (1987), President of Indiana University, said, "Lawyers are trained to take a problem, break it into its component parts, work through the issues, and put it all back together again" (p. 13). Ehrlich added that lawyers do not have "a monopoly or special lock on these qualities."

Indeed, nursing deans need these same qualities! The survival of colleges of nursing is at stake, since survival is more and more dependent on the leader's reputation for good management skills, broad pragmatism, and effectiveness in a job that is much more complicated than ever before. In the search for a dean, the tendency is still to select someone who starts out as a faculty member and who has progressed up the career ladder, steeped in academia. Central administration expects the dean to provide direction and to exhibit the courage to stand up for what the school really is good at. Meeting this expectation requires being able to make sound, deliberate choices and stick to them — keeping an eye on the large goal, while adjusting to altered circumstances that arise along the way. Above all, it requires being principled and confident.

Over the past decade, the number of practical administrative and political problems that a dean has to face has increased enormously. The most conspicuous result is that expectations and demands for academic leadership in this changing environment have also changed. These expectations and demands result in organizational power, which was defined by Kanter (1977) as "the ability to get things done, to mobilize resources, to get and use whatever it is that a person needs for the goals he or she is attempting to meet" (p. 166). Some of these expectations and demands include thinking globally, setting an example, being accountable and able to confront problems squarely, keeping up to date, and setting priorities. These are the characteristics of today's successful nursing dean that set a value tone, an ambiance.

While dreaming the dream of what might be, it is easy to get bogged down with specific details before their place in the blueprint is clear. Moreover, it is easier for people to consider specifics rather than abstract concepts. To develop strategies, leaders must master the art of synthesizing and applying knowledge appropriately to the context at hand. Nitpicking has a time and place, but rarely when goals and directions are being developed.

Effective leaders inspire followers. They do it by conveying an appealing vision of a better future; they do it through principled and courageous actions; they do it by their job performance and subtle political skills. A mark of a good leader is that she or he motivates others to achieve their full potential as professionals and as human beings. A good leader unlocks the aspirations of others and encourages the expressions of their needs, concerns, and hopes through constructive actions. It then follows that individuals typically take measure of themselves by comparison with their leaders and how the leader prepares to deal with different situations. It is proper and reasonable to expect leaders to give evidence of their preparation to deal with different situations through their performance.

Similarly, talented, motivated people have the ambition to advance in their areas, and good leaders accept and support that ambition. It requires that leaders regularly look for opportunities for others to grow professionally. It also means, of course, that some talented people successfully recruited will be lost, and the leader must constantly bring new, less experienced persons into the organization. The dividends for doing so are that the process creates high morale and the dynamic state of affairs so necessary for effective organizations.

A good staff does more than dump problems in the leader's lap. It offers specific or alternative solutions for problems. And, once agreement is reached on desired solutions, the leader expects staff to follow through with the resolution of the problem presented, with assurance that the task will be carried out with skill and precision. However, the leader is accountable for her or his work as well as that of staff and faculty. In the case of the dean, the leader is accountable to the faculty and staff as well as to administrative superiors. In the case of faculty and staff, the leader must have a systematic way for keeping in touch with what they do and know the results of their efforts. It is part of leadership responsibility to offer constructive criticism and advice when others' efforts can be improved or the direction of their efforts modified.

The leader must find ways to maintain a sense of direction and a concern for the future of the organization. Such sense of direction requires knowledge of the enterprise as well as enthusiasm and a positive attitude about the future. Among ways to do this are exchanges with counterparts at conferences and seminars, identifying role models, seeking reviews—both from within and without the organization—of one's effectiveness as a leader, pinpointing areas for improvement, and taking blocks of time to reflect on the state of the enterprise. Such reflection results in questions such as: "Where are we going? Where should we be going and why? What principles are we using to get there? In what ways are my efforts enhancing or impeding the vitality of the enterprise?"

Not surprisingly, high levels of energy and endurance are among the most commonly cited characteristics of effective leadership. The leader can take maximum advantage of a strong sense of priorities in the use of time by resisting acceptance of too many responsibilities. Without this sense one can easily not only fritter away time, but reduce one's levels of energy and endurance. However, in the final analysis, these levels cannot be positively manipulated unless the leader continues to be enthusiastic about the importance of the leader's role in what is going on. Moreover, it is not enough for leaders to have a dream—they must be able to communicate the vision in ways that uplift and encourage people to go along with them.

The presumption is that being a forward-looking and inspiring leader (and therefore a successful leader) should bring great satisfaction because the leader has passed a stringent test. What the leader has to offer has been revealed to colleagues, and they have replied, in effect, "We like what you say and do. You are worthy of our trust. We are therefore willing to join with you in our common purpose. Lead us!"

A NATIONAL TREND IN STRENGTHENING EDUCATIONAL STANDARDS

During the mid-1980s, educators began examining substance, style, and comparative quality of education. They concluded that there was a need to establish basic academic competencies in reading and writing, speaking and listening, science and mathematics, reasoning, and foreign language skills (American Association of Colleges of Nursing, 1986; Bennett, 1984, 1987; Bok, 1986; Boyer, 1986). Increasingly states have undertaken vigorous initiatives to improve curricula, as well as admission and graduation standards, in both high schools and colleges. At the same time, colleges and universities are changing basic requirements for the academic credits that students must earn in high school in order to gain admission to colleges or universities.

Most often, revised high school requirements include 4 years of English and language arts, 3 years of mathematics, 3 years of natural science, 3 years of social science, and 2 years of one foreign language. These requirements, most recently reinforced by former Education Secretary Bennett (1987), have been recommended for all high school graduates whether or not they plan to attend college. It is understandable that universities want enrollees to be ready for a university education with a minimum of remedial instruction, since they seek students who are likely to complete work on a degree and then exit successfully into a highly complex world under extremely competitive conditions. Parenthetically, American students, from even the highest ranking universities in the United States, must work hard to keep up with still better-prepared students from many foreign countries (Fiske, 1987).

The initiatives to raise college and university curriculum standards recognize a twofold challenge to graduates of tomorrow. These graduates will need skills not only for sorting and absorbing the massive amounts of information that will be available at a finger's touch, but also they will desperately need intellectual skills to translate the bewildering array of information into knowledge and understanding. This strong base of knowledge and skills will be needed to make critical judgments, to reason, to decide and act, and to communicate in a responsible and effective way.

The raising of educational standards in colleges and universities also has an inextricable relationship to teaching. On the one hand, analysts of undergraduate experiences in the United States call for substantially increased emphasis on teaching, while providing little constructive comment on the constant flow of intellectual and creative discoveries necessary to nourish good teaching at an advanced level. On the other hand, some of the more vigorous proponents of faculty research seem resentful of the time spent in the classroom. They use the phrase "released time" as if it meant release from a kind of penal servitude. All too often a presumed incompatibility between teaching and research is used to account for many of the miscellaneous ills that beset higher education, nursing included.

Academic nursing, at its best, has made a pact. Only a faculty that embodies in its own work values intellectual inquiry at the highest level—welcoming the risks of exploration, questioning, review by peers, and public scrutiny—is capable of inspiring students to undergo the searing processes of discovery, testing, and mutual criticism in their own intellectual development. When students work in an atmosphere of manifest devotion to research and continued learning, they prepare themselves for continuous, unbroken learning for the rest of their lives. They are preparing for the changes in career, in profession, or in outlook that are essential to society and to a continued robust school.

Thus, in an environment that emphasizes development of new knowledge, students learn more than the content of the courses they take. They also learn a way of life. They learn an ethos of learning, analytical thought, organization, and self-discipline. They learn enthusiastic commitment to the advancement of knowledge. That is why undergraduate education in a research university starts with such a great advantage.

RACIAL DIVERSITY IN HIGHER EDUCATION
Diversity and Educational Excellence

The underrepresentation of minority students in higher education has become a national problem of catastrophic proportions. This problem has grave long-term consequences not only for this country's economic and social well-being, but also for the educational development of students who have grown up in predominantly white communities. The Amer-

ican Council on Education (Higher education, 1985) has warned that allowing declines in minority participation to continue unchecked will return society to an elitist system of a highly educated upper and middle class, mostly white, and a seriously undereducated working and poor class, mostly nonwhite. The same warning is reiterated by the Urban League (1988; Allan, Nunley, & Scott-Warner, 1988).

In some states, students may not have encountered persons of other races in situations designed to foster learning, and thus have not considered nor analyzed issues arising from different perspectives among various racial, ethnic, and cultural groups. Immersed in such a monochromic universe, they may not even suspect that something may be missing from their view of reality. There has been the belief that extension of educational and employment opportunity to more minority students and faculty is sound educational policy, enriching the educational environment for everyone. However, many of the nation's most prestigious and wealthy universities now are calling for sweeping new initiatives to broaden and diversify the faculty and student body to make them more representative of North American society. This means that diversity is considered an important asset in the academic community. This is so not only because colleges and universities prepare students for lives and careers in a complex and constantly evolving world of many cultures, and because the opportunity to join the community must be available to all who are able and willing to meet its standards, but increasingly because it is an essential step in the pursuit of academic excellence. In short, enriching racial and ethnic diversity is essential to education in its broader sense.

By the year 2000, it is predicted that 28% of the college-age population will be black and Hispanic; and that within 15 years, one third of the work force will consist of members of minorities (Darling-Harvard, 1985; Lee, 1985). Compounding these statistics, the number of minority students graduating from college with the qualifications for graduate school is still relatively small. Conspicuously, blacks and Hispanics are losing ground at most levels of higher education—undergraduate, graduate, and professional student and faculty (Urban League, 1988).

In nursing and other sciences, one of the main reasons blacks and Hispanics are underrepresented is that they participate less often in precollege academic programs, advanced mathematics courses, and science courses. Records indicate, for example, that blacks and Hispanics are considerably less likely than whites and Asians to have taken courses in calculus, algebra, geometry, trigonometry, and chemistry. They may also lack the capability to read well enough to cope with our technological society.

Decisions about majoring in a science obviously need to be made as early as junior high school. However, black and Hispanic students may be steered away from college preparatory tracks by their peers and counselors. Furthermore, reductions in federal student aid cause problems of access to college. Consequently the growing proportion of minorities and low-income persons in college-age populations increases the urgency of assuring higher education opportunities for minorities. However, unless present trends are reversed, we will be a significantly less educated society by the year 2000 than we are now. If these trends continue over time, a significant population of blacks and other minorities will simply be lost to higher education, a potentially tragic loss for society. A direct loss will be in personal fulfillment and increased incomes that additional degrees might have brought. The loss to society is that the professional, higher-income stratum will remain overwhelmingly white, while the large and largely uneducated, lower-income class grows ever more black, more separate, and more unequal.

The Paucity of Minority Teachers

One explanation for the size of minority student enrollment may be the lack of minority faculty representation. As a matter of fact, the ranks of minority teachers in academia are shrinking (Darling-Harvard, 1985; Jaschik, 1987). The consequences are that all students do not come in contact with minority teachers, students do not see societal representativeness in positions of authority, and there are fewer role models for minority students to pattern

their performance and career aspirations. Most importantly, the number of blacks and Hispanics on school faculties is thought to be the most significant predictor of success in recruiting minority students for professional and graduate schools.

Some universities recently took several significant steps toward creating a more welcoming environment for minorities. These included such actions as making the Office of Affirmative Action directly responsible to the Office of the President and establishing a coordinated program of outreach to outstanding minority faculty (Fiske, 1987; Jaschik, 1987).

At my own university the following actions are being implemented. Faculty are urged to identify outstanding senior and entry level minority professors. There is commitment to aggressive recruitment of junior faculty through competitive financial inducements and opportunities toward tenure. Established minority scholars will be vigorously sought for tenured positions, including an endowed chair to honor a distinguished minority alumnus. Minority faculty will be provided moving expenses, salary supplements, professional travel accounts, research help, research fellowships, an accelerated faculty leave program, lighter teaching loads, protection from major committee responsibilities, and a mentoring program. Minority faculty will be identified by faculty, alumni, and friends of the university, as well as through special ties to historically black colleges. Additionally, collaborative study and research opportunities will be sought for faculty at historically black colleges. In actively seeking qualified minorities and making persuasive offers, the university will give attention to job advertisement language to remove subtle suggestions of bias. Furthermore, plans include tending to operationalization of what makes a job offer persuasive—namely salary, teaching assignment, developmental leaves, research assistants, equipment, and so on.

Nationwide, in the belief that talented minorities are likely to respond to efforts to increase the general pool of faculty, educators have suggested other ways to reverse the decline in minority teacher ranks, such as college loan forgiveness programs if students choose teaching. Discussants of the topic are quick to add, however, that the problem cannot be solved without general improvements in the previous education of minority students. Finally faculty commitment to affirmative action cannot be left to vague rhetoric of general approbation. Without full discussion and consensus based on explicit and detailed understandings, the record of action will continue to be dismal.

RECRUITMENT AND RETENTION OF MINORITY STUDENTS

Hand in hand with identifying minority faculty are special efforts to identify and attract black, Hispanic, and Native American student applicants (Higher education, 1985; Allan et al. 1988). Intensified recruitment initiatives are being directed to increase the enrollment of talented minority students through activities such as adding a director of minority affairs; providing financial aid in the form of grants and gifts rather than loans based on need as well as academic achievement; expansion of academic support services, including remedial and counseling programs; definition of the problems that minority students face; creation of a sense of community among black students; formation of coordinating councils for minority issues to institutionalize the university's efforts in lending support to minority student groups and activities; creation of a black alumni directory; mentoring efforts to raise the sights of minority students; and insistence on commitment to successful completion of a demanding, high-quality undergraduate curriculum. Burris (1987) maintains that underlying all these efforts must be faculty commitment and involvement, and the belief that a quality undergraduate curriculum is a key to minority success.

Minorities in Nursing Education

In the process of increasing the diversity of university programs and students, nursing education has to address the needs of minority students and faculty, as well as the needs of their neighboring communities. Unfortunately issues associated with continuing recruitment, retention, and graduation of members of minority groups at postsecondary levels

of education remain even more of a problem in nursing. Minorities are as unrepresented in the discipline of nursing as they are seriously underrepresented in American colleges and universities. Superimposed on these problems are a number of other obstacles: financial difficulties; lack of educational aspirations; lack of tested academic ability before college; voluntary and involuntary withdrawal before completion of the degree; and the image of nursing as a low-status occupation, with conditions of work and rewards inconsistent with modern lifestyles and expectations associated with a professional degree. Nonetheless, nursing college programs must reflect the transcultural and demographic characteristics of society at large, as well as commitment to equity and access as a social goal.

Unfortunately, efforts to increase participation by minorities in nursing higher education are distressingly stalled. Even so, concern about the number of minority students in nursing has caused the establishment of all kinds of programs for minority students, for economically and educationally disadvantaged students, and for students from culturally divergent backgrounds. These include precollege enrichment programs, better coordination between high schools and colleges, tutoring for standardized tests, early admission and financial notification programs, better orientation for incoming minority students, and attention to representation of minorities among faculty. Other initiatives include special recruitment, counseling and advising, remedial courses, tutorial systems, cultural centers, and development of more constructive relationships with faculty and staff. One strategy not exploited in nursing is a system in which colleges and universities work in partnership with both high schools and the private sector to target and track black, Hispanic, and Native American students. This strategy is a possibility, since at 80 colleges and universities and 60 community colleges, TRIO Programs (that is, Upward Bound, Talent Search, Student Support Services, Educational Opportunity Centers, Training Authority, and Ronald McNair Scholarship Program) are funded under Title IV of the Higher Education Act.

An example of one such partnership, Career Beginnings, was developed by the Commonwealth

Fund in New York as an outgrowth of a project begun 3 years ago at Hunter College and now managed by the Center for Human Resources at Brandeis University's Heller School (President Handler, Brandeis University, personal communication, December 1, 1987). The goal of Career Beginnings is to enhance aspirations of high school students from disadvantaged backgrounds. A major aspect is to target young people who demonstrate good attendance records and average academic ability—young people who might be overlooked by other programs such as those aimed at high achievers or school dropouts. Students in the Career Beginnings program come from families who live either below the poverty line or marginally above it. They may be in families in which college education is not regarded as a realistic choice or in which parents have limited abilities to help their children find places in the work world. These disadvantages usually are aggravated by gaps in a support system that high school students need to help them fulfill their college or employment potential.

At the heart of Career Beginnings is a mentor system. Students are assigned mentors with whom they meet on a monthly basis to discuss career and college planning. Mentors include business executives, government officials, owners of small businesses, educators, lawyers, physicians, technicians, professional athletes, and key community leaders. Scholastic Aptitude Test (SAT) and American College Testing (ACT) preparation, academic development, social skills, career planning, and team building are all part of the range of activities in which Career Beginnings' students participate. Programs also are needed at the elementary and preschool levels in order truly to make a difference. Nursing colleges could certainly model the Career Beginnings program.

Needs in Higher Education in General

In nursing and in higher education elsewhere, we will need to protect graduate students generally and our doctoral students in particular in order to minimize some of the frustrations that doctoral candidates face. Students cannot be left to fend for themselves and bear the onus of seeking advice and counseling from a faculty that does not see itself as having this responsibility. Students need advice, particularly between the time of passing qualifying examinations—advancing to candidacy—and before proceeding with the dissertation. It is during this trying period that students most need mentoring.

More than half the students who start doctoral education never finish. It is unreasonable to dismiss these students as being simply not smart enough or otherwise incapable of independent scholarship. Of those who complete the degree, most recognize that the process may be seriously deficient as a mechanism for training future scholars and leaders of society.

Universities in general, and graduate faculties in particular, have to take responsibility for ensuring that mechanisms required to meet the national need for scholars and leaders change to achieve this goal. We cannot continue to do things the same way. Graduate students deserve a nurturing environment as part of the intellectual stimulation they experience during their graduate career. It is the faculty that must meet the challenge to provide that environment, or the entire enterprise will falter.

THE NURSE ACADEMIC

Nurse educators, as others in a college or university, usually are required to teach courses relevant to their discipline and to their own professional and scholarly interests; nonetheless, they have relative autonomy and academic freedom. These educators also have committee work responsibilities, with a wide range of discretion, however, regarding the committees on which they serve and the degree of commitment to committee work. Moreover, universities expect faculty to obtain funding for research, and do scholarly research, writing, and publishing. When faculty choose to use their discretionary time for scholarly writing and research, the university supports their choice in a variety of ways—with office space, library services, secretarial help, materials, laboratory, computer time, assistants, and travel. If the faculty are successful, the university rewards them with increased pay, promotion, and a variety of ceremonial honors.

Thus it can be seen that the proper role of an educator requires not only teaching, serving the community at large, and serving the profession, but also research and consulting. Most universities have policies that consulting can be carried out only with an explicit proviso that it will not interfere with the regular full-time duties of the faculty member, although obviously one will find some abuses. Deans and department heads are instructed to monitor and enforce this policy. Conversations with colleagues in other institutions suggest that this is generally the position of many universities, although the degree of monitoring and enforcement may vary substantially. The key point is whether consulting is handled as a kind of de facto released time or whether it is handled as an incremental activity. There is also a value judgment relative to consulting. Some hold the view that, in most cases, the best interests of the academic community are served by broadening the professional involvement of the faculty member. The implication is that consulting provides an added degree of "real work involvement," which feeds back into improved research, public service, and instructional responsibilities of faculty.

Faculty consulting also is an important asset to research in both government and private-sector institutions. There are many research and development situations in which the nature of the work and the aggregate time involved simply are not amenable to the standard contractual relationship, if one wishes to be cost-effective. The availability of university faculty members for special consulting provides an important professional resource that would be more difficult to obtain by other mechanisms. It may not be the dollar that compels educators to maintain relevancy (although money is important); it is the experience. Many contend that those who are engaged in the education of others should have ongoing operating experience as a balance to their academic pursuits. Thus most nursing faculty, as do other university faculty, have the option to receive other earnings, such as honoraria from consultations and speeches, and royalties from book publications. These opportunities come with the passage of time.

College and university professors have long been active in private business (Pinchot, 1985). Their numbers, however, have increased rapidly in recent years with the intensified commercial interest in electronics and biological research. According to an unpublished survey by the National Science Foundation, some 3000 full-time science and engineering faculty members—more than 1 out of every 25—own, or are major shareholders in, outside companies where they also work.

All of this is good for nursing, if we accept that when teaching and research are separated, the results are detrimental to both. This means that nursing must do all we can to foster the interaction between teaching and research, not only in the institution but also within the lives of individual members of the faculty. We must encourage nurse colleagues to enter their careers with a well-developed and stimulating line of investigative activity. We must recognize that it is very difficult, once a person is appointed to a faculty position and becomes involved in day-to-day requirements of formal teaching, to develop lines of independent investigation if they are not already well-established.

Equally damaging to the nursing learning community is an imbalance in the opposite direction—the situation in which a faculty member enters an academic career so captivated by investigative zeal that teaching on any level becomes a distraction. We need to retain a sense of obligation to our students. Meanwhile, under constant review and attention is whether academia can find a place for the faculty member who is primarily devoted to teaching, as well as the faculty member primarily devoted to research (National Institute of Education, 1984).

CONCLUSION

Some crucial issues that are discussed elsewhere in the text have not been addressed in this chapter. Specifically, these are the nurse manpower shortage and the decrease in the number of students who choose nursing as a career option. The explanation for these omissions here is that I believe attention to the issues addressed is indeed part of the solution to the problems of nurse manpower and student choice.

Caring is the essence of nursing work. However, we are finding that nursing is not only what we do and what we aspire to do, or even the demonstration of our working relationship between will and intelligence, it is also how we present ourselves to the public and how we create and maintain conditions that permit caring to flourish. Meanwhile, we must have sufficient confidence in ourselves to frame and hold our opinions in the face of opposition, make courageous decisions, determine what can be trusted, and learn to take—rather than relinquish— control of our lives. That is what this chapter is about.

This is the best of times for nursing for many reasons, especially in the way that we wish to present ourselves to the public. There is now more than ever a strong emphasis on intelligence and caring; on linking nursing interventions to the basic scientific subculture of phenomena; on clarification of the conceptual bases of nursing care; on extension of scientific competence and the quality, range, and power of nursing research; on evaluation of nursing practices as they relate to patient outcomes; and on forecasting health care delivery system needs that can be contributed to by nurses. What nursing strives for is to describe the present properties of nursing care, how care differs, how general the care is across various groups, how nurses' roles and functions are generalized across different contexts, and finally how all this rationalizes the academic training and supervised clinical experiences of the nursing student. Such emphasis is at the heart of the survival of nursing, as we dream it should be, and how we wish to look from the outside.

I know nursing will survive. It will survive by dint of ability and hard work in a nation that prizes these virtues, by competence and honesty, by perseverance, by unspectacular courage, and an optimistic spirit. All we need is self-discipline and the conviction to bring out the best in each of us.

REFERENCES

Allen, M., Nunley, J., Scott-Warner, M., (1988). Recruitment and retention of black students in baccalaureate nursing programs. *The Journal of Nursing Education, 27*(3), 107–116.

American Association of Colleges of Nursing (AACN). (1986). *Essentials of college and university education for professional nursing.* Final report. Washington, DC: Author.

Bennett, WJ (1984). *To reclaim a legacy.* Report based on the National Endowment for the Humanities' Study Group on the State of Learning in the Humanities in Higher Education. *Chronicle of Higher Education, 29–30*(24), 16–21.

Bennett, WJ (1987). *James Madison High School.* Washington, DC: Department of Education.

Bok, D (1986). Toward higher learning. *Change, 18*(6), 18–23, 26–27.

Boyer, ED (1986). *College: The undergraduate experience in America.* Report issued by the Carnegie Foundation for the Advancement of Teaching. *Chronicle of Higher Education, 33*(24), 16–22.

Burris, BM (1987). Reaching educationally disadvantaged students. *American Journal of Nursing, 86*(10), 1359–1360.

Darling-Harvard, L (1985). *Equality and excellence: The educational status of black Americans.* New York: College Board Publishers.

Ehrlich, T (1987, December 25). The law. *The New York Times,* p. 13.

Fiske, EB (1987, November 18). Colleges open new minority drives. *The New York Times,* p. 86.

Forni, PR, & Welch, MJ (1987). The professional versus the academic model: A dilemma for nursing education. *Journal of Professional Nursing, 3*(5), 291–297.

Higher education and national affairs. (1985). *American Council on Education, 34*(11), 4.

Jaschik, S (1987). Major changes seen needed for colleges to attract minorities. *Chronicle of Higher Education, 13*(A), 1, 3.

Kanter, RM (1977). *Men and women of the corporation* (p. 166). New York: Basic Books.

Lee, V (1985). *Access to higher education: The experiences of blacks, Hispanics, and low socio-economic status whites.* Washington DC: American Council on Education, Division of Policy Analysis and Research.

National Institute of Education. (1984). *Involvement in learning.* Final report of the Study Group on the Conditions of Excellence in American Higher Education. Washington, DC: US Department of Education.

Pinchot, G (1985). *Intrapreneuring.* New York: Harper & Row.

Urban League (1988). *The state of black America* [Annual report]. New York: Author.

✳   **EDITOR'S QUESTIONS FOR DISCUSSION**   ✳

What are the advantages and disadvantages of having one faculty, not separate faculty, for undergraduate and graduate programs in terms of unification of a school, programs, curricula, quality, research, student outcomes, faculty satisfaction, and productivity? What are the major issues related to quality in education and academia? What are processes by which many of the ideals advocated by Felton can be attained? How can a leader most effectively communicate a vision? What are specific strategies by which the needs of minorities — students and faculty — may be more effectively met? What might be included in a recruitment program for minority students and faculty? Discuss the extent that remedial courses and work should be offered in schools of nursing for various educational and faculty development programs.

What aspects of the faculty role as an educator, a researcher, and a professional practitioner most concern faculty, administrators, and students? How may the concerns most appropriately be addressed? What expectations of faculty regarding support services should be in place in schools of nursing? What accountability should faculty have for their discretionary time in schools of nursing? What specific strategies might be offered to foster the interaction between teaching and research in schools of nursing?

62

Politics, Economics, and Nursing Education

Rosalee C. Yeaworth, Ph.D., R.N., F.A.A.N.

*Politics, economics and health have converged
towards a crossroads. This means that health is
clearly becoming a function of politics and
economics. In other words, we find a growing
amount of cases where bad health is the product of
bad politics, and of bad economics, or of both.*

(Manfred A. Max-Neef, 1987, p. 125)

In 1986, Lasswell's book, entitled *Politics: Who Gets What, When, How* was published. In the opening to the book, Lasswell stated, "The study of politics is the study of influence and the influential. . . . The influential are those who get the most of what there is to get" (p. 3). Illness care is not something that most of us think about, as something we are eager to get a lot of, until we are ill. The high cost of advanced health care technology, the high incomes of some health care providers, the decreasing amount of health care cost covered by Medicare and Medicaid, and the increasing numbers of Americans who have no health care coverage are making an impact. We are becoming acutely aware that health and illness care, which many view as a basic need and right, are increasingly becoming something that the influential can "get the most of what there is to get."

Health care is becoming a scarce resource. Decisions have to be made about who gets scarce resources. Politics may be defined as the authoritative allocation of scarce resources (Kalish & Kalish, 1982). Pirages (1976) stated, "Political institutions determine the rules within which individuals compete for or conflict over scarce resources and positions" (p. 14).

Nurses, as the most numerous of the health care professionals, have the potential to play an increasingly major role in the health and health care of this nation. A scarce resource, however, is more valuable than a widely available one, and therefore there are many interest groups who question the amount and type of health care that nurses can provide and, likewise, how they are reimbursed. Many nurses, especially in the past, have tried to avoid political involvement or economic concerns. These nurses have clung to the belief expressed in the *Code for Nurses* that they provide care without discrimination in regard to social or economic status (American Nurses' Association, 1976). However, as it has become painfully clear that political influence is imperative to receiving a share of resources and positions, nursing organizations and individual nurses are becoming more politically astute and active.

Nursing education must prepare nurses to participate intelligently in the political arena, to anticipate needed changes, and to take part in developing public policy. For in the final analysis, public policy influences what can be included in nursing, by whom it can be practiced, and how it can be reimbursed. Politics and public policy influence the content and resources of nursing education. Nursing education is also influenced by higher education and is a product of the institutions within which it takes place. This chapter presents background on the changing economic and health care scene and on the political system in which nursing education is embedded. Some specific examples of nursing's political situations are provided, and some strategies for maximizing political influence are suggested.

THE CHANGING ECONOMIC AND POLITICAL SCENE

During the 1950s, 1960s, and early 1970s public policy emphasized access to health care. Federal money was made available for building hospitals and health education facilities, for health care research, and for training large numbers of health care professionals. Medicare and Medicaid were enacted to provide health care for the elderly and the indigent. General societal attitudes and behaviors were in line with federal and other third-party payors' policies of reimbursing what was done or used. Such policies led to excesses in emphasis on, demand for, and provision of medical care.

By the late 1970s and the beginning of the 1980s, the cost of health care was escalating much more rapidly than other aspects of the economy. Although more than 10% of the gross national product was being spent on health care, public health indices (like infant mortality rates) showed the United States falling behind other nations that spent proportionately less on health care. The leading causes of death in the United States were problems that were more amenable to prevention than to cure. Thus the emphasis

of federal policy for health care for the 1980s turned to cost containment and health promotion.

Just as scarcity made health care more political, cost containment made economics and business primary concerns in health care. Fitzgerald (1977) stated that the "ultimate purpose of politics is to meet human needs" (p. xiv). Max-Neef (1987) reflected a similar perspective in regard to the economy in stating that "the purpose of the economy is to serve the people" (p. 129). The present American economy is serving some people well, but the contrasts are uncomfortably obvious. For example, a recent newspaper article stated that 16 million Americans live in households with incomes above $75,000, while more than double that number (an estimated 33 million) live below the poverty line ("America's Contrasts," 1987). Twenty percent are above the official poverty line, but below the middle income bracket. This latter 20% often do not have health insurance. They are unable to pay for health care, but they are above the income limits to qualify for indigent care.

Max-Neef (1987) listed nine fundamental human needs, stating that all are interrelated and interact and that, with the exception of subsistence, there are no hierarchies within the system. Two of these fundamental human needs are protection (for which cure, prevention, and health systems in general are satisfiers) and understanding (for which education is a satisfier). He believes that any unmet, fundamental human need is a poverty, and each poverty generates pathologies. When health care is geared more to meeting a budget than to meeting human needs, when more than 75% of college freshmen list "being very well off financially" as one of their top personal goals, and when being able to get a better job and make more money are listed as major reasons for going to college, it appears that a collective pathology exists (Hirschorn, 1988).

THE POLITICAL SETTINGS OF NURSING EDUCATION

Nursing has not been able to establish the baccalaureate degree as the minimal level of educational preparation, and therefore nursing educational programs exist under public and independent control in community and technical colleges, in small liberal arts colleges, in large universities, in academic health centers, and in hospitals. While this broad-based, diverse educational system may help to guarantee that nursing education in some form is likely to survive economic upheavals, educational reforms, and social changes, it makes nursing education unbelievably political. Each type of nursing educational program has its vested interest groups who will immediately lobby their political representatives.

Nursing education is the subject of repeated study by committees of the state legislature, coordinating bodies for postsecondary education, and higher educational systems. As a health science administrator, who wishes to remain anonymous, stated somewhat in jest, "Nursing education is too important to be left to nurses!" Hospital and nursing home administrators; physicians; presidents of colleges, universities, and various other educational organizations; librarians; media writers and even health care consumers feel qualified to speak for the what, where, and how of nursing education. These same people usually defer to the experts in other professional education.

History of Settings of Nursing Education

Some of the politics of nursing may be better understood by examining some of the history and characteristics of the settings where nursing education occurs and the economics at stake. Nursing schools began in the United States in 1873, and "for almost the entire first century of organized nursing in the United States, the diploma schools were nursing" (Bayldon, 1973, p. 33). In the early years, nursing students were the primary work force of hospitals. Students had most of their clinical experiences in the parent hospital, so they were well oriented to the hospital's setting, policies, and procedures, as part of their learning experience.

Symbolism and ceremony were used to build a sense of identity with and commitment to not just nursing, but to the particular school of nursing and the parent hospital for which the school was named.

Uniforms, caps, and pins identified the students with the school. Capping ceremonies and other activities aided this socialization to the group. Students lived in nursing homes or dormitories on the hospital property, attended classes in groups, ate meals together, and had a high proportion of faculty who had graduated from the program. Even when students attended university courses or had experiences at other hospitals, they often traveled in groups, transported by hospital-provided buses identified with the hospital's name. Nursing educators are only recently becoming fully aware of the loyalty and identification built by these combined elements of socialization. Thus hospitals with nursing schools had a ready supply of nurses who did not require much orientation and who possessed a sense of commitment to the hospital.

Influence of Nursing on Hospital and Higher Education Economy

Nurses make up a very high proportion of the work force of hospitals; therefore, their salaries have a major influence on hospital economy. Without nurses, hospitals have to close beds. Closed beds are lost potential income to hospitals and can restrict physicians' abilities to admit patients. Thus the availability of nurses influences the profits of both hospitals and physicians. Nurses' salaries directly influence the amount of money available to be used for the equipment and capital expenditures that tend to attract physicians to the staff. More physicians on staff mean more physicians admitting patients to the hospitals. A study of nonprofit hospitals has shown that their nonprofit status is of primary benefit to their staff physicians (Herzlinger & Krasker, 1987). Is it any wonder that discussions of putting nursing education in the mainstream of higher education or of adopting "comparable-worth" standards for nursing salaries evoke so much response from so many sources?

In February 1988, organized medicine offered its solution to the nursing shortage. With availability of nursing care in hospitals so related to many physicians' abilities to practice, the American Medical Association (AMA) put forth a plan for registered care technologists (Salahuddin, 1988). These workers would learn the techniques of "basic bedside nursing" in 9 months. Moreover, they would be licensed and regulated by physician licensing boards, similar to the way physicians' assistants are licensed and regulated. This is a clear effort to put basic nursing practice under direct medical control. It would undercut organized nursing's efforts for a long-range solution to recurring nursing shortages through economic and professional incentives sufficient to attract and retain people in nursing careers. The symbiotic relationship between hospitals and physicians and the economic hope of a less costly, even though less prepared, worker are probably sufficient to provide hospital support for the AMA proposal, despite the added risk entailed. The suggestion that community and technical colleges provide the educational courses for the registered care technologists will align the politically powerful community and technical college organization behind the proposal. This organization is already fighting some of the American Nurses' Association's recommendations about associate degree nursing education. It is reported that the AMA has begun efforts at the state level to investigate licensing registered care technologists. Nursing must seek social and political support through coalitions with health care consumers to resist these efforts. The threat to safe care created by minimally prepared people in high technology settings has to be continually stressed.

The availability of federal monies for nursing helped to make nursing education good economics for public and private universities and colleges. Special project grants could often be obtained from the Division of Nursing, Department of Health and Human Services (DHHS), U.S. Public Health Service to provide for the start-up costs of programs. Capitation money helped to provide ongoing support and federal scholarships, and loans made it possible for people who might not have been able to afford college to attend a collegiate nursing program. Nursing leaders and professional organizations were trying to move nursing into the mainstream of higher education. These influences led to a growth in the number of colleges and universities starting nursing programs.

As long as federal money for nursing education was readily available and hospitals and physicians were concerned about nursing shortages, colleges and universities viewed starting or continuing a nursing program as a positive economic and political move. Once federal funding for nursing education lessened, concerns began to be expressed in many academic settings. Some university faculty and administrators were concerned that the lack of nursing faculty with doctoral degrees would weaken standards. The low student/faculty ratios required for clinical teaching made nursing seem expensive, and periodically, from some locations there was concern that nursing faculty were not held to the same standards for rank and tenure.

Changing Economics of the 1980s

The changing economics of the 1980s has put nursing at particular risk in university settings. The attitude in most settings has not been one of decreasing the size of colleges proportionately with decreased economic resources and declining enrollment. The argument has been that across-the-board cuts weaken the overall organization. Vertical cuts (eliminating certain colleges or programs entirely) preserve the excellence of the remaining program. Instead of fostering efforts to operate economically, share resources, and develop innovative ideas, the vertical-cuts approach pits colleague against colleague as each discipline or college shores up to protect its turf and budget. Nursing's lower proportion of tenured faculty (compared with other colleges), its predominantly female faculty and students, the clinical nature of its practice and research, and the present reduction in its enrollments make it especially vulnerable in university settings.

The health policy and philosophy of increasing access to health care and health care education in the 1950s, 1960s, and 1970s blended well with the community college movement, which was providing access to postsecondary education for many nontraditional students. Community and technical colleges welcomed associate degree programs in nursing. Many community colleges were located where they were the proximal source of nurses for small hospitals and nursing homes in more rural areas. These associate degree programs were provided political support by the rural area institutions and their communities. Students in these programs were usually goal-oriented, attracted by the quick route to RN licensure and an almost guaranteed job, and they did well in the general studies courses. The scarcity of nursing faculty with doctoral degrees was not a particular hindrance in community and technical colleges. Associate degree education in nursing grew much more rapidly than baccalaureate education in nursing. It is the community and technical colleges that are exerting the major political force today to prevent organized nursing's efforts to standardize and upgrade nursing education. Community and technical colleges are demanding to keep the title of RN for associate degree graduates and to keep the scope of practice as it is today.

Competition Among Health Science Disciplines

Academic health centers *should* provide an ideal setting in which the various health science disciplines can share in interprofessional and multidisciplinary endeavors. The university hospital exists as a setting for clinical teaching and research. Each discipline *should* appreciate the unique contributions of the others to the overall advancement of health sciences and care and understand the demands and limitations of clinical teaching and research. Like most human undertakings, academic health centers operate according to the "shoulds" some of the time. However, since most health professions have adequate to surplus numbers of practitioners, there is an increasing overlap of roles, with disciplines trying through licensure laws to lay claim that certain procedures lie solely within their scope of practice.

There is little denying the dominance of medicine in academic health centers, with some still retaining the name of "medical centers" and most having a physician as the chief administrative officer of the center. The symbiotic relationship between the college of medicine and the hospital is particularly obvious as hospitals undertake strategic planning for their specialty niches in the "prospective payment"

scene. University hospitals are finding it difficult to compete as "preferred provider" organizations. As medical colleges lose federal support for education and university hospitals have difficulty competing under prospective payment, there is a very real threat of sacrificing the educational programs of other health science disciplines to build the strength of colleges of medicine and hospitals in academic health centers. While nursing is indispensable in the complex tertiary care scene of university hospitals, power issues and economic motives exist to attempt to reduce nursing's power and resources.

The competition for monetary resources within and among institutions is not new information. The increasing competition for *additional* sources of financial support is more recent. Independent schools are seeking state funds or increased state funds, and state schools are increasing their efforts for private gifts, foundation monies, and grants.

A much more recent happening on the health care scene is the competition for students. Applications to almost all health science programs are decreasing—and decreasing dramatically, at present, in nursing. The decreased numbers of college-aged persons; the increasing numbers of women entering schools of medicine, dentistry, pharmacy, and other academic fields; and the proportional decline of nursing salaries, compared with other health care disciplines have combined to create large decreases in the number of applicants to nursing schools. The competition for clinical learning settings, for access to patients for practice and research, and for access to role models and preceptors is becoming increasingly serious. University hospitals, once viewed as existing primarily as teaching sites, are becoming less appropriate for lower level students, as these hospitals become more specialized and intense in nature. Many health care organizations view having students as antithetical to their cost containment and enhanced productivity efforts. Nursing educators must compete effectively with other disciplines and among the various nursing schools.

The competition for political influence and support is becoming much more overt. The American Association of Colleges of Nursing, the American Nurses' Association, and the National League for

Nursing have lobbyists or government relations persons. Political action committees serve as vehicles for directing money and manpower to support political candidates. Receptions, awards, and recognitions are also a part of the political scene. In spite of the power of numbers in nursing, the amount of money spent on political influence by nursing organizations is still decidedly less than that spent by medicine.

Brower (1984) cited as a trend the increasing "number and stridency of interest groups active in the political arena, all using increasingly sophisticated techniques to move their agendas" (p. 92). She further indicated that such fierce competition now exists that individuals or organizations are "cast as fools" if they decrease their energies or give higher priority to goals that focus more on the good of the overall society than on the interests of their own group. This describes what has been happening with the issues of educational preparation for entry into practice. There has been an effort to bring together major nursing organizations for a united stand, but with nursing education existing in such diverse types of institutions, there are still related interest groups taking opposing stands. There is a need for a negotiated position that allows for some gain for all groups, without sacrificing the basic issues.

Closing of Colleges of Nursing

College closings or mergers have been proposed in several states that have been faced with financial difficulties. Jaschik (1987) recounted some of these efforts and indicated that aggressive campaigns by small groups of citizens have prevented most proposed closures. He indicated that state and higher education officials believe that the planning process for higher education has been made less logical and more political by protests against college closings. This may be a matter of whose perception of what is logical. Writing on political influence Banfield (1961) stated:

> No matter how competent and well-intended, a decision maker can never make an important decision on grounds that are not in some degree arbitrary or nonlogical. . . . Matters come before high officials for decisions precisely when it is not clear which value premises ought to be invoked. (p. 329)

Banfield contended that when social choice (a decision reached as a result of interest groups exercising their influence) takes place rather than a central decision made by a university president or governor, the social choice process may aid correct weighting of values in the choice.

Example 1: University of Nebraska, Lincoln Division of the College of Nursing. When the chancellor of the University of Nebraska Medical Center (UNMC) made the decision in May 1985 to close the College of Pharmacy and the Lincoln Division of the College of Nursing, he readily admitted that, in the final analysis, it was a value judgment. One of the criteria openly used was the "Student/Community/Employee Sensitivity," which translated to the amount of political concern likely to be aroused by the decision. (See the June 1986 and September 1986 issues of *Nursing and Health Care* and the Summer 1986 issue of *Image* for articles on this event.) Being unable to influence the central decision, the only choice for the involved colleges was to take the issues to the public for a social choice.

After the UNMC College of Nursing had successfully defended the existence of the Lincoln Division in the summer of 1985, the university president once again called for cutting the Lincoln Division in January 1987. The logic of that decision was especially difficult to discern. The mass media was beginning to carry stories about the nursing shortage, and area publications had extensive advertisements for nurses—not just local but from across the country. Discussions with the university president revealed that his expectations were that there would be less political support for nursing than from some other colleges. Even the decisions classed as logical have political components and political implications.

Example 2: Boston University School of Nursing. As nursing enrollments decline, the independent versus public issues intensify. President John R. Silber of Boston University credited public nursing education with being the cause of his decision to close the Boston University School of Nursing. In a widely copied letter to Governor Michael S. Dukakis and others, Silber wrote:

> Unfortunately, the Board of Regents of Higher Education has embarked on a policy of destroying existing, high-quality programs for the education of nurses. The Board of Regents has established or enlarged a number of expensive taxpayer-subsidized programs in nursing at the state colleges and universities which make prospective nursing students an offer they can't refuse: to provide a bachelor's or master's degree in nursing at approximately one-tenth the price of the same degree at Boston University. . . . In consequence, undergraduate enrollment in state-owned nursing schools in the Commonwealth has increased by nearly 1,000 in the past six years, while enrollments have been decreasing sharply in the independent schools of nursing. (Personal communication, April 29, 1987)

Federal funds allowed for the development and expansion of many independent nursing schools and permitted students to afford independent tuition through federal scholarships, traineeships, and loans. With the decreased availability of federal funds, private schools are turning to the state and to private donors for scholarships and other assistance. As competition for recruitment, clinical agencies, and money increases, it is likely that relationships between independent and public schools of nursing will become more strained. When the University of Nebraska College of Pharmacy and Lincoln Division of the College of Nursing were threatened with closure, private universities stated in the media that they could accept the students who could no longer be served by these public colleges. Furthermore, during the 1987 threat, the dean of another private nursing program wrote a letter to the editor of the local paper stating that the University of Nebraska College of Nursing should offer graduate programs only. Moreover, a concerted effort is being made by the executive director of the Association of Independent Colleges and Universities to convince the legislature that independent colleges can provide all undergraduate nursing education and do so at less cost to the state.

Example 3: RN second license to perform MT procedures.   Licensure laws are political means of controlling turf and limiting other disciplines. In Nebraska, medical technologists (MT) are lobbying for a licensure law to restrict nurses from performing procedures claimed by medical technologists. The version in the legislature at the time of this writing would require RNs to obtain a second license or permit for a fee of $40, plus an additional $25 fee every 2 years for renewal. It also requires RNs to have 16 hours of continuing education in laboratory technology for each 2-year renewal period. Once the RN obtains this permit, she or he is permitted to perform only 10 very simple tests. Physicians' assistants and respiratory therapists are exempted (Legislature of Nebraska, Legislative Bill 760, 1987).

POLITICAL STRATEGIES FOR SCHOOLS OF NURSING

Space allows for only brief suggestions regarding issues most frequently reaching political forums. Schools of nursing will have to do better jobs of defining and defending their costs. Schools should seek out opportunities in which student/faculty exchanges, consortiums, or some type of joint arrangements can improve educational quality and make better use of scarce resources. Curricula and transfer of credit policies must be more defensible to nursing's publics, including state legislatures. Faculty should spend less time trying to promote and defend their special interest in curriculum and choice of learning experiences; more focus should be given to collaboration across schools to promote student educational mobility, while maintaining quality and maximizing economy. It is problematic that nursing is asked for more of this than the other health science disciplines, but this is not persuasive with legislators.

While all alliances must be entered into and maintained carefully, with political implications taken into consideration, nursing should form alliances that demonstrate its value—not just to the health sciences and the university, but to the larger community. Nursing schools need to be able to document what they bring into a community through jobs, grants, and related spending. For example, when the Montana University System studied closing various colleges, they discovered that Eastern Montana University, with only slightly more than 4000 students, brought $61 million into its locale in 1984–1985 through the spending of students, faculty, and visitors (Jaschik, 1987). This type of information should be available for all nursing schools.

Lest the following suggested strategies appear defensive, nursing must use every opportunity to demonstrate its contributions to health care and research and to promote its image as a scholarly discipline. Clinical learning experiences should be selected to allow students to meet learning objectives, but they can accomplish this and also be selected to increase the visibility of nursing's contribution to an important group or organization. A school that is in an academic health science center may need to concentrate learning experiences in that setting in order to demonstrate faculty's and students' contributions and thus be able to exert more influence in the setting. Alternatively, special efforts may be developed to provide services to an undeserved population, to work with groups concerned about the health and well-being of the elderly, or to provide health promotion in business and industry. The health care system is rapidly moving to a consumer-controlled system. Nursing must form alliances with consumers to meet their needs. Faculty and students can design learning experiences to develop nursing's role in systems of managed care.

All nursing faculty, not just administrators, need to assume more responsibility in keeping informed about politics and in influencing public policy. The most benign bill being considered by the legislature can become the route for some interest group to attempt to limit nursing practice, to force articulated curricula, or to otherwise exert power over nursing and its resources. There must, however, be organization and leadership for political influence efforts.

Negotiation and compromise are often necessary to make some gains. It is almost never possible to accomplish all one wishes in a political situation. Individual nursing educators must join and participate in nursing organizations, and nursing organizations must collaborate to exert a united influence.

Political influence is promoted more covertly through a school's publics. Alumni, students and their parents, important business leaders who serve on a school's board, and other community persons may be solicited to contact legislators on behalf of salary increases, program support, scholarships, building projects, and policy matters.

Public relations and marketing experts are becoming a necessary part of administration. College catalogs, newsletters, brochures, magazines, and other media materials are being planned and designed like advertising campaigns for business and industry. Just as the politically influential "get the most of what there is to get," schools with the largest budgets have the most with which to try to generate more influence. Even so, the most attractive and informative printed material is proliferating much faster than the capacity of not only the influentials, but also the general public, to read it.

Political involvement can be exciting and energizing, but it is also hard, fatiguing work. Since it cannot be avoided, it must be participated in with judgment. As Banfield (1961) has indicated, the amount of influence that individuals or groups are willing to spend is a measure of the value of what it is they seek. Like money, influence should never be squandered.

REFERENCES

American Nurses' Association. (1976). *Code for nurses*. Kansas City, MO: Author.

America's contrasts: The very rich and the nearly poor. (1987, November 15). *Omaha Sunday World-Herald*, pp. 1E, 6E.

Banfield, EC (1961). *Political influence*. New York: Free Press.

Bayldon, MC (1973). Diploma schools: The first century. *RN Magazine, 36*, 33.

Brower, LA (1984). Mental health policies and psychiatric-mental health nursing. *Proceedings: Psychiatric-mental health nursing before the year 2001* (pp. 89–98). Chevy Chase, MD: National Institute of Mental Health.

Fitzgerald, R (Ed.). (1977). *Human needs and politics*. Elmsford, NY: Pergamon Press.

Herzlinger, RE, & Krasker, WS (1987). Who profits from nonprofits? *Harvard Business Review, 65*, 93–106.

Hirschorn, MW (1988, January 20). Freshmen interest in business careers hits new level and money remains a top priority, study finds. *Chronicle of Higher Education*, pp. A31, A34.

Jaschik, S (1987, June 24). Citizens' campaigns are foiling state plans to shut down or merge public colleges. *Chronicle of Higher Education*, pp. 1, 34.

Kalish, BJ, & Kalish, PA (1982). *Politics of nursing*. Philadelphia: JB Lippincott.

Lasswell, H (1986). *Politics: Who gets what, when, how*. New York: Meridian Books.

Legislature of Nebraska. Ninetieth Legislature, First Session, *Legislative Bill 760* (January 23, 1987).

Max-Neef, MA (1987). Economics, politics and health: The challenge of future trends (a think-piece). In D. Schwefl (Ed.), *Indicators and trends in health and health care* (pp. 125–131). New York: Springer Publishing.

Pirages, D (1976). *Managing political conflict*. New York: Praeger.

Salahuddin, M (1988, May 9). AMA seeks new nursing job category. *Health Week*, p. 1.

✳ EDITOR'S QUESTIONS FOR DISCUSSION ✳

What implications and relationships exist between the discussion in Chapter 6, by Wakefield and this chapter for nursing education? How has the political setting nationally affected nursing education? How might nurse educators more effectively influence the political, economic, and nursing environment? What are the multiple opportunities for interprofessional and multidisciplinary endeavors in health science settings for nursing? What power issues and economic motives are involved in health science settings that impact nursing? How can the nursing community more effectively influence a health science setting?

What are the steps in developing a legitimate and ethical retrenchment program that might be established for a university? What criteria are critical to be included in retrenchment programs? What issues need to be addressed in a retrenchment program? What are the advantages and disadvantages of having a planned retrenchment program policy in place for a university?

63

The Search and Screen Committee for Selecting Administrators:
Values, ethics, structure, and process

Norma L. Chaska, Ph.D., R.N., F.A.A.N.

The selection of executive administrators and leaders is one of the most crucial decisions in the corporate world of service and academic institutions. Many service institutions, such as hospitals and academic campuses, have utilized the temporary system of a search committee to choose key personnel. For some persons who have chaired or served on such a committee, the work was fraught with agonizing difficulties and the learning experience essentially one of a trial and error nature (McLaughlin & Riesman, 1985). For others, it was a first-time experience that decidedly became an *only*-time experience. For a few, the final result was rewarding; the members were keenly and happily aware that they had participated in one of the most vital functions of an institution.

This chapter builds on the collective wisdom, practices, and findings derived from the literature, from colleagues and institutions who have participated in or utilized search committees, and from the experience of this author. The author has served as both chair and member of search committees and as consultant for administration in both academic and service institutions. Values and ethics form the base of a successful search process.

Information is offered in this chapter in the form of suggestions and guidelines for an *effectively* functioning structure and process of a professional search and screen committee. Although consulting firms are increasingly being effectively and successfully used today for executive searches in both service and academic institutions (Kaplowitz, 1986), the predominant choice is to utilize search and screen committees. Much of what is addressed can be applied or easily adapted to service settings. However, the focus in this chapter is predominantly directed to their use in academia. Emphasis is placed on exploring aspects of the search and screen process in which uncertainty exists and problems are most likely to occur.

PURPOSE OF THE COMMITTEE

There are at least three purposes that search committees aim to fulfill in the selection of executive administrators or leaders. The first is to recruit a large pool of qualified applicants. The second is to provide for a consistent process by which candidates are recruited, evaluated, and one candidate is finally selected for a specific position. The third purpose is to ensure that all affirmative action and equal opportunity requirements are followed in all phases of the process. In essence, the intention is to make sure that all applicants for a specific position receive the *same* and *equal* treatment in the review of their qualifications and applications for the position (Kaplowitz, 1973, 1986). Each of the purposes of the search committee warrants discussion although, in reality, the purposes interrelate.

Applicant Pool

Most often, a large group of persons such as exists on a search committee are able to draw on various resources for a pool of applicants. The resources include a network of colleagues in one's institution and external to the institution, membership lists of major professional organizations, professional contacts at meetings and conferences, and alumni and associates from educational programs. In addition, an applicant pool may be developed through advertising in professional newspapers and publishing notices at major conferences.

The wisdom of promoting executives from within versus hiring managers from the outside has long been debated. The view that "troubled" organizations should hire outsiders—to alter existing modes of operating—and that successful institutions should select insiders—to sustain superb performance—has only recently been empirically tested (Chung, Lubatkin, Rogers, & Owers, 1987). These researchers studied the effects of leadership origin (insider vs. outsider) on corporate performance in the context of high- and low-performing firms. Their findings reveal a "momentum effect" of presuccession performance that is stronger than the effect of leadership change on corporate performance (p. 326). Principles of organizational behavior state that an organization has a tendency to continue its present course. The findings of Chung et al. suggest that, although a new leader may attempt to reverse an adverse trend, a new leader alone is not strong enough to counteract the momentum effect; "only an *exceptional* leader" might succeed (p. 327). On the other hand, insiders were found to make good exec-

utives for high-performing firms, but the insiders in this situation were not necessarily superior to outsiders.

In conclusion the authors advise that searches be left open to both insiders and outsiders (Chung et al., 1987). The candidate should be selected who is the most qualified to guide the organization effectively in the years to come, whether the person is an insider or outsider. In an open search, the scope of the selection process should be known, for purposes of enhancing the image of the successful applicant and the confidence of management thus reflected.

A Consistent Process

The second purpose of the search and screen committee is to provide for a uniform process in selecting new personnel. The assumption exists that few universities and institutions have structured, consistent processes for the recruitment and hiring of executive administrators and leaders (Kaplowitz, 1986). There are great differences and variations among institutions, universities, colleges, schools, and departments regarding how a search and screen process is carried out. It is the literature, essentially from higher education, that makes a strong plea for following uniform procedures (Kaplowitz, 1973, 1986; Rodman & Dingerson, 1986).

The committee purpose of consistency in process is one that also relates to the application of affirmative action principles. Although these will be specifically addressed later, it is important to emphasize here that all applicants or candidates are to be governed by and undergo the same process. Differences in views as to treatment of internal versus external candidates have been expressed (Kaplowitz, 1986). In the final analysis, however, the conclusion must be that it is inappropriate for internal applicants to be treated any differently from external applicants. Special treatment is never advisable or justifiable. For example, under the guise of so-called courtesy treatment, a member or members of a search committee may seek out an internal applicant (potential or actual) either to ask the person to apply or to otherwise encourage the person. Sometimes, too, a potential internal applicant is viewed as being "owed" different treatment, because of years of service the person may have provided an institution. Unfortunately courtesy treatment more often than not results in violation of equal opportunity and affirmative action policies. Furthermore, courtesy or preferred treatment jeopardizes the integrity of the committee. It most often results in negative feelings and beliefs regarding the committee's functions and process.

Sometimes an internal applicant is believed to have an advantage in knowing more about the institution than does an external applicant. On the other hand, however, an internal candidate usually has had years of exposure in an institution and is thus more vulnerable in a review. The principle remains that internal applicants should go through the same step-by-step process as any other applicant, with communication occurring on the same basis, in the same form, and at the same stage as for external candidates. A prime function of the search and screen committee is to ensure fairness. Any breach in a consistent process puts the committee's ability to provide fairness at high risk.

Another aspect of consistency involves internal and operational procedures of the search and screen committee. It is critical that the committee rigorously follows procedures that were either mandated or agreed on at its initial meeting. As one example, consider a situation in which the "charge" by a higher level administrator was for the committee to recommend three persons for a position. In this case, it would be assumed that three recommendations would be made *provided* that there were at least three candidates who held the essential qualifications. A lesser number could be recommended, or no recommendations offered if no candidates owned the qualifications. In this example, it would not be appropriate to indicate a preferred rank order of the recommended candidates, since that request was not included in the initial mandate. Nor would it be appropriate to indicate strengths and limitations of each recommended candidate, unless that too was stated in the mandate.

Procedures for voting on issues, candidates, or other agenda are established at the beginning of the search and screen process. Lutz (1979) found in his examination of search and screen practices that in the elite type of councils, such as search and screen committees, decision making essentially occurs through consensus. Consensus means that the decision of the group was made by general, mutual agreement and not by the act of taking a formal vote. It is appropriate to use this type of decision making only when there is reasonable certainty that group solidarity in sentiment and belief exists. After the work of the committee has started, it is inappropriate to switch from approval by consensus to a simple majority vote of the group.

It is usually advisable for the search and screen committee to make known its chosen basic decision-making procedures to the constituent groups for whom it is seeking to fill a position. This practice helps to establish the legitimacy of a *professional* committee as well as to facilitate trust. To alter the "rules" or procedures that were initially agreed on and made known to constituents erodes the basic integrity of the committee; this should be avoided at all costs.

Equal Opportunity, Affirmative Action Regulations

Issues concerning affirmative action are the overriding concern of the search and screen committee. It is neither the focus nor intent in this chapter to detail the policies and procedures that contribute to an effective affirmative action office. Rather, the purpose here is to highlight some aspects of affirmative action practices. Completion of an affirmative action form is required of each applicant and the institution. This form is usually processed at the time an applicant either has withdrawn or has not been approved to progress further in the search and screen process. The applicant's file is then formally closed. Notations that reflect the rationale for elimination must be made in the files of those not selected. The affirmative action form for the final, successful candidate is completed at the end of the search process. The total files of the search and screen committee, including all affirmative action forms, are closed with the committee's final adjournment. Files should be given to the appropriate administrative officer to retain for at least 3 years.

The intent of all affirmative action programs is to provide *equal* consideration for all applicants, regardless of race, sex, age, or other extraneous factors (VanderWaerdt, 1982). Consequently the essential basis of the committee's function is to provide for fairness. To achieve effectively its goals and purposes, a committee must function and make decisions on the basis of *facts*—not on opinions nor hearsay. The reputations both of institutions and of individuals have been known to be irreparably damaged by the "search and destroy" process, creative terminology attributed to David Riesman (American Council on Education, 1986, p. 6). Injustice in evaluating candidates frequently can occur when opinions, not facts, are the basis for decision making. The premise *always* should be that opinions are acceptable *Only* when they can be substantiated by specific example(s).

INHERENT VALUES FOR A SEARCH AND SCREEN COMMITTEE

It is impossible to isolate the essential values for a search and screen committee from the purposes of the committee. Values are innate to the ethics and effective functioning of a professional committee. Some values overlap with the purposes of the committee, for example, consistency and fairness. Consistency is inherent to fairness. Fairness is critical to equal opportunities and affirmative action guidelines. Other values of equal importance are confidentiality, thoroughness, courtesy, respect, honesty, and above all—integrity. Although consistency was previously addressed as a *purpose* of the committee, it warrants further discussion as an underlying *value* for equal opportunity and fairness.

Fairness

Fairness, in the sense that each applicant must be given equal chance and opportunity when being reviewed for the position, is mandatory. For example, if one applicant was given an opportunity to clarify questions regarding materials submitted for review, the same opportunity should be given to others. It is not uncommon that curriculum vitae's or resumés are insufficiently clear. Should a question arise regarding the written presentation of one candidate and clarification be requested, similar opportunities are due all other applicants.

The same principle should apply to checks on references for the applicant. The process should be the same for verification of or follow-through on the number and names of persons submitted as referees by an applicant. Following are illustrations of situations that should *not* occur. Suppose each candidate submits five reference names—for one candidate, all five references are followed up and obtained; yet for another candidate, only two persons are contacted. In another situation, choices might be made to contact only those reference persons who are expected to present the most favorable view of the applicant's qualifications. Or, in another case, decisions might be made to choose only the least potentially favorable reference persons. All these types of practices should be avoided. Clearly such "procedures" foster a biased review and violate the basic purpose and integrity of the committee.

Confidentiality

It is commonly understood that each applicant is assured of confidentiality until the point in time that the individual is invited to come for a formal interview. Information needs to be confined to the search group. Nevertheless, it is at times difficult to maintain confidentiality when persons express curiosity or raise questions regarding the applicants. One strategy, to protect confidentiality and yet respond to questions, is to present periodic progress reports to the various interested groups (Bayne, Parker, & Todd, 1982). Such reporting should be done without revealing names or identifying characteristics. Another method, often used in combination with the first, is to refer or redirect the questions to the chair of the committee. Providing information from a centralized source not only assists monitoring the quality (accuracy and amount) of the information, but also adds to the consistency dimension of the committee's function.

In spite of efforts to maintain confidentiality, leaks occur from search committees, caused by a number of factors. Potential causes are internal politics; institutional culture; conditions in which there are serious problems related to the search—such as massive budget cuts; conditions under which the previous person in the position departed; loyalties to constituencies outside the search committee; existence of internal candidates; and the pleasure or displeasure with the direction that the committee appears to be going (Kaplowitz, 1986). It takes time to develop a cohesive committee, in which individual members become committed not only to the purposes and values of the committee, but also to other members of the group. Furthermore, it takes time for individual members to become committed to confidentiality itself.

According to Kaplowitz (1986), to have it be known or rumored that someone is a potential candidate may work positively. It could be interpreted as affirmation of the person's prominence—thus a search committee could be pleased that their institution attracted such a highly qualified applicant. On the other hand, if internal candidates become known, they may have to confront a nebulous future should the position be filled by a new person arriving on the scene. The successful candidate may or may not be comfortable with an unsuccessful applicant still in the institution. In conclusion, confidentiality issues present themselves throughout the process of the search and screen committee. The earlier that confidentiality becomes an internalized value by committee members, the more effective the committee will be in its work.

Thoroughness

Thoroughness is another quality to be valued highly by a search committee. It also is a value that is underestimated in terms of the extent it facilitates an effective committee. First, there needs to be thoroughness in the search for potential applicants. Some potential applicants who are highly qualified may not necessarily be in the public eye and may be

relatively unknown. Other potential applicants may have well-established reputations, but for one reason or another have not considered a different position—and may not, until they are asked.

Thoroughness most often shows itself in the follow-through of a committee. Follow-up is critical in pursuing potential candidates—both those who have applied directly and those referred by others. Questions need to be raised regarding unclear information that has been submitted verbally or in writing, such as on a resumé or vita. Follow-up is essential in the data validation of "opinion-type" statements offered regarding an applicant; such statements require concrete examples. Follow-up is a must in the documentation of evidence, completing reference checks, and in clarifying questions and their responses during the interview (Heller, Okolowski, O'Driscoll, Frain, & Brody, 1982).

During an interview, candidates may not always be aware that they are being asked a specific question. Often questions may not have been stated or phrased sufficiently clear so as to elicit a *direct* response or indicate that such a response was expected. Usually one or the other party is aware of some dissonance between what is being asked and what is answered. Thoroughness and follow-through are critical in such a situation, whereby an immediate opportunity to clarify the situation likewise may immediately resolve the dissonance.

A simple statement might be made to the effect that what is being asked is not clear, or that the response is not specific enough. The question may then be rephrased or redirected for clarity. Of course, a candidate could choose to be very general in responses for numerous reasons. However, not to follow up such situations of uncertainty allows error-prone, premature conclusions to be drawn and puts the validity of the interview at high risk.

Honesty, Courtesy, and Respect

The values of honesty, courtesy, and respect are implicated throughout the search and screen process. These values cannot really be separated from the process and purposes of a committee, any more than those values previously discussed. All are inherent to an effective, professional committee. Various aspects of one or more of the values may come into focus at one stage of the committee's work more than at another. For example, honesty, courtesy, and respect always must be shown in verifying and validating references, in obtaining and providing information, and in communicating in general. These values are discussed further, in relation to some specific tasks and common concerns for all search and screen committees, presented later in the chapter. In that discussion, these values are noted to be crucial in communications with applicants and the documentation of references.

STAGES IN THE SEARCH AND SCREEN PROCESS

The search process may be divided into a series of somewhat overlapping steps and stages. The flowchart (Fig. 63-1, p. 550) provides a sequential summary of the stages as well as a context for additional discussion of areas and concerns that transcend the committee's work. Some of the stages shown in the flowchart warrant more explanation than others. In the following discussion, areas that prove to be somewhat troublesome are highlighted.

Search and Screen Process Deadlines

The members and chair should be selected a minimum of 1 year before a high-level administrative position is expected to be filled. It takes approximately 2 months for the committee to complete its organizational tasks and assume the characteristics of an effective, cohesive group. However, it is highly advisable that universities initiate their search and screen committees far earlier than a year. They should allow for an orderly process to occur and also take into account time for certain expectations to be met and possible legitimate delays. For example, sufficient time should be planned in the search process to allow a tenured professor to resign a position in accord with standard expectations established by the American Association of University Professors (AAUP). University system delays are increasing in approval processes. A university system may require

the approval of candidates from a Board of Regents or Board of Trustees *before* final position offers are made. Thus, significant delays can occur and the time may be very limited between a candidate's notification and actual resignation from a position and acceptance of another. The academic integrity of tenured professors is questioned and subject to jeopardy when insufficient time notification is provided. Therefore deadlines that are established by search and screen committees should be realistic.

Composition of the Committee

The size and composition of the committee varies, depending on the level of the administrative position that is the object of the search. Searches for top executive level positions such as for presidents, chief executive officers, and vice-presidents will have larger committees than those for mid-level executives such as provosts, deans, associate deans, and assistant vice-presidents. Searches for department chairs or heads will have even fewer members on a committee. More often than not, search committees are too large and unwieldy (American Council on Education, 1986; Bayne et al., 1982; Kaplowitz, 1986). The range in numbers of committee members may be a minimum of 5 for a lower level administrative search, 9 for a mid-level executive, and 13 to 15 members for a top executive search.

The composition of a committee is crucial for establishing a high-quality, professional committee and a successful search. In general, the *major* constituents for which the successful candidate will be responsible should be represented on the committee. For example, in a college or university, an equal number of representatives from the different programs should be on the committee. It is quite helpful also to have a student as a committee member, for students may often provide more input than faculty regarding concerns of the student body and its perceived criteria for an effective administrator. However, according to ethical guidelines in many universities, students are not allowed to be present, or vote, when the credentials of an internal applicant (faculty member) are discussed and reviewed. Other members who might offer valuable contributions are alumni, persons from the community and professional organizations with whom the academic unit has affiliations, and peer administrators of other related academic units.

The committee should be designated shortly after there is official notification that an administrative position will be open. The committee may be elected, but more often it is appointed by an administrative officer. Recommendations for the appointments might be obtained from various constituents and interested groups, but the selection usually is determined by administration. The chair for the committee also is usually selected by a high-level administrator. Frequently a person who represents a different but related academic unit will be chosen to chair the committee. This strategy may ensure that the basic values of the committee—in particular, fairness and objectivity—are protected. However, unless the person from a related academic unit has sufficient familiarity with the primary academic unit filling the position, has long-standing tenure and respect in the university, and has had previous successful experience in chairing *search* committees, the strategy can be very ineffective. Superior knowledge of the institution and position, excellent interpersonal skills, unquestionable integrity, various experience related to the position, previous experience as a search committee member, and stamina are highly desirable qualities for a chair. It is also imperative that the chair own exceptional ability and skill for making sound judgments.

Chair and Committee Roles

When the search and screen committee is first convened by the chair, the formal mandate (charge) is stated, and the functions and responsibilities are clearly defined. The mandate usually has been explicitly defined for the chair by a high-level administrator, before the first committee meeting. The chair, in turn, delineates the role of the committee for its members. This role is specified in terms of communication with the appropriate high-level administrator, the potential and actual applicants, the interested constituent groups, and the public, as well as with regard to its decision-making function.

The chair rarely has a vote in committee discussions, in reviews of applicants, or in decisions. The chair usually casts a vote only in the case of a tie.

The search committee does not participate in salary negotiations and extraneous benefits for a candidate; however, the members frequently provide data to the appropriate administrator regarding regional salaries, along with salary ranges, for various administrative positions. It is inadvisable for a committee to be concerned with salary issues in its search. Some highly qualified potential applicant might be overlooked or be discouraged if salary is prematurely addressed. Nonetheless, the chair of the committee may be mandated to provide general "salary range" type of responses to salary questions raised by prospective applicants. In this same vein, the committee also may obtain general information from an applicant about his or her salary expectations.

It is common and highly preferred that, in advertising the position, all letters of inquiry and applications are specifically directed to be addressed to the chair of the search committee. To advertise that applications and other correspondence be addressed to a high-level administrator rather than the chair when it is indicated that a search and screen committee is to be involved erodes the role of the chair and the basic purposes and functions of the committee itself. Moreover such a practice conveys a double message regarding the real role intended for an appointed search committee and the sincerity of the appointment. The commitment thereby is compromised—or at least highly open to question—regarding the extent of adherence to principles and practices of affirmative action and equal opportunity in the selection process that should be expected by a candidate.

Most search and screen committees play an advisory role to administration. They recommend qualified candidates for the position and in essence represent the faculty in the case of academic administrative appointments, and the nursing staff in the instance of administrative nursing service positions. The American Association of University Professors (AAUP) recognizes that the president makes the final choice for academic administrative appointments. However, the AAUP strongly asserts that

The Search Process

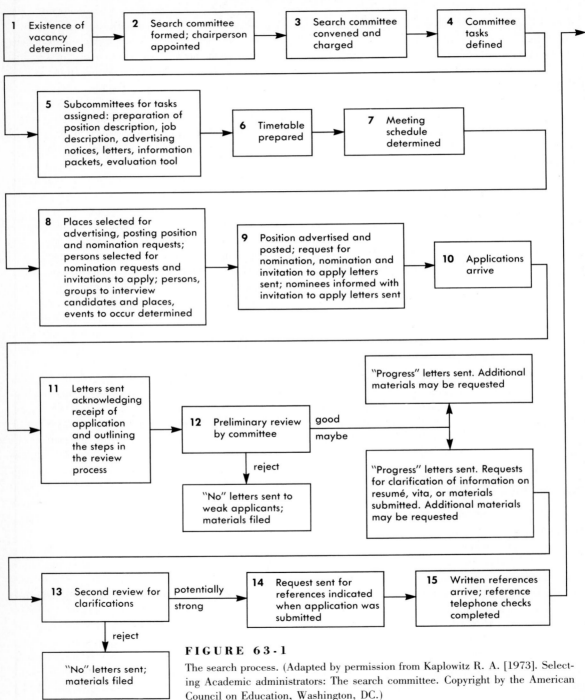

FIGURE 63-1

The search process. (Adapted by permission from Kaplowitz R. A. [1973]. Selecting Academic administrators: The search committee. Copyright by the American Council on Education, Washington, DC.)

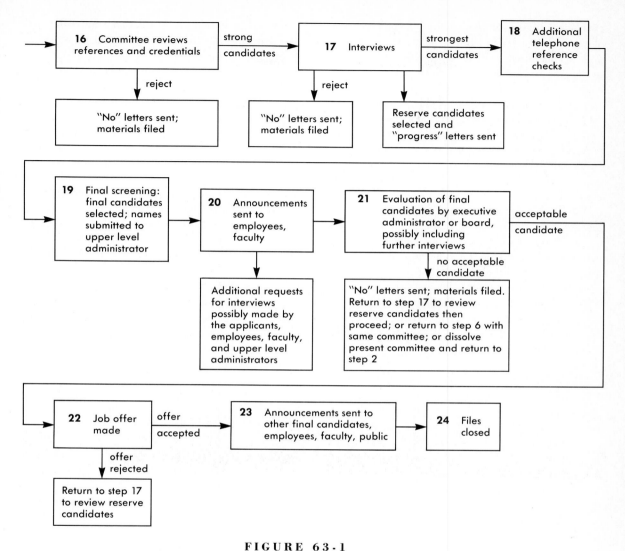

FIGURE 63-1

The search process—cont'd.

"sound academic practice dictates that the president not choose a person over the reasonable opposition of the faculty" (AAUP, 1981, p. 324).

Organizational Tasks

The voting procedure that is to be used throughout the committee process needs to be discussed and established at the first meeting. In addition, the tasks of the committee should be clearly defined. Adequate resources for the search must be allocated. Items to be considered include secretarial assistance; materials; budgetary support for long-distance telephone calls, possible travel for committee members, and interviewing costs. In some instances, site visits by one or more committee members to the institution where a candidate is employed may be very helpful.

The committee spends considerable time in assessing the institution's needs in the position, establishing criteria for the position, and prioritizing the criteria (Goldsmith & Flynn, 1983; Sagaria & Krotseng, 1986; Tucker, 1984). The job description is evaluated, redefined if necessary, and formally approved by the appropriate higher level administrator. It is helpful to establish subcommittees to complete organizational tasks, for approval later by the committee.

Advertising information has to be developed, in the form of a position description; a job description is rarely circulated. Notices announcing the position must be prepared, places and persons need to be selected to promote the position, information packets must be prepared for applicants, and evaluation tools should be developed. The latter are developed to compare each candidate to established criteria and are used by the committee and by constituent groups, who may be selected to interview candidates.

There are three tasks that warrant some elaboration. The first is establishing a communication procedure and process, with applicants and others, to provide needed information in a timely and courteous manner. The second is conducting reviews and background reference checks of applicants, and the third is planning for the interview of selected applicants.

Communication

A clear, consistent, timely, and courteous system of communication needs to be established early in the search process. Careful and detailed record keeping is essential, both for the efficiency of the committee and for providing information, should legal or other questions be raised during the search process. A file should be maintained for each applicant. This file should contain the initial application, additional application materials, records of telephone calls made, notes of telephone conversations, decisions made by the committee at each stage of the search, interview records, copies of all correspondence between the institution and the applicants and candidates, written recommendations, evaluations of the candidate submitted by others at the time of the interview, and a summary of the evaluations for each applicant and candidate (Higgins & Hollander, 1987).

Letters

Communication with applicants and others can be facilitated by preplanning a number of different types of form letters. These may later be adapted for personalized application. Some of these letters are presented in the box, Preplanned Types of Letters.

Guidelines for letters. Prompt, honest, courteous, and appropriate letters to applicants and candidates are essential. The image and reputation of an institution may be either positively or adversely affected by written communications. Time frames for each stage of the review process should be provided to applicants, and written communications should occur at each stage as the application progresses through this process. Applicants and candidates should never be left hanging in uncertainty because of ambiguous, inadequate, insufficient, or no information.

Here, rights of individuals may be very much involved. In this litigious age, committees well may be cautious as to how a negative view or vote to discontinue progression of the applicant to candidacy is communicated. On the other hand, trite statements such as, "You do not meet the needs of this institution (organization, or department) at this time," are to be avoided. Such statements may be considered demeaning, impossible to document objectively as being true, nor have any positive value. Committees may be tempted to some extent out of fear to fabricate "rationale" for rejecting an applicant. In fact, committees may err in underestimating an applicant's ability to hear and accept the truth without reprisal.

To the extent that open, honest communication with applicants is viewed with alarm by a committee, chances are great that the rights of the candidate and the principles of affirmative action and equal opportunity already have been violated. There are many legitimate reasons why persons who meet the criteria for a position and hold the basic qualifi-

Preplanned types of letters

1. Requests

Purpose: For nominations of qualified applicants and for *potential* applicants to *consider* applying themselves or to nominate qualified applicants.

Content: Provides basic information such as a brief position description; indicates criteria for the position; and furnishes a brief description of the location, facilities, personnel, programs, or services.

2. Nomination

Purpose: Informs a person of nomination as a possible candidate; invites the person to apply.

Content: Provides basic information such as a brief position description; indicates criteria for the position; and furnishes a brief description of the location, facilities, personnel, programs, or services.

3. Announcement

Purpose: Informs deans of accredited programs and heads of major organizations, departments, and members of professional organizations of the position availability and requests nominations of applicants.

Content: Provides a position announcement statement, criteria, and other basic demographic information.

4. Acknowledgement of application

Purpose: Informs and serves as a receipt for the application.

Content: Provides information that the application was received and appreciated; indicates the next specific steps in the review process and the approximate time the applicant can expect to receive further communication.

5. Reference list

Purpose: Persons as referees indicated by the applicant.

Content: Request sent to the applicant to provide the names and addresses of persons to be contacted *by* the search committee for a written reference.

6. Reference requests

Purpose: Informs the referees and sent by the committee to persons indicated by the applicant.

Content: Provides a copy of the position announcement and qualifications; personalized to elicit the information desired about the individual applicant.

7. "Thank you" draft copy

Purpose: Prepared for persons who provided references.

Content: Extends an appreciation for the time taken by the reference person and the "review" provided; later, personalized to reflect something regarding the occasion or content of the review.

8. "No" draft copy

Purpose: Informs persons of a terminal status for the application.

Content: Possible responses prepared by the committee for applicants who clearly do not meet qualifications, for those applicants who do not progress further in the process, and for those who are not chosen to be interviewed; later, personalized to reflect the situation or needs of the individual applicant.

---

cations may not be successful in their candidacy. Directness and honesty with applicants and candidates who were not successful is not only warranted, but most often is appreciated. Openness, frankness, and above all, veracity can be quite helpful to the applicant and may leave a positive tone in the interactions between the person involved and the institution.

The Application

The application process itself can be a source of confusion for potential applicants. An application should include an indication of interest, a current copy of a curriculum vitae or resumé, a formal statement regarding the position, and possibly other information such as critical examples of work related to the position. The latter two items may be found in the applications of the most sophisticated applicants, but usually are provided only on request.

A great deal of uncertainty exists regarding the submission of references. An applicant should always obtain the permission of a potential reference person (referee) to present that individual's name as a referee *before* submitting the application. Professional courtesy requires that the reference person be formally acknowledged by the committee as being willing to respond. Furthermore indication of the outcome of the application should be given later to the reference person. The request for the specific reference itself is to be made *only* by the committee. Such requests are to be sent by the committee directly to the persons named by the applicant at a time that the applicant has specified.

Because of time constraints and advertising costs for numerous advertisements, it is common practice in the initial advertising to request that names of referees be included with the application. However, institutions are strongly advised against this practice (Higgins & Hollander, 1987; Kaplowitz, 1973, 1986). Should a committee advertise that reference names be submitted *with* the application, the applicant definitely should be informed that the references will *not* be obtained until a later date—when the applicant progresses in the review process. It is inappropriate to request references until, at least, after a first major screening has taken place. However, at the time the receipt of the application is acknowledged, applicants always should be informed of *when* this request for references may occur and the process entailed.

The above recommendations are made for several reasons. In the absence of such provisions, for example, qualified potential candidates for an administrative level position may be hesitant to submit applications. They may be "wary of letting potential referees know that he or she is considering a change in position" (Higgins & Hollander, 1987, p. 31). Additionally, unnecessarily burdening "the committee, the candidates, those serving as candidates" references, and placement offices should be avoided" (Kaplowitz, 1973, p. 17).

Most persons have an adequate idea of what should or should not be included in a curriculum vitae and resumé, the differences between the two, and the appropriateness of combining both types of review in one document. Some points may be emphasized (Vecchio, 1984). Regardless of the format, the document should be accurate and complete, particularly in relation to the position for which the person is applying. The area of experience related to the position being applied for should be explicit and thorough. Similar to what would appear on a resumé, some narrative description regarding previous experience (which is usually just listed on a vita) should be included.

The sophisticated applicant will always include a formal statement regarding the position for which he or she is applying. This presumes some knowledge of the institution, but at a minimum it should indicate something further in terms of the individual applicant and possible match with the institution. For example, statements regarding the individual's philosophy pertaining to administration and being an administrator are valued highly and advisable for inclusion in an application—whether or not such information actually is requested in an application advertisement. Pointing out previous experience that is known to be highly valued by an institution is also valuable.

Reference Checks

After the applications are received a number of reviews usually occur. The preliminary review is for evaluating candidates relative to the basic established criteria and for evaluating the application in regard to completeness and accuracy of information submitted. Requests for clarifications may be sent to applicants should there be ambiguous information.

Once the application passes the preliminary review and the applicant has shown evidence that he or she holds the basic criteria for the position, references are sought. Requests are sent to the applicants for their reference lists, if this was not submitted with the application. Written references are then obtained by the committee. When telephoning persons named by the candidate as a reference, it is appropriate to indicate that the call is being made to verify information given to the committee (Kaplowitz, 1986).

Kaplowitz (1986) offers a wealth of valuable information and recommendations regarding the checking of references. It is necessary to research a candidate discretely, carefully, and thoroughly, but in so doing it is essential to respect confidentiality. Search committees often seek additional information from other sources, independent of the reference list submitted by an applicant. These sources may confirm or raise questions about the information already gathered. Information may be obtained on an informal basis, such as interactions at meetings, or formally, such as by telephone interview. Courtesy and respect for applicants demands that "the committee . . . ascertain with each candidate, whether and when referees may be contacted" (Kaplowitz, 1986, p. 67). This policy is recommended both for those references suggested by the candidate *and* for those from others *not* so named. The policy, from a professional ethics stance, particularly should be enforced in formal telephone checks. Information offered or obtained by informal, chance encounters with peers and others also needs to be treated with the utmost of ethical discretion and respect.

Kaplowitz further states that "if a candidate has indicated that a supervisor may be contacted only if the candidate is a finalist for the position," that request "needs to be respected" (1986, p. 67). If and when the candidate becomes a finalist, for example one of three candidates, then it is appropriate and necessary to inform him or her of that status and to ask for permission to contact persons on the home campus or office.

Should a candidate never give permission to contact a present superior nor provide explanation for not granting such permission, a committee is left to draw its own conclusions. It may occur that the candidate is not willing to provide an adequate explanation for a refusal. However, it may be very possible to verify the basis for the refusal. For example, the candidate may be asked whether there are other persons who might verify information related to the explanation that was given for the refusal by the candidate.

It is not uncommon to ask candidates about how they would feel if other persons were to be contacted as a referee. This type of question not only conveys the openness and permission that should exist in reference checking, but it also allows the candidate to provide any number of responses that should be quite helpful to a committee. Other persons that the committee might request permission to approach include specific individuals who have reported to the candidate—*both* some of whom are still with the organization *and* others who have left. Kaplowitz (1986) points out that such persons can present a key issue and question often overlooked, which is highly related to "administrative effectiveness: How well does the candidate build a team and develop the people reporting to him or her?" (p. 68). He also strongly suggests that a candidate's former executive secretary or administrative assistant may be able to provide more thorough and accurate information than any vice-president can.

Finally, in order to assure a uniform approach and process in reporting back to the committee, one member is recommended to do the reference checking for each candidate. It usually is preferred that this task be performed by the chair. Some committees may involve several members in this process. In the case of telephone reference interviews, it is highly recommended that these be structured, yet with sufficient open-ended questions to allow for good discussion. If several different callers are involved, formal structure is essential; otherwise, the treasury of known horror stories related to the checking of references is bound to be increased (Kaplowitz, 1986).

The Interview Process
Preparation

After the committee selects the persons to be interviewed, additional materials and information may be shared, and the formal interview schedule is planned. A comprehensive packet of information regarding the location and city; various reports related to accreditation, faculty and personnel, budget, programs, and services; bylaws; constitution; and statutes—all may be sent to the candidates to be interviewed. In return, the committee may request specific samples of the work and achievements of each candidate. Both parties might indicate key issues, questions that they would like addressed during the interview. The interview is a time for *mutual* assessment by the candidate and the committee. There should be an exchange of questions, responses, and information between both parties. Thus it is critical that both have sufficient information *before* the interview to facilitate an effective interview process.

Arrangements for the interview visit include not only planning for specific events to occur, but also for certain amenities to be provided. Arranging for prepaid travel vouchers or travel tickets to be mailed to the candidates is highly desirable. The billing for hotel accommodations and other costs, such as meals, should always be sent directly to the institution. These are demonstrations of excellent foresight and thoughtfulness. Such arrangements are always appreciated by candidates, particularly since it usually takes a minimum of 1 month for a person to be reimbursed for professional travel expenses. More significantly, the candidate will have a permanent, positive impression of the institution, regardless of the interview outcome.

Meeting the candidate at the place of arrival and returning to the travel site with the candidate are always provided by a search committee member. The same expectation exists for transporting and escorting the candidate from one interview point to another. For an executive level administrative position, 2 to 3 days are usually allocated for the initial interview process. Social events and receptions may be scheduled. Additionally the candidate may be asked to make a formal presentation or otherwise speak formally to groups. In planning the interview schedule, significant persons and groups are designated for interviewing each candidate. Each person and group interviewing the candidate should always be provided, or have conveniently available, a copy of the candidate's curriculum vitae (or resumé, if that was requested) *and* the candidate's *formal* statement regarding the position. The list of reference names and actual references are to be seen only by the search and screen committee. The higher level administrator who appointed the search committee may review the references of the final candidates.

Process

A search and screen committee usually initially meets briefly with the candidate on the first day. The agenda for the meeting includes introductions, a brief orientation to the setting, and key preliminary questions. Most often this initial contact sets the tone and stage for the remaining interviews (McVicker, 1986). Sufficient time should be allocated for the candidate to meet with the higher level administrator to whom the successful candidate will report, as well as those persons or groups for whom that individual will be responsible and accountable. Additional time might be requested either by the candidate or by persons or groups in the institution. (Two or more interview visits usually are scheduled for the final screening of the strongest candidates). The search committee normally plans to interview the candidate formally as a group, with this being last on the interview schedule (Palmer, 1983). Finally interview evaluation forms should be completed by each person and group who interviewed the applicant. The committee then summarizes the data and meets to formalize its recommendations for submission to administration.

A reserve list of final candidates, from those who completed the *initial* interview process, may be prepared by the committee. This may be helpful if some unforeseen event were to occur that ruled out the final one or two candidates. However, in such an event, it may be that administration would request or the committee recommend that the search be reopened. In that case, the present committee may be requested to begin again the search and screen process, or that committee might be abolished and a new committee named.

The conclusion of a successful search and screen process announces the beginning of a new era for an institution. The committee may make suggestions regarding the initial transition, before disbanding. Since this committee is responsible for "introducing" the successful candidate and institution to each other, the former committee members informally may prove to be very helpful in the transition process.

SUMMARY

In summary, the search and screen committee may serve to (a) attract a highly qualified group of applicants; (b) provide a consistent, fair, objective process for selecting administrators; and (c) help meet affirmative action and equal opportunity requirements. Furthermore a cohesive committee may facilitate the appreciation for values and ethics as the base for administrative decision-making and the selection of personnel. Finally, when search and screen committees are utilized, it seems likely that much time, effort, and expense may be spared and that superior candidates may more easily be located, screened, recommended, and hired for key leadership positions.

REFERENCES

American Association of University Professors (AAUP). (1981). Faculty participation in the selection, evaluation, and retention of administrators. *Academe, 67* (5), 323–324.

American Council on Education. (1986). *Deciding who shall lead: Recommendations for improving presidential searchers.* Washington, DC: Association of Governing Boards of Universities and Colleges.

Bayne, M. V., Parker, B., & Todd, A. (1982). The search committee process. *Nursing Outlook, 30* (3), 178–181.

Chung, K. H., Lubatkin, M., Rogers, R. C., & Owers, J. E. (1987). Do insiders make better CEO's than outsiders? *Academy of Management EXECUTIVE, 1* (4), 325–331.

Goldsmith, M., & Flynn, K. J. (1983). Chairman recruitment: One hospital's success. *Hospital and Health Services Administration, 28* (5), 35–45.

Heller, B. R., Okolowski, R. S., O'Driscoll, R. M.,

Frain, M., & Brody, J. K. (1982). The search interview. *Nursing Outlook, 30* (3), 182–186.

Higgins, J. M. V., & Hollander, P. A. (1987). *A guide to successful searches for college personnel.* Asheville, NC: College Administration Publications.

Kaplowitz, R. A. (1973). *Selecting academic administrators: The search committee.* Washington, DC: American Council on Education.

Kaplowitz, R. A. (1986). *Selecting college and university personnel: The quest and the questions (ASHE-ERIC* Higher Education Report No. 8). Washington, DC: Association for the Study of Higher Education.

Lutz, F. W. (1979). Deanship selection and faculty governance in high education. *Planning and Changing, 10* (4), 238–245.

McLaughlin, J. B., & Riesman, D. (1985). The vicissitudes of the search process. *Journal of the Association for the Study of Higher Education, 8* (4), 341–355.

McVicker, M. F. (1986). The seven deadly sins of interviewing. *Pace, 13* (12), 67–69.

Palmer, R. (1983). A sharper focus on the panel interview. *Personnel Management, 15* (5), 34–37.

Rodman, J. A., & Dingerson, M. R. (1986). University hiring practices for academic administrators. *Journal of the College and University Personnel Association, 37* (2), 24–30.

Sagaria, M. A. D., & Krotseng, M. V. (1986). Deans' managerial skills: What they need and what they bring to the job. *Journal of the College and University Personnel Association, 37* (2), 1–6.

Tucker, A. (1984). *Chairing the academic department: Leadership among peers.* New York: Macmillan.

VanderWaerdt, L. (1982). *Affirmative action in higher education—A sourcebook.* New York: Garland.

Vecchio, R. P. (1984). The problem of phony resumes: How to spot a ringer among the applicants. *Personnel, 61* (2), 22–27.

✳ EDITOR'S QUESTIONS FOR DISCUSSION ✳

What are the various methods by which personnel may be selected? How can an organization be encouraged to utilize a consistent process in the use of search and screen committees? Indicate specific strategies to increase objectivity and fairness on the part of the search and screen committee. What responsibilities, obligations, and options does a committee member have if there is a breach in the procedures that the committee agreed to follow? Discuss the policies and procedures that can contribute to an effective affirmative action office or practices. How can the rights of the candidate best be protected from the time of application through to the interview process and closure of the search?

What ethical dilemmas may be encountered in the obtaining and verification of references? How may such ethical dilemmas be appropriately resolved? How can a cohesive committee best be developed that is committed to a set of values and ethics in the search and screen process? What issues are involved in being open, direct, and honest with applicants and candidates who are not successful candidates? How should these issues be most effectively and ethically resolved? How can the most valid and reliable information possible be obtained about the candidate during the interview process? To what extent and on what basis can the responses of the candidate to questions posed during the interview be shared within the organization? What are types of questions that a candidate should ask the organization and vice versa, in order to assess the match between the candidate and the organization?

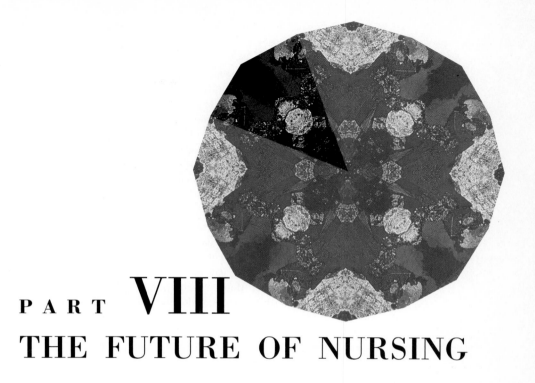

PART VIII
THE FUTURE OF NURSING

Through a kaleidoscope, one can imaginatively glimpse beyond tomorrow. Intrigue, excitement, brilliance, splendour, and refreshment are perpetually in motion as the kaleidoscope is turned. These features are intrinsic to nursing. Tomorrow is always on the horizon and in various stages and forms of becoming.

Significant projections for each aspect of the profession and the future of nursing are shown in the chapters of this section. Sisters Rosemary Donley and Mary Jean Flaherty in Chapter 64 organize the literature of predictions about nursing and future health care systems. They project two scenes reflecting the transformation of the profession to the year 2020.

Colleen Conway-Welch in Chapter 65 explores the present multiple education routes that lead to the same outcome—the RN. Five turning points that generate new ideas and designs about nursing education are highlighted.

In Chapter 66 Claire Fagin brings into focus the evolving maturation of nursing education in the academic environment. She describes the changing picture of academic expectations and forecasts the developments that are critical to ensure that nursing achieves the professional state desired in academe.

Nursing of the future holds numerous types of collaborative models in which nursing education and practice are merged. Kay Andreoli and Jane Tarnow in Chapter 67 analyze three existing collaborative models at academic health centers. Innovative models will increase nursing's ability to provide quality patient care.

Joanne Stevenson in Chapter 68 demonstrates that the transformation of nursing into a scientific field is imminent. A systematic master plan will accelerate the pace of nursing science. Stevenson proposes a model for the progression of research in the science of care.

Knowledge development is the central focus of nursing scholars who are furthering nursing as a science. Virginia Kemp in Chapter 69 reflects on the themes and future trends unfolding in the kaleidoscope of nursing theory. Points of agreement and divergence are shown among theorists. Progression is evident in the evolution of nursing to a science.

Joyce Clifford in Chapter 70 succinctly summarizes the essentials of a professional nursing practice model of the future. Major restructuring of institutional nursing practice is emerging. Redesigning models within and for nursing practice will accelerate desirable outcomes for the health care system and the nurse professional.

In Chapter 71 Edward Halloran provides a framework that nurse administrators might use for implementing future, quality nursing services. The boundaries for nursing services are to be challenged by future administrators.

Patricia Starck in Chapter 72 reveals the uncertainty as well as opportunities that are integral to the administration of academic programs. She describes how visionary deans can capitalize on predicted changes for the future of nursing academic administration.

A brilliant image of nursing can be molded tantamount to the bright moving points of light seen in a kaleidoscope. Many possible patterns of nursing exist. To choose the image that is best and to make the image real depends on the individual nurse and the profession.

64

The Future of Professional Nursing

Sr. Rosemary Donley, Ph.D., R.N., F.A.A.N.
Sr. Mary Jean Flaherty, Ph.D., R.N., F.A.A.N.

It is always difficult to bring coherence to visions of the future. The authors' task is complicated further by a vision of a complex profession with diverse work settings, competitive levels of education, and conflicting beliefs about practice.

Weisbord's "six-box model" (1983) for managing complexity (Fig. 64-1) is employed in this chapter to organize recorded predictions about nursing's future. Originally designed as a diagnostic framework for organizational analysis, Weisbord (1983) proposed six areas for examination: purpose, structure, rewards, leadership, helpful mechanisms, and relationships. His analytical model also poses questions that can be raised about the future of nursing.

PURPOSE: WHAT "BUSINESS" ARE WE IN?

The idea of nursing as a business is not a dominant theme in contemporary nursing literature. While most health care writing promotes hospitals as industries and medicine as entrepreneurial activity, nursing literature approaches the competitive health environment of the late 1980s expressing self-doubt, what Stevens (1987) describes as "a struggle between romance and power" (p. 1607).

Nursing's ability to define and market its business and find its niche in the health care marketplace has been hampered by prolonged and bitter battles over the education of its entry level workers. The official positions of the major nursing associations, the American Nurses' Association and the National League for Nursing, are not endorsed by the majority of their members, and more significantly, they are opposed by nonaffiliated nurses. Most reports in the literature discussing the business of nursing become passionate appeals to settle the "entry into practice controversy" and get on with more significant concerns: poverty, human despair, incomplete and unequal health care, discrimination against women and minorities, ignorance and repression (Styles, 1987, p. 229).

It is not surprising in this climate that even senior nurse leaders as Schlotfeldt (1987a) and Aydelotte (1987) emphasize the educational dilemma in their futuristic writings. Schlotfeldt says that lack of agreement about the knowledge base associated with the discipline of nursing and the licensure of generalist practitioners prevents a desirable future (Schlotfeldt, 1987b). Aydelotte (1987) ends a provocative essay on future health systems in 2010 with three of six recommendations centered on nursing education.

It can be argued that lack of clarity about nursing's educational and credentialing processes makes

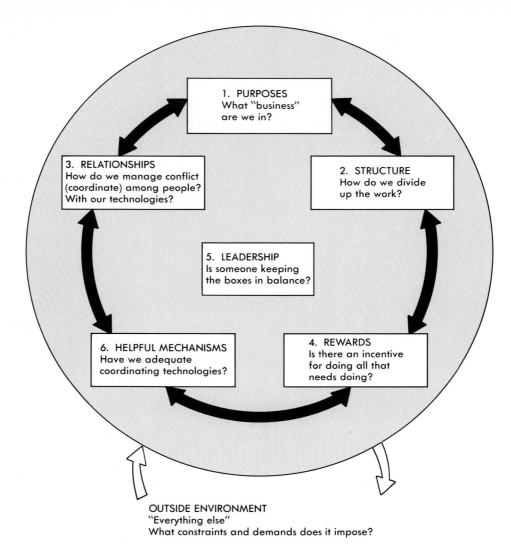

FIGURE 64-1

A six-box model. (From Weisbord, MR [1983]. *Organizational diagnoses: A workbook for theory and practice* (p. 9). Reading, MA: Addison-Wesley. Copyright 1978 by Martin R Weisbord. Reprinted by permission.)

the business of nursing noncompetitive and unattractive. These sentiments may well explain the Cassandra-like warnings of Stevens (1985a) and Goertzen (1987), who argue that if nursing does not define its product and services in real-world terms, other, less qualified health workers will be created.

In the real world, corporate executives plan, analyze, and select options from a spectrum of competitive strategies. Nursing's leaders, however, embroil themselves in intraprofessional and intraorganizational conflicts aimed at perfecting the product or protecting their own turf.

Futurist literature offers a glimmer of hope as writers suggest that nursing ventures will emphasize health promotion, self-care, and high-tech practice. Andreoli and Musser (1985) address the "greying of America," health care costs, technology, health promotion, self-care, and the oversupply of physicians as factors to be considered in future businesses. The increased number of women in the work force and the number of women who head families will influence health care delivery. Spitzer and Davivier (1987) suggest that as more women make decisions about spending money for health care or selecting a health provider, women's health care will emerge as a popular specialty for nurses. They also propose health promotion, occupational health, and the development of alternative care arrangements (e.g., sleep disorder clinics, pain control centers) as nurse-managed businesses of the future. While the aging and the continued increase of women in the work force of America are noted in most discussions of the future, less attention is given to the shifting ethnic balance and the number of young blacks, Hispanics, and Asians in American cities (Ginsberg, 1987).

The Delphi panelists who speculated on the year 2020 emphasized health promotion (Sullivan et al., 1987). They spoke of nurses as case managers, clinical decision-makers, and advocates for patients' rights. Naylor and Sherman (1987) note the promotion of nursing markets; they emphasize public-private partnerships, and propose entrepreneurial and intrapreneurial models of contract, institution-based nursing services.

Christman (1987) emphasizes science and technology in nursing's future. He acknowledges three outcomes of a high-tech future: computer assistance in clinical management and care, technological evaluation of clients and health care providers, and lessened demand for all health care workers.

The use of information technology to improve patient care has already been demonstrated by monitoring systems. These systems screen documented patient events against indicators that signal high-risk situations. Donoho and Mascar (1987) predict that creative analysis of data collected by monitoring systems will transform patterns of quality care and challenge practitioners.

In summary, the literature suggests that nursing will be in the business of health promotion and health maintenance, with practices enhanced and occasionally threatened by automation and technology. Care settings will be in industry, home, and hospitals, and the majority of clients will be older and nonwhite.

STRUCTURE: HOW DO WE DIVIDE THE WORK?

Weisbord's question about structure, or how the work is divided, is approached in projections of nursing's future by new role delineations and descriptions of the workplace. These discussions are influenced by another preoccupation of the 1980s — the nursing shortage. Most analysts of the shortage in the nursing work force and the lessened attractiveness of nursing as a field of study address the issues of salary, status, and the structure of the work. The National Commission on Nursing Implementation Project (1987) proposes the differentiation of practice as a way of creating meaningful career staging and of distinguishing the levels of work. Discussions about case management emphasize autonomy, power, and the authority to make clinical decisions. Maraldo and Solomon (1987) suggest that work should be structured so that nurses are in competitive positions with other health care providers. The Delphi panelists speak of nurses admitting and referring patients to a variety of health care centers, counseling patients and families, and offering alternative care services to the terminally ill (Sullivan et al., 1987). Aydelotte (1987) urges nurses to assume self-governing and power mentalities because nurses' work will encompass the presidencies of universities, corporations, and boards.

Regulatory and financing structures play a role in defining nurses' work. Most practicing nurses are not recognized as providers of services and are categorically ineligible to bill insurers. To the degree that demand is influenced by ability to pay for services, the work of nursing is limited by financial structures. The influence of regulations on nursing's future work is most evident in the long-term care industry. The Institute of Medicine's index (1986) of federal nursing home regulations, conditions of participation in skilled nursing facilities, standards in intermediate-care facilities, and surveys of state health facility licensure and certification provide a framework for understanding how federal and state regulations set the tone of the work environment. A recent study in long-term care by the Research Triangle Institute (1987) described nurses' work in long-term care as observing care practices and documenting activities. Future scenarios about nurses' work need to address how practice has changed to match American demographics.

Most futurists agree that financial and regulatory structures must be modified to enable professional work. There is also consensus in the literature that some accommodation and shared authority must be achieved with medicine. Spitzer and Davivier (1987) note that as more women practice as physicians, opportunities for collaboration increase.

RELATIONSHIPS: HOW DO WE MANAGE CONFLICT?

Three groups (nurses, hospital boards and administrators, and physicians) emerge in discussions of professional relationships. The high cost of failure to manage conflict is evident in the time and energy expended on intraprofessional conflicts. The energy dissipated over educational and licensing issues limits nurses' ability to chart their future. Havighurst (1987) suggests that deregulation of all health care providers may clear the air and permit the survival of the fittest. Christman (1987) says that if nurses would refuse to teach anything less than baccalaureate nursing, the educational dilemma would be resolved. Brown (1987) offers a vision of the future that promises new social contracts between nurses and patients, similar to contracts between physicians and patients. Older (1983), a behavioral psychologist, warns that concern for professional status—the plague of the past—will likely infect the future. He recommends that the hours nurses have spent talking about professional status should be "stacked in the bottom of a deep cave and sealed with a meter-thick concrete plug" (p. 78).

Although the nursing literature emphasizes an autonomous future-oriented practice, other health literature reflects an increased number of individual physicians employed by hospitals and health maintenance organizations. The evolution of health care systems in the seventies and the interest of proprietary groups in acute care hospitals, home care agencies, and nursing homes support Aydelotte's prediction (1987) that the health care industry will be controlled by a few dozen national or international companies by 2010. Health boards and administrators of health services will be significant forces in nursing's future.

Future health care conglomerates, of which the modern health care system is a prototype, will need to include nursing into their management if nursing practice is to have any institutional base for its activities. The woman's movement has advanced women on corporate and civic boards and commissions. However, nurses have not been major players on health and policy boards. The typical hospital or health care system does not have a nursing affairs committee, and ordinarily nurses do not sit on governing boards. Gender is a factor to be overcome in future-oriented business-social establishments.

The bittersweet relationship between nursing and medicine, reflected in both literatures (Iglehart, 1987) has its own history of conflict. The deep feeling about the paternalism of the American Medical Society expressed in the language of its support for bedside nurses and easy affiliations with groups who oppose change in the professionalism, education, or clinical authority of nurses leads Barbara Stevens (1985a) to remark: "The present nursing leadership is not interested in turning out a physician's handmaiden even if society decides that is what it wants or can afford" (p. 127). Relational conflict will be in nursing's future.

REWARDS: IS THERE AN INCENTIVE FOR DOING ALL THAT NEEDS TO BE DONE?

It is interesting, given the importance of salary in recruiting and retaining nurses (Aiken, 1987), that so little attention is given in the future literature to resource allocation. Aydelotte (1987) mentions the

legislators, Abdellah (1987) stresses fund raising in the private sector, and McBride (1987) emphasizes the policy arena as environments able to reward nursing activity. Maraldo and Solomon (1987) say the shortage provides a window of opportunity to restructure resource allocation. These notions of a bright economic future are tempered by fears that elitism may price nurses out of competitive ranges (Goertzen, 1987). Stevens (1985b) offers a "resource driven model" as a guide to practice. She suggests that resources should be assessed before goals and methods are determined (p. 28).

If statements that support better salaries are deleted, the allocation of health care resources is a minor theme in nursing literature. However, the effects of reducing health care costs and the ethical and social problems related to the allocation of scarce resources dominate the literature in the federal and private health care sectors. Competition in the industry has been offered as a strategy for lowering costs and rewarding the best health care providers. Competition has changed the landscape of health care. There are fewer individual providers of institutional or professional health care, more integrated institutions that bring together single services (as psychiatric hospitals), and continuums of care. There is major growth in the home health care industry and modest growth in long-term and ambulatory care centers. There are more physicians and a shortage of nurses. There is no evidence that health care costs have been lowered. There is concern noted in the nursing literature that the poor and the rich, the insured and the uninsured, receive different quality of care and that access to care has been limited for poor, minority populations (Aydelotte, 1987; Donley, 1988). The literature suggests that competition rewards those providers who limit their care of the poor and uninsured.

Futurists who write in the nursing literature assume that current modes of financing health care will continue into the next century. Their reflections address microallocation of funds among future providers, hospital-based nursing services, and contract nursing groups. It is assumed that nurses will engage in fee-for-service care. Prepayment models, regionalized capitation programs, nationalized health care services, or novel patterns of funding are given less attention by nurse futurists.

LEADERSHIP: IS SOMEONE KEEPING THE BOXES IN BALANCE?

The leadership question is discussed often in the literature under the rubric of nursing associations of the future. There is speculation about whether existing organizations can maintain control of their own constituencies and project an image of power and unity. There is some evidence of a nursing power elite. The presidents and executive directors of four associations (the American Nurses' Association, the National League for Nursing, the American Association of Colleges of Nursing, and the American Organization of Nurse Executives) met as a tricouncil to set national policies and advance legislative agenda. However, Hegyvary et al. (1987), reporting for the American Academy of Nursing, project the need for more centralized strategic planning, cooperative stances, and national mechanisms to address credentialing, education, and standards. They do not think that the current array of specialized nursing associations or the TriCouncil can meet future challenges. They argue for a restructuring of organized nursing around one of five models: the existing mosaic, the professional, the federated, the corporate, or the ministerial. Schlotfeldt (1985) emphasizes that transformational leadership is needed to exercise options for the future. She is particularly concerned about another collective, namely, academic nursing and its commitment to responsible resolution of recognized social problems. She believes that academic leadership is the key to organizing consensus about nursing's body of knowledge, regulating preservice education, and developing antonomous professional schools. Curtin (1986), on the other hand, sees the future as the stimulus for individuals to create and achieve. To advance this future, Arista '87, a national conference on the nursing shortage, concluded that better public education about the nature of modern nursing is essential to attract a sufficient number of committed nurses (Beyers, 1987).

HELPFUL MECHANISMS: HAVE WE ADEQUATE COORDINATING TECHNOLOGIES?

The nursing literature conveys an excitement about new technologies. Nursing protocols are computerized, and telecommunication and robots facilitate assessment, analysis, monitoring of patients, and patient care (Christman, 1987). The Delphi panel (Sullivan et al., 1987) raises the dark side of high-tech's future. In their predictions, they reflect an Orwellian skepticism:

> A growing societal movement toward humanizing health care, begun in the 1990's, has increased the financial support for nursing research that focuses on human responses to health and illness problems. (p. 235)
>
> Nursing, in 2020, is also in the forefront of the patients' rights movement. All hospitals and communities are required by federal mandate to have active humanistic impact study groups to assess the impact of biomedical technology/genetic engineering on patients' rights to freedom of choice and to death with dignity. (p. 235)
>
> Nursing's role in patient advocacy, in general, has become highly visible and widely recognized. . . . Nursing roles in advocacy also include consumer education, patient counseling regarding alternative treatment options, and nursing support for dying patients who choose to forego heroic lifesaving measures. (p. 235)

In summary, writers on nursing's future envisage a world in which educated professionals practice as colleague/competitors of physicians. Specializing in health maintenance and prevention, nurses use technology to improve access, quality, and efficiency, and they provide services at lower cost. Nurses are recognized for their expertise and they enjoy status, esteem, and income. They ignore or overcome relational conflicts with physicians, disenfranchised nurses, or health care administrators. Their clients, now elderly, learned to relate to nurse health-care providers in kindergarten. Nursing organizations behave rationally and assure that nursing's leadership is exerted in health care and policy environments.

Futurists often express their views by creating scenarios. Two worldviews developed for this discus-

sion were suggested by an analysis of America's response to the energy crisis. The scenarios are based on John Coleman's recollection of a speech that Robert Bellah suggested to President Carter (Coleman, 1982):

> Look, we have had a great history, we've satisfied a lot of needs, we've done a lot of terrible things too, but by and large we've been one of the more decent societies in human history . . . and we've done it all by combining an ethic of deep concern for other human beings with an ethic of everybody looking out for number one. And it's worked. But it is not going to work anymore. We're up against a new set of limits—ecological, political, economic—and we are not going to be able to afford the totally unlimited self-indulgence and the kind of economic system that feeds that self-indulgence any longer. Our choices are two: either we're going to solve it by authoritarianism or we're going to solve it through reorganization of our society along voluntaristic lines in accordance with our long tradition of democratic process. It's not going to be easy, because most of the basic interests of our society will have to be reoriented. . . . it's not going to be like it was! And we'd better start thinking about what it's going to be. The best thing is to involve the whole nation in some kind of serious consideration of what the options are as we move into a different world! (pp. 184–185)

There may be little relationship between the energy crisis and the nursing shortage, or between spiritual malaise and the competitive health environment of the eighties. However, the work of the future is the resolution of the tension between "looking out for number one," and the alternative ethic of "deep concern for other human beings."

Scenario One: The Nurse of the Future

Viewers of transistor television are not only informed about Wellness International, the newest nurse affiliate in Los Angeles, they can also use their portable sets to speak directly with their nurse health-care providers. When the nurses need more data, this handy transistor can also become an assessment device for the transmission of audio and visual images. While this style of assessment is not

exactly a hands-on experience, it saves time and money.

Nurses have adapted to high-technology diagnosis and treatment more quickly than other health care providers. Their ability to incorporate new informational systems and meet their clients where they are has given nurses a competitive edge in the overpopulated world of health care providers. The old adage—a nurse is a nurse is a nurse—seems more descriptive of flexibility in the primary care marketplace than a pejorative reminder of historically undifferentiated nursing practice. The deregulation of the health care industry has made nursing care accessible and affordable to everyone insured by privately or publicly managed insurance-provider groups.

This utopian portrayal of innovative, autonomous work masks the controversies that still divide the profession. It is ironic that nurses struggle with some of the issues that eventually diminished the influence of physicians. These controversies can be quickly summarized by a review of emergent professional organizations, Association to Promote Women in Nursing and the Committee for Nursing Insurance, or by a survey of recently released audiotapes and videotapes. Themes in the trade news include debates about financial reimbursement for television case managers, the merits of two types of nurse extenders—para nurses and robots, strategies to avoid claims of malpractice by health conglomerates, and promotion of aerospace nursing.

Because customers now design their health care service packages, propaganda (the 21st century word for advertising blended with health education) plays a significant role in marketing providers and services. There are ever-changing alliances among the "Big 10" multinational conglomerates who own the institutionalized spectrum of health care; the international pharmaceutical and equipment houses; satellite, ambulatory, and home-based services; and government and private insurers. The Big-10 provider groups compete for their market shares by creative delivery organizations, high-tech advertising, quality of care, customer choice initiatives, price sensitivity, and promises to assist business and purchasers in developing tax incentives. Because large

businesses are health-insured (the yellows), they join traditional insurers (the blues), commercial firms (the reds), and the government (the whites) in negotiating health packages with Big-10 and professional firms. Solo practitioners, health professionals, or small institutions have little influence in establishing patterns of service delivery. In response to this trend, nurses have joined or developed professional health firms. The names of the professional firms sound like the law firms of the 20th century. Some partnerships represent uneasy alliances among pharmacists, nurses, physicians, and physical therapists. Other partnerships are along traditional professional lines. Status is achieved by becoming a partner. Partners recruit clients, usually by designing creative, price-sensitive service packages for one of the conglomerates. Universities and private associations play significant roles in assisting their constituents in business. These functions rival the more traditional educational and affiliative roles that used to be played by schools.

Scenario Two: The Nurse of the Future

The great plague is over. Cataclysmic tragedy, war, famine, and plague lead to the restructuring of the social order and the recreation of its values and institutions. Health care delivery is a humanitarian service exempt from entrepreneurial excesses and freed from competitive pressures to get clients, capture market shares, and control the enterprise through national and international mergers and acquisitions. Informed choice rather than competition is the hallmark of 21st century health care systems. Clients have personal and financial rewards for good health practices. Insurers support memberships in spas, health clubs, and spiritual renewal centers, in addition to more traditional health care services. People can access computerized data systems in supermarkets, pharmacies, and department stores. These user-friendly systems provide annotated directories to nutrition centers, exercise clubs, health care providers, health care settings, and common diagnostic tests and therapies. Health care is supported by a sophisticated blending of public and private dollars. People can register in a confidential

computerized health bank that enables them to identify personal health risks and receive suggestions for self-help and professional or social remedies. Implanted devices enable health care providers and patients to monitor the effects of motor activity, chemical and hormonal changes, and cardiac and respiratory rates. Incentives to select less costly therapies and use primary and preventive health care services are realizable because preventive health services are available from a spectrum of health care providers.

The American system better approximates the welfare states of Western Europe in recognizing that housing, food, transportation, and social support are as essential as diagnosis and treatment of acute illnesses. Architects and builders play minor roles in health by designing housing, restaurants, schools, churches, health centers, and shopping centers that support the age and ethnic diversity of 21st century Americans. Recognition and enhancement of the dignity of clients, their families, and health care providers is, however, the distinctive attribute of the modern American health care system.

It is difficult to reconstruct the roots of this transformation. There are three factors to be considered. The malpractice insurance crisis reached a point where there was a leveling of expectations of entrepreneurs—medical providers, consumer-clients, and health lawyers. The ability to harness technological and genetic research enabled policymakers to control technological imperatives and make ethical choices about what should be done in an environment sensitive to quality, justice, and cost. When acquired immunodeficiency syndrome (AIDS) and the effects of chemical and nuclear waste threatened the general population at the end of the 20th century, expensive investment in hospitals and acute care was brought under scrutiny. Competition among professional and institutional providers did not address the ravaging effects of AIDS or the less dramatic, but equally fatal, environmental toxins. The failure of the systems designed to support high-tech treatment evoked an examination of preventive and educational strategies and a return to spiritual and humanistic values in health care. Nursing was transformed in the process.

REFERENCES

Abdellah, FG (1987). The federal role in nursing education. *Nursing Outlook, 35* (5), 224–225.

Aiken, L (1987). The nursing shortage: Myth or reality. *New England Journal of Medicine, 317,* 641–646.

Andreoli, KG, & Musser, LA (1985). Trends that may affect nursing's future. *Nursing Health Care, 6*(1), 46–51.

Aydelotte, MK (1987). Nursing's preferred future. *Nursing Outlook, 35* (3), 114–120.

Beyers, M (1987). *The nursing shortage—Nurses and the delivery of health care services now and in the future* (Arista '87 monograph). Indianapolis: Sigma Theta Tau International.

Brown, B. (1987). From the editor. *Nursing Administration Quarterly, 11*(2), vi–vii.

Christman, LP (1987). A view to the future. *Nursing Outlook, 35*(5), 216–218.

Coleman, JA (1982). *An American strategic theology*. New York: Paulist Press.

Curtin, L (1986). Nursing in the year 2000: Learning from the future (editorial). *Nursing Management, 17*(6), 7–8.

Donley, R (1988). Health care system in the U.S., Catholic. In B Marthaler (Exec. Ed.), *New Catholic Encyclopedia*. (pp. 187-190). Chicago: Jack Heraty and Associates, Inc.

Donoho, BA, & Mascar, GA (1987). *Nursing Administration Quarterly, 11*(2), 63–69.

Ginsberg, E (1987). Nursing for the future facing the facts and figures. *American Journal of Nursing, 87*(12), 1596–1600.

Goertzen, IE (1987). Making nursing's vision a reality. *Nursing Outlook, 35*(3), 121–123.

Havighurst, C (1987, June). *Practice opportunities for allied health professionals in a deregulated health care industry*. Paper presented at the meeting of the American Society of Allied Health Professions, Washington, DC.

Hegyvary, SR, Duxbury, ML, Hall, RH, Drueger, JC, Lindeman, CA, Scott, JM, & Scott, WR (1987). *The evolution of nursing professional organizations: Alternative models for the future*. Kansas City: American Academy of Nursing.

Iglehart, J (1987). Problems facing the nursing profession. *New England Journal of Medicine, 317,* 646–651.

Institute of Medicine. (1986). *Improving the quality of care in nursing homes*. Washington, DC: National Academy Press.

Maraldo, PJ, & Solomon, SB (1987). Nursing's window of opportunity. *Image, 19*(2), 83–86.

McBride, AB (1987). Shaping nursing's preferred future. *Nursing Outlook, 35*(3), 124–125.

National Commission on Nursing Implementation Project. (1987, February). *NCNIP encourages development of differentiated practice* [News release]. :Author.

Naylor, MD, & Sherman, MB (1987). Wanted: The best and the brightest. *American Journal of Nursing, 87*(12), 1601–1605.

Older, J (1983). Choices for the future of nursing. *Journal of Advances in Nursing, 8*(1), 77–78.

Research Triangle Institute. (1987). *Analysis of the environment for the recruitment and retention of registered nurses in nursing homes*. Rockville, MD: U.S. Department of Health and Human Services.

Schlotfeldt, RM (1985). Classics from our heritage. A brave new nursing world: Exercising options for the future. *Journal of Professional Nursing, 1*(4), 224–251.

Schlotfeldt, RM (1987a). Resolution of issues: An imperative for creating nursing's future. *Journal of Professional Nursing, 3*(3), 136–142.

Schlotfeldt, RM (1987b). Reflections on nursing. *Nursing Outlook, 35*(5), 226–228.

Spitzer, RB, & Davivier, M (1987). Nursing in the 1990's: Expanding opportunities. *Nursing Administration Quarterly, 11*(2), 55–61.

Stevens, BJ (1985a). Does the 1985 Nursing Education Proposal make economic sense? *Nursing Outlook, 33*(3), 124–127.

Stevens, BJ (1985b). Tackling a changing society head on. *Nursing and Health Care, 6*(1), 27–30.

Stevens, R (1987). Nurses for the future, the yo yo ride. *American Journal of Nursing, 87*(12), 1606–1609.

Styles, MM (1987). The tarnished opportunity: A wish for the future. *Nursing Outlook, 35*(5), 229.

Sullivan, TJ, Lee, JL, Warneck, ML, Green, L, Lind, J, Smith, DS, & Underwood, P (1987). Nursing 2020: A study of nursing's future. *Nursing Outlook, 35*(5), 233–235.

Weisbord, MR (1983). *Organizational diagnoses: A workbook for theory and practice*. Reading, MA: Addison-Wesley.

✳ EDITOR'S QUESTIONS FOR DISCUSSION ✳

Of the two scenes portraying the future, which do you believe is most likely to occur? What factors are critical for the development of nursing as a profession in the future? What evidence is there of a nursing power elite? What may be the basis or cause of a power elite within the profession? What type of leadership in nursing is needed for the future?

How can nurses and nursing impact positively the future of health care? What effects has competition had on health care delivery and the provision of nursing services? What will be the settings for health care delivery and services in the future? What strategies might be offered to increase the professionalization of home health care and the long-term care industry?

65

Turning Points in Nursing Education

Colleen Conway-Welch, Ph.D., R.N., C.N.M., F.A.A.N.

Rapid change in our society has forced nursing to examine, one more time, two painful issues: (a) the confusing educational routes to becoming a registered nurse, and (b) the decreasing interest in nursing as a career. These concerns are also highlighted in the *Sixth Report to the President and Congress on the Status of Health Personnel in the United States* (1988).

DISCUSSION OF ISSUES
Folly in Educational Routes

Nursing is the only discipline that encourages people to be educated in three different ways (associate degree, diploma, and baccalureate degree in nursing) in order to obtain the same license—the RN license. These varied educational routes have continued to educate people in three different ways to do the same job, carry the same accountability under the same nurse practice act, access the same salary opportunities with the same salary compression after 8 to 10 years of practice, be evaluated by the same tools, adhere to the same practice standards, and be responsible for the same malpractice liability.

Decreasing Interest in Nursing as a Career

Since the 1984–1985 academic year, the number of students admitted annually to basic nursing education programs has declined. Preliminary data for 1985–1986 indicate that about 99,300 students were admitted to basic nursing education programs, a decline of 20% from the 123,800 admitted in 1983–1984. ("Sixth Report," 1988).

These two issues—confusing educational routes and declining applications—demonstrate to the world that the old ways and the old solutions are not working. The old ways of educating nurses are immersed in bias, shackled by tradition, and founded on rickety assumptions.

FLAWED ASSUMPTIONS

The old ways are based on four flawed assumptions:

The first of these is that the current so-called nursing shortage can be solved by recruiting large numbers of students and giving them multiple program choices for a nursing education—a licensed practical nurse (LPN) program, an associate degree (AD) program, a diploma program, or a baccalaureate (BSN) program. This flawed assumption requires one to believe that all of these nurses who (except for the BSN) have virtually no curriculum content in

leadership, management, public health, or psychiatry can deliver cost-effective care—of a similar quality—in home health care settings, public health settings, acute care tertiary settings, and psychiatric settings.

The second flawed assumption is that both a liberal education in the arts and sciences and a professional education in nursing can be adequately achieved in eight undergraduate semesters, or their equivalent. A further fallacy involves the notion that it is acceptable to graduate generalists from baccalaureate degree programs and then require them to function immediately in a specialist setting—in spite of the fact that the days of the general, medical-surgical, garden-variety hospital units are gone.

The third flawed assumption is that the student body of tomorrow will continue to be white, young, dedicated, and full-time, in spite of overwhelming demographics to the contrary. The fourth flawed assumption is that the workplace will continue as it is, with little computerization and voluminous amounts of paperwork and with patient care tasks being performed by a myriad of nursing personnel with different levels of expertise, all supervising each other in a kind of hierarchical minuet, in spite of many futuristic predictions to the contrary.

TURNING POINTS

These flawed assumptions have triggered a number of turning points in higher education in nursing in 1988. Consumer vulnerability and economic professional survival *demand* that they be replaced with reasonable, cost-effective alternatives.

Professional and Technical Levels of Practice

The first turning point in nursing education is the inevitable acceptance that the nurse of tomorrow—the professional nurse—will follow the educational model of the other health care delivery professions. The complexities of our health care system and patients' needs require a professional nurse and a technical nurse—just as, for example, physicians utilize physician's assistants; attorneys use paralegals; social workers, who are prepared at the master's level,

have social work clerks and assistants; and dentists work with dental assistants.

The recommendations of the National Commission on Nursing Implementation Project (NCNIP, 1986), which in 1988 is in its third year of a 5-year Kellogg-funded project, address the need for recognition of these two levels of practice. NCNIP's overall responsibility is to shape the future of nursing by identifying emerging trends and consensus on these trends and then taking action today to effect this future. Two benchmark documents generated by NCNIP, the *Timeline for Transition into the Future: Nursing Education System for Two Categories of Nurse (1987a)*, and *Characteristics of Professional and Technical Nurses of the Future and their Educational Programs (1987b)*, provide a blueprint for change (see Appendix 65-1).

There could have been a turning point in 1965, when the American Nurses' Association issued a position paper stating that all nursing education belonged in institutions of higher learning. At the time, however, nurses and hospital administrators were caught up in a great egalitarian vortex and were unable to deal with the fact that different levels of education result in different knowledge and skill levels and thus necessitate different job descriptions. Today, associate degree and diploma nurses are working beyond their educational abilities, and baccalaureate and master's degree nurses are restrained by the confines of their job descriptions and work environments.

It becomes obvious that the marketplace must differentiate skill levels and that nurses must be paid at different levels, commensurate with their skills. Today, associate degree, diploma, and baccalaureate degree nurses are still paid at virtually the same scale—and usually at an hourly rate with overtime. This causes all nurses to be paid at a common denominator level—the technical level. Income has risen very slowly, in part in response to the difficulty of attracting baccalaureate degree nurses. While income has edged up in grudging acknowledgement of the need for baccalaureate skill levels, salary compression still occurs for all RNs.

Employers must be able to pay both a technical wage (which may or may not be hourly based) and a professional salary (which is *not* hourly based), and all nurses must be able to delegate nonnursing tasks to lower-paid employees. Since many staff nurses today are still treated as hourly wage earners, and "clock in" as do other hourly workers, it is confusing to argue that some nurses are professionals and should be professionally salaried because of their different educational backgrounds and abilities.

Nursing Shortage Versus Increased Demand

The second turning point is the dawning realization that the so-called nursing shortage of 1987 and 1988 is related to an increased *demand* for nurses, not a shortage. Nurses have been flexible, inexpensive, and disposable, but nurses are realizing that a background in nursing can also be a launching point for many other career interests. This increased demand has both a positive and negative side. In 1984 and 1985, the United States graduated more RNs than ever before in our history, and yet demand rapidly outstripped supply.

On the negative side, nurses have been relatively cheap labor, can perform a variety of nursing and nonnursing tasks, are frequently not hampered by union restrictions, are available 24 hours a day, and are expected to work in difficult environments because of their calling. On the plus side, many employers in the health care and other industries are discovering that nurses are very versatile and ideal employees. Hospitals are also finding that the increasing acuity levels of hospitalized patients' conditions are resulting in an increased need for well-educated nurses who can carry a greater level of responsibility and accountability.

Future of the Bachelor of Science (BSN) Degree in Nursing

A third turning point is the recognition of the complicated dilemma of how to provide *adequate* professional preparation for baccalaureate degree nurses. The original BSN programs were 5 years (or a minimum of 10 semesters) in length, and many of the early nurse leaders had a college education before they entered a diploma school of nursing. How-

ever, in face of competition and marketplace realities, BSN programs were gradually shortened to eight semesters. This allows approximately four semesters to be devoted to liberal arts and sciences and four semesters to general nursing courses. This results in BSN graduates having an introductory and superficial exposure to the liberal arts and only a generalist background in nursing. The reality in the world of work is that there are very few "general" nursing units; BSNs work in specialty-focused settings immediately on graduation. They then need extensive orientation to specialist content, which must be given by the somewhat disgruntled employer.

The BSN program also creates a "professional" whose appreciation of history, philosophy, geography, science, cultural differences, and language is marginal. These nurses must perform in a world and in a profession in which increasingly complex moral and technical issues will cause them to examine themselves, their value systems, and their world daily. Nurse educators are beginning to focus on the increasing need for a sound foundation in the liberal arts before pursuing graduate study (Carter, 1986; Conway-Welch, 1986; Sakalys & Watson, 1986).

The half-life of much of the technical information taught in schools of nursing is less than 5 years. Many businesses (although few health care businesses) are recognizing this and are seeking broadly educated employees rather than those who are trained in technologies that will rapidly become obsolete. The recent publication *Essentials of College and University Education for Professional Nursing* by the American Association of Colleges of Nursing (1986) supports this concern. Even a cursory examination makes nurse educators wonder how this essential content can be achieved in eight semesters!

Other disciplines that educate "professionals" at the baccalaureate level are also questioning the validity of their efforts. For example, engineers are examining the wisdom of an engineering education at the baccalaureate level (Gray, 1986; Keyser, 1987; Walker (1987).

Historically nurses prepared for leadership positions at the baccalaureate level only because the vast majority of nurses were diploma-prepared. With the rapid increase in science, psychosocial, and bio-medical knowledge, nursing education moved into academic settings. Nurses prepared in this academic setting were generalists. Since 4 collegiate years are utilized to prepare a nurse to function as a generalist in a variety of settings, preparation for leadership and specialization has necessarily become a function of the graduate level.

The Student of Tomorrow

A fourth turning point is the changing student body. Students are questioning the tuition costs of obtaining a BSN versus the salary compression now faced in the workplace, since they can become an RN by a shorter, less expensive route. Since 1980, the cost of attending college has risen at twice the inflation rate. The American Council on Education predicts that college fees will continue to outpace inflation by as much as 30% for the next few years (Brimelow, 1987).

Schools of nursing are beginning to recognize that nontraditional or adult learners constitute the largest future applicant pools. In the decade 1975 to 1985, the undergraduate rate of growth for the 18 to 22 age-group (22%) was exceeded by almost twice that rate by the older 25 to 34 age-group.

Finally, many future nursing students will be older and nonwhite. Hodgkinson (1985) expresses concern that by 2005, one in three Americans will be a minority—black, Hispanic, or Asian. Tomorrow's students will come with varying levels of skills and interest. They will make the decision to enter technical or professional schools of nursing from a career point of view. They will recognize that a change from technical nursing to professional nursing is a career change, requiring a different educational experience.

For years, nursing has spoken of "articulated" programs, in which a licensed practical nurse program constitutes about half of an associate degree program, and an associate degree program is about half of a baccalaureate program. Harsh examination indicates that the "articulation" concept exists only in the minds of educators, and that it is virtually impossible to give an associate degree in four semesters, followed by a baccalaureate degree in four more semesters. Students have been advised into educational paths that have involved costly rework, because lower division, associate degree nursing courses are not automatically transferrable as upper division baccalaureate courses. One realization that must be drawn from this dilemma, however, is that such devices as alternative learning experiences, credit by examination mechanisms, and others, which allow a student to achieve advanced standing by demonstrating knowledge—regardless of how that knowledge has been obtained—are critical to our future professional education pathways.

Professional Level of Practice

A fifth turning point is the realization that the future pathway to nursing on the professional level is not the BSN. The BSN is neither fish nor fowl—it produces neither a liberally educated citizen nor a specialty-oriented professional. The future of nursing belongs to the following two categories of nurses: (a) the technical nurse, educated at the associate degree level (with curriculum content refurbished to provide less of the liberal arts and more of the essential technical knowledge base needed for hospital, nursing home, and home health care); and (b) the professional nurse educated at the specialist postbaccalaureate (liberal arts and science) level.

The future may also see liberal arts colleges teaming up with professional schools of nursing to offer 5-year programs leading to an MSN as the first professional degree. The professional nurse of tomorrow will first and foremost be at the patient's side, well-grounded in patient care skills. Additionally this nurse will possess the management and communication skills needed to care for the patients and families of tomorrow.

Moribund Titles

A sixth turning point is the acceptance of the fact that the complex and rapidly changing patient-care acuity levels of today's multisetting health care delivery systems has caused the old titles of clinical nurse specialist (usually hospital-bound) and nurse practitioner (usually found in ambulatory settings) to become meaningless. Nurses with the titles of clinical nurse specialist are already working in community settings and have already developed the nurse practitioner skills of health assessment and physical diagnoses. At the same time, the nurse practitioner utilizes assessment and physical diagnoses skills to care for acutely ill patients in hospitals. The graduate curricula of today are moving toward a graduate who has expertise in *advanced practice roles*, one who moves freely among a variety of roles including the traditional clinical nurse specialist role and the traditional nurse practitioner role.

The Workplace of the Future

The seventh turning point is the changing workplace. At the NCNIP conference, "A View of the Immediate Future" (1986) there were identified five major forces that will shape nursing's role in the future health care environment: (a) shifting payment systems; (b) increasing aged population; (c) increasing competition among health care providers; (d) increasing complexity of patient needs and acuity; and (e) increasing government involvement in cost containment. These are discussed in more depth in the document itself.

CONCLUSION

As the complexity of care requirements increased, the ratio of registered nurses to other staff has increased ("Sixth Report," 1988.) The need for broadly educated nurses prepared for advanced practice roles, assisted by technical nurses and other types of workers who are assigned to the nurse, not the task or patient, seems obvious.

The turning points in the nursing profession are coming together, demanding change. If we do not differentiate nursing practice in both clinical agencies and educational institutions, others will implement models of care delivery that will continue the fragmented patient care system that now exists and nursing's contributions will be further reduced and confused.

REFERENCES

American Association of Colleges of Nursing. (1986). *Essentials of college and university education for professional nursing: Final report*. Washington, DC: Author.

Brimelow, P (1987). The untouchables. *Forbes, 140*(12), 7–11.

Carter, M (1986). The professional doctorate as an entry level into practice. In *National League for Nursing Perspectives 1987–89* (pp. 49–52). New York: National League for Nursing.

Conway-Welch, C (1986). School sets sights on bold innovations. *Nursing and Health Care, 7*(1), 21–25.

Gray, P (1986, December 3). *Chronicle of Higher Education*, p. 42.

Hodgkinson, H (1985). *All one system*. Washington, DC: The Institute for Educational Leadership.

Keyser, SJ (1987, July 19). Future engineers getting more humanities requirements. *The New York Times*, p. 26.

National Commission on Nursing Implementation Project (NCNIP). Invitational conference. (1986). *A view of the immediate future*. Milwaukee: Author.

National Commission on Nursing Implementation Project (NCNIP). Invitational conference. (1987a). *Timeline for transition into the future: Nursing education system for two categories of nurse*. Milwaukee: Author.

National Commission on Nursing Implementation Project (NCNIP). Invitational conference. (1987b). *Characteristics of professional and technical nurses of the future and their educational programs*. Milwaukee: Author.

Sakalys, J, & Watson, J (1986). Professional education: Post-baccalaureate education for professional nursing. *Journal of Professional Nursing, 2*(2), 91–97.

Sixth report to the President and Congress on the Status of Health Personnel in the United States (Publication No. HRP0907200). (1988). Washington, DC: US Department of Health and Human Services, Public Health Service.

Walker, E (1987, December 2). Our engineering schools must share the blame for declining productivity. *Chronicle of Higher Education*, p. A52.

✳   EDITOR'S QUESTIONS FOR DISCUSSION   ✳

What critical factors are in play that may be associated with the declining enrollment in schools of nursing? What effects and impact have the increase of part-time students had on curricula, the quality of nursing education, the preparation of the nursing student for professional practice, attitudes, and values held by those graduating from programs? How valid are the four "flawed" assumptions indicated by Conway-Welch?

How can some nursing programs resolve the issues concerning the influence and impact of state legislatures and higher education commissions on the type of nursing programs and curricula that are offered? What specific strategies can be offered to educate legislatures and politicians concerning professional requirements for nursing practice and appropriate nursing education needs? What data would be valuable to maintain and offer for effective discussions, and negotiations with higher education commissions, politicians, and state legislatures? To what extent is there an increased demand for nursing services and not a nursing shortage? What evidence is there that the demand has increased? What are the factors contributing to an increased demand?

Compare this chapter with those written by Rapson (Chapter 10), Duffy (Chapter 12), Fitzpatrick and Modly (Chapter 13), and Watson and Bevis (Chapter 14) regarding the types of programs and models that provide the best preparation for entry into professional practice. What data are available for support of Conway-Welch's statements concerning articulation programs? What is the difference between articulation programs and alternative learning experiences, as suggested by Conway-Welch? What are the advantages and disadvantages in offering the first professional degree in nursing at the graduate level? Might this type of model be discussed as a "bypass" (baccalaureate) master's degree? What assumptions and implications are inherent to and critical for the development of nursing as a profession in bypass-type programs? What is the rationale for expecting a shortage of baccalaureate-prepared nurses and an oversupply of associate-degree-prepared nurses? What specific measures should be implemented to prevent the decrease of nurses during a transition period from multiple types of programs for entry into professional practice to one type of program? How can new models of care delivery be a basis for demanding new types of educational programs for entry into professional practice? How can two separate levels for the practice of nursing be developed and implemented and an effective transition period be planned and implemented? What strategies and processes can be offered to differentiate preparation for professional practice, outcomes of programs, skills and knowledge base that are developed, job descriptions, and licensing examinations?

Appendix

TIMELINE FOR TRANSITION INTO THE FUTURE NURSING EDUCATION SYSTEM FOR TWO CATEGORIES OF NURSE

The Timeline for Transition into the Future Nursing Education System for Two Categories of Nurse graphically projects (1) nursing education programs today and their transition into the 21st century and (2) a timeline which reflects changes that have been in process and the timing needed to complete the process while maintaining an adequate supply of qualified nurses.

As noted on the timeline, there are presently four types of preparation leading to two types of licenses to practice nursing. Today, preparation for LPN or LVN licensure is currently at the vocational level. Preparation for RN licensure includes the associate degree program with a two-year completion, the diploma program, a three-year course of study usually associated with a hospital, and the college programs offering nursing preparation at the baccalaureate, masters, or doctoral level.

Predictions of the future suggest that there will be dramatic changes in the nature and intensity of nursing care to be delivered. Expansion of technology, a multiplicity of health care settings providing care, and an increase in the aged population with needs for multisystem care, will all affect the type of nurse who will be needed. It is within this framework that the two categories of nurse will evolve from that which now exists.

The expectation that two categories of nurse will evolve from the present four is based on the socio-economic health care picture that calls for the creation of more cost-effective systems of education. At present the four types of educational programs for nurses are costly because the system prepares nurses in programs with significantly different outcomes and varying levels of ability. These graduates are then employed in a health care delivery system which uses them as if their abilities are the same. The consumer is unaware of the qualifications of the nurse caring for him/her and the health care system is often not using each nurse to the level of his/her ability. An educational system which consists of four programs that prepare four categories of nurse, only to provide care either as a registered nurse or a licensed practical nurse, is not cost-effective from either the educational or service perspective. The current nursing education system is inefficient and inadequate to meet future health care needs.

Description of the Timeline

The graph entitled "Timeline for the Transition into the Future Nursing Education System for Two Categories of Nurse," illustrates systematic transition from the present nursing education system to a nursing education system of technical and professional programs for the future. It identifies timelines for transition or closure of programs, including time for curriculum development and transfer of resources while maintaining an adequate supply of nurses. These timelines are approximate, recognizing that transitional periods will vary from state-to-state.

According to the plan, licensed practical/vocational nursing programs are expected to continue their transitions. Programs now in existence will determine the best use of their resources. This may include developing an associate degree program or closing the program and diverting the resources to another nursing education program. The transition period also allows time for nursing faculty to seek advanced education, if needed, and to prepare for teaching in other programs. The transition of licensed practical/vocational nurse programs is expected to be completed by 1992.

Diploma programs in nursing are expected to continue the transitional phase that has been underway for many years. The timeline projects the conclusion of this process before the end of the century. Present programs will determine the best use of their re-

Timeline for Transition into the Future
Nursing Education System for Two Categories of Nurse (continued)

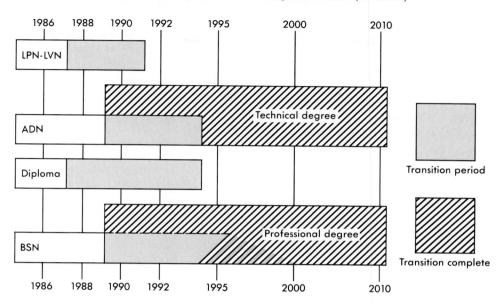

sources. It is recognized that these programs have a proud history of preparing nurses for their communities. The strengths of these programs should be considered when determining the best mode of change. For some, transition to an associate degree or baccalaureate program in cooperation with a junior or senior college may be feasible. For others, use of the clinical resources and faculty by associate or baccalaureate degree programs may be an option.

Present associate degree programs will determine the best use for their resources. The plan for transition will allow for present programs to design curricula to prepare the technical nurse, as described in "Characteristics of Technical Nurses of the Future." In other instances, depending upon the institutional resources and mission, nurse educators may see a need to phase out an associate degree program and develop a program leading to a baccalaureate or graduate degree in nursing.

The transition, reflected in the timeline, will require national and regional coordination to assure that the changing needs of clients and health care systems will be met by qualified nurses. The transi-

tion period will afford nursing faculty the time and opportunity to seek advanced degrees where necessary.

The professional educational programs of the future will be different than the baccalaureate programs of today. The timeline for transition allows time for the present educational programs to design curricula to prepare the professional nurse of the future as defined by the needs of the practice setting and reflected in the "Characteristics of Professional Nurses of the Future."

It is possible that additional time and degrees beyond the baccalaureate may eventually be required for education of professional nurses as described by the future professional nurse characteristics. Some baccalaureate programs may choose to refine and extend their programs to develop those characteristics more fully in their students. Some schools may choose to institute generic masters or doctoral programs.

Critical to any change in the nursing education programs of this country is the assurance that nurses, particularly professional nurses, will be prepared in sufficient numbers to meet the nation's needs. It is imperative that an adequate supply of professional and technical nurses be maintained according to need projections and that individuals are allowed an opportunity to advance through the education system.

CHARACTERISTICS OF PROFESSIONAL AND TECHNICAL NURSES OF THE FUTURE AND THEIR EDUCATIONAL PROGRAMS

The characteristics of professional and technical nurses are basic descriptors of the graduates of nursing programs of the future. These characteristics follow from the nursing needs of patients and the health care environment of the year 2000.

Professional Nurses
Education

Educational programs to prepare professional nurses of the future will be different than those of today. They will consist of liberal education and nursing education components. Changing health care needs, an increased knowledge base and the impact of technology will stimulate the change in these educational programs. Professional nurses of the future will be graduates of baccalaureate or higher degree programs with a major in nursing.

Knowledge

The graduates of professional nursing programs of the future will have an understanding and appreciation of various disciplines; a broad perspective which will be achieved through study of multiple content areas. The knowledge base of the professional nurse will include the ability to think logically, analyze critically and communicate effectively. Professional nurses' scientific background will provide a distinction between observation and inference in scientific investigation. As liberally educated individuals, professional nurses will understand the influence of personal and social values on human behavior.

Nursing knowledge which incorporates all perspectives of nursing science as well as other disciplines will include theory, methods, processes and ways of knowing and understanding, analysis and study of human events and issues that are of importance to nursing. Professional nurses will integrate knowledge from liberal education and nursing and apply this knowledge in client situations.

Practice

Skills, values, accountability. Professional nurses will assume primary responsibility for assisting individuals, families and groups to attain their maximum health potential. Professional nurses will be skilled in nursing practice as caregivers, case managers, and problem solvers. These professionals will analyze health care data and diagnose problems for clients in all types of care settings.

Professional nursing practice will include direct care to clients in any setting as well as case management. Encompassed in the direct care of patients, professional nursing practice will include counseling, health education, and the delegation and evaluation of nursing practice. In coordinating care between patients and existing health care services, professional nursing practice will include adjusting plans for the delivery of nursing care and engaging informal support systems and necessary resources. Professional nursing practice will also include nursing administration, education, and research. Professional nurses will make decisions regarding nursing care and develop policies, procedures, and protocols as guidelines for the provision of nursing care.

The Code of Ethics developed by the profession will provide the framework that guides the decisions and behavior of professional nurses in the clinical situation. Professional nurses will develop systems and ethical standards that govern professional and personal behavior.

Professional nurses will be accountable for all aspects of nursing care and evaluating the outcomes of care delivered. Professional nurses will be directly accountable and responsible to the patient for the quality of nursing care delivered.

Technical Nurses
Education

Educational programs to prepare technical nurses of the future will be different than those of today. They will consist of general education courses and natural and behavioral sciences which support the nursing component of the program. Changing client needs, increased knowledge base and the impact of technology will stimulate the change in the educational programs. Technical nurses of the future will be graduates of associate degree programs in nursing.

Knowledge

The graduates of technical nursing programs of the future will have an understanding of the common effects of attitudes, beliefs and values of health behavior. The knowledge base of technical nurses will be used for understanding patient's problems from biological, social and psychological perspectives. The knowledge base of technical nurses will emphasize facts, concepts and principles, demonstrated relationships and verified observations. Nursing content for technical nurses will include a well-defined body of established nursing skills and knowledge which is applied in a problem solving way as technical nurses care for individuals and their families experiencing usual, well-defined problems.

Practice

Skills, values, accountability. Technical nurses will be caregivers and participants in developing the plan of care for patients with well-defined health or illness problems.

Technical nurses will be responsible for organizing the individualized care of patients, prioritizing client needs effectively and implementing care efficiently. Coordination and direction of nursing care will be facilitated through the use of policies, procedures and protocols developed by professional nursing. Technical nursing practice will include providing patient care in a structured environment, implementation of the teaching plan, management of an individual plan of care and data collection for the evaluation of nursing care. Technical nurses make decisions about the care of individual clients by applying tested criteria and norms.

The Code of Ethics developed by the nursing profession will guide the actions of technical nurses in the clinical setting.

Technical nurses will be accountable for their own actions in the care of patients within the total context of the nursing plan of care using protocols or standards developed by professional nurses. Technical nurses will be responsible and accountable to the patient for nursing care delivered.

The entire Appendix is reprinted with permission by Vivien DeBack, Ph.D., National Commission on Nursing Implementation, 3401 South 39th St., Milwaukee, WI 53215.

REFERENCES

American Nurses' Association (1981). *Educational preparation for nursing: A source book*. Kansas City. ANA Publication No. NE-105M 4/81.

American Organization of Nurse Executives Staff. (1986, July/August). Maine passes model legislation on educational requirements. *The Nurse Executive*, 9–10.

Council of Associate Degree Programs. (1978). *Competencies of the associate degree nurse on entry into practice*. New York. National League for Nursing No. 23–1731.

Council of Baccalaureate and Higher Degree Programs. (1979). *Characteristics of baccalaureate education in nursing*. New York. National League for Nursing.

Hanner, MB (1985). Associate and baccalaureate degree preparation for future clinical practice in home health care. *Journal, NYSNA, 16*(4), 31–37.

Johnson, DE (1966). Competence in practice: technical and professional. *Nursing Outlook, 14*, 30–33.

Midwest Alliance in Nursing. (1985). *Associate degree nursing: Facilitating competency development, defining and differentiating nursing competencies*. Unpublished report. Dr. P Primm, Project Director.

New York State Nurses Association. (1978). *Report of the task force on behavioral outcomes of nursing education programs*. Unpublished by the Council of Nursing Education. Albany.

North Dakota Board of Nursing. 1986. *Administrative rules, article 54-03.1, requirements for nursing education program*. Bismark.

Stevens, BJ (1985). Does the 1985 nursing education proposal make economic sense? *Nursing Outlook, 33,* 124–127.

Styles, MM (1985, July). *The future market place, regulation of health care providers and education of nurses.* Paper presented at the conference on nursing in the 21st century sponsored by AACN, AONE, Aspen, CO.

Texas Nurses' Association. (1983). *Directions for nursing education in Texas 1983–1995: An operational plan.* Unpublished report of the council on education. Austin.

The Professional Preparation Project. (1986). *Seven liberal outcomes of professional study.* University of Michigan, Ann Arbor, MI.

Vermont Nurses' Association. (1985). *Vermont Registered Nurse, 51*(4).

Wisconsin Task Force. (1982). *Competencies of two levels of nurses.* University of Wisconsin-Madison.

66

The Maturing of Nursing Education in the Academic Environment

Claire M. Fagin, Ph.D., R.N., F.A.A.N.

This chapter serves as an overview of the important elements relevant to nursing's fit in academia. The principles that are discussed (and they must be looked at as principles rather than prescriptions) are chosen because they can be operationalized flexibly, in terms of the organization in which the academic leadership takes place. Rules for one institution may differ markedly from those of another. Discussion in this chapter is limited to college and university settings granting at minimum the baccalaureate degree. While principles having to do with fit and growth of the nursing enterprise exist in any setting, it is in the university that maturity problems are the most pressing. Thus stress is placed on this setting. The most salient points of the chapter have to do with assessment of the organization and of the nursing subset within it. To that end the author explores issues of where we were, where we are, and where we need to go.

WHERE WE WERE

During the first half of the 19th century, nursing's development in academia focused on the preparation of leaders of educational and service programs. In addition, "postgraduate" training for specialties such as public health and psychiatric nursing received emphasis after 1946 when the National Mental Health Act was passed. Nursing's fit in the academic environment was most appropriate in teachers' colleges. The few schools in colleges and universities that offered the baccalaureate degree in nursing had difficulty arranging for appropriate clinical experiences for students and attempting to "fit in" to the academic environment with other curricula in their institutions. In some institutions nursing faculty suffered from questioning of their credentials vis-à-vis other faculty and from derogatory views about the quality of their curricula compared with other disciplines. In other institutions, however, the credentials of faculty in general had not yet progressed to include the doctoral degree, and there was less certainty about curriculum issues. There the place of nursing was not as much of an issue and in some instances, because of nursing faculty's preparation in teachers colleges, their curriculum knowledge provided status.

In those institutions with nursing programs in which there were severe problems, issues surrounded not only the academic preparation of faculty but also a number of other concerns. These included questions of the body of knowledge that was the basis of the nursing curriculum, autonomy in control of curriculum, faculty scholarship, and relative achievement of faculty in nursing as compared with other faculty when reviewed for tenure. One or another of these issues pertained to all types of institutions; however, in institutions in which faculty credibility was not a concern, nursing programs and students were well accepted and nursing's equality could be established. This acceptance, seen in specific institutions with fewer pressures on faculty, should not cloud the main point of this chapter: the maturing of nursing education in the academic environment. The absence of pressure on the nursing faculty to move forward in scholarship affected the entire profession, since it limited the building of a group of accomplished investigators and scholars so necessary to a new and advancing discipline. This is particularly important as one recognizes that the majority of collegiate nursing programs were and are in small liberal arts secular and sectarian colleges rather than in universities.

Major changes took place in academic environments during the 1960s that significantly increased pressure on all faculty to engage in scholarly work and to publish. In the late 1960s, deans and directors of nursing programs were asked about their greatest problems and needs. In 1978, Hagopian reexamined these questions and found that over the 10-year period between investigations, the matter of obtaining and retaining faculty continued to be the single most frequently cited problem. The second-ranked problem was financial support and fiscal concern (Hagopian, 1979, p. 50).

This period was characterized by intense competition for the limited supply of credentialed faculty. The market for doctorally prepared nursing faculty was, and continues to be, excellent. However, until recently the demand for leadership positions in academic environments had to be met before widespread faculty development could occur. The development of the profession imposed a wide variety of leadership roles on the doctorally prepared nurse. Only when an institution could develop a cohort of such nurses was it possible to begin the process of maturing that was required for the nursing component to achieve equality.

Nursing has been underfunded in its academic development. Federal funding of the 1960s and 1970s helped schools to develop faculty and programs and to expand enrollment. However, Lysaught (1981) stated that

> fiscal problems remained a high priority for educational administrators. The reasons are many and complex, but among the causes are these: the unpredictability of federal funds and decisions; the higher costs attached to clinical teaching generally; [and] the long history of 'deprivation' in nursing education. (p. 109)

This list does not mention the need for support for nursing research, nor the absence of nursing research from public and private priorities as recently as 10 years ago.

Indeed as recently as 1980, the number of nurses who could devote themselves to a research career, rather than to the many other needs of a developing profession, was miniscule. Although recognizing its responsibility to provide for the teaching of a new, very different generation and improvement of the profession through higher education, faculties were less appreciative of the concomitant responsibility for both development of new knowledge and improvement of practice. As nursing became integrated into university life, faculties became aware of this latter responsibility, with all its ramifications; and in many university schools, nursing faculty set about both to prepare themselves and the next generation of investigators.

WHERE WE ARE NOW

Of the more than 643 nursing programs in the United States, 410 are members of the American Association of Colleges of Nursing (AACN, personal communication, August 30, 1989). Of the total number of nursing programs in the Fall, 1988, 84 were in academic health centers (overlapping colleges and universities), 243 were in 4-year colleges, 340 were in universities, and 7 were in external degree programs or consortium schools. Fewer than one-tenth of the university nursing programs have doctoral programs. (The small number of doctoral programs is fortunate, since even among these existing programs, some are ill-equipped from the standpoint of nursing faculty research and university graduate strength). Nursing's current fit in each of these academic settings varies widely, as do the requirements for faculty permanence.

As of the Fall, 1988, 38.9% of 7857 nursing faculty in baccalaureate and higher degree programs hold the doctoral degree (AACN, personal communication, August 30, 1989). This compares with 65.1% of faculty in general in 4-year colleges in 1984, as reported by the Council of Graduate Schools whose data were gathered by the Carnegie Foundation (American Council on Education, 1987). These data suggest that from the standpoint of credentials nursing is far from mature in the academic environment, as compared with faculty at large, despite having made considerable progress in the past decade. These data also pose serious implications for the possibility of scholarly research by large numbers of college and university faculty when the majority are themselves engaged in doctoral study. Ten years hence the picture will be very different, but nursing at this time, although maturing, is far from mature academically.

What percentage of nursing units in higher education require the doctoral degree for tenure or other permanent status is unknown at this time. However, among the faculty there is a growing group of leaders who provide excellence of teaching and leadership in the profession. Faculty development and the development of deans are major agenda items for national organizations, and nursing's acceptance of the need for such development is apparent.

The extent to which particular institutions value teaching varies. Some of them place less value on teaching, more on research; others have the opposite values. For nursing to mature as an academic discipline, nursing faculty must increase and improve their research capability. Nursing units in the major universities not only require the doctorate for consideration for tenure, but increasingly are requiring a substantial record of research accomplishment, including funding ability through some peer-reviewed

process. There is growing competition for faculty with such credentials, and capability for producing them through governmental initiatives is growing moderately. A recent foundation program focusing on postdoctoral training in clinical collaboration, research, and practice was exceedingly successful. This was evidenced in the output of its graduates, their current positions, and the competition that occurred to attract them as faculty. However, for the most part, the competition for the scholars who completed the program took place among a core of university schools that recognized the importance of the training and the need for expert clinician researchers in their settings.

In institutions in which teaching is valued highly in the reward structure, nursing faculty have demonstrated considerable achievement and are at least comparable with their nonnursing colleagues. The marketability of these faculty, despite fine teaching records, has been sharply reduced in recent years, however, as research credentials have become an imperative. It might be said that requirements for tenure have matured in academe before nursing's maturity level has reached comparable status. In too many instances up to this point, even when faculty members in nursing have achieved the doctoral degree, the weak research emphasis in their programs has limited their subsequent research activities. Faculty differences in scholarly qualifications among the institutions offering baccalaureate and higher degree programs in nursing mirror the diversity in the nursing population in general. It seems that multiple educational preparation levels confound nursing in all its aspects.

Currently nursing educators are showing great interest in enhancing their clinical skills and finding ways to retain and reward expert clinicians. At the University of Pennsylvania a clinician educator track has been developed for fully credentialed (doctorally prepared) faculty whose major interests lie in clinical practice and who also make a significant contribution to the educational program. These individuals must be promoted to the associate professor rank and maintain a significant role to achieve permanence. A great deal of interest has been generated by this "standing faculty" position, judging by the quantity of correspondence asking for the job description.

Other types of appointment are utilized at Penn and other major universities for faculty who are not members of the fully credentialed, permanent staff. These include part-time appointments in clinical, or adjunct status at appropriate ranks, and short-term appointments in the academic support staff for faculty who do not hold the doctoral degree.

The problems that nursing is currently facing with regard to the drastic decline in its applicant pool must be mentioned in the context of maturing in the academic environment. Between the academic years 1984-1985 and 1988-1989 there was an approximate 31.9% drop in enrollment of baccalaureate students. During the same time period there was a 5.6% decline in full-time and a 14.7% increase in part-time enrollments of master's degree students (Division of Research, National League for Nursing, personal communication, August 30, 1989). The administrator's latitude and flexibility are sharply reduced in such a climate. Difficult decisions must be made in the nursing unit, and the college and university administrations are concerned about nursing's viability over the long haul. Several important schools and programs are closing or have closed, and others are examining changes that will have long-term implications for their own settings and for the profession. Gasping to stay alive may hinder or help the maturing process, depending on one's point of view and particular location. In an unfriendly atmosphere, the decline of the nursing population will cause some actions to take place that would have been delayed or deterred in a successful climate. In other situations, the decline in student numbers may present opportunities to rethink the mission of the nursing unit. Likewise strategies for accomplishing this mission may be considered to maximize the school's survivability and excellence during a downturn in enrollment. Seeking more stable sources of funding and increasing the faculty's research capability are high priorities during this time. This entire subject requires very careful analysis and planning in specific schools and in national forums. Nevertheless, it is mentioned here since it is in no way separate from the topic of the chapter.

Assessment of the fit of the educational program in its specific environment, integration of students in university life, and participation of faculty in governance of the school and the university are all indicators of the current level of maturity of the nursing unit.

WHERE WE NEED TO GO

First, the present state of the discipline of nursing demands the minimum of a baccalaureate degree as preparation for entry into professional practice. University programs basing their clinical course content on a broad liberal arts and science foundation prepare nurses for generalized practice and access to advanced preparation in clinical specialties. Second, the majority of faculty teaching at all levels, whether the school has a doctoral program or not, must hold the doctoral degree. In a clinical field such as nursing, it is to be expected that expert clinicians prepared at the master's level will be a vital part of the clinical education of students. However, those faculty in the permanent classification of the college or university must hold the recognized academic credential for teaching at that level. Third, the dean plays a major leadership role in moving the school and its faculty forward in its maturing process. The dean is a planner, energizer, and initiator who takes actions, accepts risks, and is accountable (Claus & Bailey, 1977). Fourth, all faculty—but particularly the senior faculty—have a role in planning for the future and in helping the school actualize these plans. Fifth, the maturing of nursing in the academic environment requires that nursing faculty develop and maintain a significant research agenda; this includes engaging in research, seeking and gaining funding for this work, and publishing results.

To get where we ought to be in the coming years requires looking hard at all the components of our academic environment and developing a rationalized way to prepare for the desired future. At the same time, a minimum set of essential goals must be established, since all the goals we would *like* to meet may not be possible to achieve. Planning should not be a wish list, but rather a clear statement of objectives as they relate to the components of the organization and the intellectual directions essential for the school. Furthermore the strategies for meeting these goals need to be described, and a realistic calendar for their achievement stated.

A consensus generally has developed regarding planning in higher education, which has been codified by Millett (1977). Millett assumes that human beings can modify their environment and react to it in rational ways, leading to improved institutions. Elements involved in planning are applicable to all organizations, including nursing units in specific academic environments as well as the nursing profession as a whole. In a university setting, it is assumed that faculty will be part of planning for the future and that there will be considerable consensus building concerning the unit's goals, objectives, and strategies. Nursing's maturing in academe is a natural focus for strategic planning, since the component parts of the planning process will lead to a recognition of the strengths and weaknesses in the current programs and a practical, intellectual look at the possibilities for change.

For example, every planning document proceeds from the statement of a mission that overarches the institution. Is the nursing mission of the future congruent with the parent institution? Does it go beyond the mission of the parent institution? Is it too limited? What does the recent history of the nursing unit tell planners in terms of improvements for the future? To what extent are our hopes reasonable, in light of the background of the institution? Demographic and societal trends are important external factors in planning, as are the internal factors stated above. Clear statements of program objectives as they relate to the components of the organization, of strategies, and of budgetary strengths or weaknesses for accomplishing the objectives and operationalizing strategies must be examined at the start.

A detailed plan with realistic and documented strategies for academic nursing units, or for the profession, can be of enormous use in eliciting the interest of others, outside of nursing, in helping to accomplish the stated goals. The necessary condition for this to be effective, of course, is that the goals are consonant with others' views of nursing—its

problems, strengths, and needs—and are appropriate for meeting societal needs.

For the nursing faculty to reach maturity in its academic environment, it is important for the faculty and administration of the school to have similar goals and commitments that are also congruent with those of the parent organization. Tenure, other faculty tracks, reward systems, and programs must fit in the institution and be calculated to advance the nursing unit toward meeting its goals. Regardless of the particular institution, nursing's goals must include the identification and development of leaders because of "the shortage of leaders required to accomplish nursing's agenda in research, practice, and education" (Fagin & McGivern, 1983, p. 210). Furthermore the need to focus on superior teaching—including maintenance of clinical expertise when this is related to the teaching area—is crucial in the coming decades, whether or not the faculty member is actively involved in a research agenda. A refocus on the importance of senior faculty involvement with undergraduate students is in order as we look ahead. During the past decade, there has been a growing tendency among senior, doctorally prepared faculty to prefer teaching assignments on the graduate (preferably doctoral) level. Fagin and McGivern (1983) assert:

> This is a pernicious problem with potentially dire long-term effects. . . . Steps to alleviate this problem must be identified if . . . expectations include the offering of high quality programs at every level and the recruitment of students into graduate programs from an undergraduate population. (p. 211)

The clinician educator role in the permanent faculty was discussed previously. This type of appointment is extremely important for academic nursing programs. The demands of a clinical profession often militate against the development of a research career, as is common in other academic disciplines. Regardless of its quality, substitution of clinical or descriptive writing for research will not advance the profession in many academic settings, particularly in university centers. Yet learning experiences for nursing students demand the expert clinician who has significant faculty status and power. It is important for nursing to develop a wide spectrum of collaborative models to "facilitate the sharing of practice and teaching roles," (Fagin & McGivern, 1983, p. 213) and research.

Changes in the size of the nursing unit, because of downturn in enrollment, provide opportunities for strategic planning. Choices are either to downsize the faculty component or to strengthen the faculty capability to obtain external funding for research and educational programs. It is crucially important that the downturn in student interest does *not* lead to a lessening of requirements for the student body, since the principle of fit with the parent organization must be maintained. Thus far, the schools of nursing that have closed have been those that showed not only a drop in numbers, but also those whose students were said to be of lower quality than the parent institution. Admitting a class with markedly lower standards may seem like an attractive option to maintain size, but should be avoided. Instead strategies for handling the reduced numbers should be developed.

Unless there are significant changes in national priorities, the competition from well-received proposals for program funds will continue to exceed available dollars. Downsizing the faculty will give some schools welcome opportunities to strengthen the faculty and programs in light of current and future needs; for this, there must be some latitude among the faculty for qualitative retrenchment. Each program should be carefully examined from the standpoint of professional, societal, and school needs, and faculty should be helped to assess their own careers and be guided to subsequent choices. Internally, faculty development must include discussion of priority areas for development both of the nursing unit and of individual faculty. Likewise the reward system for achieving these priorities needs to be made explicit. Rewards that may be available to further goals are promotions, tenure, salary increases, work load reductions, space, and leaves to pursue scholarly work. Deans may be less or more free to use such rewards, depending on the parent institution. In the case of promotion and tenure, most deans have considerable latitude in choosing whether to support recommendations of the school committee. It would be hard, if not impossible, to make a case for granting tenure to a nursing faculty member without a doctorate (unless Florence Nightingale were to be reincarnated) in the coming years. Furthermore, more universities will expect evidence of scholarship in the form of research and publications in refereed journals. Fagin and McGivern (1983) state that "permanence in one's position should be granted only under the most exceptional circumstances which provide evidence that one will continue to grow and produce" (p. 255).

Throughout the country, schools of nursing in major university settings must develop independently funded investigators. The development of research will alter nursing's image both within the university and external to academia; the latter is essential to attracting bright women and men to the profession. Nursing's possibilities for research funding have improved recently, although the level of available support may become problematic as nursing's competence increases. The advent of the National Center for Nursing Research (NCNR) was a wonderful accomplishment for nursing and its congressional advocates. However, given the needs of the field, the Center is insufficiently funded if it is to build its research enterprise to an appreciable extent. (In 1989 the appropriation for NCNR totaled over $29 million. Dental research received $130 million, and the newest institute established in 1989—the Institute of Deafness and Other Communicative Disorders—received over $92 million.) Until recently, it was close to impossible for nurses to compete successfully in the National Institutes of Health (NIH) and at the National Institute of Mental Health (NIMH). In recent years, task forces were appointed for both NIH and NIMH to examine nursing research. In both instances the task forces were interested in ways of increasing nursing's participation in the extramural activities of the Institutes. Strong recommendations were made to focus on preparing nurse researchers, supporting research careers, and providing linkages for current nurse researchers through existing and new mechanisms. These recommendations, if operationalized and coupled with funding available from the NCNR, should assist in the maturing process of the nursing faculty in the academic environment.

Several foundations have shown interest in promoting nursing's academic maturity. However, there have been no large-scale efforts directed at nursing research. Apparently, many foundations see the need for extensive support of medical research; this is evidenced in the breadth of the research topics fundable, the depth of institutional support, and the dollar amounts granted. Foundation support, added to the enormous federal support for medical research, has helped our medical colleagues to mature in the academic environment and to achieve respect equal to basic scientists. When criticisms of nursing's achievements are made, compared with the achievements of medical and basic science research, the lack of financial support from federal and private sources rarely is taken into account. Clearly the academic leaders in nursing must make their case both within the institution and external to it, in order for the nursing investigator to be appreciated within the profession and better supported by external groups. Clarity in the message of nursing research is a crucial aspect of this leadership role.

SUMMARY

The past, present, and future of nursing education's maturing in the academic environment have been examined in this chapter. A brief view was presented as to how nursing developed in academia, the problems of a practice field, underfunding, and the way the profession has had to use its small number of prepared leaders to develop itself further and to meet societal needs for nursing personnel. Further the author has examined where nursing is currently in its quest for academic equality, by discussing qualifications of faculty, the numbers of schools and

where placed, and the downturn in student interest in nursing. The clinician educator track for permanent faculty is emerging as an important trend. Finally necessary developments were posed for the future, to ensure that nursing matures in academe, specifically in the major university settings, which are the hallmarks of excellence in the United States. Major issues are the changing picture of academic expectations in the 1990s, the importance of strategic planning, reward building to advance goal achievement, and the importance of the clinical and research faculties. At least comparable quality in the educational offerings of the profession at all levels and in the research accomplishments of nursing faculty and administrators must be apparent in the coming years. It is essential that nursing programs and people achieve parity with other groups in university settings for the survival of each nursing unit, for the development of the profession, and subsequently for society.

REFERENCES

American Council on Education. (1987). *Fact book on higher education 1986–1987*. New York: Macmillan.

Claus, K.E., & Bailey, J.T. (1977). *Power and influence in health care*. St. Louis: C. V. Mosby.

Fagin, C., & McGivern, D. (1983). The dean and faculty development. In M.E. Conway & O. Andruskiw (Eds.), *Administrative theory and practice* (pp. 207–229). Norwalk, CT: Appleton-Century-Crofts.

Hagopian, G.A. (1979). *The nursing deanship: Administrative problems and educational needs*. Unpublished doctoral dissertation, The University of Rochester, Rochester, NY.

Lysaught, J.P. (1981). *Action in affirmation: Toward an unambiguous profession of nursing*. New York: McGraw-Hill.

Millett, J.D. (1977). *Planning in higher education*. Washington, DC: Academy for Educational Development.

✳ **EDITOR'S QUESTIONS FOR DISCUSSION** ✳

What mechanisms might be offered for increasing the number of doctorally prepared faculty in universities? What ethical obligations are there regarding faculty who are on a tenure track, have provided substantial quality service to a university, but are not doctorally prepared? How can doctorally prepared faculty continue to develop their clinical competency? Should there be different and separate criteria for tenure for faculty whose major expertise is clinical and major interest is clinical practice rather than research? What tenure criteria might be suggested for faculty who have or prefer clinical expertise more than research expertise that would be equitable with the rigorous research criteria commonly expected for faculty? How may dichotomous expectations most effectively be resolved that exist concerning the requirements for heavy teaching loads and establishing strong research programs? How can the issues regarding doctorally prepared faculty preferring teaching assignments at the master's or doctoral level rather than at the undergraduate level be resolved?

What potential issues or problems may need to be addressed in employing only doctorally prepared faculty for undergraduate programs?

What obligation and accountability does a dean of an academic unit have in establishing support systems, accountability mechanisms, and realistic standards in a school? How is planning most effectively developed for an academic university and for a school of nursing program? How can faculty be helped to increase their efforts in scholarship? What are the critical aspects of a faculty development program? What should the priorities be in planning faculty development programs? How might such programs be established, provided, and evaluated? How can strategies and mechanisms be encouraged or developed to establish realistic expectations for performance, productivity, and scholarship in academic settings? Who is primarily responsible for the establishment, development, maintenance, and evaluation of professional expectations and outcomes in academia?

67

Collaborative Models in Nursing Education and Practice-Service

Kathleen G. Andreoli, D.S.N., R.N., F.A.A.N.
Jane E. Tarnow, D.N.Sc., R.N.

Nursing has been challenged to implement creative models of effective leadership for nursing education and service. Now that challenge is even more intense, linked to nursing's ability to survive. Nursing must cope with a national nurse shortage, an unstable economic base, diminished student applicants, and minimal amounts of nursing research. In reviewing historical precedents for possible solutions to the forgoing problems. Mundinger (1988) found that the merits of reviving the formal partnership between nursing service and nursing education are apparent. Clearly the separation of service and education was essential during the first half of this century to prevent the then common exploitation of students in the service sector at the expense of their education, and to move nursing education into the mainstream of higher education. The academic respectability of nursing education, however, has become a reality. Now it is time once again to plan, develop, and implement a formalized organizational relationship between service and education on a national scale, since such systems have been proved to impact successfully on the problems mentioned above. In this chapter, three integrated models of nursing education and service are described and analyzed. Recommendations for future goals are provided.

THREE COLLABORATIVE MODELS

In the United States, there are over 400 schools of nursing within senior colleges and universities, yet only three academic health centers have emerged with experience operating organizational models of cooperation between nursing service and education. These three models have similarities and differences. For example, all are located in privately owned (as opposed to federal or state regulated) academic health centers, a major resource in this country for defining patient needs and for generating the knowledge, health manpower, and service models to address these needs. Two academic health centers own their teaching hospital, whereas one affiliates with an established separate teaching hospital. This ownership has major implications for the kind of organizational model that is successful, as noted below.

1. *Collaboration model*. This model supports separate administrations for the school of nursing and hospital nursing service. The agencies are owned separately; however, they function in-

Special thanks to Sheila A. Ryan, Ph.D., R.N., F.A.A.N., Dean and Medical Center Director of Nursing at the University of Rochester.

teractively. The collaboration model exists between Case Western Reserve University and the University Hospitals of Cleveland in Cleveland, Ohio.

2. *Unification model*. In this model the school of nursing and hospital share ownership; therefore, one administrator is appointed for the school of nursing and the hospital nursing service. The administrator of nursing interacts functionally with the administrators of medicine and administration. This model exists at the University of Rochester Medical Center in Rochester, New York.

3. *Unification and matrix model*. The ownership in this model is like the unification model in supporting one administrator for the college of nursing and the hospital nursing service. The administrator of nursing functions interdependently with the administrators of medicine and administration. This model exists at Rush-Presbyterian-St. Luke's Medical Center in Chicago, Illinois.

The history and progress of the foregoing models are described below.

Case Western Reserve University and the University Hospitals of Cleveland

In 1961 Case Western Reserve University and the University Hospitals of Cleveland initiated a project to develop and test new interinstitutional relationships that would effect change in the patterns of organization and function within each of the two institutions. The concept underlying the project was termed academic leadership for nursing. Case Western Reserve University set forth a trend of excellence in nursing leadership that would not be repeated again for the next 10 years. This concept held that all leaders of nursing in an academic health center must meet standards of academic credentials that were not usually required of nursing service leaders. This meant that academically qualified leaders in nursing were operational in setting standards of quality nursing care and for serving as role models within the service setting. The resultant change in leadership skill fostered the development of superior clinical settings, which in turn provided

an academic learning environment and a research climate for both staff and students. A unique organizational model was developed that provided a structure in which neither institution relinquished its independence, governing board, administration, or budget. Efforts were directed toward collaboration and mutual reinforcement.

The interinstitutional model increased interaction through three types of joint appointments: (a) *shared appointment*, with salary and division of time and responsibilities apportioned between the two institutions; (b) *associate appointment*, with the primary appointment in the school of nursing and an associate in nursing appointment in the hospital. There was no sharing of cost between the two organizations; the salary was paid by the school. (c) *Clinical appointment* for nurses in "mutually agreed upon" leadership positions in the hospital. There was no sharing of cost. The salary was paid by the hospital. The nurse was responsible for maintaining the quality of care to patients on units used for nursing student experiences (MacPhail, 1981; Schlotfeldt, 1981).

At this time the organizational chart for this collaboration model is not available since the model is in a state of transition. The organizational independence of the two nursing agencies is clear and the titles and appointments represent interinstitutional functional cooperation. In this model, however, there is no involvement of the medical school organizationally.

The University of Rochester Medical Center

In 1972 the University of Rochester established a unification model by changing the organizational structure to integrate the School of Nursing into the University and the Medical Center, with nursing leadership assuming authority and accountability for nursing education, practice, and research within both. In this model, the Dean of the School of Nursing is also the Medical Center Director of Nursing. The unification of practice, education, and research is represented by a system of academic, clinical, and associate appointments for faculty who have authority in both practice and education. It provides and supports an environment for faculty to participate fully

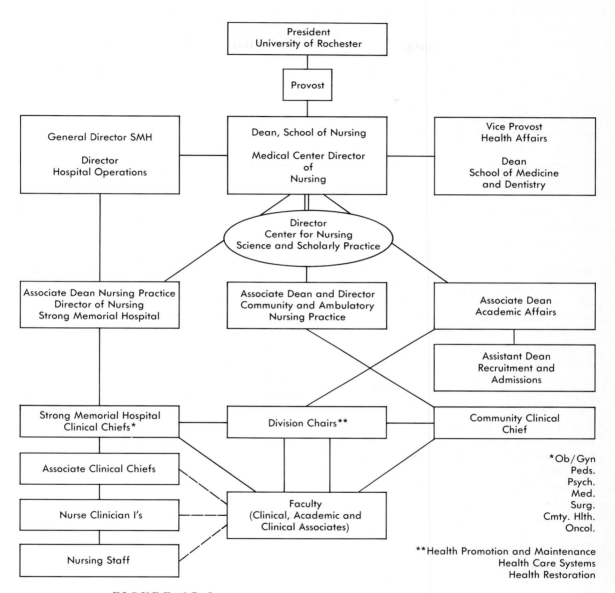

FIGURE 67-1

Unification model, University of Rochester. The authors are grateful to Sheila A. Ryan, Ph.D., R.N., F.A.A.N., Dean and Medical Center Director of Nursing at the University of Rochester, Rochester, New York for permission to reproduce the University of Rochester organizational chart.

in the clinical setting, patient care, and clinical nursing research of the university teaching hospital.

This change in organizational structure of the School of Nursing was designed to elevate the school to full status among the university's other schools and, particularly, to encourage articulation with the School of Medicine, by promoting joint decision-making at comparable levels within the hospital and medical center management structures. These disciplines share a common mission and have the common objectives of excellence in practice, education, and research, all at controlled costs. This common mission and support from both medicine and administration have created a climate for a center of excellence in nursing practice, education, and research at Rochester (Ford, 1981).

A recently modified organizational chart for this unification model (Fig. 67-1) suggests a new movement for clinical practice, research, and nursing science. Additionally, clinical faculty and chiefs may hold appointments throughout the community in primary care settings and in ambulatory and long-term care facilities.

Common features of the unification model that are peculiar to the University of Rochester and Rush-Presbyterian-St. Luke's Medical Center address faculty and nursing staff relationships. For example, nurses prepared at the master's level and above are eligible for faculty appointments. This means that a nursing budget for 1200 positions may include 200 faculty and 1000 staff nurses, thereby allowing for the provision of a large and diversified faculty for students. Budgetary differences do not inhibit collaboration and respect in the practice setting. On the contrary, the model provides for advanced clinical practice and research in the clinical setting.

Rush-Presbyterian-St. Luke's Medical Center

In 1972 Rush University, comprising a College of Nursing, Medical College, Graduate College, and College of Health Sciences, was created at the Rush-Presbyterian-St. Luke's Medical Center. Concomitant with the creation of the academic institution was the creation of the unification and matrix model for the administration of education and service across nursing, medicine, and administration. The unification of practice and education is reflected in the parallel titles of the administrators of nursing and medicine as the Vice President for Nursing Affairs and Dean of the College of Nursing, and Vice President for Medical Affairs and the Dean of the College of Medicine. The matrix management of the medical center is focused on health care delivery; authority for setting health care policy is relegated to, and shared by, the Vice Presidents for Nursing, Medicine, and Administration. In other words, these three administrators are coequal partners in management decisions. A vertical and horizontal administrative structure reflects position counterparts in nursing, medicine, and administration at the levels of vice president, associate vice president, chairperson of clinical departments, and unit leadership. Fig. 67-2 depicts the relationships that ensure nursing's access to articulation, decision making, and accountability across the disciplines.

Nurses with advanced preparation hold strategic positions utilizing the teacher and practitioner role. Doctoral preparation is required for positions from chairperson to the top of the organizational chart, and master's degrees are required (doctoral degrees preferred) for unit leaders. The decentralization of decision making, moreover, facilitates interdisciplinary communication, negotiation, and cooperation.

The Rush unification and matrix model assures that those who teach nursing also practice nursing, and this combination offers a substantive contribution to six essential components of a successful nursing program:

1. Quality of patient care
   a. Increases quality patient care directly by access to the best prepared practitioners, as well as indirectly through advanced-level teachers and researchers.
   b. Assures patients that their care is provided by professional nurses and is continually analyzed and updated through research.
   c. Assures comprehensive nursing care for patients and families, with understanding and self-involvement of those receiving care.
2. Quality of student education

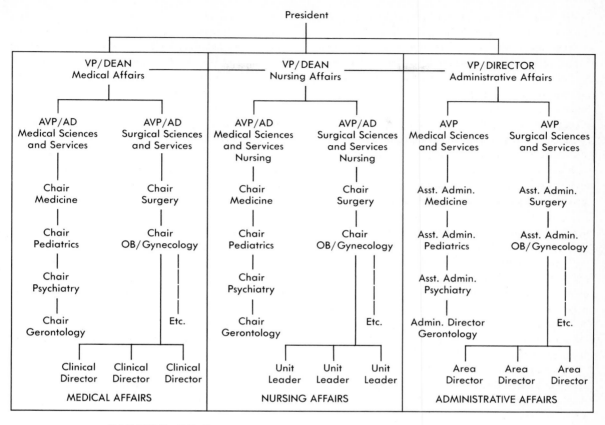

FIGURE 67-2

Unification/matrix model, Rush-Presbyterian-St. Luke's Medical Center. (AVP, Associate Vice President; AVP/AD, Associate Vice President/Associate Dean.)

a. Provides students direct access to patients for clinical experience. Patients are selected and cared for by faculty.

b. Enhances learning with clinically proficient faculty.

c. Affords a means to maintain a diverse and qualified faculty with low student to teacher ratios.

3. Opportunities for clinical nursing research projects on unidisciplinary and multidisciplinary levels

a. Makes available reality-based nursing problems for nursing research.

b. Provides opportunities for interdisciplinary research projects.

c. Offers opportunities for faculty, staff, and students to solve research questions together, as well as develop grants for support.

d. Facilitates the discovery of and dissemination of new knowledge.

e. Supports the testing and validation of new knowledge, thereby improving nursing practice.

4. Credibility of nursing faculty

a. Allows for expression of the full professional role of service, education, research, and consultation.

b. Provides the opportunity for students to observe and participate in quality nursing care with faculty as role models.

c. Implies that faculty can practice what they profess.

d. Keeps curriculum and faculty updated.

5. Development and productivity of nursing faculty and staff

a. Encourages team participation in curriculum development and research projects.

b. Encourages team participation in professional development conferences.

c. Provides built-in resources for consultation across clinical nursing specialties.

d. Supports and offers opportunities to pursue an advanced degree in a supportive environment.

6. Productivity and cost-effectiveness of academic health centers

a. Provides a mechanism for nursing service revenues to contribute to the educational program.

b. Makes academic consultation immediately available at no extra cost.

c. Sets expectations for nursing care innovations to be created and tested for effectiveness.

d. Allows for shared resources for budget, human resource services, marketing, recruitment, office space, and others.

Nature of Noncollaborative Models at Academic Health Centers

Major responsibilities of academic health centers are manifold: medical education, nursing education, hospital administration, nursing service, and research across all disciplines. In these centers the university and hospital may be under one board of trustees, administration, and budget. Alternatively, the teaching hospital may be affiliated with, but not owned by, the university. In academic health centers with noncollaborative models, nursing education programs and nursing services have separate organizational structures. Moreover, in these models, the school of nursing is often geographically distant from the hospital. That is, the school is often one to several city blocks away from the hospital. The dean in the school of nursing is responsible for the education of practitioners and administratively reports to the president of the university. The vice-president or director of nursing in the hospital is responsible for the provision of nursing care and administratively reports to the president or administrator of the hospital. Successful collaboration between these two nursing leaders, therefore, may be limited because there is no administrative tie and frequently no ideological unity. Since education and service are isolated, each develops separate statements of its mission, although some common features may occur between the two. Although there are examples of schools of nursing and hospitals that have shared interprofessional committees for nursing service and education, their programs for accomplishing the mission and goals of their respective institutions are often not synchronous. Herein lies the potential break in the collaborative relationship. Clearly, one administration facilitates unified planning, change, and growth in nursing education and service.

RECOMMENDATIONS

With only three formalized collaborative models in nursing education and service functioning over the last 16 years, one would assume that there has been no incentive for academic health centers to change their nursing administrations. The health care crises of the late 1980s give reason for a renewed interest in such models. Change is everywhere—new regulations, delivery systems, health manpower technology, financing mechanisms, and competition. Although decreasing admissions and length of stay have affected hospital revenues, the overwhelming problem to economic survival appears to be the nursing shortage. Hospital beds can only be open if there are enough nurses to staff them. Closed beds mean decreasing business for physicians and hospital administrators. Keeping nurses in the work force and assuring that there are adequate numbers of nurses coming through the educational system is the solution to this crisis.

Although a number of factors have been identified as causing the nursing shortage, the two that continually appear as the most influential are professional prestige and wages. The professional prestige for nursing associated with a unification model has been established in the previous pages. Moreover, the economic advantages of merging education and practice are (a) decreased expenditures through reduction of the number of nursing administrators; (b) the involvement of faculty in the delivery of patient care services and clinical research; and (c) shared support services. Such a system allows for efficiency of scale and thereby better wages for nurses. Moreover there is a high likelihood that the improvement of nursing's professional image and salaries will influence nurses to remain in the profession, as well as draw more applicants. With adequate numbers of nurses, hospitals will be able to meet their demands for bed occupancy; physicians will be able to admit patients to the hospital at a time convenient to them and to the patient; and the health care of the public will be assured. In addition, this projected scenario has positive ramifications for the noninstitutional sectors of health care where patients need nursing services, as well.

As noted earlier, academic health centers are the obvious site for such innovative change. The most logical places to begin are the nongovernment-regulated academic health centers that incorporate their own hospital and college or school of nursing. The choice of the unification model to be used (Rochester model or Rush model) would depend on the administrative politics, history, resources, and future plans of the organization. Whatever gives the best fit should be used.

In an academic health care setting in which the hospital is owned by another corporation, some form of a collaborative model may be the best solution. An innovative partnership for nursing education and service should be implemented. The Case Western Reserve University model has proved effective and should be considered and tested, if appropriate, in these settings.

With no other plausible solutions on the horizon for resolving the critical nursing shortage, there is good reason to embark on a plan for merging nursing service and education. Beyond being a solid fiscal and management decision, it will offer a means for providing a collaborative environment for clinical research, and trend-responsive high-quality nursing care that will satisfy patients and nurses alike.

REFERENCES

Ford, L. (1981). The University of Rochester model. In T. Kunan, L. Aiken, & L.E. Cluff (Eds.). *Nurses and doctors—Their education and practice* (pp. 69–83). Cambridge: Oelgeschlager, Gunn & Hain, Publishers.

MacPhail, J. (1981). The Case Western Reserve University model. In T. Kunan, L. Aiken, & L.E. Cluff (Eds.). *Nurses and doctors—Their education and practice* (pp. 95–101). Cambridge: Oelgeschlager, Gunn & Hain, Publishers.

Mundinger, M.O. (1988). Three-dimensional nursing: New partnerships between service and education. *Journal of Professional Nursing*, 4(1):10–16.

Schlotfeldt, R.M. (1981). The Case Western Reserve University model. In T. Kunan, L. Aiken, & L.E. Cluff (Eds.). *Nurses and doctors—Their education and practice* (pp. 85–94). Cambridge: Oelgeschlager, Gunn & Hain, Publishers.

✳ **EDITOR'S QUESTIONS FOR DISCUSSION** ✳

What are the differences in planning and decision-making processes for clinical practice and curriculum in the three collaborative models? What issue must be addressed and resolved in maintaining joint decision-making at comparable levels by two institutions? How is innate conflict that usually exists between professionals and bureaucracies effectively resolved through collaborative models? What indicators of quality could be suggested for measurement and evaluation concerning the six essential components of a successful nursing program? What evidence exists in the literature regarding the six essential components? Given the advantages indicated for collaborative practice, what data may be available to provide a method for costing out the direct and indirect care provided by nursing staff? How might unified planning, change, and growth be facilitated in nursing education and service for noncollaborative-type models at academic health care centers? What other types of collaborative models can be proposed? Why have there been only three formalized collaborative models in nursing education and service over the last 16 years? What data might be available to confirm or discredit hypotheses concerning the existence of collaborative models? What kind of support services might be shared when education and practice are merged? How might the number of nursing managers or administrators be reduced or increased when merging education and practice?

To what extent do collaborative models imply or require that one person is fulfilling the work and roles of two persons. How can burnout, and unrealistic expectations and demands be prevented in collaborative models? What criteria does a nurse use in a collaborative model for establishing and meeting priorities to fulfill multiple roles? What are the critical variables that need to be considered and addressed in planning, developing, implementing, and evaluating a collaborative model? How may an institution determine the fit of the model for its setting? To what extent should people determine the structure, or should structure determine what roles evolve and how people are to fulfill them?

68

The Development of Nursing Knowledge:
Accelerating the pace

Joanne S. Stevenson, Ph.D., R.N., F.A.A.N.

The development of knowledge for nursing has had a tortuous history. From the earliest dawn of human existence, physical care has been provided to women during childbirth and to infants, children, ill or injured adults, and the very old. From the beginning, women assumed the major responsibility for health care. It is still that way today. Historians suggest that this was a natural outgrowth of pregnancy and mothering (Ehrenreich & English, 1973; Jamieson & Sewall, 1942).

Women in early times invented many techniques of health care. They made discoveries about plants with medicinal properties, modalities to soothe or heal injuries, and techniques to relieve pain. Their approach was largely trial and error, but over a period of many centuries, a knowledge base slowly accumulated. The body of knowledge thus amassed was handed down by word of mouth and role modeling from the wisest of the older generation to the most promising young women of the next generation. In this manner, some women became the designated specialists to whom other women looked for expertise about birthing and care of the ill and infirm.

In the cultures that devised techniques for writing and preserving records, the content of the records is knowledge developed generally by men. These records focus almost exclusively on men's responsibilities including hunting, fishing, building, and mastery over dangerous animals or the elements. Perhaps because the activities and discoveries made by women were considered so mundane or natural, they much less often became part of the permanent cultural record. Through the golden ages of Greece and Rome, the Dark Ages, the Middle Ages, and even into the industrial era, women's contributions to society were not considered of equal significance to the contributions of men. Women did not receive education equal to that of men and consequently the knowledge amassed by women was not recorded for posterity. The outcome of this historical fact was that knowledge about health care throughout the ages has been considered a noncognitive activity. Deeply imbedded in the cultural legacy of humankind is the belief that the knowledge base for caring (including health care) comes from an inborn or intuitive sense. It is assumed that this intuitive sense is innate in all women, or most women to some extent, and to a greater extent in especially gifted women who "have the touch." This appears to be a very deeply ingrained belief, shared by both men and women.

Florence Nightingale is perhaps the exemplar of the fallacy of this myth. Nightingale was educated by her father as if she were a male offspring (Woodham-Smith, 1983). She was exceedingly privileged, for a woman, to receive a solid grounding in history, mathematics, and other classical subjects. Florence Nightingale used her unusual education coupled with her own superior intelligence to make numerous contributions to the development of knowledge about care and caring and to the professionalization of care providers, or nurses. However, she too was a victim of her culture, with its discriminatory attitudes toward women and toward the knowledge base for nursing. Nightingale did not leave any followers. In the programs she developed for nursing students, she did not select women of high natural intelligence and then educate them to be scholars, scientists, or innovators. Instead she developed an apprenticeship-training program for nurses and concentrated on producing trained personnel who would implement care modalities based on knowledge generated by others, tradition, and authority. These training programs were set in the apprenticeship mode of the trade occupations. When transferred to the United States, they became attached to hospitals as the site of training rather than to universities.

Through Nightingale, professional nursing captured the opportunity to become a recognized technical occupation requiring specialized education and apprenticeship. Simultaneously through Nightingale, nursing missed an opportunity to shift knowledge about nursing care from a secondary, knowledge-acquisition mode to a primary, knowledge-development mode.

The history of knowledge development in American nursing began to make a slow shift at the turn of the 20th century with the appointment in 1907 of Adelaide Nutting to the faculty of Teachers College, Columbia University (Jensen, 1955, p. 200). Progress was extremely slow; it was concentrated on improvement of the teaching and training of nurses to become beginning practitioners. The actions of the professional and educational associations in nursing exerted considerable influence on nursing education to improve curriculum and teaching practices. However, the science of care still was not recognized as a focus for nurses. Most of the nursing content continued to be obtained from other fields,

intuition, personal experience, tradition, and authority figures. This state of affairs persisted until the late 1940s.

DAWNING OF THE SCIENTIFIC ERA

The post–World War II years saw the dawning of a new age for nurses as scholars and for a new philosophical orientation toward care as a unique scientific field. The details of the massive changes in the collective self-concept of nurses, the multiple programs, the policy changes, the impact of forward-thinking individuals, the group networks, and the publications that brought the new age to fruition are discussed elsewhere (Stevenson, 1987). There was a slow evolutionary dawning of awareness that nursing care requires cognitive, rather than only intuitive, effort. Eventually the awareness emerged that new knowledge about care parallels the development of knowledge about any other phenomenon. This insight came too late for nursing, and its concern with the development of knowledge about care, to be included in the early period of the scientific activity of the other health sciences in the United States. Most notably, the development of knowledge about nursing care was not a designated component of the National Institutes of Health (NIH) during the first 98 years of its existence.*

Between 1982 and 1985, a massive informational-educational-political campaign staged by organized nursing came to fruition and a law was enacted (Health Research Extension Act of 1985, P.L. 99-158). This law transferred the nursing research program and predoctoral and postdoctoral fellowship programs from the Division of Nursing in the Department of Health and Human Services (DHHS) to the NIH in a semiautonomous unit called the National Center for Nursing Research (NCNR). The NCNR was officially established by Secretary Bowen of the Department of Health and Human Services on April 18, 1986 (Merritt, 1986). These actions signaled

---

*Briefly during the 1960s, the Nursing Research Grant Program was housed in the NIH's Institute of General Medical Sciences. However, it was moved shortly thereafter to the Health Resources Administration, Bureau of Health Professions, Division of Nursing, where it remained until 1986.

that development of knowledge about care belonged in the mainstream of the health science establishment.

BACKGROUND ON KNOWLEDGE DEVELOPMENT IN NURSING

Two long-standing criticisms about knowledge development in nursing have been the lack of systematic building of knowledge and the dearth of research utilization in practice. The remainder of this chapter addresses potential solutions to these two problems. If they can be solved, the pace of scientific work on care problems will accelerate and findings will be implemented in practice.

If one accepts the definition contained in the American Nurses' Association's *Social Policy Statement* (ANA, 1980) that nursing is "the diagnosis and treatment of human responses to actual or potential health problems," certain targets and parameters for nursing research logically follow. If, in addition, one accepts the Donaldson and Crowley statement (1978) that nursing is a practice discipline and that improved practice is the aim of knowledge building, scenarios that feature research utilization follow.

Weaknesses Inherent in Past Research Efforts

A criticism often voiced by NIH and other Public Health Service personnel is that nursing does not do "substantive" research. Many nurses refuse to take this criticism seriously. They argue that this criticism simply reflects a bias against a field that infrequently does bench research or animal research and does not concentrate on the "disease of the month."

There is another interpretation of these criticisms. It touches the core of a fatal flaw in nursing's past research. Jacobsen and Meininger (1985), in their 1956 to 1983 survey, found that 49% of the studies in three nursing research journals measured one point in time and 36% used questionnaires. These findings are only one form of corroboration that nursing research often has not been substantive. For too many years unvalidated paper and pencil instruments superficially skimmed the surface of nursing phenomena. In other studies, a morass of statis-

tics produced such a tangled complex of interrelationships that much heat but no light was shed on the phenomena of nursing. Still another problem has been the dearth of efforts at theory building that would provide the context for interpreting findings. Jacobsen and Meininger (1985) found that most published studies were one-time efforts rather than progress reports of long-term programs of research.

Many groups and organizations have developed priorities for nursing research (ANA, 1981; ANA, 1985; Brower & Crist, 1985; Dodd, 1987; Lewandowski & Kositsky, 1983; Lindeman, 1981; Marchette & Faulconer, 1986; McBride, 1987; Raff & Paul, 1985; Stevenson & Woods, 1986; Thomas, 1984). Unfortunately, many of these priority lists were not built on state-of-the-art assessments of extant knowledge. Most of them came from Delphi surveys or consensus-generating meetings; hence they were written at a broad level of generality. However, these priorities explicate major foci that make up the phenomena of concern to nursing (Stevenson, 1988).

A few people are currently engaged in doing critical reviews in nursing. Critical reviewers, especially those whose work appears in the *Annual Review of Nursing Research*, evaluate the extant knowledge and make recommendations about voids in knowledge that merit scientific attention. There is need for more clarity and consensus about the next logical stage in the evolution of research following a critical review.

MODEL FOR NURSING SCIENCE

A model is proposed that shows the progression of programs of research from the earliest phase of exploratory work to the most advanced stage of verification. It implies progressive development and crystallization of knowledge in a designated content area. The model continues through additional stages of evaluation in practice settings toward the end of widespread utilization by clinicians.

A schematic representation of the model is shown in Figure 68-1; it can provide a master plan and logistical map for investigators and critical reviewers to use. This model can be used to pinpoint the current stage of evolution in an area and give direction for the next logical phase of work. Career researchers would enter the stairway at a particular point in the evolution of their target-problem and be able to map out objectives and strategies for the next several steps. Critical reviewers could determine the current state of the art and recommend next steps toward the ultimate goal of use in practice.

Exploratory Research

Step 1, at the far left side of the Figure 68-1, represents an initial condition wherein very little knowledge has been developed in a problem area. It may be an old care issue or a new one produced by technology, or simply one that was not deemed important heretofore. Under these circumstances, qualitative approaches are posited as more appropriate than quantitative approaches. Qualitative research is best suited to separating the undifferentiated whole of the phenomenon into subsets (e.g., themes) of more

meaningful components as distinguishable from less meaningful components. The criterion for meaningfulness in a practice discipline such as nursing is any condition or situation potentially amenable to change through nursing actions.

Valid and reliable qualitative research promotes progress from the undifferentiated whole phenomenon to a beginning sense of what is more and what is less important for the science of care. Replications, perhaps using different qualitative approaches, different investigators, and different respondent groups, are equally necessary here as at any other step in the model. Once a "trustworthy" (Lincoln & Guba, 1985) set of findings are available, movement to Step 2 becomes appropriate.

Descriptive Research

The next stage is perhaps the most complex and lengthy stage of knowledge development. The ap-

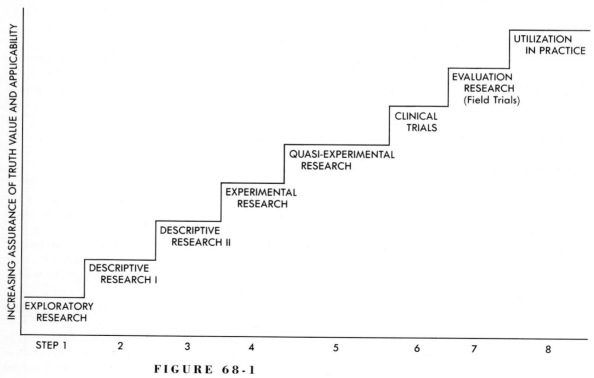

FIGURE 68-1

Steps of research development toward utilization in practice.

proaches that seem to be most fruitful at this stage are classic descriptive methods. Qualitative approaches remain valuable. However, since the goal is to build on findings from Step 1, increased specificity of the research questions is appropriate (unless there is reason to discount previous findings). Hence, qualitative studies should not reinvent the wheel, but should focus on potentially fruitful components of the whole. As shown in Figure 68-1, two steps were allocated (Step 2 and Step 3) to descriptive research. This choice was made to emphasize the complexity and critically important role of descriptive research. During Step 2, progress beyond the exploratory stage is evident but there is still too little known to trust purely quantitative methods. Therefore, more qualitative or open-ended forms of descriptive designs are in order during Step 2. In the second phase of descriptive research (Step 3), designs that feature more specificity, more quantification, larger samples, and attention to statistical analysis become appropriate. Correlational designs, ex post facto designs, regression approaches, or path models can be useful to test emerging theory and to determine how well it holds up with different subject groups and in various situations. Descriptive research can sometimes be speeded along through multisite studies or other forms of simultaneous-parallel work by two or more investigators. More systematization and orchestration of this stage of research is needed in nursing.

Descriptive studies serve the critically important purpose of differentiating the more or most important factors, characteristics, patterns, or variables from the less or least important ones. In studying phenomena at the complex levels with which nursing deals, the effort spent on descriptive research is extremely important. The quality, rigor, and completeness of work performed at this stage will make later stages much less vulnerable to major setbacks from contradictory findings.

Experimental Research

Eventually, descriptive research becomes redundant. After descriptive studies have uncovered sufficient knowledge and replications have shown relatively consistent results, it is time to move to the next phase. It then becomes appropriate to develop and test therapeutics, that is, new care protocols. The exploratory and descriptive phases should have produced predictive theories or theoretical propositions that can be further tested through experimental and quasi-experimental studies. The transition from descriptive studies to experiments requires decision rules. Often a critical need for therapies by a subpopulation or an economic imperative speeds decisions along (e.g., note the case of urinary incontinence in elders, Hadley, 1986). In ideal situations, a timely critical review can provide the impetus to move from description to experimentation.

Weaknesses of past experimental efforts

During the 1950s and early 1960s, experimental studies in nursing often resulted in conflicting or uninterpretable results. One explanation for this outcome is that many of these studies actually were "exploratory experiments." One observant professor at The Ohio State University called them "black box" experiments. He meant that the treatments were merely fishing expeditions that emanated from conventional wisdom or tradition. They were not built on adequate predictive theory derived through descriptive research. Hence, there was not an adequate base of theory to guide the formulation of the experimental phase of research. The most vivid examples in this author's memory were the many experiments testing myriad treatments for decubitus ulcers in the absence of adequate basic research about the nature of the underlying condition (Berecek, 1975).

Many challenges must be faced to implement the ambitious master plan in Figure 68-1. One major challenge is the development of valid measurement approaches. Most of the methodological work on paper and pencil instruments in nursing has focused on tools for exploratory or descriptive research. Minimal work has been done to create and validate instruments that measure effects of therapeutic interventions. Instruments borrowed from the social sciences are generally designed to measure static or trait attributes and are virtually useless for experiments. They are insensitive to the effects of nursing interventions. For example, the most frequently used instruments to measure anxiety, depression, life satisfaction, morale, self-esteem, self-concept, or health perception are rarely specific or sensitive enough to detect changes produced by nursing intervention.

Instruments borrowed from the biological sciences are sometimes sensitive to the effects of nursing interventions and sometimes not. For example, instruments developed for use with young adult athletes would require major redesign to be sensitive enough to detect changes in strength and flexibility in persons over 85 years old.

Developing new or redesigning existing instruments for nursing science is a time-consuming and expensive task. However, it is a challenge that must be met for the master plan in Figure 68-1 to be fully implemented.

A new era of experimental studies

Experimental testing of new care modalities is a goal of the immediate future in nursing science. The driving force of science is the constant discovery of new knowledge and the consistent creation of uses for this knowledge. The social mandate for a practice discipline dictates that new or untested therapeutic protocols be rigorously tested.

In Figure 68-1, Step 4 refers to experimental research and Step 5 is designated as quasi-experimental research. True experimentation is shown as preceding quasi-experimental studies. In general, more tightly controlled work precedes less tightly controlled work. Nevertheless, there are times when either or both designs may be adequate or appropriate depending on what is feasible within human subject considerations and administrative constraints. The essential idea is to achieve internally and externally valid studies of independent variables (to the extent that it is possible for quasi-experimental designs). These independent variables would be theory-based and descriptive research–based therapeutic interventions.

Another important research activity, although it does not explicitly appear in the model, is meta-analysis. The chapter in this volume by Devine describes this important approach to reviewing experimental research (see Chapter 24). Meta-analysis is particularly important for a practice discipline like nursing. The effect size of the experimental treatment across studies is critical to decisions for or against eventual adoption in practice. The cost-benefit question can be answered in a more logical and valid manner through meta-analyses of multiple studies.

One sophisticated and complex experimental design merits special attention in this discussion because it has rarely been used in nursing. This specialized form is the randomized control clinical trials method. Clinical trials are a natural next step on the stairway shown in Figure 68-1 as Step 6. Assume that moderate-sized experimental and quasi-experimental studies showed relatively consistent positive findings with different investigators, samples, and geographical locales. A clinical trial is the customary next step before widespread utilization. This is a safety precaution for the public. The use of clinical trials is well developed in certain medical specialties (Friedman, Furberg, & DeMets, 1985). Nursing, possibly through an NCNR funding mechanism, will doubtless become increasingly involved in clinical trials in the near future. The recent successes of five clinical trials of behavioral approaches to decrease urinary incontinence in the elderly bodes well for more general use of this approach in nursing (Burns, 1984; Fantl, 1984; Hu, 1984; O'Donnell, 1985; Schnelle, 1984).

Another strategy rarely used by nursing is multisite studies and consortium arrangements. This topic is addressed under Step 6 because it often is used by NIH in clinical trials. However, as a strategy to achieve rapid progress in uncovering unknowns in an area of high priority (e.g., acquired immune deficiency syndrome [AIDS]), it is equally appropriate during the exploratory and descriptive steps of the model. A fuller discussion of the significance for nursing and strategies to implement multisite studies and research consortiums appears elsewhere (Stevenson, 1988).

Evaluation Research

The final stage of research shown in Figure 68-1 as Step 7 is arbitrarily called evaluation research. Evaluation research refers to applied studies wherein investigators attend to the efficacy, utility, cost-benefit, and operational feasibility of a given protocol or program of care during day-to-day use in field settings. Even a comprehensive series of successful exploratory, descriptive, and experimental studies is not enough. There remains a question about the feasibility, pragmatic utility, and cost benefit of any therapeutic protocol in a specific type of setting such as a tertiary center compared with a community or rural hospital. There are also questions to be addressed about the numbers and sophistication level of clinicians required to implement the protocol successfully. Hence, evaluation of feasibility and local efficacy are necessary to the overall effort.

Evaluation research often depends on single-group experimental designs that Campbell and Stanley (1963) called preexperimental designs. Most such studies lack the controls built into quasi-experimental designs (Cook & Campbell, 1979). However, this situation is not really a weakness, since the goal is to determine whether the innovation works in one targeted setting. Generalizability is not the purpose of such studies.

KNOWLEDGE DISSEMINATION

Progress along each step of the staircase depends on many resources not explicitly stated in Figure 68-1. Some important resources include availability of a cadre of well-prepared expert scientists to do the work at each step; creative minds to derive theoretical formulations; monies, equipment, and other resources to support the effort; communication and networking so that persons working on the same problem can keep up to date on other researchers' work; and an adequate dissemination system for findings at each step.

There are several components to an adequate dissemination system: (a) a reasonable number of high-quality refereed journals that publish the findings in a timely fashion; (b) an adequate number of conferences, seminars, and other opportunities for neophyte scientists to practice giving presentations, for adequate networking to occur and for seasoned scientists to present work on the cutting edge and receive immediate critique; (c) a comprehensive,

valid, user-friendly literature searching system to facilitate rapid access to the full repertoire of past publications on a topic; (d) a reasonably up-to-date series of comprehensive and specific critical reviews; and (e) a reasonably comprehensive set of meta-analyses. While this list is idealistic, it is presented as part of the master plan. To visualize the full scope of the plan is important, even if the full complement of components may never be totally in place.

A historical review of nursing's dissemination system appears elsewhere (Stevenson, 1987). Much progress is evident in the maturation of research societies and sections, the growth of research journals and methods textbooks, and the use of newsletters to inform the nursing research community about research-related opportunities.

A significant stumbling block that remains to be addressed is the computer access to the literature. Too much of the nursing literature is not on-line and therefore not accessible through computerized searching services. A second problem is that the literature on-line has been categorized into a medically oriented thesaurus. Hence, natural nursing language cannot be used to scan the data base. This problem merits attention in the immediate future.

KNOWLEDGE UTILIZATION

The ultimate goal of scientific work in a practice discipline is use of the knowledge on behalf of clients. This step is shown as Step 8 in Figure 68-1. The literature on research utilization in nursing is relatively large. Unfortunately the impact of this literature on the practice of nursing has been nearly inconsequential.

The ideas espoused in the nursing utilization literature can be distilled into three major models. The oldest model postulates that staff nurses who participate in the conduct of research will be more likely to use research in their practice. This model formed the philosophical basis of the Western Interstate Commission on Higher Education in Nursing (WICHEN) research development program of the 1970s (Kreuger, Nelson, & Wolanin, 1978; Lindeman & Kreuger, 1977).

A second approach involves utilization research and is exemplified by the Conduct and Utilization of Research in Nursing (CURN) project conducted in Michigan (Haller, Reynolds, & Horsley, 1979; Horsley, Crane, & Bingle, 1978). In the CURN approach, a team of trained persons critically reviews the literature to determine areas of research that are judged to be ready for the development and testing of therapeutic protocols in practice settings. In the CURN project, the research team actually created and tested 11 therapeutic protocols in hospitals throughout the state of Michigan. The CURN project is an exemplar of how to do Step 7 of Figure 68-1.

The third approach is a high-tech model used to implement the results of the Nursing Child Assessment Satellite Technology (NCAST) program conducted at the University of Washington. The team (King, Barnard, & Hoehn, 1981) used satellite television to teach the NCAST assessment technique to maternal-child nurses in major cities throughout the United States. This project exhibited one way to implement Step 8 of Figure 68-1.

These three models are good ones and they worked well during the original projects that funded them. The problem with all three approaches is that there is no self-perpetuating subsystem in nursing to finance the program beyond the research grant period.

Strategies from Other Fields

Nursing is not the only practice field that wishes to reduce the culture lag between research and utilization in practice. Agriculture, engineering, dentistry, medicine, and pharmacy are fields in which research findings need to be translated into practice. The lag between research and practice in these fields is reduced most effectively when academic, industrial, and business partnerships exist to form the bridge between research outcomes and innovations in practice.

Research and development departments in corporations employ a research staff of scientists, technicians, and support personnel. These persons scan reports of research conducted in academe and either follow the natural evolution of work or actively engage in accelerating it through grant or contract mechanisms. The ultimate goal is to produce a marketable product or service that can be made available to the grassroots consumer in a minimum of time. In medicine, the time between the discovery of a way to perform a new surgical technique and the widespread training of practicing physicians to perform that technique is minimized by medicine's sophisticated interrelationship with the medical, industrial, and business complex.

Nursing could foster development of an analogous subsystem (Stevenson, 1977). It could be designed to bridge the gap between experimental research (Steps 4 to 7) and utilization in practice (Step 8). There are nurse-run businesses that could begin to expand and become brokers for research utilization. Examples include private continuing education corporations, nurse-consultant businesses, and independent nursing practices. There are also not-for-profit organizations that could expand their repertoire of strategies to include strategies such as those used in the CURN and NCAST projects. Examples here include the San Francisco Consortium and sponsors of research-utilization newsletters, such as *Nursing Research Review*, edited by Linda Cronenwett.

Centers and offices of nursing research in schools of nursing and major hospitals serve as one example of a new subsystem that has had a significant impact on the conduct of nursing research (Stevenson, 1987). A second new subsystem in nursing, one similar to the academic, industrial, and business subsystems that interrelate with medicine, agriculture, or engineering could have a significant impact on research utilization in nursing.

SUMMARY

The goal of this chapter was to explicate a master plan to accelerate the pace of knowledge development in nursing. A model was proposed for the systematic, efficient, and sufficient progression of knowledge development. Between 1955 and 1985, progress in nursing scholarship primarily was focused on developing a cadre of nurse scientists (Stevenson, 1987). The challenge facing nursing now and in the immediate future is to produce valid new knowledge about care (Stevenson, 1988) and put it into use for the benefit of nursing clients in a minimum of time at an acceptable cost. The model presented herein was designed to promote the orderly progression of development of research and theory from the earliest exploratory stage of work to later stages. In later stages variables are well defined, theoretical connections are tested and verified, predictive theory leads to therapeutic protocols, and these in turn are tested through experimental designs. The model went beyond experiments into the real world of practice. Field-based evaluation research was espoused as a strategy to test the efficacy and cost-effectiveness of nursing therapeutics. Finally a plan was proposed to bridge the gap between the development of new knowledge and its use by nurse-clinicians.

Nursing is the oldest of the health care fields; it predates such fields as medicine, dentistry, and pharmacy. Unfortunately the historical development of nursing as a woman's enterprise caused it to lag behind other health care fields in scientific productivity. The opening of the National Center for Nursing Research at the National Institutes of Health is the benchmark of a new era in the evolution of nursing science. The future will be less tortuous as nurses straighten out the path through clarity of purpose, consensus about priorities, collaboration toward solving the many inherent methods and measurement problems, and systematic progression of work in long-term programs of research. The moment in the history of humankind has arrived when nursing care can no longer be considered a mundane, intuitive, naturalistic phenomenon. Care and caring have been propelled into the mainstream of sociopolitical and economic concerns in the wake of an aging population that poses myriad challenges for science-based innovations in health care. Nursing is the discipline with the social mandate to meet these challenges.

REFERENCES

American Nurses' Association (ANA). (1980). *Nursing: A social policy statement* (Report No. NP-63). Kansas City, MO: Author.

American Nurses' Association, Commission on Nursing Research. (1981). *Research priorities for the 1980's: Generating a scientific basis for nursing practice*. Kansas City, MO: Author.

American Nurses' Association, Cabinet on Nursing Research. (1985). *Directions for nursing research: Toward the twenty-first century*. Kansas City, MO: Author.

Berecek, K.H. (1975). Treatment of decubitus ulcers. *Nursing Clinics of North America, 10*, 171–210.

Brower, H.T., & Crist, M.A. (1985). Research priorities in gerontological nursing for long-term care. *Image, 17*, 22–27.

Burns, P.A. (1984). *Stress or mixed incontinence: A behavioral intervention* (Grant No. 5U01 AG-05260, 1984–1988). Buffalo: State University of New York, Department of Nursing.

Campbell, D.T., & Stanley, J.C. (1963). *Experimental and quasi-experimental designs for research*. Chicago: Rand-McNally College Publishing Co.

Cook, T.D., & Campbell, D.T. (1979). *Quasi-experimentation: Design and analysis issues for field settings*. Chicago: Rand-McNally College Publishing Co.

Dodd, M. (1987). Problems, approaches, and priorities in oncology nursing research. *AARN Newsletter, 43*(3), 13–14.

Donaldson, S.K., & Crowley, D.M. (1978). The discipline of nursing. *Nursing Outlook, 26*, 113–120.

Ehrenreich, B., & English, D. (1973). *Witches, midwives, and nurses: A history of women healers*. Old Westbury, NY: The Feminist Press, SUNY at Old Westbury.

Fantl, J.A. (1984). *Behavioral therapy for urinary incontinence in females* (Grant No. 5U01 AG-05170, 1984–1988). Richmond: Virginia Commonwealth University, Medical College of Virginia, Department of Obstetrics and Gynecology.

Friedman, L.M., Furberg, C.D., & DeMets, D.C. (1985). *Fundamentals of clinical trials* (2nd ed.). Littleton, MA: PSG Publishing.

Hadley, E. (1986). Bladder training and related therapies for urinary incontinence in older people. *Journal of the American Medical Association, 256*, 372–379.

Haller, K.B., Reynolds, M.A., & Horsley, J.A. (1979). Developing research-based innovation protocols: Process, criteria, and issues. *Research in Nursing and Health, 2*, 45–51.

Health Research Extension Act of 1985, P.L. 99-158.

Horsley, J.A., Crane, & Bingle, J.D. (1978). Research utilization as an organizational process. *Journal of Nursing Administration, 8*, 4–6.

Hu, T.W. (1984). *Cost effectiveness evaluation of bladder training* (Grant No. 5U01 AG-05268, 1984–1988).

University Park: Pennsylvania State University, Institute for Social Policy Research and Evaluation.

Jacobsen, B.S., & Meininger, J.C. (1985). The designs and methods of published nursing research: 1956–1983. *Nursing Research, 34,* 306–312.

Jamieson, E.M., & Sewall, M. (1942). *Trends in nursing history: Their relationship to world events.* Philadelphia: W.B. Saunders.

Jensen, D.M. (1955). *History and trends of professional nursing* (3rd ed.). St. Louis: C.V. Mosby.

King, D., Barnard, K.E., & Hoehn, R.E. (1981). Disseminating the results of nursing research. *Nursing Outlook, 29,* 164–169.

Kreuger, J.C., Nelson, A.H., & Wolanin, M.O. (1978). *Nursing research: Development, collaboration and utilization.* Germantown, MD: Aspen Systems Corporation.

Lewandowski, L.A., & Kositsky, A.M. (1983). Research priorities for critical care nursing: A study by the American Association of Critical Care Nurses. *Heart and Lung, 12,* 35–44.

Lincoln, Y.S. & Guba, E.G. (1985). *Naturalistic Inquiry.* Beverly Hills, CA: Sage Publications.

Lindeman, C.A. (1981). *Priorities within the health care system: A Delphi survey.* Kansas City, MO: American Nurses' Association.

Lindeman, C.A., & Kreuger, J.C. (1977). Increasing the quality, quantity and use of nursing research. *Nursing Outlook, 25,* 450–454.

Marchette, L., & Faulconer, D.R. (1986). Perioperative nursing research: A study of priorities. *AORN Journal, 44,* 387–394.

McBride, A.B. (1987). Developing a woman's mental health research agenda. *Image, 19,* 4–8.

Merritt, D.H. (1986). The National Center for Nursing Research. *Image, 18,* 84–85.

O'Donnell, P.D. (1985). *Biofeedback therapy of urinary incontinence* (Grant No. 5U01 AG-05267, 1985–1988). Little Rock: University of Arkansas for Medical Sciences, Department of Urology.

Raff, B.S., & Paul, N.W. (1985). March of Dimes Foundation. Birth defects (Original article series). *Proceedings of NAACOG Invitational Research Conference, 21,* 1–110.

Schnelle, J.F. (1984). *Behavioral management of urinary incontinence* (Grant No. 5U01 AG-05270, 1984–1988). Murfreesboro: Middle Tennessee State University, Department of Psychology.

Stevenson, J.S. (1977). Nursing research and the industrial community. *Image, 9,* 3.

Stevenson, J.S. (1987). Forging a research discipline. *Nursing Research, 36,* 60–64.

Stevenson, J.S. (1988). Nursing knowledge development: Into era II. *Journal of Professional Nursing, 4,* 152–162.

Stevenson, J.S., & Woods, N.F. (1986). Strategies for the year 2000: Synthesis and projections. In G.E. Sorensen (Ed.), *Setting the agenda for the year 2000: Knowledge development in nursing* (pp. 38–40). Kansas City, MO: American Nurses' Association.

Thomas, B.S. (1984). Identifying priorities for prepared childbirth research. *Journal of Gynecological Nursing, 13,* 400–408.

Woodham-Smith, C. (1983). *Florence Nightingale.* New York: Atheneum.

What are the issues regarding the lack of substantive research being conducted in nursing? How might these issues be most effectively addressed? What should be the components of an effective mentoring research relationship or program? What are the advantages and disadvantages for nursing as a profession to develop a master plan for nursing research? What master plan can you propose and implement to develop a program for nursing research? What developmental stages may be appropriate for your individual research interests? What issues need to be addressed in developing your research program? What strategies can be proposed to address and resolve the issues concerning your research development?

What are the advantages and disadvantages of developing research through a group endeavor? What steps and decisions need to be defined and established before the initiation of group research? How and what consortium arrangements might be established and developed for multisite studies? What examples are available on how research questions can be identified through teaching in undergraduate programs that may be developed as an area or program of research for a faculty member? How can curriculum be developed in each type of nursing program on the basis of research and research findings? How might brokers for research utilization be established in nursing? How might the clinical nurse researcher in the health care setting become a broker for nursing research? What are the relationships between the content offered by Haller (Chapter 26) and Stevenson?

69

Themes in Theory Development

Virginia A Kemp, Ph.D., R.N.

As nursing has evolved into a science, theory development has become a central focus of nursing scholars. While it may be argued by purists that nursing has not achieved scientific status, the position can be advanced that nursing meets criteria for classification as a science. According to Parse (1987) nursing is a science because it (a) is an intellectual discipline with knowledgeable researchers; (b) has some cumulative knowledge and competing paradigms (overriding ideas that define a field's phenomena) that provide direction to research; and (c) the phenomena is specified or inherent in the paradigms. As a science with researchers concentrating on expanding nursing's empirical knowledge, theory development is a priority. The importance of theory is evident when its connection to science is explicated. Science is actually a collection of isolated and disjointed principles with theory providing science with coherence and continuity (Jennings, 1987). Numerous nurse theorists have emphasized that theory provides definition for nursing knowledge and gives direction to research and practice (Chinn & Jacobs, 1978; Walker & Avant, 1983).

It is useful to reflect periodically on and analyze the status and future of theory development in nursing. An examination of nursing theory can provide a sense of the present state and future trends unfolding in nursing literature. Although a variety of techniques may be used to analyze the status of theory,

in this paper the focus will be on examining themes in theory development. The term *theme* is used to represent subjects and issues that recur frequently in the literature addressing theory. An examination of themes should provide a sense of specific aspects of theory development that are currently important to nurses and the future status of theory development in nursing. Themes identifying areas of agreement among theorists, points of divergence, current predominant theoretical issues, and evolving topics are explored.

Before proceeding to evaluate themes, some specific terms must be defined. A problematic area for nursing is theoretical terminology. Preciseness is essential in defining terms that can be assigned numerous meanings. The term *theory* itself has many connotations. In scientific literature as well as scientific practice, theory refers to a specific set of related doctrines (commonly called hypotheses, axioms, or principles) that can be used in making specific predictions and detailed explanations of natural phenomena (Laudan, 1977). In contrast, Laudan also states that theory is used to denote more general, less easily testable sets of doctrines or assumptions. In nursing these more general types of theory described by Laudan are often labeled as conceptual models or conceptual frameworks. Flaskerud and Halloran (1980) note that although nurses identify formulations in nursing as simply models or concep-

tual frameworks, they are not reluctant to label frameworks from other fields, such as psychology and sociology, as theories.

Although there are semantic differences between models, conceptual frameworks, and theories, arguments among theorists about the precise distinctions have not resulted in less confusion or specific answers regarding definitions. According to Adam (1985) in seeking a common denominator, it may be argued that frameworks, theories, and conceptual models may all be defined as abstractions, conceptions, mental images, and ways of looking at, or conceptualizing, reality. Since the purpose of this paper is not to clarify theoretical terminology, distinctions are be made in references to theories, conceptual frameworks, or conceptual models. The term *theory* is used to describe the conceptualizations (theories, models, and frameworks) that have been proposed by theorists.

AREAS OF AGREEMENT IN THEORY DEVELOPMENT
Theme 1: Acceptance of the Need for Theory

One area of accordance is the general acceptance among nurses of the need for nursing theory. Important historical events occurred in the early 1970s when the American Nurses' Association acknowledged the significance of theory development and the National League for Nursing made theory-based curriculum a requirement for accreditation (Meleis, 1985). These two events gave credibility to theory development. As evidence of nurses' focus on and acceptance of the value of theory, Chinn and Jacobs (1983) found that between 1964 and 1981 at least 22 conceptual models or theories of nursing were published.

There has been skepticism voiced about the emphasis on model development in nursing. In discussing the National League for Nursing requirement concerning conceptual models, Siegel (1983) pointed out that there is no real evidence that the emphasis on conceptual models is accomplishing anything. Diers (1984) stated that "creative research does not need an artificial framework to help it make sense" (p. 192). The nurses who have voiced these

criticisms have defined conceptual models and theories in different ways. The term *conceptual model* has been applied to broad conceptualizations that are not given to empirical testing, while theory has been used to represent specific, testable ideas. Nurse scholars seem to agree on the need for developing specific, testable theories but question the usefulness of generating untestable conceptual models.

The value of theory in guiding research is clearly recognized by nurse researchers. In reviewing issues of journals publishing nursing research, it is apparent that the majority of researchers are using a theoretical base to guide their studies. There is evidence of general acceptance of multiple levels and foci of theoretical perspectives rather than a concentration on embracing one overall theory for nursing. Examples of studies testing propositions based on grand nursing theories, theories borrowed from other disciplines and adapted to nursing phenomena, and middle range theories can be found in the nursing literature (Silva, 1986).

Although nurse researchers advocate the testing of nursing theory, Silva (1986) states that the true testing of nursing theory has remained outside the mainstream of nursing research. She believes that the reason for this situation is a lack of clarity about what constitutes theory testing in general and testing of nursing theory in particular.

In supporting this point, Silva (1986) performed extensive searches of nursing research from 1952 to 1985 for reports that incorporated nursing frameworks in their discourse. She located 62 empirical studies that used the nursing models of Johnson, Roy, Orem, Rogers, and/or Newman. She identified three ways that investigators used nursing models as a framework for research: (a) minimal use of models, in which the investigator identified a particular model for research and then did little more with the model in the study; (b) insufficient use of models for theory testing, in which the investigators basically used the nursing model to organize their studies; and (c) adequate use of models for theory testing, in which aspects of the model were explicitly used to test nursing theory. Silva concluded that only 9 of the 62 studies really tested aspects of nursing the-

ory. Silva's findings emphasize that although the value of theory development in nursing has been accepted by nurses, problems remain in terms of defining and testing theory.

Theme 2: Acceptance of the Domain of Nursing

A second point of agreement among nurses is the general acceptance of the basic concepts of the domain of nursing. The domain of a field consists of the phenomena of central interest, the areas of socially ascribed authority and responsibility, and the targets of research (Parse, 1987). The nursing domain does not simply encompass results of research, nursing theories, or nursing practice; it also includes the knowledge of nursing practice that is based on philosophy, history, former practice, common sense, research findings, theory, and genealogy of ideas (Meleis, 1985).

The domain of nursing was addressed by Yura and Torres in 1975 when they described the major concepts or the domain of nursing as being man, society, health, and nursing. Newman (1983) identified the concerns of nursing as nursing, client, environment, and health, while Meleis (1985) indicates that nursing client transitions, interaction, nursing process, environment, nursing therapeutics, and health are domain concepts. Conway (1985) questioned the inclusion of nursing within the domain, but most nursing theorists accept nursing as a domain concept.

Although there are slight variations in terminology among theorists, there is general agreement that the domain of nursing is person, environment, health, and nursing. By specifying the domain of nursing, research and practice should reflect common goals of providing nurses with knowledge within these four conceptual dimensions. This is an important step in theory development because it signifies that nursing has developed to the stage of identifying major ideas that guide common lines of inquiry (Fawcett, 1984; Jennings, 1987).

AREAS OF DIVERGENCE
Theme 3: Disagreement on Meanings of Theoretical Terms

According to Adam (1985) in reviewing multiple ways that certain terms are used in the nursing literature, one notes the lack of agreement among authors and even a number of contradictions in the writings of the same person. She indicates that confusion surrounds the meanings of the terms *theory*, *conceptual framework*, *conceptual model*, *philosophy*, *discipline*, *profession*, and *science*. While this may not seem to be a critical area of disagreement, the lack of clarity in semantics creates confusion among nurses attempting to understand the use of theory and conceptual models in research and practice.

Nursing scholars have advocated numerous definitions of the terms *theory* and *conceptual model (framework)*. Some authors tend to use theory and theoretical framework as synonyms for conceptual framework (Peterson, 1977), while others have defined them in different ways. Reilly (1975), for example, states that a conceptual model does not constitute reality and simply provides a way of looking at nursing. In contrast she believes that a theory constitutes reality since it has a scientifically accepted base. Newman (1979) defines theory as testable and alterable, while stating that a conceptual model (framework) specifies only a focus of inquiry.

According to Flaskerud and Halloran (1980), the concentration on specifying the differences between models and theories has deterred theory development. Meleis (1985) notes that the confusion surrounding the meaning of terms has delayed seasoned theoreticians and researchers in their attempts at knowledge development, has kept the novice from getting involved in the process of theory building, has confused those outside of nursing who have not understood what nurses are quibbling about, and has stood in the way of nurses understanding, contributing to, and improving patient care.

Theme 4: Disagreement on What Constitutes Nursing Theory

In addition to arguments about the precise definitions of theories, conceptual models, and conceptual

frameworks, there have been numerous debates concerning what constitutes nursing theory and what types of theory should be developed and tested. Meleis (1985) states that "nursing needs theories to describe and explain phenomena that are significant in the act and process of nursing, to prescribe effective strategies of care, and to predict outcome" (p. 102).

One continuing debate among nurse scholars has been the place of borrowed theories in theory development and research. Borrowed theories are theories that are developed in disciplines such as psychology and sociology and are used by nurses to guide their research. Examples of borrowed theories that are frequently used by nurses in their research studies include family theory, systems theory, and stress or coping theories. Some nurse scholars believe that the use of borrowed theories hinders nurses from developing their own unique theories based on the domain concepts. However, Meleis (1985) believes that theories developed in other disciplines are useful to nursing if they go through a process of derivation, integration, and synthesis with the nursing perspective. Adam (1985) contends that the day may come when nursing theory will be as useful to related disciplines as existing theories, developed in other fields, are today useful to nurses. This viewpoint seems to be gaining acceptance based on the numbers of published examples of borrowed theories that have been used as frameworks for nursing research.

Disagreements center on whether nurse scholars should concentrate on the development and testing of basic or applied theory. Arguments also focus on the development of theory for practice and the application of existing nursing theories for clinical situations. Aggleton and Chalmers (1986) indicate that there exists tension between those who argue for theory development out of the everyday experiences of practicing nursing (Dickhoff & James, 1968) and those who argue for its development from the rigorous testing in nursing contexts of hypotheses derived from nursing theory and from existing fields of natural and social inquiry. Contentions such as these appear to be useless since there is no one correct position. Multiple levels and types of theory can advance the knowledge base for nursing.

CURRENT THEMES IN THEORY DEVELOPMENT
Theme 5: Holism and Particularism

Holism is a popular concept in the nursing literature. Numerous nurse theorists advocate a holistic perspective, and there seems to be a concentration on holism with an exclusion of particularism. Kim (1983) defines holism as a conception of an object or a situation "as having meanings as a totality" (p. 15). The concept of holism is more than the addition of subparts since the subparts do not give a full understanding of the whole object, situation, or person (Roy, 1980). In contrast, particularism means breaking down characteristics of persons or events into discrete parts for study.

Most of the references in nursing literature advocate viewing persons and situations from a holistic perspective as the optimum way of gaining insight into people and events. Holism is labeled as being a positive perspective, while particularism is often viewed as negative. Conceptualizing holism as good and particularism as negative is a simplistic and impractical way of addressing many nursing phenomena. Holism is a valuable theoretical idea, but it is very difficult to address in a practical sense.

Research strategies for testing holism are limited. Viewing the particular cannot be rejected outright, and a holistic approach cannot be wholly adopted until adequate research methodologies and designs are developed to represent both (Meleis, 1987). To adopt both particularism and holism allows for temporary acceptance of the limitations in existing modes of inquiry, but it does not preclude the need for the future development of other modes more congruent with the emerging shared beliefs of nurses (Meleis, 1986).

Theme 6: Shifting Philosophical Base

There has been a growing awareness by nurse scholars of the need to accept both the received view and the perceived view of science. In some of the nursing literature, the received view is referred to as logical positivism or empiricism and the perceived view is called postpositivism or historicism. The received view is characterized by adherence to the scientific method in which "reductionism, quantifiability, objectivity, and operalization" are essential (Watson, 1981, p. 414). In contrast, the perceived view takes into account other epistemic factors related to the context of discovery and accepts values, subjectivity, intuition, history, tradition, and multiple realities (Meleis, 1985).

Silva and Rothbart (1984) attribute the philosophical shift in nursing from positivism to historicism because of the inadequacy of empiricism to deal with certain phenomena in nursing, in particular, humanism and holism. They state that by exploring alternative philosophies of science, it is possible to study nursing phenomena in a more meaningful and creative way and to help bridge the gaps among philosophies of science, nursing theory, and nursing research.

The shift in philosophy in nursing from a rigid received view to an allowance for a perceived perspective is in process. The most desirable outcome would appear to be an acceptance of both views with different expressions, and different sources within a discipline (Laudan, 1977).

Theme 7: Gender-Sensitive or Feminist Knowledge

"The scientific enterprises in many disciplines have reflected a masculine culture, bias, and ideology while women and their traditional female values have been conspiciously invisible" (Meleis, 1987, p. 10). Meleis advocates a gender-sensitive approach for nursing. The term *gender-sensitive* is broader than feminism and is based on removing the barriers that exist between the subject matter and the researcher, between the subject and the researcher, and between the practice and the research roles (Stacey & Thorne, 1985). Chinn (1987) concurs with Meleis's view of incorporating gender-sensitive awareness into research but believes the term *feminism* is more appropriate terminology. By feminism Chinn means the experiences and reality of women. However, gender-sensitive, as a term, seems to truly embody a caring view of both men and women's issues rather than an exclusive focus on women's health concerns.

According to Meleis (1987) there has been an emergence of interest in topics significant to women in the nursing literature. Since nursing primarily consists of women, this is understandable. Sherwin (1987) points out that the majority of women in the world suffer from both poverty and low status, with these conditions resulting in poor nutrition, reduced strength, and diminished self-esteem. Thus women's health is a critical area for nursing theory development and research. Meleis (1987) cites examples of osteoporosis during menopause (McPherson, 1985) and patterns of support of chronically ill lesbian women (Browne, 1985). Articles concerning women's health from cross-cultural and global foci are appearing in nursing journals. For example, *Health Care for Women International* provides numerous examples of topics regarding women's health from a cross-cultural, global perspective.

Sherwin (1987) states that the health care system is almost entirely controlled by men who retain the positions of authority in the system as administrators, legislators, and physicians. She advocates theory and research that addresses the quality of the interactions that the health care institutions foster, including the attitudes of women who come in contact with the health care system, and the attitudes expressed by the system toward the women who use and provide its services.

EVOLVING THEMES
Theme 8: Relevance to Humanity

Meleis (1987) has advocated that nurses consider what difference nursing research makes to humanity. Humanity encompasses topics related to cultural and global concerns of people. Ostergaard (1987) encourages deliberate efforts on the part of nurses aimed at understanding the living conditions of people and the development of global strategies for improving health. Achieving goals such as these would require groups of nurses from varied cultural and ethnic backgrounds to develop theory foci and research programs to address global, cross-cultural concerns of health care. Leininger (1978) has identified as a goal of nursing "to make professional nursing knowledge and practices culturally based, culturally conceptualized, culturally planned, and culturally operationalized" (p. 12). She has emphasized the important place of transcultural nursing (a major area of nursing that focuses on a comparative study and analysis of different cultures and subcultures in respect to their health care) in the future of nursing. Leininger (1978) believes that for nursing to be relevant to the world, transcultural nursing knowledge will be imperative.

It is critical that theory development and nursing research be relevant to social and health issues. In the past much nursing research has been at the descriptive level, with the focus being on describing phenomena of interest to nursing. As nursing evolves its science, research foci must be expanded to include intervention models that demonstrate relevance to health. If nurses clearly direct their goals toward theory development and testing that are congruent with the domain of nursing, then social relevance will occur. With the competition among sciences for research funding, nurse researchers must design proposals that clearly demonstrate an impact on health.

Theme 9: Acceptance of Diversity

Many theorists are advocating a pluralistic, eclectic approach to theory development in order to embrace the entirety of human behavior to give nursing its richness and complexity (Jennings, 1987; Newman, 1983). The scientific knowledge base of nursing is expanding by the use of diverse theories, research strategies (qualitative, quantitative, and triangulation), and tolerance of multiple topics for research investigations.

Diversity in approaches toward theory development and testing in nursing signals a growing maturity in the profession. Scientific progress for Laudan (1977) means a reduction in the number of unsolved problems within a discipline. Therefore, the assessment of progress in nursing theory development and testing will be a tolerance for diversity, a concentration on promoting theory development that addresses the domain of nursing, and a focus on expanding the knowledge base of nursing.

Theme 10: Theory for Practice and Clinical Modeling

The true application of theory to clinical and practice settings has not been a primary focus of nurses. One reason for this is that many nurse researchers and theorists are detached from clinical practice (Dracup & Weinberg, 1983). Another difficulty in developing practice models or applying existing nursing theories in clinical settings is due to the diversity and complexity of practice arenas. For example, attempting to apply only one nursing theory to the numerous kinds of situations in a hospital may be frustrating since a specific theory may not have been developed to meet these multiple foci. However, with more nurses having knowledge of nursing theory and its usefulness in organizing phenomena, the development of clinical models and the application of existing nursing theories to practice is an evolving issue in theory development.

Although application of nursing theory to clinical settings has occurred, it has generally involved isolated, specific instances. The use of nursing theory in practice has not enjoyed the attention of nurses when compared with the emphasis that the application of theory in educational settings has received.

An example of the application of nursing theory to practice can be found in the literature on Roy's theory (1984). Extensive work has been performed on applying Roy's model by Roy and others. It is a valuable theory for nursing practice because it includes a goal that is specified as the aim for activity and prescriptions for activities to realize the goal (Roy, 1984). The two-level assessment is unique to Roy's model and is well suited to the nursing process that is widely used in practice settings (Blue, Brubaker, Papazian, & Riester, 1986). The model has been used in outpatient settings (Wagner, 1976), by nurse administrators in a practice setting (Blue et al., 1986), and with hospitalized pediatric patients (Galligan, 1979).

Models specifically designed to address the delivery of health care in practice settings are also being advanced. An example of a practice-derived model is the McGill model of nursing (Gottlieb & Rowat, 1987). This model is based on the assumptions that the health of a nation is its most valuable resource;

that individuals, families, and communities aspire toward better health; and that nursing exists in order to assist families in developing their potential for health. The McGill model of nursing gives the profession a distinct and unique role within the health care system. The salient concepts of the model include health, person, environment, and nursing. Both assessment and implementation phases are specified in the model. According to Gottlieb and Rowat (1987) the model has been applied in various practice settings such as ambulatory care, intensive care units, and communities with positive client outcomes identified as reduced stress, increased satisfaction, improved problem solving, and increased involvement in health learning. This model is continuing to be evaluated and revised, but it provides a clear example of the usefulness of theory in practice settings.

SUMMARY

There are many themes in nursing literature that provide evidence of the progress, concerns, and future issues surrounding theory development in nursing. There has been progress achieved in defining the domain of nursing and in identifying theory development as an important area for nursing. Disagreements still exist among nurses regarding what precisely constitutes nursing theory and theoretical terminology. Current themes in theory development seem to be focused on holism, the shifting philosophical base of nursing science, and gender-sensitive issues.

It is encouraging that future themes demonstrate a progression from a concentration on the process of theory development to more substantial concerns for the health of humanity, a tolerance for diversity, and application in practice. These evolving themes demonstrate the continuing maturity of the profession in its approach to theory development and research.

REFERENCES

Adam, E. (1985). Toward more clarity in terminology: Frameworks, theories, and models. *Journal of Nursing Education*, 24, 151–155.

Aggleton, P. & Chalmers, H. (1986). Nursing research, nursing theory, and the nursing process. *Journal of Advanced Nursing*, 11, 197–202.

Blue, L.B., Brubaker, K.M., Papazian, K.R., & Riester, C.M. (1986). Sister Callista Roy: Adaptation model. In A. Marriner (Ed.) *Nursing theorists and their work* (pp. 297–312). St. Louis: C.V. Mosby.

Browne, S. (1985). Supportive and nonsupportive interventions for the lesbian chronically ill. Unpublished doctoral dissertation, University of California at San Francisco.

Chinn, P.L. (1987). Response: ReVisions and passion. *Scholarly Inquiry for Nursing Practice: An International Journal*, 1, 21–24.

Chinn, P.L., & Jacobs, M.K. (1978). A model for theory development in nursing. *Advances in Nursing Science*, 1, 1–11.

Chinn, P.L. & Jacobs, M.K. (1983). *Theory and nursing: A systematic approach*. St. Louis: C.V. Mosby.

Conway, M.E. (1985). Toward greater specificity in defining nursing's metaparadigm. *Advances in Nursing Science*, 7, 73–81.

Dickoff, J., & James, P. (1968). A theory of theories: A position paper. *Nursing Research*, 17, 197–203.

Diers, D. (1984). Commentary on three research articles using conceptual models of nursing as frameworks. *Western Journal of Nursing Research*, 6, 191–192.

Dracup, K., & Weinberg, S.L. (1983). Another case for nursing research. *Heart and Lung*, 12, 3.

Fawcett, J. (1984). *Analysis and evaluation of conceptual models of nursing*. Philadelphia: F.A. Davis.

Flaskerud, J.H., & Halloran, E.J. (1980). Areas of agreement in nursing theory development. *Advances in Nursing Science*, 3, 1–7.

Galligan, A.C. (1979). Using Roy's adaptation model: Testing the adaptation model in practice. *Nursing Outlook*, 24, 682–685.

Gottlieb, L., & Rowat, K. (1987). The McGill model of nursing: A practice-derived model. *Advances in Nursing Science*, 9, 51–61.

Jennings, B.M. (1987). Nursing theory development: Successes and challenges. *Journal of Advanced Nursing*, 12, 63–69.

Kim, H.S. (1983). *The nature of theoretical thinking in nursing*. Norwalk, C.T.: Appleton-Century-Crofts.

Laudan, L. (1977). *Progress and its problems: Towards a theory of scientific growth*. Berkeley: University of California Press.

Leininger, M. (1978). *Transcultural nursing: Concepts, theories, and practices*. New York: John Wiley & Sons.

McPherson, K.I. (1985). Osteoporosis and menopause: A feminist analysis of the social construction of a syndrome. *Advances in Nursing Science, 7,* 11–22.

Meleis, A.I. (1985). *Theoretical nursing development and progress.* Philadelphia: JB Lippincott.

Meleis, A.I. (1986). Theory development and domain concepts. In P. Moccia (Ed.), *New approaches to theory development* (pp. 86–94). New York: National League for Nursing.

Meleis, A.I. (1987). Revisions in knowledge development: A passion for substance. *Scholarly Inquiry for Nursing Practice, 1,* 5–19.

Newman, M.A. (1979). *Theory development in nursing.* Philadelphia: F.A. Davis.

Newman, M.A. (1983). The continuing revolution: A history of nursing science. In NL Chaska (Ed.), *The nursing profession: A time to speak* (pp. 385–393). New York: McGraw-Hill.

Ostergaard, L. (1987). Role of women as a motivative and collective force in international development. *Health Care for Women International, 8,* 219–229.

Parse, R.R. (1987). *Nursing science: Major paradigms, theories, and critiques.* Philadelphia: W.B. Saunders.

Peterson, C.J. (1977). Questions frequently asked about the development of a conceptual framework. *Journal of Nursing Education, 16,* 22–32.

Reilly, D.E. (1975). Why a conceptual framework? *Nursing Outlook, 23,* 566–569.

Roy, C. (1980). The Roy adaptation model. In JP Riehl & C Roy (Eds.), *Conceptual models for nursing practice* (2nd ed., pp. 179–188). New York: Appleton-Century-Crofts.

Roy, C. (1984). *An introduction to nursing: An adaptation model* (2nd ed.). Englewood Cliffs, NJ: Prentice-Hall.

Sherwin, S. (1987). Concluding remarks: A feminist perspective. *Health Care for Women International, 8,* 293–304.

Siegel, H. (1983). Misconceptions about conceptual frameworks — A point of view. *Nursing and Health Care, 1,* 16–17.

Silva, M.C., (1986). Research testing nursing theory: State of the art. *Advances in Nursing Science, 9,* 1–11.

Silva, M.C., & Rothbart, D. (1984). An analysis of changing trends in philosophies of science on nursing theory development and testing. *Advances in Nursing Science, 6,* 1–13.

Stacey, J., & Thorne, B. (1985). The missing feminist revolution in sociology. *Social Problems, 32,* 301–316.

Wagner, P. (1976). The Roy adaptation model: Testing the adaptation model in practice. *Nursing Outlook, 24,* 682–685.

Walker, L.O., & Avant, K.C. (1983). *Strategies for theory construction in nursing.* Norwalk, CT: Appleton-Century-Crofts.

Watson, J. (1981). Nursing scientific quest. *Nursing Outlook, 29,* 413–416.

Yura, H., & Torres, C. (1975). *Today's conceptual frameworks with the baccalaureate nursing programs* (NLN Publication No. 15-1558, pp. 17–75). New York: National League for Nursing.

What is the connection between theory and science? What evidence is there that a conceptual model has had value as a basis for curriculum development? What evidence is there that theoretical perspectives have specifically guided the studies being conducted by the majority of nurse researchers? How does the discussion by Deets (Chapter 20) relate to Kemp's comments concerning the domain for nursing research? What points made by Newman (Chapter 30) regarding the use of terms are further supported by Kemp? What evidence is there that concentration on specifying the difference between models and theories deterred theory development? What is the difference between applied theory and theory for practice? What is the difference between the development and testing of basic and applied theory? How important is it to teach nursing students the difference in concepts used in arguments regarding practice theory, applied theory, and how theory is developed rather than trying to resolve the issue?

Discuss the received and perceived views of science. To what extent do these views constitute two mutually exclusive perspectives within the philosophy of science? How then can both views be advocated within a discipline? How does Laudan address this issue? What has been or is the contribution of nursing research to humanity? How are theory development and nursing research relevant to social and health care issues from a broad perspective? What type of questions should be addressed in nursing research that might have an impact on health?

70

The Future of Nursing Practice

Joyce C. Clifford, M.S.N., R.N., F.A.A.N..

As we turn the corner and enter the last decade of the 20th century, speculation abounds over the future of nursing practice. Especially, questions flow concerning its ability to survive the multiple societal and health system issues that have contributed to a shortage of well-prepared nurse professionals at a time when society may need them the most. Such speculation suggests that radical changes are required in the delivery of health care services in this country. The response of the health care system to the issues faced by nurses in clinical practice signals the turning points that will bring nursing practice well into the 21st century. Turmoil within the entire health care industry is complicated by the return of a significant nursing shortage in the last half of the 1980s leading to another examination of the problems of the nursing profession.

Yet, at the same time, and slowly over the last quarter of the 20th century, remarkable change within nursing has actually occurred. Because the centrality of nursing practice within the health care delivery system itself became clear to many as a result of two major nursing shortages occurring back to back, practice emerges as the area holding the most potential influence within the nursing profession. Nursing's opportunity for the future is therefore in place. What is now needed is for the resources and the work environment to be designed in a manner that fully demonstrates the capacity of nurses to be cost-effective contributors to the health care of this nation's people. In doing so, nursing as a career opportunity will become better recognized and viewed as an attractive choice.

The directions that must be taken to achieve this outcome have been articulated frequently and in many ways. Certainly the findings and recommendations of two national nursing commissions occurring in the same decade—one supported by the private sector (National Commission on Nursing, 1983) and the other by the public sector (Department of Health and Human Services, Secretary's Commission on Nursing, 1988)—provide a very large blueprint for use in the design of nursing's future practice systems. Both commissions identified the need for issues related to nursing to be examined within the context of the larger health care system, a system that has and will continue to undergo significant change as a result of the many social, political, technological, and financial forces now shaping the environment.

Everyone involved in establishing policy, whether at an institutional or national level, must assume some level of responsibility for ensuring the future accessibility of nurse professionals in the health care system. However, a major burden of this responsibility continues to lie with nurses themselves. Bold strokes must be taken. Unified approaches to practice need to be presented to the public in order for nurses to actualize the leadership role they potentially have within the larger health care system. The decade of the eighties demonstrated both the need for professional nursing in the health care delivery system and the possibility for broader leadership by nurses; the decade of the nineties must solidify the progress made and provide opportunities for expansion of nursing as a professional, clinical discipline with an accepted, recognized mission to provide cost-effective health care services to society.

WHERE WE ARE: THE CURRENT STATE OF THE FIELD

The future always depends on the past and the evolution of nursing practice into the 21st century is no exception. There is probably general agreement that in this country the field varies widely in the application of professional practice models. Among nurse executives, there is probably just as much agreement that over the last two decades hospital nursing practice systems have made tremendous change in the way professional nurse staff are used in the delivery of nursing care to patients. Riding the crest of large nursing school enrollments in the mid and late 1970s, nursing practice systems, especially those of hospitals, expanded their use of the registered professional nurse in the delivery of nursing care. With a better-prepared health care provider available, substantive changes in the clinical practice system began and expanded services within the hospital were possible. Although only a few hospital nursing service departments report that they have a single practice system in place for the care of all patients, most hospitals identify specific nursing care delivery systems being used, suggesting that an attempt to improve the context within which nurses practice is in place (American Hospital Association, 1987).

The context of practice is clearly an essential element in determining the possibilities for practice. The variables are many, but of great significance is the overall value system of the institution, the nurse executive and, of course, the marketplace from which nursing staff are recruited. The ability to develop a professional model of practice is thwarted, for example, when institutional values related to pa-

tient care are focused singularly on cost efficiency and basic safety outcomes. Unfortunately, since the implementation of the federal prospective payment system for Medicare, many believe that the financial environment has fostered health care agencies, hospitals, health care institutions and other based solely on values of cost efficiency. Ginzberg in a description of the changes in the health care system warns:

> During this time of destabilization, there is risk that important values may be lost. Whether they are lost will depend on the quality of the . . . leadership and the response of the public. (Ginzberg, 1986, p. 760)

Leadership becomes the essential element then, not only in sustaining the advances made but also in moving forward in a time of great uncertainty for the health care industry.

At this point in time, it is generally acknowledged that the challenges facing the leadership of the industry include the effective retention of experienced nurses. These challenges encompass (a) the organization of clinical services within hospitals and health care agencies; (b) the support services provided; and (c) the perception of and value given to the work of the clinical nurse. Once again, the way each of these is addressed in a given institution will depend as much on the values held by the leadership of that institution as anything else. Thus one of the critical issues for the future of nursing practice is the priority that the nursing profession places on the development and mentoring of administrative as well as clinical leaders.

Alexander (1988) indicates that the role of management and administration in changing organizational conditions has often been discounted when examining the reasons for nursing turnover. The need for organizations to become more porous in terms of their information systems and participation in decision making by all staff is also frequently cited as issues leading to nursing staff turnover. Development of such practice systems is directly related to the leadership of the chief nursing officer and nursing administrative staff. The need for this group of professionals to operate from a commitment to leadership for a clinical discipline, as well as executive management leadership, is critical for the successful implementation of effective practice models.

Many health care professionals predict that there will be a continuing change in the balance of where people receive their health care. The reliance on the hospital as the primary organizational unit for health care is diminishing and increasingly more health care is provided through outpatient and community-based services (American College of Healthcare Executives, 1987). Few disagree, however, that hospitalized patient care will continue to grow in its intensity, as will the need for well-prepared nurse professionals to meet these requirements (American Hospital Association, 1987; Department of Health and Human Services, 1988). The demand for nurses in hospital-based nursing practice will continue; consequently the hospital will remain the largest employer of professional nurse staff.

Hospital practice today is perceived by some as the administration of a number of unit routines and tasks to be accomplished for patients. A routinized, unit-based organizational structure that focuses predominantly on how to get the work done diminishes the potential of nursing and detracts from the real contributions that can be made by nurses in the care of patients. Routines need to be substituted by individualized care planning done by nurse professionals. The organization of the unit-based nursing system should be such that the professional nurse is provided the opportunity to render her or his services directly to patients. This direct relationship with patients and their families is the essence of practice, and nurses have expressed this preference in many different ways (Kramer & Schmalenberg, 1988). The success of those practice models using the delivery system of primary nursing is in large measure related to their support of a direct nurse-patient relationship (Clifford, 1988). What has been learned from these successful systems is the need to relieve the nurse from nonessential tasks related to the care of patients, decreasing their stress and in-

creasing their work satisfaction (Betz & O'Connell, 1986).

In addition to the nursing shortage, the issues of cost-effectiveness, quality of care, and changing patterns of hospitalization occurring since the implementation of the federal prospective payment system in 1982, have dominated the field during this decade. As a result, experimentation in the hospital nursing practice setting has occurred and new organizational patterns for professional practice have been developed. Primary nursing remains the fundamental design for delivering care in each of these new organizational systems, but models such as case management (Zander, 1985), group practice, and the contract model (York & Fecteau, 1987) have modified some aspects of primary nursing and are now being tried in many other hospitals. More experimentation is expected to occur as hospital nursing practice systems attempt to become more efficient in the delivery of nursing care and services. The intent of all, however, is to increase the professionalism of nursing by providing increased autonomy, decentralization of decision making, and participation in determining the standards of practice and outcomes expected for patient care. The continued development of a professional model of nursing practice through the restructuring of multiple organizational relationships becomes the major challenge of the future for nurse leaders.

THE FUTURE

Predictions for the future suggest that the changes faced by the health care system during the past decade are only representative of those yet to occur. Efforts to curtail the costs of health care will continue to dominate the environment, as will the issues of a declining pool of health care professionals. Clearly a reoccurrence of a nursing shortage at the end of the decade—similar to that which opened the decade in 1980—signals the industry that major restructuring of institutional nursing practice may be the single most important factor for achieving a balance between the issues of cost and quality of care in the future.

Hospital nursing practice is expected to lead the

way in this restructuring process, because of its historical employment of two-thirds or more of the available registered nurses. This is expected to continue. Nursing is and will remain a personal service profession. The increasing intensity and complexity of hospital services and the acuity of illness presented by patients mandate that well-prepared nurse professionals are present at the bedside in order to coordinate, provide, and expedite the care of seriously ill patients. As hospitals continue to focus on shortening the length of stay, there is the growing additional need for more highly qualified nurse professionals to function independently in the increasingly intense, acute-care community-based practice settings. These settings demand practitioners who are also extremely competent, flexible, and capable of independent judgment. They are not the place for the novice. Thus hospital nursing practice will remain the major employment setting for the new nurse graduate, while it also increases its own demand for well-prepared, competent nurse professionals.

Restructuring Hospital Practice

As the leadership in nursing and institutional management struggles with the environmental forces of the decade ahead, the conditions cited above provide an unusual opportunity for major restructuring of the practice setting. Acknowledging, through organizational design, the need for hospital nursing practice to serve as the basis for all other practice settings may begin to relieve the current built-in turnover factor now experienced by many hospitals. The question becomes, Is there a way that the development of novice nurses can be achieved in hospitals while controlling the traditional turnover? To do so would seem to be in the best interest of patients and staff, as well as the health system as a whole. Perhaps hospital-based nursing practice should be developed to provide a supportive and developmental environment for the novice nurse, using an organizational structure similar to the medical housestaff programs now in teaching hospitals. These nursing programs will require a different organizational structure than traditionally found in hospitals. They

will necessitate the reorganization of experienced and advanced nursing practice to provide clinical leadership for the novice nurse, as well as to direct patient services. This highly differentiated clinical practice model requires many expert practitioners to accept the challenge of becoming careerist in the direct care of patients.

Career development must be conceptualized as an articulated pathway in nursing, rather than the current career by chance, luck, or occasionally good planning. The notion of the nurse as a careerist needs to be established in the early phases of a nurse's socialization into the profession. In addition to the responsibility of the educational system for initiating this notion, the first work experience becomes a critical juncture for the early stages of career development, and a change from highly bureaucratic hospital organizational systems is required. Within the hospital organization, self-managed, senior nursing practice groups can be used to make this area of practice more attractive to advanced and expert practitioners. In this organizational model, hospital nursing practice becomes more flexible, and nurses are not limited in their practice to single, individual patient care units. The time and space constraints historically placed on nurses in hospital-based practice become less prominent, and practice can extend across units as well as settings. In this way, the juxtaposed issues of the need to have competent, independent thinkers who are clinically expert in hospital nursing practice systems, as well as in outpatient and community-based systems, is more likely to be resolved. Self-managed work groups of nurses, providing clinical leadership and consultative services for the novice, establish a career model that can become an incentive to the young professional. Obviously the incentive for hospital practice systems to be designed with a career development approach for the nurse is the potential for better retention of the nurse in their system.

Self-managed (autonomous) work teams hold much promise for assisting in the cure for hospital turnover of experienced and well-prepared nurse professionals. The group approach to the work load stressors found in hospital nursing practice may allow for more effective allocation of resources, particularly at times when extreme variances occur (Susman, 1976). The possibility of extending one's expert practice across multiple systems becomes an enticement for the nurse who enjoys the rigors of complex clinical situations, yet seeks the opportunity to provide care on a continuum. Certainly the health care system can benefit from having available nurse professionals who have a broader view of the whole context of health care delivery.

Nurses are needed who can support the continuum of care for patients, especially the elderly who rely on the hospital as an important health care agency. Even without the radical organizational change suggested here, the need for clinical practice systems to focus on placing nurses in the mainstream of health care delivery so that care to patients can be qualitatively and expeditiously carried out cannot be overestimated. Primary nursing and case management embody these principles. At the very least, they each monitor, coordinate, and evaluate services needed and those provided for the patient and family throughout the episode of hospitalization and often following it.

Transcending the walls of individual institutions, or parts thereof, may assist in preserving scarce and increasingly expensive nursing resources. More consortiums of hospital-based practices are likely to occur in the future, as a way of assuring patients and staff accessibility to needed resources. Regional centers of expert practice are envisioned, just as there are regional specialty institutions. Nurse experts may be available to other institutions on loan, closing the gap between the haves and have-nots of teaching and nonteaching institutions, urban and rural hospitals, and acute and chronic care facilities. The need for nurses to be linked to a central base, however, is critical for the continued development of the careerist role.

Support Systems Required

It is clear that developing a strong clinical model for nursing practice that uses nurses with advanced preparation in the direct delivery of care and promotes practice that transcends the boundaries of inpatient, outpatient, and community will require a change in the traditional hospital support services and management systems. For example, a resurgence of the nonnurse unit manager may occur, who becomes a member of the *nursing* support system rather than an extension of the hospital administration. Nonnursing assistance for transportation, dietary trays, receptionist, and clerical activities all require rethinking in the future practice system. Conversely, changes in these management systems have implications for the clinical leadership and administrative role of nurse managers.

The overwhelming need to preserve the valuable time and talent of registered professional nurses is well documented (DHHS, 1988; Fagin, 1988; Friss, 1988). Future models of nursing practice will feature fewer registered nurses with an increase in support personnel to assist in carrying out a multitude of activities. The need for the delineation of nonnursing tasks has already begun and the implementation of multipurpose, support personnel, some of whom are called "nurse extenders" is expected to continue (Donovan, 1988). The critical element in assuring the success of these roles is to have the individual nurse or group of nurse professionals maintain control over their own practice, by determining for themselves what component of the health care activity with which they wish to have assistance. This will differ of course by patient and by nurse as well, but the criterion that must be maintained is that determination of delegated responsibility remains under the direction of the registered nurse.

Automated information systems will also support practice. Bedside information systems and expert systems will provide the practice environment supplemental resources to offset the decline in the numbers of nurses available. Through these systems nurses will be able to manage large amounts of information about patients, a necessary element in complex practice settings (Schank, Doney, & Seizyk, 1988). Continuity in care planning and evaluation, as well as accountability for that care, is more likely to occur when information is complete, accurate, and accessible. Nurses in clinical practice will come to rely on these information systems in the future in the same way that they now rely on the stethoscope.

COLLABORATION

Collaborative relationships, especially with medical colleagues, is frequently stated to be a goal of restructured practice systems. For the most part, these relationships are little more than cooperation and good communication between professionals. Parallel goal setting has been the norm. The proposed future model suggests the possibility that true collaborative practices, which integrate planning and goal setting for the patient, may finally become an achievable goal and serve as another mechanism for balancing the issues of cost and quality in care (Mowry & Korpman, 1987). As groups of expert practitioners become available across the system of health care services, the contributions of these practitioners to patient outcomes will become well recognized and their expertise more frequently sought. New partnerships between and among groups of professionals, nurses, doctors, social workers, and others are expected to develop as a result of better definition of professional and expert nursing practice.

COMPENSATION

The need to conceptualize compensation for nurses in the broadest terms does not negate the need also for continued development of salary and wage programs that adequately compensate nurses for the responsibilities they hold (McDonagh & Sorensen, 1988). The need to move nurses into an exempt, salaried compensation model becomes more critical as change toward a professional practice model that clearly differentiates novice from expert practitioner occurs. Benner's model is likely to be used as a framework for changing the clinical advancement programs currently in place in many institutions (Benner, 1984). In doing so, the development of more rigorous evaluation methods that will examine how practice actually advances in these programs and the differences that might be expected in patient outcomes should also result. As nursing demonstrates its willingness to accept accountability for the outcomes of practice, the more likely the health care system and the public will support increased compensation for nurses.

SUMMARY

The complexities of the health care system call for nurses to be very clear about their mission. Clinical practice is the essence of the profession and future practice systems must be designed to promote the centrality of this role. The way in which nursing practice is organized to deliver service will become increasingly more critical as the issues of declining resources frame the future direction of health care services. Leadership in nursing cannot be limited to individual positions within an organizational hierarchy, but must encompass all professionals working in a synergetic way. In some institutions, the organization of nursing services to deliver effectively care to patients in an ever-increasing complex environment will be radically different than it is today. It is imperative that sufficient numbers of nurses prepared at the professional levels of baccalaureate and master's education be available to provide direct care, and that publicly recognized accountability systems are established. These professionals must be supplemented with excellent support systems, which include nonlicensed ancillary support personnel as well as state-of-the-art information systems. Most of all, universal acceptance that clinical practice must be experientially and empirically based, calling for the development of career models that provide nurses the opportunity to remain in direct patient care, is needed as we move closer to the 21st century.

REFERENCES

Alexander, J.A. (1988). The effects of patient care unit organization on nursing turnover. *Health Care Management Review*, 13(2), 61–72.

American College of Healthcare Executives. (1987). *The future of healthcare: Changes and choices.* Chicago: Arthur Andersen & Company.

American Hospital Association. (1987, December). *Report of the 1987 Hospital Nursing Demand Survey* (Catalog No. 154753). Chicago: American Hospital Association, Center for Nursing.

Benner, P. (1984). *From novice to expert: Excellence and power in clinical nursing practice.* Menlo Park, C.A.: Addison-Wesley.

Betz, M., & O'Connell, L. (1986). Primary nursing: Panacea or problem? *Nursing and Health Care*, 7(7), 457–460.

Clifford, J.C. (1988). Will the professional practice model survive? *Journal of Professional Nursing*, 4(2), 77.

Department of Health and Human Services. (1988). *Secretary's Commission on Nursing. Final Report, Vol. I.* Washington, DC: U.S. Government Printing Office.

Donovan, M.I., Slack, J., Robertson, S., & Andreoli, K.G. (1988). The unit assistant: A nurse extender. *Nursing Management*, 19(10), 70–76.

Fagin, C.M. (1988). Why the quick fix won't fix today's nurse shortage. *Inquiry*, 25, 309–314.

Friss, L. (1988). The nursing shortage: Do we dislike it enough to cure it? *Inquiry*, 25, 232–242.

Ginzberg, E. (1986). The destabilization of health care. *New England Journal of Medicine*, 315(12), 757–760.

Kramer, M., & Schmalenberg, C. (1988). Magnet hospitals: Part II. Institutions of excellence. *Journal of Nursing Administration*, 18(2), 11–19.

McDonagh, K.J. & Sorensen, M.A. (1988). Restructuring

nursing salaries: A mandate for the future. *Nursing Management*, 19(2), 39–41.

Mowry, M.M., & Korpman, R.A. (1987). Hospitals, nursing, and medicine: The years ahead. *Journal of Nursing Administration*, 17(11), 16–22.

National Commission on Nursing. (1983, April). *Summary report and recommendations* (Trust No. 654200). Chicago: Author.

Schank, M., Doney, L., & Seizyk, J. (1988). The potential of expert systems in nursing. *Journal of Business Strategy*, 18(6), 44–47.

Susman, G.I. (1976). *Autonomy at work: A sociotechnical analysis of participative management*. New York: Praeger.

York, C., & Fecteau, D.L. (1987). Innovative models for professional nursing practice. *Nursing Economics*, 5(4), 162–166.

Zander, K. (1985). Second generation primary nursing: A new agenda. *Journal of Nursing Administration*, 15(3), 18–24.

✳ EDITOR'S QUESTIONS FOR DISCUSSION ✳

How is the context of practice an essential element in determining the scope for nursing practice? What are the issues involved in developing administrative and clinical ladders in the professional practice of nursing? How might Benner's model be used as a framework for changing clinical advancement programs in institutions? What are alternative types of models for professional nursing practice in acute care settings? What is the difference between primary nursing, case management, group practice, and contract models in hospital nursing care? What has been learned from those departments of nursing in which primary nursing has been the major model for providing care? What are strategies that can be used to promote the value of hiring expert practitioners from the highest academic

program levels by hospital administrators and executives?

How might hospital nursing practice lead the way in restructuring models of health care for a balance between cost and quality of care? What factors or variables must be considered or included in designing a department of nursing for professional hospital nursing practice to serve as the basis for all other practice settings? How can career development in nursing be conceptualized as an articulated pathway? How might hospital practice systems design or use a career developmental approach as a means for retaining their nurses? What type of consortiums of hospital-based practice might be developed for the future? How might regional centers of expert nursing practice be developed and for what purposes?

The Challenge for Nursing Administrators:

Nursing care, quality, and decision support for future delivery systems

Edward J. Halloran, Ph.D., R.N., C.N.A.A., F.A.A.N.

FUTURE NURSING SERVICES

Any consideration of nursing administration must begin with a description of what nursing care (i.e., what is administered) is designed to achieve. Henderson and Nite describe nursing as:

> helping people, sick or well, and the performance of those activities contributing to health or its recovery or to a peaceful death that they would perform unaided if they had the necessary strength, will, or knowledge. Likewise, it is the unique function of nursing to help people be free of such assistance as soon as possible. (1978, p. 34)

One need only ponder this description of nursing for a while to realize how essential nurses are to our modern Western society. When there were few medicinal or surgical remedies for ills of body and mind, nursing was used to give solace to those afflicted. Over the past century, modern medicine, in conjunction with society, evolved to the point where many had expectations of being free of these maladies. In reality, medicine can only do so much for a mortal human body. Nursing care is acutely needed more now than ever. After medical management has

been concluded, patients are now frequently left on their own to manage chronic illness. Nurses will increasingly be left with them, helping them be as independent of such assistance as is possible and as soon as possible.

Assistance from nurses in the future will come in two basic forms: institutional and noninstitutional nursing services. First, and most familiar, is the acute care nursing now associated with hospitals. It is unlikely that future acute care will vary appreciably from what is provided in hospitals today. Hospitals will continue to provide high-technology, high touch services to patients to establish disease causation and to initiate treatment, especially surgical, for those illnesses amenable to treatment. Medicine and nursing in the acute care setting will continue to complement each other, for the patient needs the services of both.

A second level of hospital-based patient service will develop as a direct consequence of acute episodes of illness. Thirty years ago the Loeb Center for Nursing and Rehabilitation (Vladek & Alfano, 1987), was established at the Montefiore Hospital in New York City. The Loeb Center provided a very clear distinction between the new service offered to patients and that available in the acute care hospital. This successful, early model treated patients with chronic illness, often the frail elderly, who had a recent acute illness episode. The average length of stay for the individuals treated at the Loeb Center was 14 days, which followed a hospital stay of 7 days. The Loeb Center was relatively small in relation to the Montefiore Hospital, serving only 60 of 1000 patients at any one time. Every rehabilitative effort was made to bring the patient back to a level of activity that the patients experienced before the onset of illness. Particular emphasis was placed on returning the patient home and preventing nursing home placements.

In the absence of this second type of service patients are transferred from the acute care hospital to a long-term care facility. Unfortunately, not much nursing in the sense advocated by Henderson and Nite (1978) of helping individuals be free of assistance as soon as possible takes place in nursing homes. If patients have rehabilitation potential, it is clear that their care must take place in a nursing unit where nurses provide rehabilitative care. The Loeb Center had an all-RN staff. In the future, units of the Loeb type will be established and administered by nurses in conjunction with patients. The specific intent of these institutions will be to prevent long-term care hospitalization. Because nurses do not have the capital to establish this type of institution, hospitals may use their excess capacity to establish Loeb-type units in conjunction with nurses.

Currently 5% of the United States population over the age of 65 is institutionalized for long-term care (Kane & Kane, 1987). If this age-adjusted use rate were projected onto the population reasonably expected in the year 2020, our society would have to double the number of nursing home beds it has at the present time to accommodate the patients. Good nursing administrators will help prevent doubling the number of nursing home beds by designing and initiating Loeb-type alternate care programs.

Noninstitutional nursing services, most commonly associated with visiting nurses, will also become much more available to the American populace than they are at present. Home visits will increasingly be designed to help people manage chronic illness. These highly professional nursing services will encompass little of the procedure-oriented care now deemed by regulatory bodies to be an essential component of home nursing care. Rather, the services will be oriented toward patient and family support and education, that is, education and encouragement designed to help the patient and family be free of any assistance from organized health care services as rapidly as possible. Working with the chronically ill to help maintain a good balance between exercise, nutrition, and the use of medicinals will enable these patients to decrease the use of higher cost, acute institutional care. Such services would be directed toward decreasing hospital readmission rates, particularly for those with chronic heart disease, respiratory disease, cancer, and chronic mental illness. These visiting nurse services are apt to be organized either as they are now, through exemplary visiting nurse agencies providing the service contractually with patients recently discharged from hospitals, or hospitals themselves may choose to employ nurses who are capable of treating patients both within and after they leave the hospital.

The institutional and noninstitutional nursing service described above both now exist to some degree. It is expected that these services will grow substantially as nurses convey more clearly the expected effect of having good nursing services.

CONCERNS OF NURSING CARE QUALITY

Nearly all measures of nursing care cost fail to account for the result of having had good nursing. The outcome of nursing provides an essential measure to balance against its cost. The relationship between dollars and nursing care may be placed in the familiar economic context of supply and demand. However, in the case of nursing care the supply to meet the demand depends on the need for nursing rather than the desire for it. The supply of nurses to meet the demand for nursing depends on how best the need can be met; that is, the need can be met by professional nurses or it can be met by someone with less skill. Furthermore the need for nursing care can be met by the family, or by the persons themselves.

It is this choice of health care provider that perplexes those who administer the costs of nursing care. If disability alone were the measure of need for nursing, then known levels of disability (from epidemiological studies) would equate with the need for nursing. Health Care Financing Administration actuaries have long known that many disabled now care for themselves or arrange for the needed care through family (Kane & Kane, 1987). Concern has been expressed that if the responsibility for care is shifted from the patient or family to the government, the cost would be prohibitive. Such a view implies that recipients of health care are naturally dependent. Even if such a perverse view of human nature was more evident, Henderson and Nite and the nursing profession come to the rescue by declaring that the objective of providing nursing care is to help people be independent of nursing as soon as possible.

There are many constraints that militate against consideration of nursing practice issues in progressive nursing administration. The most important of these is the lack of agreement on what constitutes good nursing care. Nursing offers many varied types of practice in the United States, and even greater variation is seen internationally. Although nursing has been described as being what nurses do, to some extent this definition has only been useful in light of the wide expectations of nurses in various settings. The utility of such description wanes when one considers that nurses and nonnurses alike perform seemingly identical functions. Henderson and Nite's is a more fitting description of nursing function: "acting for the patient where he lacks knowledge, physical strength, or the will to act for himself." (1978, p. 34) This unique function of nursing is based on the application of physical, biological, and social sciences for problem solving using a systematic method or process. This definition necessitates a knowledge base in practice that is now present in widely (and wildly!) varying degrees.

Meeting basic health care needs, ideally done by people themselves, is shifted to nurses when people lack strength, will, or knowledge. Conditions in patients that always effect the shift form self-care to a nurse's care include age, temperament, emotional state, social or cultural status, physical and intellectual capacity, as well as pathological states (as contrasted with specific diseases) that modify basic needs (Henderson, 1966). Henderson points out, however, that:

> the assessment of patients' needs demands among other things sensitivity, knowledge and judgments. Modifying nursing procedures, even simple ones, according to the individual needs of the patient often requires a high degree of competency. (p. 49)

Henderson further stresses that:

> while giving basic nursing care, the qualified nurse has an opportunity to listen to the patient or client, to identify with him and his family, to assess his needs, and to build up the helpful, personal relationship essential to the most effective nursing; that which helps the individual gain independence as rapidly as possible. (1966, p. 49)

Effective nursing care delivery systems must function at every level to enhance the adequacy and efficiency with which nursing care needs are met. Skillful management is predicated on (1) clearly identifying patterns of nursing needs; (2) knowledge of the nursing products required to meet these needs; and (3) awareness of the resources that must be allocated to provide the necessary nursing products. Patient-centered nursing information systems assist nurse administrators to be the driving force underlying decision making for the organization of nursing care delivery and the allocation of nursing resources.

THE NEED FOR COMPUTER DECISION SUPPORT FOR NURSES

Crucial to the development of future systems of health care that meet the needs of patients are tools that assist nurses and nurse administrators to make decisions, in conjunction with patients, about who should give care and where nursing care should be given. Such decisions are the resource allocation decisions of the future, much as nurse staffing methodologies are resource allocation decision aids of the past. The need for such computer-based decision support has been known for some time.

Florence Nightingale, in her efforts to explain and predict morbidity and mortality rates in London hospitals, advocated the adoption of a statistical system incorporating nurses' daily observations of patients, as well as medical diagnostic and treatment information and demographic data. In Nightingale's words:

> They would show subscribers how their money was spent, what amount of good was really being done with it, or whether the money was not doing mischief rather than good: they would tell us the exact sanitary state of every hospital and of every ward in it, where to seek for causes of insolubility and their nature; and if wisely used, these improved statistics would tell us more of the relative value of particular operations and modes of treatment than we have any means of ascertaining at present. (1863, p. 176)

For many years the International Classification of Diseases (ICD) has been employed to classify hospital inpatients. More recently the ICD data has been grouped into diagnosis related groups (DRGs) and computer programs have been developed to relate this clinical information to cost data that are used to evaluate the cost benefit of hospital care. These data-based systems, however, do not account for a crucial dimension of patient status related to quality of life, that is, patients' functional abilities and integration into the larger social community. In short, these medical data systems fail to incorporate the nurse's assessment of patients as well as the patient's progress to independence that results from good nursing (and medical) care.

The degree of patients' dependence on nursing care is of considerable importance in their clinical management and the management of nursing resources. The nursing dependence must be ascertained for two reasons: first, to ensure effective patient management, and second, to utilize nurses more efficiently, the costs for whom make up 20% to 30% of total hospital expenses. The contributions that nurses make in patient care management are not well understood because nursing is often blurred together with medicine and the outcome of nurses' activity sometimes is attributed to physicians.

The development of the DRG concept facilitated the melding of two seemingly unrelated hospital activities: medical care and financial management (Thompson, Averill, & Fetter, 1979). In addition, the DRG concept helped explain the considerable variation in treatment costs from one hospital to another by citing differences in the medical diagnoses and treatments provided for hospitalized patients (Shin, 1977). All hospitals now can be differentiated by their medical case mix; some hospitals treat more medically complex (and therefore, more expensive) patients than others.

Medical case mix alone, however, does not explain all variability in the cost of treating hospitalized patients, nor do physicians direct all of the clinical services that a patient receives in a hospital. Clinical attributes of patients including demand for nursing care and social services have been associated with variations in the case cost and length of hospital stay (Berki, Ashcraft, & Newbrander, 1984; Halloran & Halloran, 1985; Horn, Sharkey, & Bertram, 1983). The nurse individualizes the care provided a patient, and this, too, may vary according to a nurse's experience and education. The momentum of the diagnosis related group and prospective payment has caused hospitals to examine case costs, for which the nursing provided is a substantial part. Case-specific examinations of the nursing care patients received have shown a high degree of association between length of hospital stay and the amount of nursing care provided patients (Catterinicchio & Davies, 1983).

To manage optimally a patient's hospital course, data explanatory of patient nursing care dependency are required. A nurse management information system, based on patient case mix and nurse capability, enables those responsible for allocating nursing resources to manage patient care more effectively and efficiently. This nursing case mix management system complements the DRG medical data system, the social service data system, and together these three discipline-related data sources provide information highly predictive and explanatory of patient resource use, cost, and length of stay.

THE HOSPITAL STAY

The hospital length of stay has been employed as a surrogate measure of the use of hospital resources. Berki et al. (1984) have shown that there is considerable variation in patient length of stay that is not explained by medical diagnosis. This is not surprising, since provision of medical care (or nursing care for that matter) does not depend on hospital status. The complexity of the patient's medical problem (as defined by DRGs), the degree of the patient's functional incapacity (nursing dependency), as well as the patient's social and economic resources, determine the setting for patient care (hospital, nursing home, or home) and the amount of nursing care provided.

Nurses contribute to the management of a hospital patient's care by diagnosing and treating human responses to actual or potential health problems. When registered nurses diagnose and treat nursing conditions, they act in synergy with patients, physicians, and social workers to ensure that the patient's hospital course is optimum in length, in resources consumed, and in placement for aftercare consistent with functional and social independence.

Wennberg, McPherson, and Caper (1984) observed differences in admission rates for various illnesses and attributed the variability to physician behavior. Yet the decision to admit or not admit a patient is in large part due to the patient's dependence on services that they would ordinarily perform for themselves if they had the necessary strength, will, or knowledge. The dependence of patients on nurses constitutes a rationale for hospital admission, the effect of which was not measured by Wennberg et al., yet it is an alternative explanation for variability in admission rates to hospitals for patients with particular medical conditions.

DEVELOPMENT OF A COMPREHENSIVE PATIENT CLASSIFICATION

Only recently has retrievable information about nursing care become available. While patient classification schemes, indicative of nursing dependence, have been employed in American hospitals for many years, such information about patients has either been discarded, stored separately from patients' hospital records, or been in a form that is neither retrievable nor possible to relate to other patient information (Giovannetti, 1978).

Patient classification schemes traditionally con-

ceptualize nursing as the completion of some standard work complex, or task pattern (defined in time intervals) associated with selected patient demand attributes. Assumed in these staffing methodologies is the existence of a standard value that defines the nurse-patient ratio and is applicable to all situations. Acceptance of the assumption underlying these methods means the considerable variability observed from one hospital to another in size of nursing staff is related to the staff-patient interaction alone. Differences among nurses, in organizational support systems, tradition (past practices), and economics play no part in determining staff size and composition in these methodologies. While these task-time methods may be used by nurse managers to support staffing decisions, the results so obtained are often incongruent with the decision-making processes employed by bedside nurses. Furthermore, the current methods do not distinguish nurses from nonnurses. When patient demand attributes are identified, staff allocations, often in full-time equivalent (FTE) units, are made with little distinction between registered nurses, licenses practical nurses, student nurses, or aides as caregivers. Such distinctions are not made because there is no standard minimum competence required for performing any nursing task or procedure. The illogical extreme in using a time- and task-oriented nurse staffing system can be observed in the efficiency-based American nursing home industry. All of the care procedures are done for patients primarily by well-intentioned aides but the quality of living conditions and the forced dependence are a national and international scandal (Miller, 1985; Vladek, 1983).

Nursing is as much an intellectual endeavor as it is a physical one. To decide what to do for a person requires considerable knowledge applied in some orderly manner. A nurse assesses a person's need for nursing care, plans the care, implements the planned care, and evaluates its result in resolving the patient's problem. Patient assessment is a most crucial step because all health care flows from assessed patient need.

Nursing diagnosis terminology is used to summarize more comprehensively the nurse's assessment. The diagnoses describe patient conditions and situations that are amenable to nursing intervention. In this manner, nursing care, in one sense, is being defined by specifying problems in patients that nurses have the knowledge, skill, and experience to treat. The nursing diagnosis is a sound method of operationally describing patient problems in terms that are meaningful to nurses.

PATIENT INFORMATION AND USE

A nursing diagnosis–based patient classification system is used to describe all patients on a daily basis to capture information about nursing dependency. The data are used to help clinicians optimize how patients receive nursing care both during and after the hospital episode and are thus related to their future nursing services, described earlier. The options for care include movement within the hospital (transfers from one unit to another, particularly to and from intensive care units), and after discharge (self-care, family care, visiting nurse, assisted living, rehabilitation or extended care facility).

Data used to support the nurse's resource allocation decision at the bedside include a comprehensive view of the patient's condition at specified time intervals. Because of the dynamic nature of a hospitalized patient's requirement for nursing, a "snapshot" is obtained every 24 hours.

The conditions are not weighted with time values, since it has not been determined, for example, that the treatment for grieving is more or less time-consuming than that for incontinence. Furthermore society depends on the nurse to establish priorities (to treat an impaired airway before treating body image disturbance), and allocate self (care time) in the most effective and efficient manner possible. The nurse involves the patient and often the patient's physician in establishing short- and long-term treatment goals. The nurse may also combine treatment methods, thus giving a bed bath may support good hygiene, provide comfort, manage immobility, and treat grieving, all at the same time. The measurement device is used to help allocate nursing resources and supports the judgments that bedside nurses are required to make. The nursing diagnosis–

based patient classification scheme supports the resource allocation decisions made by bedside nurses.

RESULTS

The data system has been used to quantify the incidence (among 31,326 inpatients discharged from four hospitals in 1986) of the 61 patient indicators on the instrument (Table 71-1). These variables were shown to be associated with length of hospital stay [$R^2 = .609$, $F(57,31269)=776.34$. $p <.0001$]. The nursing dependency index derived from the incidence of these conditions was not substantially correlated to the DRG index of relative cost weights [$R^2 =.16, F(2,29216)=750.57$, $p <.0001$].

Based on these observed relationships, it was concluded that nursing care was not determined by DRG category. Nursing care was provided on the basis of the nurse's judgment about the level of patient need. The following admonition, lost for over a century, sums the implications of these findings:

> Experience teaches me now that nursing and medicine must never be mixed up. It spoils both. (Florence Nightingale, in a letter to Sir Henry Wentworth Acland, 1869/Cope, 1958, p. 121)

FUNCTIONAL STATUS AND QUALITY OF LIFE IMPLICATIONS

When a subsample of the 31,326 inpatients, those 336 who underwent an elective surgical procedure for a major joint (hip, knee, or shoulder) replacement, were compared with the total sample using the nursing diagnosis framework, by comparing columns 2 and 4 from Table 71-1, a number of differences were observed. The joint replacement patients were more dependent on nurses as measured by the nursing dependency index, the mean number of nursing diagnoses per stay in the hospital. Furthermore nurses observed these patients to have greater potential for injury (nursing diagnosis no. 1 from Table 71-1), infection/contagion (3), bleeding (12), skin impairment (16), body temperature alteration (19), constipation (22), activity intolerance (25), impaired home maintenance management (35),

TABLE 71-1

Incidence* of nursing diagnoses for all patients discharged in 1986 from an urban health science center hospital (Columns 1,2), a subset of those having elective major joint replacement surgery (column 3,4), and a subset of joint surgery patients transferred from hospital to extended care facility (columns 5,6)

	ALL HOSPITAL PATIENTS (N = 31326)		MAJOR JOINT REPLACEMENT SURGERY PATIENTS			
			ALL JOINT SURGERY PATIENTS (N = 336)		DISPOSITION: EXTENDED CARE FACILITY ONLY (N = 21)	
COLUMN NUMBER:	1 INCIDENCE	2	3 INCIDENCE	4	5 INCIDENCE	6
NURSING DIAGNOSES	#	%	#	%	#	%
HEALTH PERCEPTION–MANAGEMENT						
1. Potential for Injury	22796	72.7	329	97.9	20	95.2
2. Noncompliance	5668	18.0	63	18.8	13	71.4
3. Infection-Contagion	18416	58.7	289	86.0	18	85.7
4. Prolonged Disease/Disability	19415	61.9	334	99.4	21	100.0
5. Instability	8740	27.9	53	15.8	5	23.8
6. Impaired Life Support Systems	3052	09.7	13	3.9	1	4.8
7. Sanitation Deficit	1926	06.1	14	4.2	2	9.5
8. Socio-cultural–Economic Considerations	7191	22.9	58	17.3	8	38.1
NUTRITIONAL-METABOLIC						
9. Excess Fluid Volume	9181	29.3	83	24.7	11	52.4
10. Fluid Volume Deficit	7242	23.1	84	25.0	11	52.4
11. Potential Fluid Volume Deficit	17366	55.4	198	58.9	12	57.1
12. Bleeding	14101	45.0	271	80.7	15	71.4
13. Less Nutrition Than Required	18948	60.4	218	64.9	15	71.4
14. More Nutrition Than Required	2988	09.5	95	28.3	5	23.8
15. Potention for Excess Nutrition	3276	10.4	52	15.5	3	14.3
16. Actual Skin Impairment	21291	67.9	336	100.0	21	100.0
17. Potential Skin Impairment	19914	63.5	335	99.7	21	100.0
18. Alterations in Oral Mucous Membrane	6746	21.5	54	16.1	7	33.3
19. Altered Body Temperature	10964	34.9	253	75.3	12	57.1

*Incidence is the number of cases in which the nursing diagnosis occurred sometime during hospital length of stay.

TABLE 71-1

Incidence* of nursing diagnoses for all patients discharged in 1986 from an urban health science center hospital (Columns 1,2), a subset of those having elective major joint replacement surgery (column 3,4), and a subset of joint surgery patients transferred from hospital to extended care facility (columns 5,6)—cont'd

			MAJOR JOINT REPLACEMENT SURGERY PATIENTS			
	ALL HOSPITAL PATIENTS (N = 31326)		ALL JOINT SURGERY PATIENTS (N = 336)		DISPOSITION: EXTENDED CARE FACILITY ONLY (N = 21)	
COLUMN NUMBER:	1 INCIDENCE	2	3 INCIDENCE	4	5 INCIDENCE	6
NURSING DIAGNOSES	#	%	#	%	#	%
ELIMINATION						
20. Urinary Incontinence	3598	11.4	62	18.5	14	66.7
21. Other Altered Urinary Elimination Patterns	8303	26.5	184	54.8	16	72.5
22. Constipation	10601	33.8	319	94.9	20	95.2
23. Diarrhea	5127	16.3	75	22.3	7	33.3
24. Bowel Incontinence	2819	08.9	44	13.1	11	52.4
ACTIVITY-EXERCISE						
25. Activity Intolerance	20047	63.9	322	95.8	20	95.2
26. Ineffective Airway Clearance	8650	27.6	73	21.7	7	33.3
27. Altered Breaching Pattern	9539	30.4	65	19.3	8	38.1
28. Impaired Gas Exchange	7149	22.8	70	20.8	7	33.3
29. Altered Tissue Perfusion	9562	30.5	136	40.5	10	47.6
30. Decreased Cardiac Output	5434	17.3	77	22.9	7	33.3
31. Diversional Activity Deficit	17732	56.6	246	73.2	18	85.7
32. Altered Health Maintenance	11293	36.0	110	32.7	11	52.4
33. Impaired Mobility	19745	63.0	336	100.0	21	100.0
34. Self-Care Deficit	21294	67.9	334	99.4	21	100.0
35. Impaired Home Maintenance Management	9533	30.4	274	81.5	20	95.2
COGNITION-PERCEPTION						
36. Altered Comfort: Discomfort	26111	83.3	336	100.0	21	100.0
37. Altered Comfort: Pain	18033	57.5	334	99.4	20	95.2
38. Altered Level of Consciousness	4304	13.7	48	14.3	8	38.1
39. Altered Thought Processes	4991	15.9	56	16.7	13	61.9
40. Impulsivity/Hyperactivity	3662	11.6	45	13.4	7	33.3
41. Altered Sensory Perception	8255	26.3	107	31.8	14	66.7
42. Knowledge Deficit	24446	78.0	334	99.4	20	95.2
43. Growth and Development Deficit	6595	21.0	31	9.2	5	23.8
44. Sleep Disturbance	19219	61.3	259	77.1	16	76.2

Continued.

TABLE 71-1

Incidence* of nursing diagnoses for all patients discharged in 1986 from an urban health science center hospital (Columns 1,2), a subset of those having elective major joint replacement surgery (column 3,4), and a subset of joint surgery patients transferred from hospital to extended care facility (columns 5,6)—cont'd

	ALL HOSPITAL PATIENTS (N = 31326)		MAJOR JOINT REPLACEMENT SURGERY PATIENTS			
			ALL JOINT SURGERY PATIENTS (N = 336)		DISPOSITION: EXTENDED CARE FACILITY ONLY (N = 21)	
COLUMN NUMBER:	1 INCIDENCE	2	3 INCIDENCE	4	5 INCIDENCE	6
NURSING DIAGNOSES	#	%	#	%	#	%
SELF-PERCEPTION/SELF-CONCEPT						
45. Anxiety	23959	76.4	308	91.7	21	100.0
46. Disturbed Self-Concept	8065	25.7	159	47.3	12	57.2
47. Depression	8124	25.9	138	41.1	9	42.9
48. Fear	12975	41.4	262	78.0	18	85.7
49. Powerlessness	14692	46.9	281	83.6	19	90.5
ROLE RELATIONSHIPS						
50. Grieving	5271	16.8	48	14.3	1	4.8
51. Altered Family Process	15436	49.2	190	56.5	13	61.9
52. Altered Parenting	6967	22.2	28	8.3	3	14.3
53. Social Isolation	7507	23.9	61	18.2	8	38.1
54. Impaired Verbal Communication	6552	20.9	35	10.4	13	61.9
55. Potential for Violence	1513	04.8	9	2.7	3	14.3
SEXUALITY-REPRODUCTION						
56. Sexual Dysfunction	2126	06.7	113	33.6	3	14.3
57. Rape-Trauma Syndrome	179	00.5	0	0.0	0	0.0
COPING—STRESS TOLERANCE						
58. Ineffective Individual Coping	6722	21.4	93	27.7	11	52.4
59. Ineffective Family Coping	4920	15.7	25	7.4	2	9.5
60. Potential for Growth in Family Coping	19795	63.1	132	39.3	6	28.6
VALUE-BELIEF						
61. Spiritual Distress	3079	09.3	74	22.0	4	19.0
TOTAL NURSING DIAGNOSES	675,941		9,365		711	
NURSING DEPENDENCY INDEX	21.6		27.9		33.8	

discomfort (36), pain (37), fear (48), and powerlessness (49). This pattern of conditions separates these patients from the average hospital patient and seems consistent with a hypothesized pattern for all patients having major surgical procedures.

When the joint replacement patient sample was further stratified by discharge disposition, a somewhat revealing pattern emerged. Those 21 patients who underwent major joint replacements and were discharged from hospital to a long-term care facility (columns 5 and 6 in Table 71-1), were found to be noncompliant (2), incontinent of bladder and bowel (20,24), to have altered thought processes (39), and impaired verbal communication (54), all to a much greater degree than either the other patients undergoing the same procedure or the whole hospital sample of patients. Certainly the bodily functions of these patients and thus their quality of life had deteriorated since the surgery, as patients undergoing elective surgery are not thought likely to exhibit the nursing dependency traits found (items, 2, 20, 24, 39, and 54).

Two clinical patient-management questions were raised with the physicians and nurses who ordinarily cared for these joint replacement patients. The first question, directed to surgeons was, Were some patients selected for this surgery poor candidates? It is hypothesized from the data presented in Table 71-1 that better patient selection criteria would screen out some individuals whose functional status would not be improved by the surgery. The second question was directed to nurses: Could more have been done to clear the altered thought processes, impaired verbal communication, and noncompliance if these diagnoses had been the focus of the care plan and subsequent nursing care? Henderson and Nite (1978) in the *Principles and Practice of Nursing* provide considerable information on the reasons for, and the treatment of, these circumstances in patients. Again it is hypothesized that the rate of transfer to a long-term care facility (6.25% in this sample), could have been reduced by rehabilitation-oriented nursing care.

To the patients with adverse outcomes of surgery, these care patterns are crucial. The average stay in an American nursing home is 3.5 years. Placing the wrong patient is a serious matter. In addition, the cost to society in Medicaid payments for nursing homes are great, and are often the largest uncontrolled cost of state government. Patient, nurse, and physician must have a better understanding of each of their unique roles. Patients need physicians, patients need nurses, and patients need to know what to expect from both. There should be little overlap in the activities and responsibilities of patient, nurse, and physician lest confusion, waste, and untoward care results arise. To date, failure to develop an use retrievable information about patient functional status and quality of life along with the clinical judgment of nurses has impaired clinical, analytical processes. Such a deficit can be overcome through the use of computer-assisted decision-making aids such as the classification system employing nursing diagnosis elements.

CONCLUSION

The need for decision support data has been recognized for some time. Nightingale (1863) said:

> To the experienced eye of a careful observing nurse, the daily, I had almost said hourly, changes which take place in patients, and which changes rarely come under the cognizance of the periodical medical visitor, afford a still more important class of data, from which to judge of the general adaptation of a hospital for the reception and treatment of sick. (pp. 6–7)

One such system that offers future promise in complementing medical diagnosis and treatment information is an automated version of a patient-classification device that summarizes the judgments of nurses about their patients. The content of the system was devised by the North American Nursing Diagnosis Association. It is consistent with other efforts in patient classification in nursing (Giovannetti, 1978), the quantification of (a) patient need (Abdellah, Beland, Martin, & Matheney, 1960); (b) measures of severity of illness (Jencks & Dobson, 1987); and (c) measures of quality of life and functional status (The Portugal Conference, 1987).

Elements of this system have been incorporated

into the refinement of a nursing minimum-data set, applicable in all settings in which nurses see patients (Werley & Lang, 1988). This information aids in clinical decision-making in a range of settings, from acute hospital care to home care to long-term care. This information shows promise in predicting the outcome of high-cost medical interventions by evaluating their long-term effect on patients' functional status and quality of life. The Institute of Medicine has recommended that this type of information be systematically gathered in American nursing homes to help patients' progress assessment and the quality of their care (Committee on Nursing Home Regulation, 1986.) Progressive nurse administrators should take a hard look at the concept of recording and retrieving information from nurses about their patients. Efforts along these lines have revealed considerable potential for the involvement of nurses in designing future-oriented cost-effective health care systems based on patient need.

REFERENCES

Abdellah, F., Beland, I., Martin, A., & Matheney, R. (1960). *Patient centered approaches to nursing*. New York: Macmillan.

Berki, S.E., Ashcraft, M.L.F., & Newbrander, W.C. (1984). Length of stay variations within ICDA-8 diagnosis related groups. *Medical Care, 22*(2), 126–142.

Catterinicchio, R.P., & Davies, R.H. (1983). Developing a client-focused allocation statistic of inpatient nursing resource use: An alternative to the patient day. *Social Science and Medicine, 17*, 259–272.

Committee on Nursing Home Regulation, Institute of Medicine, National Research Council. (1986). *Improving the quality of care in nursing homes*. Washington, DC: National Academy Press.

Cope, Z. (1958). *Florence Nightingale and the doctors*. London: Lippincott.

Giovannetti, P. (1978). *Patient classification systems in nursing: A description and analysis* (DHEW Publication No. HRA 78-22). Hyattsville, MD: Department of Health, Education and Welfare.

Halloran, E.J., & Halloran, D.C. (1985). Exploring the DRG/nursing equation. *American Journal of Nursing, 85*(10), 1093–1095.

Henderson, V. (1966). *The nature of nursing*. New York: Macmillan.

Henderson, V., & Nite, G. (1978). *Principles and practice of nursing* (6th ed.). New York: Macmillan.

Horn, S.D., Sharkey, P.O., & Bertram, D.A. (1983). Measuring severity of illness: Homogeneous case mix groups. *Medical Care, 21*, 14–25.

Jencks, S.F., & Dobson, A. (1987). Refining case mix adjustment: The research evidence. *New England Journal of Medicine 317*, 679–686.

Kane, R.A., & Kane, R.L. (1987). *Long term care: Principles, programs and policies*. New York: Springer Publishing.

Miller, A. (1985). Nurse-patient dependency—Is it iatrogenic? *Journal of Advanced Nursing, 10*, 63–69.

Nightingale, F. (1863). *Notes on hospitals* (3rd ed.). London: Longman, Green, Longman, Roberts and Green.

The Portugal Conference. (1987). Measuring quality of life and functional status in clinical and epidemiological research. *Journal of Chronic Disease, 40*, 459–650.

Shin, Y. (1977). *Variation of hospital cost and product heterogeneity* (Health insurance studies contract research series, Publication No. 77-11722). Washington, DC: U.S. Department of Health, Education and Welfare.

Thompson, J., Averill, R., & Fetter, R. (1979). Planning, budgeting and controlling, one look at the future: Case mix cost accounting. *Health Service Research, 14*, 111–125.

Vladeck, B.C. (1983). Nursing homes. In D. Mechanic (Ed.), *Handbook for health, health care, and the health professions* (pp. 352–364). New York: Free Press.

Vladek, B., & Alfano, G. (1987). *Medicare and extended care: Issues, problems and prospects*. Owings Mills, MD: Rynd Communications.

Wennberg, J.E., McPherson, K., & Caper, P. (1984). Will payment based on diagnosis related groups control hospital costs? *New England Journal of Medicine, 311*(5), 295–300.

Werley, H., & Lang, N. (Eds.). (1988). *Identification of the nursing minimum data set*. New York: Springer Publishing.

✳   EDITOR'S QUESTIONS FOR DISCUSSION   ✳

What predictions suggested by Clifford in Chapter 70 are reinforced by Halloran? What might be the second-level hospital-based service to develop in the future? Who might be the persons providing these services? What implications are there for rehabilitation graduate programs in nursing given Halloran's predictions? How can nurses effectively convey the needs and development of home health care services? How might professional nurses impact the influence of the long-term health care industry? To what extent do present professional nurses practice in the mode advocated by Henderson? How might standards of minimum competence in practice be established and monitored in departments of nursing? What enforcement issues might have to be addressed in order to implement such standards?

How can nursing diagnoses complement DRGs for possible allocation of nursing resources? How can patient classification schemes be used with nursing diagnosis to determine the needs for nursing care, allocation of resources, and the potential cost for nursing services? What types of decision support data are essential for nurse administrators? What automated information systems are needed for the effective practice of nurse administrators? What strategies should be implemented to increase the use of valid and reliable data for nursing administration?

72

Academic Administration for Uncertainty:
Molding the future for nursing education

Patricia L. Starck, D.S.N., R.N.

The uncertainty of the future challenges leaders in nursing education administration to provide the vision for preparing nurses who will practice in the 21st century. The administrative challenges discussed in this chapter stem from three predicted changes. First, the value of nursing in society will undergo rapid and positive change as several economic forces come together in a consumer-based health care market. Second, the increasing sophistication of doctorally prepared nursing faculty, skilled in clinical research, is coinciding with society's readiness at long last to open all doors to women. Third, accelerated by technology and information services, the impetus for collaboration among universities, businesses, and government will beckon nursing to become a full team member. Visionary leaders can mold the future for the nursing profession to undergo a much needed renaissance. New-age executive skills include strategic planning, creating an environment in which creativity and excellence can flourish, as well as fund raising and other developmental activities. The 21st century can be a turning point for nursing.

PREDICTED CHANGES

The cost consciousness of health care is the driving force in the major shift in paradigm of America's health care delivery system. Ryan (1988) described this paradigm shift from the present focus on medical cure and illness care to a futurist model of focus on health-promoting lifestyle behaviors and chronic illness management. The prospective payment system of the 1980s gave rise to early discharge of patients from the hospital that, in turn, created an expanding need for home health care. This phenomenon will continue to accelerate as consumers learn that care in the home is safe, effective, and economical. Consumers will learn that care can often be "hospital care" in the home with miniature versions of technological devices. The cost savings of home health care will receive increasing recognition by third-party payors. Nurses are the principal providers of home health care services, and many are becoming agency owners as well.

It is only a matter of time until nurses in various aspects of practice will receive widespread third-party reimbursement. This will result from increased documentation of the nursing profession's ability and from pressure by government and business to curtail health care costs. For example, 75% of Medicare patients receive anesthesia from nurse anesthetists. In 1986, the average salary of a nurse anesthetist was $46,000; that of a physician anesthesiologist was $150,000 (Gavzer, 1988). It does not require more than common sense to realize what would happen if only physicians were available to administer anesthesia. Nurse anesthetists were granted third-party reimbursement privileges in 1989.

Alternative care delivery models, such as the Block Nurse Program of Martinson et al. (1985), which emphasized maintaining functional independence and managing chronic illness for the elderly, will be successful ventures because they meet an important need and because there is a realistic congruity between service and price. Midwifery services and hospice care are other alternative models that are in tune with the needs of society. As nurses gain more sophistication through education, they will form small businesses to meet health care needs. This author recalls a recent student, an RN with much experience, who returned to school for the baccalaureate degree. After graduation, she took a position with a well-known home health care company that provided parenteral nutrition therapy. After 1 year, she resigned, stating she had calculated that her services alone had earned the company $1 million dollars. She resigned to form her own company. Why shouldn't nurses have the potential to become millionaires? A few such examples will improve the profession's image and attractiveness to career-seeking, goal-oriented youth.

The role of nursing will also undergo positive change as a result of the focus on the hospital's financially impelled goal of early discharge. With the trend toward ambulatory care, outpatient surgery, and home care, it becomes increasingly obvious that the reason patients are in hospitals is the need for 24-hour-a-day nursing care. Likewise, a nursing shortage that forces the closing of beds and thus leads to the loss of revenues draws attention to the unalterable value of nursing to society. A new appreciation of this scarce resource is emerging among the public sector. The past practices of keeping nurses' wages low has been perceived by the public as unfair and unjust. Demands of the marketplace in a free enterprise system are stimulating salary ad-

justments, incentive benefit packages, and new professional models to prevent attrition. The wise health care administrator will have learned from the critical nursing shortage at the end of the 1980s and will restructure the workplace, as well as the salary and benefits package, to avoid a recycling of another shortage.

The improved image of nursing is long overdue and very welcome. However, it also presents challenges to schools of nursing to prepare nurses who can continue to use this leverage as a wedge into the public's perception and value of nursing so that these gains can be sustained and built on for future generations. The public is also becoming aware that more nurses will be needed as the population ages. Thus, much will be expected of the nursing education institutions.

NURSING FACULTY—INCREASING OPPORTUNITIES

It is a truism that the more educated and sophisticated the faculty is, the more challenging the role of the dean becomes. It was only a couple of decades ago that a master's degree in *any* subject qualified a nurse for a faculty position. Today, in many settings, deans are able to select from several applicants who have doctorates in nursing. Many schools have reached the state of having the majority of faculty with doctoral preparation. A bright, energetic faculty who are equipped with the latest knowledge and intellectual skills require a different kind of administrative leader than in years past. Today's faculty are more capable, as well as eager, to control budget and assume responsibility and accountability for management. A decentralized organizational structure will be needed to allow creativity and entrepreneurial approaches to education, clinical practice, and research. Not only will the structure be flatter, clear lines will disappear as new models for collaboration are developed.

Faculty practice will become the norm in the next century and historians will think it incredulous that their predecessors attempted to teach and conduct research in a clinical discipline while confining themselves to the halls of academe. This earlier period will be seen as isolationist and related to nursing's slow progress in being a significant player in shaping the health care arena in issues such as reimbursement, admitting privileges, and practice recognition. Faculty practice will generate revenues for schools of nursing that will enable them to join the big league of schools in a health science center.

This trend for faculty practice and nurse entrepreneurship is supported by a descriptive study conducted by Aydelotte, Hardy, and Hope (1988) that examined the entrepreneurial movement. Of the 361 participants, 15.6% held doctoral degrees. Most of the nurses for whom the venture was a part-time business were employed by colleges and universities. Deans will face choices of facilitating outside, independent practices (entrepreneurship) or incorporating practice into the university role ("intrapreneurship").

The establishment of the National Center for Nursing Research as part of the National Institutes of Health in 1986 legitimized clinical nursing research in the eyes of the public. Nurse scientists are on the frontier of discovering new knowledge about some of society's most distressing problems. How long has it been since a nurse made a discovery that interested the world? Sister Kenny's finding that hot packs relieved the muscle spasm of acute poliomyelitis is the last that the author can recall. In the last few years, many interesting discoveries by nurses are solving problems for society. The visionary leader must encourage faculty to challenge their minds and actualize their potential.

There has been a long-standing earning gap between men and women, and this phenomenon has attracted public attention (Griffith-Kenny, 1986). People are now working in policy areas to lessen gender discrimination. Women are moving into leadership positions in all fields in academe, business, and government. As more success is achieved in this area, new problems will surface. How will a more equitable climate affect the administration of nursing education? Will it change the gamesmanship deans have always known? What stressors will appear?

THE UNIVERSITY IN INTERACTION WITH BUSINESS AND GOVERNMENT

There is no doubt that technology will be a driving force in the 21st century. A new trend will be the relationship between the private and public sectors, specifically the relationships that universities will have with business and government. This new linkage is referred to by Smilor, Kozmetsky, and Gibson (1988) as a technopolis—the modern linkage of technology commercialization with public and private sectors, for the purpose of stimulating economic development and promoting technology diversification. Universities are beginning to establish the infrastructure for technology transfer and to capitalize on the valuable resources of the research mind. Policies regarding intellectual property, the process of marketing, entrepreneurship education, and venture capital are new topics being discussed in the halls of academe.

Nursing has traditionally had a peripheral relationship with technology. Nurses use it as extensions of their skills, but otherwise, as consumers, show little concern or interest. Nurses deal with both high technology and low technology. The number of nurses considered experts in the field of technology assessment and development is few indeed. Perhaps it is the close connection with the old procedure manuals that makes the subject of technology distasteful. It may also be the fear of dehumanization by machines that gives the subject an undignified aura. Whatever the reason, nurses as consumers have assessed technology, given sales representatives feedback for making a better model, and thus, no doubt, helped them reap the rewards of improved technology. It is time that nurses get into the business of technology development.

Nurses have made little focused effort to develop technology for commercialization. Likewise, universities' nursing schools have made few inroads in research that have led to transfer to industry. Herein lies an opportunity for the future. Who better than a nurse knows the clinical problems of caregiving? Nurses know what safety features are needed. They know what functional problems related to technology that living patients experience. If this clinical knowledge were coupled with bioengineering knowl-

edge, nurses could play a major role in the development of low technology to meet the needs of the elderly who are seeking to live independently at home, to manage chronic illness safely, to self-monitor progress, and to promote health and prevent disease. The university nursing faculty should take the leadership role in this new endeavor. The astuteness of the dean in communicating the vision as exciting, as well as providing resources and supportive networks, will help determine the outcome.

NEW-AGE EXECUTIVE SKILLS FOR THE NURSING EDUCATION ADMINISTRATOR

Nurse administrators will need sophisticated skills equal to those of corporation executives in order to flourish in the future. These skills include strategic thinking and planning, creating a culture to foster excellence, and developmental activities to ensure fiscal viability. One of the most important skills is the ability to think strategically and to plan for the future. Strategic thinking is visionary, especially in times of uncertainty. People resources are all-important and hence culture-building will be a renewed focus. The dean of tomorrow will unquestionably need financial skills that reach beyond the traditional role of planning and administering a budget. The chief administrator will spend considerable time and effort in fund raising whether in private or public institutions. Relations with community members and business leaders will be as important as those with fellow administrators. The challenges presented will require creative financing, as well as negotiating new joint ventures with business and industry. The "intrapreneurship" of faculty will call for skills never before needed by the dean.

Strategic Thinking and Planning

The Greek words for "strategic" come from "generalship" or "leading an army" and thus have a military connotation. Armies would not be very successful if they simply tried to do more of what was done last year, or even to do it more efficiently. Quantum leaps are not made by little increments across the board. Rather, the military nature of the concept

suggests that one must be ahead of one's competitors in thinking, must be in a more advantageous place, and have available newer, more sophisticated skills. The emphasis then is on having a differential advantage. Strategic planning is fundamentally a process for determining resource allocation and institutional emphasis or deemphasis. It is a proactive, externally oriented process that is especially critical in a rapidly changing environment.

There are various types of planning with different objectives. *Long-range planning*, which prepares for tomorrow using today's trends, is often upset by external changes. *Strategic planning*, on the other hand, relies heavily on assessment of internal strengths and weaknesses, and on external threats and opportunities. *Tactical planning* specifies the administrative details of strategic planning, while *operational planning* is practical, in the here-and-now, with concrete results.

Strategic planning for colleges and universities is particularly challenging when compared with that of business. Whereas a troubled business can relocate, divest its assets, or turn over its personnel, the educational enterprise is constrained by tenure systems, public expectations, and geographical location. "A president in business is paid to think strategically and to act decisively, not to be a consensus builder or moderator of opinion," argued Ryans and Shanklin (1986, p. 8). Such autocracy by the leader would not be tolerated in the academic milieu. Yet there are many similarities between educational and business enterprises and, more and more, boards of trustees are using businesslike approaches and standards to run their universities. In either case, information management is a key factor. The new-age executive needs to be a strategic thinker.

One popular model for strategic planning employs three scenarios describing the future; one for the most likely future, one for a pessimistic future, and one for an optimistic future. With the first, a master plan is developed; with the second and third, contingency plans as a modification of the master plan are developed as companion to it. The value to the scenario-based plan is the opportunity to debate in a proactive fashion what action would be appropriate. This "strategic rehearsal" in the "what-if" planning

methodology prepares administration for the future, which will most likely be some variation of the three scenarios (Ryans & Shanklin, 1986).

One of the most critical components of strategic planning is to clarify the mission of the entity, whether department, college, school, or university. In general, the answer to the question, "What business are we in?" for universities is straightforward. Universities are in the "knowledge" business. They generate knowledge (research), transmit knowledge (teach), and apply knowledge (community service, and in the case of health science centers, patient care). Strategic planning in the future for deans includes thinking through the impact of a more sophisticated nursing presence, faculty "intrapreneurship," and research linkages with business and industry.

Creating Excellence Through Creative Thinking

Excellence is a goal that can be achieved by every institution, not just the most elite institutions of higher education. The "niches" for excellence may be targeted by clarifying the mission. Obtaining excellence means having a competitive edge. Excellence rarely occurs by accident. It has to be sought diligently and with commitment. The increase in doctoral preparation of nursing faculty will strengthen the goal of excellence.

What kind of leader is needed to seek and maintain excellence among a stimulating faculty? Leaders must have vision and the ability to inspire others without intimidating them. Leaders must create the kind of culture to foster excellence, balancing academic freedom with focused centrality of mission. The right mix of idealism and practicality, as well as task orientation and people orientation, is necessary. The challenge is having teamwork with bright, independent, highly specialized professionals.

Once excellence is attained and recognized, the college, university or school cannot rest on its laurels. Competition is too fierce and progress too rapid. It is easy to be left behind without constant attention to maintaining excellence.

Developmental Attention for Fiscal Visibility

The new-age executive will spend a considerable proportion of time in development of the school, including fund raising, in order to assure resources for excellence. The reward of fund raising is generally that of helping to enrich the quality of life and to maintain excellence. Fund raising skills include planning and marketing. "Development" in its broadest sense means more than fund raising; it is helping the school attain its full potential. People skills are essential, as are communication skills.

Important factors in fund raising include honesty, integrity (honoring the verbal agreement), knowledge, willingness to work hard, and optimism. People make gifts to support goals. Goals and plans for the future are prerequisite for fund raising (Broce, 1986). Would you have a ready answer to the question, "What would you do with a million-dollar gift if it were received today?"

Skills in proposal writing are necessary in preparing a goals statement as part of the marketing process. The art of successful proposals depends on clarity and soundness. Brevity increases the chances of its being read throughly. The proposal should reflect standards of excellence, the importance of the idea, as well as the urgency.

The state of the economy will not necessarily be a predictor of philanthropy, that is, a downturn in economy does not mean an automatic decrease in giving. The school most likely to acquire funds from private gifts is one that is successful and promising, not one that is needy and of poor quality. People want their investment to pay off, and a school with a record of achievement is more likely to succeed again. An assessment of the donor's interests and a match with the school's needs will increase the chances of voluntary giving.

The dean will also be involved more intensely with the community, and particularly with industry. Joint ventures with health science agencies will be common as both institutions seek to maximize resources and recognize their inherent dependency on each other. The business community will be interested in the economic impact of the educational enterprise. Venture capitalists will be interested in nursing research that has commercial applications.

Nurse "intrapreneurs" will flourish in an environment that emphasizes alternative delivery of services. Deans will facilitate faculty practices that generate revenues and create a research arena. Special populations will be served in nursing school clinics. Faculty will have ideas for small businesses as subsidiary corporations of the school. These "intrapreneurs" will demand resources, both human and material, as innovations are actualized.

The trend toward decentralization and "intrapreneurship" will result in smaller units of the organization, shifting emphasis from the whole to the component parts. The dean's challenge will be in communicating the vision and managing the component parts, which will operate competitively as well as collaboratively. Other challenges will come in determining ways of measuring success and profitability and allocating rewards to an innovative faculty. Joint ventures with industry, limited partnerships, leased arrangements, and other financial opportunities will be activities that the dean must evaluate for realizing school goals. Nursing technology assessment and development will be a thrust for the future, requiring knowledge of intellectual property rights, invention disclosures, venture capital resources, and patent processes. Nursing research will come into its own in the years ahead.

In summary, the future is uncertain but positive changes for nursing are predicted in this chapter. The new-age executive skills needed by the dean in the future will require more knowledge of finances and tracking of societal trends in the dynamic environment. The ability to think strategically and plan accordingly will be basic to survival. Creating a supportive corporate culture and maximizing the efforts of people working toward the same goals will help to ensure excellence. The dean will need to spend considerable time enhancing fiscal viability of the school by being involved in fund raising activities. Furthermore, the dean may be heavily involved in facilitating commercialization of nursing research and technology development. All in all, the future holds a challenging vision for nursing education administrators.

REFERENCES

Aydelotte, MK, Hardy, MA, & Hope, KL (1988). *Nurses in private practice: Characteristics, organizational arrangements, and reimbursement policy*. Kansas City, MO: American Nurses Foundation.

Broce, TE (1986). *Fund raising: The guide to raising money from private sources*. Norman: University of Oklahoma Press.

Gavzer, B (1988, July 17). What this medical battle could cost you. *Parade Magazine*, p. 10.

Griffith-Kenny, J (1986). Employment discrimination. In N. Evans (Ed.), *Contemporary women's health: A nursing advocacy approach* (pp. 401–407). Menlo Park, CA: Addison-Wesley.

Martinson, IM, Jamieson, MK, O'Grady, B, & Sime, M (1985). The Block Nurse Program. *Journal of Community Health Nursing, 2* (1), 21–29.

Ryan, S (1988). *Transition from institutional to home and ambulatory care*. Paper presented at the Forum for Nursing Practice in the 21st Century, which was co-sponsored by the American Nurses Foundation and the Annenberg Center for Health Sciences of the Eisenhower Medical Center, Kansas City, MO.

Ryans, CC, & Shanklin, WL (1986). *Strategic planning, marketing, and public relations, and fund-raising in higher education: Perspectives, readings, and annotated bibliography*. Metuchen, NJ: Scarecrow Press.

Smilor, RW, Kozmetsky, G, & Gibson, DV (1988). *Creating the technolopolis: Linking technology commercialization and economic development*. Cambridge, MA: Ballinger.

✳ EDITOR'S QUESTIONS FOR DISCUSSION ✳

What differences exist in leadership and administrative styles, predominant goals, objectives, and values held by deans of the past versus the present? How have expectations for the role of the dean changed from the past versus the present and future in terms of academic preparation, professional experiences and qualifications, needed skills, and knowledge base? What factors have most contributed to these differences and changes? What are the advantages and disadvantages of having a majority of faculty with doctoral preparation in nursing versus a nonnursing discipline?

How can a dean be assured that a doctorally prepared faculty member has both expert clinical and research skills? How might two track systems in doctoral programs—clinical and research—alleviate potential problems regarding the clinical expertise needed for faculty? How might deans successfully incorporate practice into the university role? To what extent should or how can a dean resolve potential conflicts that may result in simultaneous, competing expectations for faculty work loads? Given that the faculty member is awarded funding for research, what ethics are inherent in the use of such funds? What obligations may be inherent regarding the faculty member who has been hired on the basis of "soft money?"

What applications can be made from the dis

cussion by Beyers (Chapter 55) and Farrell (Chapter 59) for the suggestions offered by Starck? What type of resources and support networks might a dean provide to encourage interaction and utilization of business principles and processes? How is strategic thinking different from strategic planning? Can strategic planning be learned? What conditions might make one type of planning more appropriate than another? How can a dean most effectively assess a community for potential fund raising opportunities, as well as services that faculty practice might provide? What standards of excellence should be evident in fund raising proposals?

What are the strategies, structures, and processes that most facilitate a culture and environment for excellence in a school of nursing? How can a culture and climate most effectively and successfully be altered in an institution? What applications and relationships exist between Baker (Chapter 60) and Starck? What is the relationship between competition, motivation, and effectiveness in academic administration? What might be the impact of competition on the culture in a particular school? How can a dean inspire others most effectively? How can the dean of the future most effectively allocate rewards for faculty? What criteria might be suggested for determining the rewards as well as their allocation?

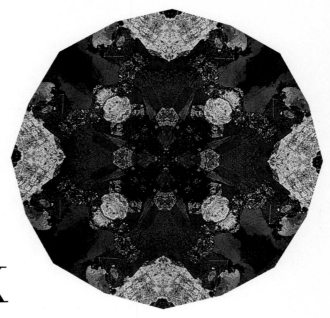

PART IX
SUMMARY

The circular design of the kaleidoscope may be thought of as symbolizing the universe, totality, and wholeness. The kaleidoscope of nursing transforms objects from individual prisms and scopes within the profession for a wholistic view. Thus each of the major facets of the profession that were focused in the preceding parts of this volume are reflected in the summary chapter by Chaska. The diversity within and among the separate areas or scopes of nursing are unified for a global image of the profession. The observations, comments, and suggestions should move others to project more questions, turning points, and changes in the kaleidoscopic view of nursing. Movement is natural and harmonious within the cylinder. There is room and a place for each individual scope and all the dimensions of nursing for a whole view of the profession. Each is vital for the transformation of nursing into a unified forward-moving profession.

643

73

The Kaleidoscope of Nursing

Norma L. Chaska, Ph.D., R.N., F.A.A.N.

Turning points and changing patterns are inherent in a kaleidoscope. Nursing may be reflected through a kaleidoscope. Numerous prisms of truth, direction, and certainty are projected on the mirrors of error, deviation, and doubt in one ever-shifting kaleidoscope. Multiple shades of vibrant images and inspiring designs are formed. The visual potential is as infinite as the colors and shapes of thoughts, beliefs, and values.

Obviously there is movement within a kaleidoscope. The changing patterns are natural, evolving spontaneously. The transformation of the old therefore becomes easy. The old is discarded and the new introduced in time. Nursing may be viewed as a historical kaleidoscope that has undergone hundreds of changing turns. Numerous changes may be exhibited through a succession of shifting phases in most every aspect of nursing—within nursing education, nursing research, nursing theory, nursing practice, and nursing administration. Depending on the viewer, there may have been multiple turning points for the particular facet under focus or for the profession as a whole. The possibility also exists that there is only one turning point—yet to come.

Whatever the perspective one sees, there is room for diverse viewpoints in a kaleidoscope of nursing. Bright colors, symmetrical figures, and objects can be seen in the kaleidoscope, symbolic of the process of change always ongoing in all the areas of the nursing profession. These are constantly altered until a form (a new emphasis, a new model) is brought into focus for varying periods of time. The kaleidoscope of nursing represents the views and beliefs of many persons and many facets of the profession. Each person creates her or his own kaleidoscope for (philosophy) nursing, selecting materials according to individual beliefs. Each aspect of the nursing profession may form a kaleidoscope of its own, as well as contribute its part to the total profession. There is also emerging a design for a universal kaleidoscope of nursing.

The kaleidoscope is an appropriate tool and prototype for the nursing profession. The word is derived from three Greek terms meaning "beautiful," "form," and "to see" (Baker, 1987). It symbolizes wholeness, the universe, and totality. The great spectrum and diversity of colors offer constant refreshment, as the individual scopes and scopes representing each aspect of the profession are transformed and merged into one. With each turn the creative flow of thought is tapped for professional inspiration.

A holistic view and holism is being advocated for the profession. The inner realm of wholeness can be difficult to understand and express. Many of life's secrets and mysteries are buried deep within a unified wholeness. Creativity comes from within before it can be shown in the external realm. Each of us has a kaleidoscope within. Each of us in nursing contributes to the various colors, shades, hues, to the cuts, facets, and gems that exist in the kaleidoscope of nursing.

Windows of the inner space within ourselves and the profession must be opened for the light of reflected thoughts and ideas. These may be like a gentle breeze to stir existing beliefs, values, and action patterns. The kaleidoscope wheel may then be turned until a spectrum of thoughts are lifted up, shared, and valued. Each particle of thought is essential, not necessarily greater or lesser in importance—but different. When there is an intuitive and empirical knowing that all the pieces are falling into place, then a true kaleidoscope for the profession will be complete. Until that exists we suggest, motivate, turn, rotate, and evaluate views to allow for the maximum in sharing, to permit a true, accurate perspective to be developed and become real.

To encourage the process of developing a kaleidoscope for nursing, this author has chosen to reflect predominantly on some of the issues and concerns that the contributing authors have raised concerning nursing education. Nursing education provides the foundation for the profession itself. Without education there is no knowledge development, research, high-quality caring practice, or human resources and effective systems to provide for, develop, and manage. Without nursing education there *is* no future in nursing. Without nursing education there *will be* no future of nursing. As viewed by many, nursing education is in crisis and—as some might perceive—near chaos.

This focus is not to imply that other aspects of the profession are less important. For example, nursing research and practice are also critical to the profession. However, these present different issues that cannot be thoroughly and meaningfully addressed until nursing education is more clearly stabilized, with clearer views and relevant responses. Only then may the profession continue to move on and forward.

For this reason, nursing education is the facet of the profession that is most emphasized in this summary chapter. First, some thoughts are offered regarding the professionalization of nurses and nursing. Next are reflections on education. Later, some issues and concerns are highlighted that the chapter authors have called to mind in other portions of this volume: nursing research, its theory, nursing practice and administration, and the future of nursing.

Regarding these, additional considerations are offered in all of the facets of nursing to portray in this volume an overview of nursing. Finally, an analogy with the kaleidoscope is offered as a means for projecting nursing in its completeness into the future.

PROFESSIONALIZATION

There are a number of recurring themes in the contributors' chapters that reflect specific facets of professionalization. These are (a) the meaning of what a profession is and what it means to be a professional; (b) resurgent emphasis on professional values for nursing; and (c) perennial concerns regarding the organization of the profession.

The Professionalization of Leadership

Throughout the contributors' writings about professionalization, as well as in other portions of this volume, there appears a subtle acknowledgement and plea for leadership—but leadership of a different kind than perhaps has ever existed within nursing. In the first eight chapters, the underlying force that warrants further emphasis is leadership. Without it the critiques, suggestions, and recommendations that are offered in those chapters will go unheeded and not be activated.

Even so, there is more to professionalization than leadership. One might suggest that today there is a call for a professionalization of leadership. Professionalization in itself is an issue that requires leadership for resolution. Nursing has been somewhat obsessed with making distinctions between professional and technical practice. Margaret Newman (Chapter 7) has suggested a most realistic and relevant resolution to those no-win discussions. She urges that differentiations be made according to the paradigm for practice one uses. The same application might be made to the professionalization of leadership.

Paradigms of Leadership and Moral Meaning

Leadership requires more than specialized expertise. There are paradigms of leadership, some more effective than others. Today, critical questions are being raised regarding the ends and values that our profession should serve and the justifiable means that leaders use to achieve their ends. Clarity of moral vision is essential in the professionalization of leadership.

Fowler (Chapter 4) emphasizes nursing's moral commitment. She shows the need for attention to nursing's emerging public roles and responsibilities. Perhaps to some extent, nursing previously applied the language of ethical responsibility to concerns related more to economic self-interest and a desire for social status than to ethical dedication. Now it is apparent, not only in nursing but in all of the professions, that the moral meaning of professionalism implies a dedication to a distinctive set of ideals and standards of conduct. This idea further calls for a moral ethos beyond that which has previously existed in any of the professions.

Sister Rosemary Donley and Sister Mary Jean Flaherty (Chapter 64) seem to caution the profession of nursing regarding the possible erosion of the moral meaning of professionalism. They alert the profession to avoid degenerating into a composite of special interest groups engaged in a socially harmful struggle for privilege, power, and position. It is imperative that nursing heed such words of discretion as the profession takes on new roles of social power and leadership.

Moral Empowerment for Leadership

Power and empowerment are inherent in the professionalization of leadership. Yet power is a controversial and much maligned word, more related to demonstrated misuse or abuse rather than positive uses. Sherry Cohen (1989) proclaims tender power as the dream of the future. Tender power is the instinctive warmth, empathy, nurturance, cooperation, connection to others—balanced and combined with intellectual and economic freedom—in play with the clout to lead, make decisions, make money, and change the world. She defines the role of the new woman as one who uses her femininity and sheds the masculine leadership style while keeping the power.

In referring to nursing as traditionally a profession almost exclusively peopled by women, Cohen cites examples of tender power. Although she does not refer to Shirley Chater—a renowned nurse—in this part of her book, Cohen later extols Chater in her present role as President of Texas Woman's University as a model of tender power in higher education. Cohen acclaims the form of management that is evident at Texas Woman's University as being highly moral, encompassing humanistic values, and the essence of professionalized leadership.

A Moral Vision for Nursing

Reflection on the words of the numerous contributors to this volume who have addressed professionalism remains insufficient. Nursing as a profession must play an even more positive social and cultural role than it has in the past. It must help sustain and revitalize the shared values and goals that inform our sense of common purpose. New kinds of social and political roles are being called upon by some contributors, such as Aydelotte (Chapter 2), Wakefield (Chapter 6), and Yeaworth (Chapter 62).

A new kind of moral vision is advocated for the profession if nursing is to play these roles legitimately and well. Nursing has shown itself to be quite adept at lobbying. However, the legitimate lobbying to protect a profession's special interests is no substitute for using the expertise and experience of the profession as a resource for policy analysis and policymaking in the public interest. Nursing possesses a distinctive kind of knowledge and experience about important areas of health, human life, and social concern. The history of the profession, its own changing values, and its special vantage points provide a unique source of insight. Nursing nurtures particular values and social priorities, but the common good is a kaleidoscope of many different goods and values. Our general sense of the common good evolves out of the multiple views of many. The insights and perspectives of numerous professional nurses can contribute to a cultural whole that is greater than its separate parts. That is the final dimension of the public duty of nursing as a profession.

Commission on Organizational Assessment and Renewal

Influential segments and intellectual ferment now at work in nursing are presenting new opportunities for the profession and professionalized leadership. The profession is creating a renewed vision of its mission and of its place in the broader society. The goal of the American Nurses' Association's (ANA) Commission on Organizational Assessment and Renewal (COAR) has been to strengthen the ANA on behalf of its members, the nursing profession, and the American people. Through study of the structure of the ANA, its function, membership base, and interorganizational relationships specific goals can be accomplished (COAR, 1989). The Commission proposed a set of 59 recommendations to strengthen the ANA internally and reinforce its role in all of organized nursing and in the health policy arena. Margretta Styles perceived the deliberations and decisions of the House of Delegates of ANA as the opportunity either to launch nursing into a new era or to stand still while time and circumstance passed by the profession (Styles, 1989). The House of Delegates of ANA acted on the COAR recommendations in June 1989. The major recommendations were approved for implementation. The profession is now entering a new era.

Multiple forums, such as provided through COAR, have been and are being advanced in which professionals may discuss and debate their public duties with one another and with laypersons. Such forums may be turning points toward a more complete vision for the future. Ethical commitments may counter economic and political pressures and mitigate against narrow professional self-interest. Today's moral aspirations for nursing may become tomorrow's expectations and society's demands.

NURSING EDUCATION

Perhaps at no other time in the history of nursing education has there been more simultaneous challenges. Provocative questions present themselves in numerous issues pertaining to students, faculty, curriculum, and the increasingly scarce resource—money. There are some obvious interfacing relation-

ships among the significant issues and some that may not be as obvious. Of all the variables that are having a strategic impact in nursing education, the one considered by many to be the most elusive is sufficient finances to provide the type of professional for the public that may best meet their nursing care needs. This author believes that if quality attention is focused on students and their needs, the other concerns (including money) will effectively be resolved.

The great majority of the chapters in the nursing education portion of this book focus on program and curricular concerns. Underlying many of these matters is an increasing consciousness of the need to recruit students. Therefore, addressed first below is the broad area of recruitment for nursing programs and the profession. Substantial attention is directed toward curricula, and models for nursing programs. Finally direction is offered as a potential suggestion for meeting the complex problems related to education and planning for the future.

Recruitment

Students are the main concern in nursing education. Marketing to draw students has become a dominant need. A critical aspect in successful marketing is to define the product not only for the consumer but also for attracting the essential resources to develop the product. For nursing education this means that students are both the essential resource to provide the product (nursing care services) and also the consumer of goods (knowledge) provided in nursing education programs. Heretofore, minimal efforts were directed at marketing strategies. Nursing students frequently entered nursing programs with some ideals about caring for people but with vague notions of the role and functions of nursing. Furthermore students previously have had even less of an idea of the opportunities that exist in nursing as a career. Consequently the profession has been crippled by not clearly defining its function and by its inattention to marketing.

In spite of the lack of clarity for the public regarding the professional role of nurses, the demand is increasing for nursing and health care services. The demand is partly related to some commonly known facts; persons (a) are waiting longer to seek care; (b) are sicker or more acutely ill when they are admitted to hospitals; and (c) frequently require more extensive services, treatment, and care while they are hospitalized.

Nursing schools are realizing the need to increase enrollments. Systematic recruitment programs are being developed. It appears that at least four major steps are essential to attract students. The first is to have valid and accurate information regarding the perceptions of the public (and potential students) concerning what nursing has to offer, what services nurses provide, and the degree to which nurses and nursing care are viewed as making a difference in the quality of health and illness care that is provided. Second, professors need to define the distinct professional role and functions of nurses. Third, education programs need to be developed further to prepare nurses sufficiently to fulfill the professional role and provide these functions. Finally, education programs should specifically define and evaluate the outcomes of its programs.

The product must be clearly and sufficiently defined. Not only must the public know what to expect from nursing service, but also potential students must be fully prepared and qualified to provide the services. To be qualified implies that students must have accurate knowledge of their professional role, functions, market demand, and availability of positions for which they are being professionally prepared. The question might be raised of where nursing and schools should start with systematic recruitment efforts.

Systematic recruitment strategies. Initially efforts might be made to ascertain the attitude, values, and beliefs of the public (and potential students) toward nursing as a career. One such study was conducted by Sigma Theta Tau International (STTI) in the state of Indiana (1988). Similarities and differences were identified between the Indiana public's perception of an ideal career as compared with nursing as a career. The findings of the study suggest approaches that may be used in recruitment. For example, the public in Indiana viewed the ideal career

and a nursing career in the same way with regard to these five aspects (STTI, 1988, p. 26):

> (a) career security, (b) intellectual application, (c) caring for people as a career attribute, (d) academic achievements, and (e) scholastic achievement as a prerequisite for career development.

Each of those five aspects should be reinforced in recruitment programs. In the Indiana study, the public perceived "autonomy in decision-making" to be a positive factor in an "ideal" career, but less apparent in nursing. In this aspect then, recruitment programs could focus on, articulate, and publicize the autonomous scope of nursing practice. Additional studies in other states might well be conducted to survey the perspective of the public in other regions regarding nursing as a career.

These studies should be followed up by an assessment of the public's knowledge and attitude concerning what nurses are professionally prepared to do, as well as how well they do it. Such studies might further enable nurses and nursing to set aside philosophical differences and declarations of "turf" in specialized areas and levels of practice. Nursing then freed from such constraining forces may focus on the one common goal of providing the high-quality, professional nursing care that the public needs and demands.

Implications of data about the public's knowledge of nursing. Such data would also be valuable in planning curricula and programs that define and sufficiently prepare the professional product that meets the public's nursing care needs. Extensive collaborative efforts between the public and the profession are needed to define health care needs and plan curricula that prepare practitioners to provide the needed care. Otherwise, efforts may be misguided and in vain.

For example, a total concentration in education programs on wellness and health maintenance—without significant content in the educational programs on illness care—is inadequate. A single-focused program limits the professional practitioner's preparation and ability to perform and the public's ability to be informed and experience the full scope of professional nursing practice. Although the public is increasingly seeking health care, the first encounter with services for many is when they are ill, not well. Until they have suffered the effects of illness, the public most often may be inclined to be unwilling to pay for health promotion or maintenance services, to ignore health practices, and to disvalue wellness programs.

A product is not marketable when it is unrecognized as a need. In the professions, as in business, it is becoming increasingly evident that success means listening to the consumer. It is essential first to listen to the needs that the public and consumer identify as being critical. Then the consumer may be more receptive to hear and see what additional services a profession may offer and what other needs may be met. Traditionally the professions have tried to tell a client or patient what is "best for them." Neither the professions nor a professional can prioritize needs for clients or patients and expect a positive response. The professions, nursing included, are discovering that this is the age of the consumer. Consumers are recognized as those persons who utilize goods; in so doing, they pay for these goods. It follows that consumers should have significant say as to what those goods should be—not only in kind and number, but also in quality and for what need or purpose.

Two-pronged approach to recruitment. The preceding discussion also has implications for recruitment programs. The point is that the public is not only a potential consumer of nursing care services, but also the public includes potential consumers (students) of nursing knowledge in nursing programs. Thus a two-pronged approach is needed in recruitment programs. First, recruitment for the profession should focus on the total person, that is, needs for care in both health and illness; furthermore specifically what nurses and nursing have to offer to provide this care should be indicated. Second, education programs need to be more appropriately designed, offered, and marketed to meet the needs of potential students and to prepare them to provide high-quality, professional nursing services. The development of nursing programs is addressed later. Additional comment is helpful here regarding recruitment efforts.

Pool recruitment needs. The pool of qualified nursing applicants is quickly evaporating, leading many institutions to cut programs. A number of factors have contributed to the alarming state of affairs, including fewer high school graduates compounded by expanding career options for women. The image of nursing that is projected by the media also has been cited as a factor (Wohlert, 1987). According to Rosenfeld (1987), shrinking applicant pools are forcing programs to lower admission standards. "The United States Department of Health and Human Services has projected a deficiency of 600,000 nurses prepared at the baccalaureate and higher levels by the year 2000" (Rosenfeld, 1987, p. 286).

Moreover, it is becoming very difficult to retain students once they are admitted (Rosenfeld, 1987). Remediation is projected to be a more serious problem than in the past. Extensive efforts are urged for educators to increase their efforts in assisting students' performance at a high level academically rather than to lower their standards, which would be disastrous for consumers and the profession.

Recruitment considerations, techniques, and mechanisms. Special considerations are urged for potential groups of recruits such as minorities, immigrants, and older students who have family responsibilities. Recruitment efforts might include offering day-care facilities, remedial courses, flexible schedules, tutoring, television and radio spots, and booths at shopping malls and health clubs (Rosenfeld, 1987).

Faculty and practicing nurses might also work with high school counselors for career days. Offering lectures about nursing in a high-school health class or courses in a high school's facility for public continuing-education groups, or lecturing to volunteer service groups and organizations, also would provide access to accurate information about nursing and programs.

As another recruitment strategy, Ellis (1989) suggests the development of an honors program for high school seniors to promote qualified applicants. Selected nursing courses or independent study projects might be made available for such seniors. Ellis (1989) further suggests the development of cooperative work study programs and more flexible curricular patterns for course and clinical experiences.

Consistent effort to develop a strong network and support system between freshman college students and upper division students who are completing their nursing major courses should be encouraged. Students who are completing liberal arts and science requirements can be motivated to excel and complete a nursing major through planned interaction and support activities, such as "sponsors" for lower division undergraduates and mentoring. Furthermore prenursing-major students also may develop more accurate perceptions about nursing through network systems. Increasing the maximum number of years for the completion of a degree program and the planning and advertising of course schedules for a number of years in advance may facilitate part-time students to persevere and complete programs.

Wohlert (1987) has suggested that nurses themselves have a responsibility in recruiting students. Volunteering to be a mentor and forming future nurses' groups, projecting a positive image, arranging a nursing career day, and speaking at school clubs or church gatherings are means for attracting potential students.

Some states and universities (e.g., Indiana University) are developing prepaid tuition programs to provide a solution for those who either cannot or will not set aside enough money for paying future college tuition. Indiana University's plan provides for the future purchase of a 15 undergraduate credit hours at current tuition rates. The Guaranteed Tuition Certificates provided the purchaser are tax deferred and transferrable. A secondary market also has been established to permit the sale of the certificates, in the event a potential student does not attend the university (Hackett, 1989). Similar payment provisions, including installment tuition plans, may be increasingly advocated as a means for recruitment into nursing programs as tuition and education costs continue to rise.

Attracting and keeping qualified students is only half the challenge. Questions and concerns further abound regarding nursing education programs. These program issues need resolution for realization of a legitimate, qualified, professional product that is marketable and for the survival of the profession itself.

Nursing Education Programs

In the chapters by Beletz (9), Rapson (10), Mundt (11), Duffy (12), Fitzpatrick and Modly (13), Watson and Bevis (14), Farrell (59), and Conway-Welch (65) it is apparent that a sense of impending chaos exists with regard to nursing education programs in general and, perhaps, particularly to those for undergraduate education. Radical changes are being advocated, promoted, and implemented. Journal publications further proclaim a turning point that is ahead and that must be achieved. An article by Ida Orlando and Anna Dugan (1989) is somewhat representative of the current literature. This and other articles lend support to beliefs that the American Nurses' Association's social policy statement and proposed definition of nursing is too general, failing to justify nursing as a distinct profession, and that it does not facilitate the understanding of differences between nurses and other professionals. Clearly nursing education has the opportunity to make a public social statement by providing programs that demonstrate what nursing is and what it has to offer the public. First, some general comments are in order.

Nursing education in the business of knowledge. Nursing education is in the business of knowledge development, implementation into practice, utilization, and evaluation (Farrell, Chapter 59). Other contributors in this book, particularly Snyder (Chapter 15) and Lenz (Chapter 16), make significant points regarding the diversity that exists within and among nursing education programs.

Although *quality* is not a tangible, it is important that nursing provides standards for its programs. Standards are evident, perhaps more so in some programs than in others. However, standards should be specifically established for admissions into programs, curriculum content, teaching methods, qualifications of faculty, and the evaluation of program outcomes. Holzemer (Chapter 17) presents an excellent stimulus for the development of standards and program evaluation. Limiting the extent of program offerings, when faculty resources are minimal or are being overextended is advisable. For example, in schools that have both undergraduate and graduate programs, it is probable that every area of concentration should not be offered in a graduate program. Multiple areas of concentration may be desirable to maintain a program; however, the areas should be selected and restricted according to the number of qualified faculty.

Universities should focus on providing education for the focus in nursing that is based on their faculty resources and the public demand for this category of nursing services. For example, if there are already sufficient undergraduate programs available in a local or state area, it may be more advisable to focus on graduate education (master's and doctoral level) rather than on undergraduate education. Or the situation could be reversed. If there is an exceeding need and demand for students prepared at the undergraduate level and there are limited resources, faculty, equipment, and clinical experiences available for graduate education, the focus might better be placed on undergraduate education. Nursing education needs to reconsider its efforts to provide every program for every need for all persons, particularly when a single school with minimal and scarce resources is involved. The quality of content in the program and its outcomes for a school and students should not be placed at high risk or jeopardized. Too often quality is sacrificed for the benefit of numbers.

Problematic Areas in Undergraduate Education

There are a number of specific problematic areas in undergraduate education. Beletz (Chapter 9) highlights many of the issues, and Rapson (Chapter 10) addresses others concerning articulation of programs. Newman's emphasis in Chapters 7 and 30 on defining one's paradigm and urging a wholistic person approach in research, education, and practice should be most helpful. As a result, the arguments concerning levels of practice and defining who is being prepared to practice "technically" or "professionally" may be put into a relevant perspective.

From the content addressed by Newman (Chap-

ters 7 and 30), it seems obvious that the philosophical base and framework for programs (research and practice) should be clearly visible and identified. However, it is far more relevant to question the extent a program is person-based rather than to argue whether a program is based on the medical model or a nursing model. Questions also should be raised on the extent that a program is focused on both wellness and illness. Health encompasses both the concepts of illnesses and wellness, but health does not include disease. The latter is *not* an appropriate framework for nursing programs that are preparing students to *provide health care* functions, but *not* curing of disease.

The "fruit" analogy, input from students, the general public, nursing professionals, and articulation programs. It was reported that in providing testimony and trying to explain some of the differences between programs and graduates of associate and baccalaureate nursing programs at a commission hearing on higher education, an analogy was made to fruit (Sherry T. Smith, EdD, RN, personal telephone communication, June 1, 1989). Apparently, a person responded to the cliché, "a nurse is a nurse is a nurse," and to the often-phrased conclusion and question, "so what difference does it make what program a nurse graduates from?"

In the response, several points were made. Although peaches, tangerines, apricots, and plums are all fruits, they are different. Different does not mean necessarily less than or better than, but unique. The "seeds" may be similar in the numerous nursing programs, but each seed does not necessarily make the same fruit. Nor can one use any kind of seed or seeds and expect a fruit. Likewise, nurses from all nursing programs are expected to be and are caregivers. However, it does not mean that they are all the same, nor does it mean that they administer care in the same way.

The analogy helps to further pinpoint what appears to be the essential problem in undergraduate nursing education programs. Nursing's distinct role and functions are *not* clearly, concretely, and sufficiently being stated, taught or reflected in the content and clinical experience offered in programs. Furthermore nursing's role and functions have never been sufficiently operationalized for job descriptions that allow for distinctions, differences, and relevance in practice settings.

Lest one is tempted to complete the analogy of fruit by advocating a generic brand, a word of caution is advised. Recently this author had a discussion with a number of undergraduate baccalaureate students from an Eastern state. Some students resented being called generic students. To them the label was not a compliment. It meant "easily available" and "worthless."

Further exploration revealed that students attributed the negative meaning as being identical to that inferred by some people who buy products labeled "generic" in the supermarket! It never occurred to them that generic could mean owning all of the valued characteristics that are inherent to a product. Nor did it ever occur to them that, as a minimum, generic could refer to the essence of something being present to develop a unique or distinct product or entity, such as a nurse. Viewpoints are always best seen from one's own value system!

However, listen to your consumers—your students—as to what they say and what they believe is essential for their knowledge and experience in programs. Student input in the planning, development, implementation, and evaluation of programs is critical. Students and graduates may be the most strategic persons in recruitment of potential students and in marketing products from programs to the public at large. Developing and producing a true professional is a process. Students can provide valuable information for the most effective process.

The concerns regarding articulation of programs will remain as long as multiple programs and entry levels for professional practice exist. There are also many questions surrounding the generic, baccalaureate program. As long as there are no distinctions made in content, outcomes, and expected roles and functions between programs, confusion and frustration will reign.

Many of the approaches advocated by the contributing authors' are in direct response to many of the questions being raised by the profession, the general public, students, and nurse executives. In completing the telephone survey done by Chaska and Alex-

ander (Chapter 57), these investigators frequently were offered additional comments by nurse executives regarding undergraduate education and the preparation for nursing practice. After this author reflected on the content presented by contributors in this volume and discussions she had with numerous executives, a number of summary statements and questions are offered for further consideration.

Evidence of crisis in undergraduate education. Undergraduate nursing education appears to be in crisis. Noteworthy are the numerous directions that are suggested for developing programs. A number of persons and schools advocate a total revolution in the baccalaureate approach to education. For example, the University of Virginia in Charlottesville offers an experimental approach whereby the generic students complete core nursing courses in the first 3 years; in the fourth year, students choose one of two areas—wellness or illness—as a focus area for *specialty* practice. For the wellness focus, students study and are placed in community health, school, and home care situations. To concentrate on illness care, students have learning focused on advanced nursing practice in specialized units of tertiary care centers.

Another approach seen is the offering of a number of specialty areas from which a student may choose for specialized clinical knowledge and experience leading to specialized future practice, while providing very limited general knowledge. A third approach is to require the baccalaureate student to complete a set of basic core nursing courses, and then focus predominantly on the child or the adult, or both in a specialty area of practice. Examples of such adult specialty areas are oncology, mental health, or gerontology.

Then, too, there are numerous types of baccalaureate programs advocated that are planned predominantly to meet the needs of "transition" students. Students who have earned a diploma or associate degree may enter these generic baccalaureate programs on review and approval of their initial educational experience.

Postbaccalaureate education for entry into practice. The professional doctorate (ND), as originally planned and implemented at Case Western

Reserve University (Chapter 13), might be considered a transition-type program since it was offered for students who previously held a baccalaureate degree. However, as it was and currently is being conceptualized for entry into professional practice, the title Doctor of Nursing (ND) is misleading. The degree is misunderstood by many and often thought to be a *graduate* degree in nursing equivalent to or in the same category as a doctoral degree. Although it is a postbaccalaureate degree, it is eligible *only* to those whose previously earned baccalaureate degree is in a discipline *other than* nursing.

The idea of a postbaccalaureate degree in nursing as the first degree for professional practice, yet *not* of the ND type of program originally planned and offered at Case Western Reserve University, has received some attention. Fitzpatrick and Modly (Chapter 13) and Watson and Bevis (Chapter 14) imply that there are universities that have implemented this idea. Conway-Welch (Chapter 65) advocates the postbaccalaureate degree for professional practice, but emphasizes that this is a specialist level. It is not clear whether or how content is built on that which was gained in a baccalaureate program. Does not the term "specialist" presume that, at some point in the education process, the learner has obtained "generalist" knowledge?

Other questions need to be addressed. What differentiates specialist from generalist content? What specifically is the difference between undergraduate and graduate level content? How might content appropriately be defined and developed for one type of undergraduate program versus another? How can one legitimately claim or refer to *any* program as preparing "advanced" practitioners for the nursing profession or offering "advanced" knowledge if the learner in that program has never had any prior nursing content and knowledge in a nursing education program? These questions need to be resolved for numerous reasons, regardless of what type of education program one is advocating.

As one example of the confusion and its effect, many persons believe "advanced" implies graduate level content and knowledge in the discipline that one is studying. It is *not* fair (and possibly unethical) to the consumer (both public and students) to

make a claim that is virtually impossible to demonstrate.

Some other types of postbaccalaureate programs in nursing are considerably different from the ND programs. Essentially students in these other programs have obtained previous nursing knowledge in a nursing program. These postbaccalaureate programs most often offer some advanced, master's level content in nursing and appropriately capitalize on the knowledge and experience that a prospective student has previously achieved. Frequently the students are originally diploma and associate degree graduates. Such programs might be referred to as the "bypass" (baccalaureate) master's program, a descriptive term for these programs that this author coined.

In a bypass program, differences in outcomes most likely would and should exist, given the diverse student background preparations and types of master's programs in nursing. Perhaps that may be a false assumption. However, another supposition is offered. One should expect distinct outcomes for those who hold a baccalaureate degree in nursing and then complete a master's program in nursing. Such outcomes might be juxtaposed for comparison with outcomes for those who had no previous type of baccalaureate or nursing education and then conceivably completed some type of condensed program labeled as a master's program in nursing. Should not one then see critical differences in the outcomes and differences in practice for the profession?

Further issues, presented by Mundt and Duffy (Chapters 11 and 12, respectively), center on the clinical experiences offered in the undergraduate curriculum and the teaching methods utilized. There is no question that both are critical areas that need extensive discussion and evaluation. In addition to the insightful and valuable ideas presented by these two authors, the reader is urged to become acquainted with an article written by Carol Lindeman (1989). Lindeman presents four cogent recommendations concerning the clinical laboratory and teaching.

International nursing education programs, as they pertain to the future, are addressed later in this summary chapter. However, the anticipated student population and care needs in the future demand significant changes and modes in the delivery of knowledge and provision of high-quality, appropriate clinical experience.

Understandably there are numerous approaches being considered in undergraduate education. Nursing as a profession is in a state of transition. Increasingly acuity in illness, hospitalization for care, technology, the content evolution of new knowledge, knowledge explosion, and the need for significant and extensive knowledge in many areas for holistic health care have resulted in a formidable situation. All needed learning cannot be accomplished in a 2, 3, 4, or 5-year program. How can the issue be resolved?

Undergraduate education might be better conceptualized as an introduction to nursing by gaining a solid foundation in liberal arts and science. Most educators insist that more liberal arts content is needed. The question is what is the best combination of liberal arts and science for nursing practice and for the vitality of the profession?

Graduate Education—Master's and Doctoral Levels

The master's graduate level in nursing education might more appropriately be planned to be a generalist preparation and the beginning of professional practice. Contributing authors writing for the nursing education portion of this book, in addition to discussing the limited time and vast knowledge needed, have provided convincing reason to believe that a true specialist level of nursing education is *not* realistic at the master's level. Specialist education and preparation is most appropriate at the doctoral level. However, it would appear that master's programs might appropriately begin to prepare a *specialist* in a *general* fashion, thus referred to as a generalist-specialty program.

Some examples may help. A student in a master's program may focus on nursing care in the general specialty areas of mental health and illness. This would be considered a generalist preparation that has sub-specialties. For example, the specialist type

of preparation at the doctoral level might concentrate on child abuse or abuse in the family. The phenomenon of concern to nurses and nursing at the doctoral level should be more specifically focused and concentrated, requiring specialized preparation.

Students who are interested in adult health might focus in a general way in that area as a general-specialty. Health promotion, maintenance, restoration, and education are general substantive areas in the field of adult health. Critical care, oncology, and gerontological nursing are others. However, caring for patients who have organ transplants; distinctive types of care needs related to radiation, chemotherapy, or terminal illness; caring for the dying or those that pose ethical issues—all of these require substantive, focused knowledge and specialized preparation that may be provided most appropriately in a doctoral program. These areas may be considered sub-specialties.

Role preparation. Preparation for specific roles in graduate education requires specialized knowledge. Snyder (Chapter 15) suggests that a general framework be developed for role preparation. Role theory could serve as the general base within this framework. However, use of the term *functional* in relation to role preparation and consequent reference to "functional role" seems redundant, misguided, and inappropriate. Role refers to expected behavior. *All* role preparation is intended to be functional, not dysfunctional. An identifier is usually attached to an index term that shows some relationship between the terms. It would seem more correct to refer to clinical specialist role preparation, management role preparation, or teacher or patient education role preparation.

Using the term *functional* attached to role also may suggest that a specific scientific base or framework is not necessary or nonexistent for the enactment of specific roles. Some might argue this point. However, there is evidence that significant effort is being advanced toward developing a substantive scientific base for a number of specific roles. The networking efforts through the Council of Graduate Education for Administration in Nursing (CGEAN) are merely one example. Moreover, to be noted is the emphasis on role preparation in some doctoral programs in nursing by means of clinical practicums that focus both on research and role application.

Doctoral Programs in Nursing

A significant amount of discussion remains focused on the differences in nursing programs that offer the two types of doctoral degrees: the doctor of nursing science (DNS) and the doctor of philosophy (PhD). The historical development of doctoral education in nursing, distinctions between these two degrees, and other salient issues have been consistently addressed in the literature. Two recent articles offered some additional strategies to resolve the issues (Meleis, 1988; Werley & Leske, 1988). Chapter 15 by Snyder and Chapter 16 by Lenz in this book offer additional substantive insight into the issues.

The need and demand for doctoral education in nursing are well documented in the previously cited works. Thus comments in this section will be limited to three currently prevalent themes: (a) the proliferation of programs; (b) consensus for one doctoral program in nursing; and (c) quality control measures.

Proliferation of doctoral programs.   The number of new doctoral programs in nursing have dramatically increased in the last 10 years. As of May 1989, 47 doctoral programs in nursing have been approved (P. Rosenfeld, personal communication, May 1, 1989). Furthermore numbers of schools are in various stages of planning and obtaining final approval. Lenz (Chapter 16) raises significant questions related to adequate resources of qualified faculty, facilities, services, and funding. It seems most reasonable and prudent wise that some consensus be developed regarding criteria for resources that should exist *before* establishing a doctoral program. Ideally the criteria might be directed at the initial assessment and planning stage for a doctoral program.

Most often the issue is what may or may not be deemed "adequate" in terms of resources and the considerations of planning for a program. More often the question is directed toward faculty resources. It is most desirable that *before* planning a doctoral program the institution has present a sufficient number of doctorally prepared faculty who have had experience in conducting research, obtaining grants, and guiding student research. What may be deemed a "sufficient number" depends on several factors, such as (a) the *areas* of clinical and research expertise; (b) the clinical and research expertise of the doctorally prepared faculty; and (c) a clearly defined and established program of research.

Areas of concentration or specialization in a doctoral program should be identified on the basis of present faculty strengths. Proposals for funding doctoral programs frequently include extensive recruitment plans for qualified faculty. Funding agencies also allow planning time to recruit and develop a program. However, it is ill-advised to propose a doctoral program if there is no qualified faculty member on board that represents the area or areas of concentration and expertise being proposed in a program. That occurrence might be rare. It happens, though, that a new major area of concentration is proposed in ongoing doctoral programs even though no qualified faculty for the subject area are present. There should be at least one (preferably two) faculty member(s) present with expertise in the proposed new area of concentration. Certainly it may be possible to recruit the essential faculty, particularly if the doctoral program has been firmly established for a period of time. However, the risks are extremely high, in terms of jeopardizing the quality of a program, overloading and overextending the present faculty, setting up unrealistic expectations of students, as well as raising serious ethical issues.

When faculty resources are scarce and it is not realistically expedient to recruit, universities might more appropriately plan doctoral programs to share faculty. Consortiums and cooperative doctoral programs exist and are thriving. One example of the latter is the program between the Schools of Nursing at the Medical College of Georgia in Augusta and Georgia State in Atlanta. Another approach might be to capitalize statewide or regionally on the expertise of potential faculty. Programs should be planned to develop expertise and an eminent reputation for a particular area of concentration or specialization. Thus different areas of concentration in nursing might be advisedly provided, promoted, and located in various parts of the country. The pooling of efforts and resources to establish excellent programs rather than struggling to compete seems wise.

Consensus in doctoral education.   Consensus to have one type of doctoral program in nursing is growing. The American Association of Colleges of Nursing (AACN) held a conference in February 1989 in which the agenda was to achieve consensus about the type of doctoral programs in nursing. Numerous participants indicated that the issue needed further discussion and consideration. It appears from that conference and others, the contributions to this volume, and other literature that consensus is nearing for one doctoral program that provides options (Meleis, 1988).

There are two main issues. The fact is that not everyone wants the same doctoral education, for career goals differ (Werley & Leske, 1988). Another fact is that the type of doctoral degree for nursing that frequently is proclaimed to be the most desirable is one that is nationally and internationally recognized, accepted, and associated with the highest standards of higher education and research. Consequently the doctor of philosophy (PhD) degree is the one most commonly advocated for nursing.

The issue remains—persons have different career goals, trajectories in education and experience, talents, and drives. The profession has many needs for sufficiently prepared leaders in practice, education, and research. For persons and the profession, a two-track option within one PhD program for nurses may be the solution. The options should include one for advanced professional clinical practice and a second for those who are committed to a lifelong career in research.

Defining the content differences between the two programs is advisable in terms of the (a) predominant focus in the two career tracks, (b) projected outcomes for students; and (c) expected future positions. There are market needs for doctorally prepared clinicians. It is becoming evident in the practice setting that these clinicians can make a difference in practice and in accomplishing relevant research (see Haller, Chapter 26). Both tracks should require common core courses pertaining to inquiry, including philosophy of science, theory development, research design and methodology, measurement, and statistics. Content could be organized around fields of concentration or conceptual areas of practice divisions as suggested by Meleis (1988).

An important concern that will need to be addressed is that some schools or colleges of nursing may find it difficult to obtain approval for a two-track PhD program. The problem involves the heavy emphasis on research in PhD programs, with traditionally far less focus on clinical content. Particularly approval may be a factor if the school or college is under the direction and control of the graduate division in a university. Furthermore it may be especially problematic for proposed clinical tracks that have indicated substantial practicum requirements or role preparation practicums in the program. Rather than reorganize such practicums under the guise of research, a more appropriate and advisable strategy is to plan and justify practicums that provide a research focus for the clinical track and practice. Both the preparation for conducting research in a clinical setting and role actualization need to be targeted in such practicums. There are numerous strong arguments that can be made for clinical practicums including examples from the discipline of psychology.

Quality control in doctoral education.   A third major theme in doctoral education is quality control. Holzemer (Chapter 17) provides directions on how to approach some of these issues. Meleis (1989) proposes a role for the National Forum for Doctoral Education in Nursing in the monitoring of doctoral programs. The Forum is a faculty peer-operated group that was established in 1977. The School of Nursing at Indiana University hosted the 13th Forum in 1989. The history of the annual forums and informal guidelines for its functioning are included in the 1989 Proceedings (Chaska & Markel, 1989). It was announced at the 1989 meeting that Sigma Theta Tau International (STTI) now has a copy of each year's previous proceedings. In addition, STTI has agreed to hold in its library a copy of the proceedings and the materials for participants in annual meetings of future years.

Voting agenda items for the Forum have included

jurisdiction over doctoral programs and potential affiliation with other organizations.* To have doctoral programs under the jurisdiction of an accreditation agency is not acceptable. This was evident in the "nay" voting results of Forum participants in recent years. Although Meleis's recommendation (1988) for monitoring doctoral programs may be a viable option, it is uncertain what future direction will surface concerning quality control.

Reconceptualizing Baccalaureate Education

Obviously there are many needs and issues to be addressed in undergraduate education. Furthermore it is possible that the conceptualization of baccalaureate education might be reconsidered. This author offers the following thoughts regarding a reconceptualization of baccalaureate education. The objective here is to contribute to the resolution of some of the present problems. It is hoped that further chaos is not a result! The public, students, and educators are confused with all the turns that have continuously occurred in nursing education. In Table 73-1 the *preliminary* reconceptualization of a model for baccalaureate nursing programs as two separate tracks is shown for discussion and reflection.

Clearly the two tracks in university undergraduate education, that is, the associate degree program and baccalaureate program, are here to stay. Nevertheless, extensive changes are being proposed, particularly in the baccalaureate program. It also seems clear that the essential focus in the associate degree program and the future role of its graduate is that of an *associate* primary caregiver. The future of the baccalaureate graduate will be predominantly in a distinct role as a generalist, clinical nurse. The major focus in such a baccalaureate program, however,

---

*Unpublished notations from the minutes of the 1987, 1988, and 1989 National Forum on Doctoral Education in Nursing. The actions related to the notations are included in the Business Meeting Minutes for the 1989 National Forum on Doctoral Education in Nursing, which was held June 7 to 9, 1989 at the School of Nursing, Indiana University (IUPUI), Indianapolis. The 1989 Business Meeting Minutes will be included with the package of materials prepared for participants who attend the 1990 National Forum at the School of Nursing, University of Texas at Austin.

would appear to be the roles of the clinical planner of care, primary caregiver as a primary nurse and case manager, and the coordinator of the health care role as in case management (distinct from a case manager). Case management, in this context, would include following patients or clients from the moment that they enter a health care system until their discharge to home care. It does not imply that these nurses necessarily provide the basic nursing care needed for clients; however, they could do so. Rather, these nurses are essentially planners of health care, assure its coordination, and follow through on all care that is provided. Case managers per se usually provide direct care to a group of patients who have the same type of nursing needs, such as patients who have organ transplants.

The associate degree graduate should have significant knowledge of direct primary care, with particular emphasis on technology and clinical skills. One type or level of nursing personnel cannot realistically be expected to provide all the nursing care that is needed for a patient. Knowledge, technology, and patient needs demand that the work and roles be divided.

A model for reconceptualizing baccalaureate education. There are a number of questions that need to be addressed should this unrefined model warrant further definition. One issue is whether to redefine the current basic baccalaureate program as a two-track option. The first track could be a clinical role track. The second could be a first-level management track.

Rationale for a two-track option. The rationale for offering a distinction between two tracks in a baccalaureate program is based on data that were obtained (See the studies by Sides, Chapter 56 and Chaska and Alexander, Chapter 57 concerning the preparation of nurse managers.) This author discussed the entry management role and preparation needed for that role with numerous nurse executives (Chapter 57). Many of the nurse executives offered additional information regarding the clinical preparation and skill competencies needed from undergraduate nursing programs. They strongly urged more general clinical content and practicum experience for baccalaureate students. The nurse execu-

TABLE 73-1
Preliminary draft in reconceptualizing baccalaureate nursing programs: a model for a two-track option

COMPONENTS	CLINICAL	MANAGEMENT
Goals	Initial preparation for first-level clinical practice	Initial preparation for first-level nursing management
Purposes	Facilitate preparation and operationalization of clinical ladders	Facilitate preparation and operationalization of nurse management ladders
Objectives	Facilitate distinct role, functions, job descriptions, and expectations for distinct levels of clinical practice	Facilitate distinct role, functions, job descriptions, and expectations for distinct levels of management practice

Core content	One year—liberal arts and science
	One year—technology
	Two years—clinical:
	  a. Nursing content
	  b. Clinical practicum
		One year—liberal arts
		One year—generic nursing
		Two years—management:
		  a. Management content
		  b. Integration of management with nursing content
		  c. Management practicum

Education ladders	1. Transition or mobility options?
	  a. Diploma, Associate graduates enter during second or third clinical years after evaluation or
	  b. No options
	
	2. Baccalaureate in Nursing with focus on clinical nursing
	3. Master's in Nursing with clinical area of concentration
	  a. Preparation as a clinical specialist
	
	4. PhD in Clinical Nursing track or Clinical Nurse Research Track
		1. Transition or mobility options?
		  a. Persons can opt for management after completing second year of the clinical track or
		  b. Transition-type students enter at the second-year level
		2. Baccalaureate in Nursing (?title of degree) with focus on nursing systems
		3. Master's in Nursing with area of concentration in nursing systems or nursing administration
		  a. Preparation for mid-level nursing management
		4. PhD in Nursing—Clinical Management track or Research Management track

Basic years of education	Four	Four
Salary	Beginning clinical level = Equitable with = Beginning entry level management	

tives understood the time constraints for these students. Some suggested deleting the management content per se from these programs. Given competing time needs, a priority for stronger clinical preparation of baccalaureate students was recommended. Furthermore a number of these nurse executives stated the belief that persons aspiring to or holding the first-level management position in nursing (charge nurse, assistant, or head nurse equivalent titles) should be prepared in a baccalaureate nursing program.

This author later reflected on the problem and the question arose as to how to simultaneously (in one degree program) prepare nurses for two beginning roles? Further discussions were held with other nurse executives, faculty, and approximately 90 nursing graduate students. The students were beginning their graduate program in the 1988–1989 academic year. Their initial nursing preparation was fairly equally distributed, representing associate, diploma, and baccalaureate undergraduate programs. As a result of these discussions and reflections, this author developed a preliminary draft of a "reconceptualized" model.

In recalling the earlier discussions with the nurse executives, it was apparent that the management content that is offered in present baccalaureate programs is grossly insufficient to prepare a beginning professional for entry level management practice. Furthermore the type of content and amount of experience in management in most baccalaureate programs are fairly superficial and often misleading. Students at times err in assuming that they are sufficiently knowledgeable and prepared to carry out significant management functions. Baccalaureate programs may be better advised to emphasize the *broad planning* and management skills that are needed in case management or primary nursing.

However, in considering all of the responses and options, it seems wise to reevaluate baccalaureate programs and possibly reconceptualize them into a two-track type of program. One track might focus on clinical education in a very broad, generalist fashion so that graduates would be prepared as a generalist in clinical nursing; alternatively, a management track might prepare students for a first-level management nursing position.

Clinical content in a two-track program option. The question remains what content might be considered appropriate in the two tracks. The clinical track content should ideally focus on extensive, didactic clinical content and clinical experience. Emphasis should be put on conceptualizing and planning basic nursing care.

Content for the clinical track in a baccalaureate program might be based on the work that has been done by the National Commission on Nursing Implementation Project (NCNIP), described by Conway-Welch (Chapter 65). The Commission's recommendations for the future stimulated this writer to reconsider the design of baccalaureate programs. From the appendix included in Chapter 65, it is apparent

that different levels of professional and technical nurses are needed to maintain future projections of nursing care needs.

This author agrees with recommendations that the baccalaureate nurse should have a strong foundation in the arts and sciences. However, the emphasis may more realistically be placed on preparing baccalaureate students for overall general clinical care, not necessarily for providing direct primary care. In the beginning clinical role for the baccalaureate professional nurse, it seems more realistic also to emphasize patient education, not faculty or staff education. Neither is it necessary to emphasize the *conducting* of research.

The emphasis for the associate (technical) nursing practice role, according to NCNIP, should be on direct care and technology. However, there does not appear to be discrete differences between the professional and technical nurse, as described by NCNIP. Clear distinctions should be made between the education preparation and outcomes expected between professional and associate (technical) nurses *if* the profession continues to plan for two specific role levels. If clear distinctions are not made, continued duplication in education and job descriptions, confusion and wastefulness in human resources, and high costs will remain and become insurmountable. In time, it is hoped that the two levels of practice will be more clearly defined.

Management content in a two-track program option. The management track might include 1 year of liberal arts content, 1 year of broad generic nursing content, and 2 years of basic management content. It would be important to emphasize that the generic nursing content should be substantially different from that provided in health management programs or hospital administration programs. The clinical content should be general nursing content. For example, focus should be on the broad professional role of nurses in clinical care—primary nursing and case management—so that the nurse in a first-level management position may understand the needs and resources of staff to provide care. Persons in the management track should have a broad understanding of nursing systems content. Such nursing systems content should include core management concepts regarding (a) leadership, (b) planning, and (c) personnel management. The predominant role to be emphasized in this track would be that of responsibility for obtaining, directing, and planning of resources for providing care in a nursing system. The emphasis in the beginning management role should be that of one who interfaces between direct nursing care, management of the nursing unit, and the department of nursing.

Mobility options in a two-track program. Another issue that needs to be addressed, before further consideration of a two-track option, is whether or not mobility options should be included for the associate degree and diploma graduate. One can argue that there should be no mobility options for the associate degree and diploma graduate, for example, in terms of those suggested in Table 73-1 for nursing graduates who are interested in the clinical track in a baccalaureate program. The profession clearly needs to take a stand if it wants to design a mobility option in a baccalaureate program. Indicators from politicians and legislators in state higher education commissions indicate that nursing most likely will be in continuing difficulty unless the mobility option remains.

A more critical question may be whether or not to design the outcomes of the associate degree programs as a terminal track program. Then two distinct levels of clinical practice need to be clearly evident in (a) the two education programs (associate and baccalaureate); (b) roles in the practice setting; (c) the basic job descriptions that are designed; and (d) compensation.

If one includes mobility options, it seems realistic that such options be offered to diploma and associate degree graduates at the second or third clinical year for the clinical track. The relevant diploma or associate degree program should be evaluated before designating the clinical year in which its graduate may matriculate. Possibly the management track would appeal more to the "transition" student; it may offer more new challenges for an experienced, more mature nursing student. Perhaps also, through this option, the frustration and anger frequently expressed by transition students may be alleviated. It would seem necessary, however, that "mobility op-

tion" students who choose the management track matriculate for 2 years of management content.

Finally, it should be emphasized that the model proposed in Table 73-1 is merely a *beginning* in the possible redesign of baccalaureate programs of the future. Many questions remain concerning the model's implementation, as well as that of others that might be proposed for initial consideration. However, without a major turning point in education—which such models suggest—there will be no future for nursing.

National Center for Nursing Education

A need for a center in nursing education is apparent. Confusion obviously exists regarding the design and implementation of numerous programs in nursing education. There are many knowledge gaps. For example, one school may evaluate and decide to change its curriculum. A second school may adopt a previously rejected curriculum that was thought to be ineffectual (but not necessarily evaluated as such) by another. Thus mistakes and errors are likely to reoccur in the process of nursing education.

Such occurrences are *not* the fault of any one school, numbers of schools, or the profession itself. Rather, the repetitive change and rejection of programs and consequent errors in implementing education programs are more likely related to many factors. Some of the variables are (a) insufficient dissemination of knowledge about education; (b) geographical distances between schools; (c) rapidity in the development of knowledge and technology; (d) differences in the cultural, socioeconomic-political factors across the country; and (e) accessibility of students and qualified faculty. It is difficult for any one school to be aware of the current effectiveness of its curriculum, let alone the suitability of its curriculum for other schools.

There also appears to be a need for some consistency among states and schools regarding the types of programs and content offered. For example, the content in the basic associate degree program should be similar throughout all schools for outcomes expected. A similar expectation might be proposed for basic baccalaureate programs. The concern therefore is that too many *different* designs are being considered and proposed for virtually all education programs, whether undergraduate, graduate, or postdoctoral. The lack of comparative evaluation of programs and the premature (without sufficient reliable and valid data) changes in curriculum, design, and programs must not continue in nursing.

Consequently it is proposed that a center for nursing education be established and federally funded in the United States. Its purpose would be to develop knowledge regarding the design, organization, implementation, and evaluation of the various types of nursing education programs from the associate degree to the doctoral degree. The proposed center should focus on all kinds of models, at the undergraduate as well as at the graduate level of education. Experimental designs should be developed whereby models for nursing education programs could then be tested *centrally* and outcomes evaluated. It could be the most effective mechanism for monitoring the quality of nursing education now and in the future, as well as evaluating present and future educational needs for the profession. Knowledge could thus be quickly disseminated. Furthermore this center should propose, design, implement, and evaluate various types of *international* models for nursing education.

A second purpose might be to monitor *other* programs that are currently being offered on a national and international basis. In so doing, a center could fulfill a third purpose and function—to be a centralized organizing unit for the ongoing implementation and evaluation of various nursing education programs for numerous schools and universities, who generally do not have the resources in personnel expertise and finances to develop and maintain high-quality, effective evaluation mechanisms and programs.

A national education center should be funded and operationalized without the control of overseeing concerns or jurisdiction of accreditation bodies. A center for nursing education might either be established minimally as an institute or as a complete center. If nursing education is indeed the foundation for the profession, it is critical that at least one national-international center be estab-

lished in the very near future for nursing education to survive and the profession to thrive.

NURSING RESEARCH

Three areas are highlighted regarding nursing research. The first area addressed is research methodologies. Then a brief discussion follows regarding the dichotomous demands in developing research programs; third, the implementation of research in the service setting is considered. There is evidence that there is a growing consensus for using multiple approaches and methods in research. The previous debates regarding the merits of qualitative versus quantitative methods for research in nursing appear to be lessening (Knafl, Pettengill, Bevis, & Kirchhoff, 1988).

Methodology and Phenomena for Study

There is no single best approach to nursing research. The contributing authors' writings on nursing research make it evident that a theory or conceptual base should direct the research questions that are being addressed. Research methods in themselves are merely ways of making observations. Thus, as emphasized by Donnelly and Deets (Chapter 21), the methods that are utilized should be appropriate to the research question being addressed. Furthermore, according to Deets (Chapter 20), serious questions should be raised regarding the use of the concepts "environment," "health," and "nursing" as the basis for nursing research. Deets's review indicates that this frequently espoused nursing metaparadigm is questionable as the conceptual base for nursing research.

Orlando and Dugan (1989) propose a more relevant direction for systematic study. These authors maintain that defining distinct functions and formulating the products for service in a clearer fashion will in turn provide the base for nursing's research efforts. They advise that carefully controlled studies that generate data about interventions with phenomena of nursing's concern are critical for the profession. These writers further point out that data about nursing interventions will show variations in the course of a person's condition, to which nurses may respond. If nurses focus on the phenomena of concern in nursing, the profession certainly should benefit, but most importantly the patient or client, as well as students in nursing education, will gain. The interventions most appropriate for nursing practice could then be emphasized in the education process.

Numerous strategies need to be considered, tested, and evaluated in developing research programs for nursing. The content offered by Ray (Chapter 23) concerning phenomenological methods, and that by Devine (Chapter 24) concerning the appropriate use of meta-analysis, should be most helpful in increasing the awareness of researchers to the possible uses of alternative methods. Stember and Hester (Chapter 22) present an additional viewpoint regarding the debate between quantitative and qualitative methods. In essence they suggest an approach that encompasses the two.

Developing Research Programs and Work Loads

A problematic concern exists regarding the development of faculty research programs. Clinton (Chapter 25) offers some concrete suggestions to resolve many of the issues. Nevertheless, the basic resolution of the dichotomous demands for nursing faculty remain. Essentially, the methods and the decisions for resolving the dilemma rest on the faculty member. However, two other suggestions are offered in an article by Megel, Langston, and Creswell (1988). These authors advocate the lightening of teaching loads of faculty who need and wish to initiate, develop, and enhance their research. They further suggest that faculty be given a blend of activities related to research, teaching, and service so that faculty are not overextended in any particular area. These writers believe that all three areas and roles should be supported and reinforced by the others.

Faculty who teach in graduate programs commonly are expected to carry the equivalent of three graduate courses per quarter or semester. This course load frequently is a portion of a total work load that includes the expectation to supervise dissertations, theses, and research projects. It appears that this is an unrealistic expectation for faculty who need to initiate, improve, or expand their research programs. Until the point in time that the faculty member is conducting a funded research project or program, a teaching load for faculty who are teaching only at the graduate level might more realistically include the equivalent of two graduate courses. Then, after the funded research has actually begun, it would seem highly advisable to have the teaching load reduced to one course. This limitation is particularly advisable for faculty who also are supervising clinical practicums in graduate programs.

For faculty who are teaching in undergraduate programs, it is imperative that the time needed for clinical practicum *teaching* always be included in the overall teaching load. In general, for faculty who are teaching undergraduate courses, the sum of the clinical teaching and didactic course load *and* student contact hours most likely should total no more than 18 hours per week. Ideally, the 18 hours per week should be inclusive of the contact time that includes counseling with students and evaluation.

The work load may vary not only with universities, but it also depends on faculty resources, size of the institution (faculty and students), and whether it is a private or state school. Regardless, it is critical to consider the following factors in determining work load patterns and expectations: (a) number of students that may be in a single course; (b) amount of faculty time needed for clinical precepting and teaching; (c) number of students a faculty member may be advising in student research; (d) program advising time for students; and (e) minimum university committee work.

Flexibility for variations and adaptations must be provided. However, a general, informal guide for an ideal distribution of work load requirements for a 5-day week might be as follows: (a) teaching, 2½ to 3 days per week; (b) scholarly endeavors (research and publication), 1 to 2 days per week; (c) service or committee work to the university, ½ to 1 day per week. These proportions are offered for a faculty member who does not have an ongoing funded research program. However, in accordance with that proposed earlier, once funding has been obtained, it appears reasonable to reduce the amount of time expected in direct teaching.

The increasing need and expectation for faculty to spend additional hours in class preparation, course preparation, and travel time to agencies and other teaching facilities continues to be a demand made on faculty in all programs. It is imperative that serious consideration be given to *realistic* expectations. Work loads need to be adjusted for faculty to be sufficiently free to initiate, develop, and maintain a research program. *Simultaneous* demands for providing challenging teaching content, enhancing excellent teaching skills—frequently while under heavy teaching loads—*and* developing an initial research program are totally unrealistic. Demoralized faculty and faculty burnout are predictable results. Academic administrators *in union with* faculty must devise ingenious approaches for their distinct settings and situations to resolve this suicidal dilemma.

On the other hand, it is unrealistic for faculty to expect that the so-called off-months during the summer should be totally free leisure time. One of the common attributes of professionals is that they maintain and further develop their professional expertise, to a great extent on their own time and with their own resources. Vacations should be taken, but faculty need to plan for some *additional* time, when they are relatively free of other academic obligations and responsibilities, to develop further their research skills, their programs, and their clinical expertise. Most professionals *seldom* function on the basis of an 8-hour day or 40-hour week. Nevertheless, it is imperative that faculty and academic administrators develop realistic expectations for themselves and each other. While so doing, they must be accountable for their own professional growth, development, and productivity whether it as teacher, researcher, clinician, or administrator.

Nursing Research in the Clinical Setting

The final area of concern addressed under the research topic is that of developing research in a practice setting. Haller (Chapter 26) presents significant suggestions for implementation of the clinical research role in the hospital or service setting. In-

creasing evidence indicates that establishing joint faculty research positions is one of the most effective ways to develop research in a service setting. Joint faculty research positions need to be further advocated and established. However, in so doing, role and accountability mechanisms for clinical researchers who have dual positions need to be clearly defined. Otherwise, the quality of their work, their effectiveness, and their productivity may be seriously questioned and in jeopardy if priorities become confused and role demands become too extensive.

In developing joint projects between service and academic settings priorities should be identified. Both clinicians and faculty members must be encouraged and utilized to develop further their research programs. These joint endeavors can be initiated by developing small, focused interest groups organized around phenomena of concern to nursing and the distinct interests of clinicians and faculty members. Development of focus groups may be the first step that leads to a potential clinician or faculty member developing an ongoing independent research program at a later stage. Periodically research groups should be encouraged to organize joint conferences for sharing concerns, methodological issues, and different approaches that might be used. Later, as funded investigators, their research findings should be shared. Collaboration and the sharing of resources, research opportunities, and adequate settings for research are imperative if nursing research is to be further developed.

NURSING THEORY*

Significant strides have been made in explaining the purpose of a philosophy of science as it relates to developing knowledge for nursing. Progress is apparent from the contributions of Fry (Chapter 28) and Sarter (Chapter 29). In comparison with 10 years ago, the higher level of sophistication now seen in the writings of numerous authors about the-

---

*The editor is indebted to Eleanor Donnelly, PhD, RN, Associate Professor, Department of Psychiatric-Mental Health Nursing, School of Nursing, Indiana University (IUPUI), Indianapolis for extensive discussions concerning the nature and development of nursing science.

ory is evident. Fry and Sarter indicate that a philosophical foundation for the discipline of nursing needs to be established.

The goals of science are the description, explanation, prediction, and control of phenomena. According to the contributor's writings about theory in this text, there is a growing consensus that each goal of science can best be met by drawing on a variety of approaches and methods to develop nursing knowledge. No one way is the single best and only way to develop nursing knowledge. The process of *how* we develop knowledge is equally important as *what* methods are used. To understand both the process and the methods, it seems imperative first to identify one's philosophical base. The writings in this portion of the book represent a trend toward identifying a relevant philosophical base in the further development of nursing theory. It is important not to think of the *proposed* (insufficiently tested) theories or models as actual theories.

Development of Knowledge in Nursing

Differentiating the terms *philosophy of science*, *philosophy of nursing*, *philosophy of nursing science*, and *nursing science* is critical. However, defining each is fraught with controversy and potential problems. The philosophy of science commonly is described as being based on a preoccupation with conceptual development rather than a preoccupation with actual events or phenomena. Menke (Chapter 27) discusses the assumption that philosophy of science speaks directly to the interest of the particular investigator. If this is so, it would be important to understand, for example, what kinds of questions a philosophy of science raises for an investigator or "tells" a researcher to address. Or conversely, what kinds of questions it tells a researcher *not* to address.

Philosophy of science in nursing must connect with other philosophical aspects of the discipline— such as metaphysics, logic, epistemology, and ethics (Sarter, Chapter 29). Much of that addressed by the nursing theory contributors in this text reflects a kind of metaphysical commitment on the part of nurse scholars, rather than actual paradigms for nursing science. This commitment may reflect nursing's eagerness to seek philosophical reference points for the real practice problems that confront us (see Kramer, Chapter 32). Fry discusses many philosophical issues in the development of nursing knowledge (Chapter 28). Her chapter is an excellent example of bringing the latest thinking of philosophy into the realm of nursing. However, this author questions the total application of the prevailing ideas in the philosophy of science to nursing without extensive examination. For example, Laudan's discussions (1977, 1984) of the problem-solving effectiveness of a theory appear to be commonly misunderstood. See Fry, Chapter 28, p. 219. Laudan is *not* concerned with the *how* of doing the practical, hands-on kinds of things in nursing nor with the usefulness of theoretical strategies that may make one nursing intervention more effective than another. For example, he would not be concerned with the most effective way to apply a bandage to reduce edema. Rather, he would be interested in trying to operationalize the *concepts* of pressure or constriction as it relates to reducing edema. Another example in which the emphasis would be on conceptual development rather than immediate practical application may be taken from physics. Some problems may not be resolvable within the realm of Newtonian physics. Laudan then would be more interested in asking which is better—Einstein's theory or Newton's theory? According to Laudan, the question to be asked is which theoretical framework—when applied to a set of conceptual problems—gives us a better focus conceptually. Thus, from his perspective it would be important to evaluate a proposed theory in terms of what *conceptual* problems are resolved in the proposed theory, what are not resolved, and how significant are these? Questions might well be raised here on whether or to what extent *any* of the theorists being cited has resolved their respective conceptual problems. Regardless of whether the conceptual problems are related to Roger's theory or Orem's theory or nursing diagnosis or taxonomy, the point is that Laudan *does not* provide direction on which proposed theory may be *useful* for practice. Therefore, it is doubtful that Laudan has relevance to the development of practice theory per se. There is need to distinguish the development of nursing knowledge per se from a conceptual point of view, contrasted with the application and relevance of knowledge for practice.

Beckstrand, Knowledge Development, and Practice Theory

A misunderstanding commonly exists concerning the frequently cited writings of Beckstrand (see, for an example, Fry, Chapter 28 p. 215). Beckstrand attempted to clarify the misunderstanding in an article published in 1984 and most recently in a telephone conversation with this writer (Beckstrand, 1984; J. Beckstrand, personal telephone communication, May 25, 1989). Beckstrand (1984) states that she was misinterpreted as saying that knowledge needed in nursing practice consists *solely* of theories and methods borrowed from the existing branches of science and ethical philosophy. Her intent was *not* to convey that the substantive scientific and ethical knowledge needed in practice must be borrowed from, or developed within, the existing branches of science and ethical philosophy. "[Her] point was that the theoretical knowledge required in *any* kind of practice activity was scientific and ethical in *form* and that practice could not be helped by a proposed new form of theoretical knowledge known as prescriptive theory" (1984, p. 190). Beckstrand also advises that knowledge from one discipline is often useful as a tool for others and that "nurses should expect to use and contribute to the development of existing areas of knowledge" (p. 196). Beckstrand further points out "what is important is that the explanations are made, or the problems are brought by people concerned with nursing" (p. 196). In this regard, Beckstrand's main thesis, however, is that *"THE UNDERSTANDING OF THE PHENOMENA THAT IS GAINED IS NOT BORROWED, BUT CREATED, AND CAN BE CONSIDERED ORIGINAL NURSING THEORY "* (p. 196). It is evident then that Beckstrand believes when knowledge is used from other disciplines to explain a phenomenon in nursing that that *understanding* is new nursing knowledge.

A question still remains about how Beckstrand defines practice theory. In discussions with Beckstrand, this author advocated that knowledge about what is useful or effective in practice contributed to the development of practice theory. Beckstrand raised the question, "If a practice theory exists, is it unique to nursing?" (J. Beckstrand, personal communication, June 16, 1989). This author responded that by Beckstrand's own argument (1984, p. 196) this is practice knowledge gained and *not borrowed* and that the result could be considered original nursing practice theory. It became clear that Beckstrand and this author define practice theory differently.

To Beckstrand, practice theory refers to *overall* practice. Therefore, a "practice theory" is a *form* of *generalized* knowledge. Scientific and ethical knowledge (and all of philosophy) are *forms* of knowledge. Questions about forms of knowledge and substantive knowledge are two different issues. To this author practice theory means theory that is developed from performing, evaluating, and testing nursing interventions, for example, the knowledge obtained by comparing two approaches in patient positioning. (The focus or phenomenon of concern to nursing is another issue.) The accumulation of such data would be *substantive* knowledge that may be tested.

Beckstrand sees the author's example as being the same as scientific knowledge. Her point is that if nursing wishes to develop practice theory that is on a par with scientific and philosophical theory as *forms* of knowledge, nursing has to show that the knowledge is different from science and ethics and that it is generalizable to the universe. This author believes that the kind of knowledge needed for nursing practice is that which is derived from both the empirical bases of the "received" and the "perceived" views of science as well as ethics. Both Beckstrand and this author concluded that the definition and clarification of terms is imperative for nursing to develop its knowledge base further. Admittedly, however, this is difficult to do with the confusion of definitions that presently exists. Further discussions are warranted regarding knowledge development and practice theory.

Paradigms and Consensus Definitions

Commitments in knowledge development may also be made to actual paradigms. However, paradigms presume a *substantive* knowledge base. Newman (Chapter 30) and Malinski (Chapter 31) propose a paradigm or theory for nursing knowledge. Theories within the discipline are derived from nursing's worldview and will be contingent, for example, on how such notions as health and illness are conceptualized. Malinski suggests one approach for a world view (see Chapter 31). Newman offers another approach in deriving theories from a world view through the development of patterns (see Chapter 30). She offers a way to conceptualize patterns of health; there is another way to conceptualize patterns for relevant understanding and applying the concept of health. For example, patterns that show an interface between the concepts of wellness and illness may be included in the overall concept of health. Such paradigms would be applicable in autonomous nursing practice (see Lyon, Chapter 34).

A further point should be made regarding the development of consensus definitions for concepts. Consensus definitions in the development of nursing knowledge may actually limit the development of knowledge. Consensus definitions may be appropriate, for example, for statements having to do with health policy for practice, but they do not allow for variations and scientific endeavors in the development of nursing knowledge. A thing becomes what it is *only* from the perspective from which one looks at it. Therefore, it would seem more appropriate to define the perspective or reality that one is using as suggested by Newman (Chapter 30), rather than impose a consensus definition.

Fawcett's use of rules (1989) in developing conceptual systems for nursing practice shows potential relevance. The link between theory, conceptual models, and rules for practice (Fawcett, Chapter 33) needs to be clearly defined as it is developed and used. The reader is referred to Fawcett's recent text (1989) for a more complete description and definition of rules and practice. As Newman (Chapter 30) advises, it is imperative that we know which paradigm is guiding our research and practice.

Holism Theory, Nursing Science, Holistic Nursing Practice, and Practice Theory

How appropriate are the philosophical underpinning and tenets of holism, as described by Kramer (Chapter 32), for practice theory? Questions regarding what is being advocated in the discussion by Kramer (Chapter 32) seem warranted. To view the patient in terms of meeting the needs of a *whole* person is one thing. Application of the tenets of holistic theory in practice or the use of tenets as a base for developing nursing practice theory is quite another. Some words of caution appear to be in order.

There is a difference between the tenets of holism subsumed within the scientific enterprise, holistic nursing practice, and practice theory. First, it may be helpful to recall that this author views practice theory as that which is developed from performing, evaluating, and testing nursing interventions.

In science one does not need to consider a particular phenomenon in relation to the whole. One never takes a "particular" in all of its "particulars" to understand a whole. Rather, one focuses only on the phenomenon of relevance. For example, in scientific research it is not a distortion to look at cells in relation to the tissue. But it would *not* be appropriate in nursing practice to look at a patient's skin lesion or what is inside of the lesion without looking at *who* has the lesion and the relationship it has to the person. Scientific theories and the tenets of holism as subsumed within the scientific enterprise do not enjoin the scientist to deal with *everything*.

The question must then be posed, Does nursing science focus on the whole person? This author's response is, "no, it cannot." Science is science. Science is concerned with particulars as representative of universals. It generalizes from particulars to universals. A nursing scientist would be interested in studying that tissue cell insofar as it represents all cells of that type for the purpose of understanding and explaining cell function. That appreciation may provide a theoretical basis from which the practitioner can draw creative interventions. At the level of a person, who is experiencing cellular dysfunction, the practitioner may choose how *best* to remove a dressing, cleanse a lesion, or apply a moist compress. Moreover, the practitioner may also choose *what* dressing to apply, what type of solution to use in cleansing the lesion, or what type of moist compress to apply.

Another example of science versus holistic practice in the real world of nursing may be posed in studying respiration as an exchange of gases. How the exchange takes place, the laws and regulating mechanisms governing the exchange, would be the "particulars" of interest to a scientist and possibly nursing science. The practitioner is interested in the exchange of gases only in relation to the whole person. The practitioner would want to know how to manage the care and comfort of a person who is experiencing respiratory distress. This is an example of a holistic approach to practice.

To illustrate that the concerns of science (nursing science) and nursing practice are different, use an orange. Sections in an orange are connected with membranes. One can easily section out a piece of the orange for in-depth study or use. In so doing, however, the investigator in science is *not* concerned whether characteristics of the *whole* orange exist any longer—only the segment. Nursing and nurses should address research questions, identify and define, and study phenomena that are empirically relevant to nursing practice. Practice people want and need answers about the "whole orange" (person). Practice has to deal with the whole area of nursing practice, not just nursing as a science. Holism and science are interested in the segments, and not distorting the segments of the orange, and being able to provide a base of knowledge from which practitioners can create application.

It appears unlikely that one can "section out" (like an orange membrane) phenomenon in nursing without distorting the phenomenon (person) itself. Nursing is and must be constantly concerned about the parts in relation to the whole. Furthermore, nursing practice must specifically focus on the connections, links, or interfaces that similarly could be compared to the membrane between the sections of an orange. These connections cannot be identified, defined, or focused on in applying the tenets of holism without distorting the phenomenon itself. Moreover, it seems that in trying to apply holistic nursing

practice the tenets of holism are not viable because scientific theory is not interested in the "particulars" of the actual world, but what appears to be empirically relevant with respect to a well-defined question. In terms of the orange, a question may be, what type of membrane exists between the sections of an orange?

If the connections could be identified in nursing science, the phenomena may have little relevance for nursing practice, since in science these connections would be studied in isolation, independent from the total person. To be relevant for nursing practice, the isolated knowledge about connections would need to be generalized to all connections that are in persons. Moreover, the knowledge must serve as a knowledge base for practice in some fashion. Even if the connections could be "holistically" included in studying the *whole* person, holistic theory does not really appear to be applicable to nursing practice theory. Kramer reminds the reader (Chapter 32) that the whole is still greater than the sum of its parts. Four further questions must then be asked: (a) What is nursing science? (b) What phenomena may be studied that have relevance for nursing science? (c) Of what relevance is nursing science? and (d) What relationship may exist between nursing practice theory and nursing science? Some comments are offered for consideration.

Holistic *nursing* practice has to do with *real* things, such as comfort measures and patient teaching. In practice, one may be concerned which is the *best* way to put on an ace bandage. The bandage is real. One may also be concerned about health status. For the practitioner, health status *in itself* is not real.

The bandage may contribute to the health status of Mr. Jones. The bandage and health status have little relevance and no real actuality for the *practitioner*, independent from the person. The practitioner is only concerned about health status as it takes on meaning from being imbedded in a whole person. To apply the tenets of holism to holistic practice as the base for developing theory suggests to the practitioner that health status as a concept is a thing "in itself," rather than a thing that derives its meaning from the theoretical framework (a person) in which it is imbedded. The tenets of holistic theory appear to be irreconcilable with nursing practice and thus not appropriate for developing nursing practice theory.

For the scientist, Mr. Jones exists with all of his "particulars" including his health status (measured by test indicators). For the scientist and nursing science, health status and its indicators may be foci independent of an interest in Mr. Jones as a person. To such an investigator, health status is a "real" actual phenomenon of concern.

Conceivably, in accumulating substantive practice knowledge that is generalizable to many patients, practice theory may be developed. Moreover, if one discovers that, for example, there is one *best* way to apply an ace bandage for *all* patients who have edema, nursing science may be created. Possibly, the phenomena—applying an ace bandage—may be a "particular" that may be generalizable and representative of all "particulars" and a universal method. Practice theory and nursing science also may be created in a similar way through the accumulation of knowledge about specific nursing interventions, such as comfort measures for stress. Further thought and discussion are needed to explicate the answers to the previously posed questions, particularly as they concern the relationship between nursing practice theory and nursing science.

Approaches and Methods in the Development of Knowledge

Comment is warranted regarding the approaches and methods that are utilized in the development of knowledge for nursing. According to the contributing authors (Menke, Chapter 27; Fry, Chapter 28; Sarter, Chapter 29; and Kemp, Chapter 69), nursing has been heavily influenced by the "received view," that is, logical positivism. Standards in positivism as a philosophy of science were based on experiences in the physical sciences. The hallmarks of logical positivism are its emphasis on empirical evidence and the notion of verifiability. Some hold that in order for nursing to become a science, nursing must follow the principles of positivism. Consequently nurse scholars may mistakenly use the principles

that evolved in positivism as a "set of directions" for *doing* science.

Positivism or empiricism emphasizes deduction and quantitative methods. Kemp (Chapter 69) points out, however, that the "perceived view" and its consequent inductive, qualitative methods are necessary to understand complex problems in nursing. Since one cannot see pain, but rather feel it, the subjective aspect as conveyed most commonly through qualitative methods needs to have an appropriate equivalent role in the development of nursing knowledge. Although there are differences between the inductive and deductive approaches in developing theory, it should be emphasized that an interplay does and should exist in the use of both approaches for the development of nursing science.

Menke (Chapter 27) examined the present state of knowledge development for nursing. She demonstrates that some progress has been made. Menke urges that mentor programs be encouraged to develop knowledge for the discipline and within the discipline.

In summary, there is a broad need for understanding the empirical world in nursing, whether the phenomenon is pain or caring. Nursing embraces a holistic and humanistic viewpoint with the fundamental ethic of caring. Thus both approaches (the received and the perceived views—as associated with quantitative and qualitative methods) for developing nursing knowledge are important for the discipline. The critical question remains *how* can inquiry produce substantive knowledge that will make a difference in health care?

NURSING PRACTICE

There are a number of themes reflected in the extensive writings of the contributing authors in the nursing practice section of this volume. The major foci appear to be (a) nursing's identity and image; (b) concepts regarding process; (c) nursing roles in practice; and (d) the settings for practice and population-specific care.

Identity and Image

In effect, Lyon (Chapter 34) uses a "zoom lens" to focus on the number one issue for the profession—its identity. Her chapter is further supported by Orlando and Dugan (1989). Lyon indicates a direction for obtaining consensus on who and what we are, both as nurses and as a profession. An issue related to the identity concern is that of defining one's identity in terms of a positive image. Porter, Porter, and Lower (1989) offer suggestions for projecting a positive image of identity through one's dress, speech, and action. We need to verbalize to the public, potential students, and other professional groups who we are, what we are, and what we have to offer.

Process Issues

A second major theme is one that may be called process. Chapters that highlight process include those by Soares-O'Hearn (Chapter 35), who focuses on nursing diagnosis; Brown and Davis (Chapter 38); and Flynn and Davis (Chapter 39), who address ethics concerns; Driscoll (Chapter 40), who discusses legal issues; and Hartigan (Chapter 46), who prescribes continuity of care.

A taxonomy of nursing diagnoses may be a valuable means for designating the phenomena of concern to nursing (Jenny, 1989). Soares O'Hearn (Chapter 35) proposes an alternative guide for developing a classification system that should be valuable to the discipline. Very often the nursing diagnosis, language, and semantics of a classification system may be a challenge to the beginner and experienced professional alike. Soares O'Hearn provides relevant examples in advancing her system.

Continuity of care through a humanistic approach to providing care, described by Hartigan (Chapter 46), is imperative. It is hoped that the nursing diagnosis movement will focus on more specific interventions that directly impact continuity of care. Continuity of care is bound to become an increasing need in the future, given the shortened hospital stays and costs of acute care.

Reilly (1989) has clarified the mandate given to educators and practitioners to address the concepts of standards and ethics that govern nursing practice. Brown and Davis (Chapter 38) and Flynn and Davis (Chapter 39) discuss the ethical issues confronted in nursing practice. Essentially the nurse in practice needs to understand her or his roles as patient advocate, professional caregiver, and participant in ethical decision-making.

A guiding question for the practicing professional nurse, with regard to making ethical decisions, might be: What is in the *best* interest of the *patient?* To use this principle as a guide the nurse needs to (a) have access to relevant, available facts; (b) imagine the *feelings* of the person involved; (c) have a disinterested stance (no vested interest); and (d) be dispassionate in interactions throughout the decision-making process. The nurse must endeavor to keep from being overwhelmed with emotion at critical times.

In discussions of rights of nurses, focus should be placed not only on what nurses should *not do* but also should include what they *may* or *should do*. In the role of patient advocate, the nurse may need to ask whose interest has priority—the patient's well-being or the nurse's conscience? Foremost is the *best* interest of the patient. A nurse may not allow personal beliefs to influence actions that would be in the patient's best interest in the event these beliefs are counter to the patient's wishes. Situations arise in providing care when a patient's wish is contrary to the personal beliefs of a nurse, such as a circumstance involving a patient's request to have a feeding tube withdrawn. In discontinuing a life support system or removing a tube for feeding, the major concern should be what is in the *best* interest of the patient and what are (or best thought to be) the wishes of the patient.

In general, the basic principle held by professionals seems to be never to abandon a patient. Rather, in the event of an ethical dilemma that the nurse cannot resolve in accord with the patient's *best* interest, the nurse is advised to arrange for a replacement. There is another general guideline that seems to be applied in trying to resolve some of the potential ethical dilemmas. The suggestion is to ask oneself, "Is the patient highly likely to be *more* comfortable with the action?" And later, in evaluating the decision: "Do the ensuing effects evidence that the patient's wishes have been respected and provided for?"

The issue regarding refusal of patient care assignments may present complex problems. In this, common sense and reasoning should prevail. For example, if a nurse is *willing* to acknowledge lack of the competence necessary to care for a particular patient, such acknowledgement is more likely to be accepted by a nurse administrator than a statement that caring for a certain type of patient, such as one with AIDS, poses a health risk for the nurse. Admittedly, numerous factors are involved. However, clear job descriptions and thorough preemployment interviews may preclude many problematic situations.

There are obvious legal concerns related to many of the ethical dilemmas, as have been expressed by Driscoll (Chapter 40) and Murphy (Chapter 5). However, it is probable that legal concerns consistently have been expressed in relation to the so-called expanded role of the nurse in practice.

Nursing Roles in Practice

Bullough (Chapter 45) looks at the legal scope of nursing practice. It appears obvious that legal research, monitoring, and analysis regarding the scope of nursing practice need to be an ongoing process within the profession. Individual nurses, nursing organizations, and boards of nursing need to mount legal challenges. Those who practice nursing without a license, act without authority to change the scope of practice, or change the scope of practice in violation of the property right that nurses have in their license need to be questioned and targeted for legal action (Northrop, 1989). Furthermore Northrop suggests that the scope of nursing practice may be targeted for change, given a continued nursing shortage and the redistribution of tasks and responsibilities among other health workers, such as registered care technicians (RCTSs).

Mechanic (1988) redefines the scope of professional nursing practice and the extended role for nursing that has application to much of the content offered by Bullough (Chapter 45). Mechanic emphasizes that in three ways contemporary nursing practice is practice in the expanded role: (a) health promotion and protection in illness; (b) collegial and collaborative relationships with other health team members; and (c) assumption of full accountability for actions while acting with autonomy and authority. Mechanic further advises that the restructuring of credentialing mechanisms to demonstrate advanced competencies at both the generalist and specialist level could potentially increase direct reimbursement opportunities for nurses.

The restrictive definition of the expanded role has limited nurses' potential for third-party reimbursement. Mechanic's focusing on demonstrating advanced competencies for both generalist and specialist practice could also facilitate the development of a clear generalist-type program at the master's level and specialist-type programs at the doctoral level for nursing education.

Yasko and Dudjak (Chapter 41) and Whitney (Chapter 43) identify further implications of the expanded role for nurses. It appears that, now and in the forseeable future, there are and will be fewer distinctions between the roles of a clinical specialist and the nurse practitioner. Reflecting on these chapters made Mechanic's article (1988) worth recommending for supplementary ideas.

To stimulate further debate regarding differentiation in roles of the clinical specialist and the nurse practitioner, the reader is also referred to an article by Feldman, Ventura, and Crosby (1987). These writers list and describe the most relevant and valid studies (56 in number), as identified through an information synthesis of nurse practitioner (NP) effectiveness. This listing should be helpful to educators, providers of nursing care, and researchers.

There is continuous emphasis on the role of the staff nurse in providing care (Chaska, Clark, Rogers, & Deets, Chapter 36). Concern regarding this role has to do not only with the status and prestige of the profession, but also with variables that affect different types of performance (Martin, 1989; McCloskey & McCain, 1988). Chaska and colleagues are expected to indicate in future articles the differences in perceptions of physicians and nurses concerning expectations of staff nurse role performance. (See

Chapter 36 by Chaska et al. for essential background information on these data.) Martin (1989) provides support for the findings and implications of the research conducted by Chaska and colleagues. There is a great need for reconciliation of differences in professional opinions, views, and beliefs regarding nurse's performance. In addition to furthering the prestige and status of the profession, role performance research also is important for understanding career commitment, education, job satisfaction, and feedback as determinants in job performance of nurses. The latter factors are advocated by McCloskey and McCain (1988) to be included in role performance studies.

Settings for Practice and Population-Specific Care

The settings for providing nursing care as well as the type of nursing practice are changing owing to many complex factors. The nursing shortage, costs of health and medical care, complex technology, and social factors such as increased stress and fast-paced living styles are some of the contributing variables.

As Sister Rose Therese Bahr notes in Chapter 42, the elderly are increasing in numbers. Furthermore as Yasko and Dudjak (Chapter 41) point out, there are increasing demands for oncology nursing specialists. Special population groups are requiring extensive and extended care. Whether one provides nursing care as a clinical specialist or nurse practitioner (Whitney, Chapter 43), or in some type of a private practice model (Lyon, Chapter 44), the scene for health care is changing.

Critical care nursing demands a humanistic approach, as illustrated by Dracup and Marsden (Chapter 37). However, for humanistic care to be provided in acute care settings now and in the future, continuity of care through exemplary discharge planning is mandatory (see Hartigan, Chapter 46). Increasing transitions for home health care must be provided, as advocated by Barkauskas (Chapter 47).

Home health care will be the hub of the future health care delivery system and the setting for the major nursing care of the future. Barkauskas notes the Medicare Catastrophic Coverage Act of 1988, indicating implications for home care in particular as well as for the nursing profession.

Hamilton and Wilson (1989) add further support to Barkauskas's statements. They point out provisions of the Act that involve skilled nursing facilities (SNF) and hospice care. Specifically an increase in allowable home health care visits will create a rise in demand for home health care nurses, as predicted by Barkauskas. Numerous opportunities for entrepreneurs in nursing are emerging as a result of the provisions of the Act.

Valuable services, such as respite care permitted under the Act, will be offered through those home health care agencies that previously only provided skilled home visits. Increased demands in long-term care for nursing care in the SNFs are bound to occur because of the elimination of the requirement for a 3-day hospital stay before admission. Thus sound discharge planning, both for extended care facilities and long-term care, as well as for home care, is bound to become even more imperative. In addition, the numbers and acuity levels of patients in long-term care facilities will most likely increase. Thus Bahr's and Barkauskas's discussion (Chapters 42 and 47, respectively) and their predictions regarding the elderly and home care may demand a shift in emphasis toward gerontological nursing in some nursing education programs. Emphasis on the elderly in nursing curricula could have positive effects for the quality of nursing care in SNFs, hospices, and home care, as well as for the care provided in acute care settings. The topic of international nursing practice, which was included in the nursing practice part of the book (Brown, Chapter 48), is addressed under the future of nursing section in this summary chapter.

NURSING ADMINISTRATION—SERVICES

There are three predominant themes in the contributing authors' writings about the administration of nursing services. These themes are (a) cost-effectiveness and high-quality care; (b) recruitment and retention of qualified nurses; and (c) the preparation of nurse managers and executives. Each of these themes are addressed below.

Cost-Effectiveness and High-Quality Care

Wolf (Chapter 49) starts this part of the book, focusing on how to balance cost with quality care. She emphasizes strategies for empowering the nursing staff. Her arguments are supported in an article by Pointer and Pointer (1989). These authors present a model that provides a framework for meeting creatively both the challenges of increasing productivity and provision of high-quality patient care.

Balancing cost and quality is emphasized further by Weaver (Chapter 53). Her emphasis concerns professional resources. The equating of services to product lines represents a business orientation that remains unattractive to many in nursing. Nevertheless, the reality *is* that nurses must be viewed as vital components of some 468 "product lines" known as diagnosis related groups (DRGs). (Staff, 1989, June 5). Omachonu and Nanda (1989) further indicate that nursing professionals should agree on the importance of outcome measures. Thus both Wolf and Weaver (Chapters 49 and 53 respectively) are supported in their arguments about nursing resources and productivity. Moreover Omachonu and Nanda provide a conceptual framework for the development of a productivity measurement model in which nursing care and the environmental context of the institution are included.

Nursing case management is probably the most effective human resources measure for quality nursing care and productivity in this decade. The emphasis is on high-quality care that is truly humanizing but at the same time balanced with cost. The Nursing Network at Carondelet St. Mary's Hospital in Tucson is one such exemplary model of nursing case management. The network is an integrated system of nursing care that spans the health care continuum. It seeks to improve the quality and cost-effectiveness of care by strengthening nurses as professionals and enabling nurses to contribute the full range of their expertise (Ethridge & Lamb, 1989). The Nursing Network appears to reflect not only the type of environment, design for case managers, re-

cruitment and accountability strategy, and potential retention factor for nurses that is strongly advocated not only by Wolf, Weaver, and Porter (Chapter 50), but also the type of design and governance structure system that is recommended by Porter-O'Grady (Chapter 51).

Porter-O'Grady clearly promotes the development of new models for nursing services. Furthermore Clifford (Chapter 70) prescribes that institutions of care be restructured for the future. Clifford is Vice-President for Nursing and Nurse-in-Chief at Beth Israel Hospital, Boston. Beth Israel Hospital is commonly known as the epitome for providing high-quality nursing care that is balanced with cost-effectiveness. The Nursing Network at Carondelet St. Mary's Hospital may well be proposed as another exemplary model not only for care, but also for the retention of nursing staff. Porter (Chapter 50) and Graham and Sheppard (Chapter 52) further emphasize the type of recruitment and retention strategies that need to be employed in nursing services.

There is considerable discussion that market-based financial plans are vital for survival of care institutions. Beyers (Chapter 55) emphasizes the need for strategic planning and forecasting in nursing services. A recent article cautions, however, that strategic planning also needs to consider the financial consequences of low-probability scenarios (Staff, 1989, May 5). It was further pointed out that the conceptual power structure of hospital institutions has changed. For example, less rather than more is considered better. Forecasting by payor for each product is appropriate for a hospital's first estimate of revenue and expenses, since hospitals now value product-use budgeting. To forecast how many patients an institution will have, what will be the patient's medical problems, and who will pay for them is a fundamentally different way to forecast. This method needs to be considered when reviewing Beyer's (Chapter 55) discussion on strategic planning.

Recruitment and Retention of Qualified Nurses

Graham and Sheppard (Chapter 52) set the tone regarding recruitment and retention strategies.

These writers emphasize the importance of shared values between nursing staff and nursing administration. In addition, they emphasize that roles must be clarified among nursing staff, management, and physicians. The study conducted by Chaska and colleagues (Chapter 36) concerning expectations of professional roles supports the beliefs of Graham and Sheppard.

The development of clinical ladders (Porter, Chapter 50) also is an excellent strategy for recruiting and retaining staff. Perhaps further discussion of curriculum models such as that posed in Table 73-1 of this final chapter might facilitate not only the development of clinical ladders in hospital institutions but also management ladders and career planning. The kind of retention and recruitment strategies discussed by Porter (Chapter 50), Graham and Sheppard (Chapter 52), and Weaver (Chapter 53) might be capsulized in a specific retention program, such as that planned by Wall (1988). Wall endorses the concept, also offered by contributors to this book, that retention of nurses begins at the time of recruitment. She strongly supports Graham and Sheppard's claim that a long-term commitment and support of hospital administration is needed to resolve the concerns and issues related to the nursing shortage.

According to data from the American Hospital Association, the severity of the nursing shortage is easing (Staff, 1989, May 5). In a survey of 813 hospitals nationwide conducted in 1989, only 13% of hospitals—as compared with 19% in 1987—were experiencing a "severe" shortage of staff registered nurses. The decrease is attributed to creative retention strategies. Even so, these investigators indicate that nurse shortages appear to remain widespread, although less severe.

Another factor to be considered in relation to retention of staff is that of increasing autonomy for the nurse, as advocated by Wolf (Chapter 49) and Porter-O'Grady (Chapter 51). Such strategies for enhancing professional environments should reduce the call for unions. Pettengill (Chapter 54) clearly presents the factors and concerns involved in unionization of professional employees. Instead of contributing to the dualism found in nurse unionization and to competition for the right to represent professional

employees, nurse administrators are in a position to prevent such problems. Nurse administrators are well advised to create positive climates and structural organizational designs for nursing staff governance and nursing service. "Moral and ethical issues underlie the argument for comparable worth for nurses," according to Christensen (1988, p. 49). The lack of comparable worth promotes subsequent consideration of unionization.

The Preparation of Nurse Managers and Executives

Many enlightened educators and practitioners believe that a management style that incorporates ethical principles will empower nurses as people (Christensen, 1988). Increasing participation of staff nurses in decision making directly affects nurses, encouraging their consideration and respect. The question is how can managers be prepared to promote such strategies for empowerment?

Sides (Chapter 56) and Chaska and Alexander (Chapter 57) have been concerned about the content offered in preparing nurse managers and executives. Sides, a practicing nurse executive at the time of her study, focused on data obtained about practice directly from the practice setting. Chaska and Alexander's data reinforce some findings of Sides. In both studies it is discouraging to note the apparent lack of recognition for liberal arts and ethics to be a foundation in the preparation of nurse administrators. However, it should be noted that the semistructured interview questions developed by Chaska and Alexander did not attempt to "lead" respondents to identify *specific* content needed, such as ethics, in the preparation of nurse managers.

Increasing attention is being given to organizational, ethical issues. Managers as individuals may intervene to end unethical organizational behaviors. Being a part of the organization, managers also may lead an ethical organizational change (Neilsen, 1989). Ethics might well provide the foundation for a framework that creates a work environment consistent with the nursing profession's beliefs about human beings, humanism, and caring as advocated by Christensen (1988) and contributors to this book such as Fowler (Chapter 4) and Brown and Davis (Chapter 38). An ethical work environment in which nurses' human welfare is promoted should be highlighted in the curriculum for preparation of nurse managers and executives.

Additionally, some type of integrated framework should be included in the conceptual base for programs preparing nurse managers and executives. Integrated frameworks and specifically the synthesis of content between nursing and management were an area for query in the Chaska and Alexander study (Chapter 57). These were originally advocated in a chapter by Chaska (1983). Jennings and Meleis (1988) significantly further discuss the relationship between nursing theory, clinical nursing practice, and administrative nursing practice. Clearly, integrated frameworks should be initiated and further developed within programs to prepare nurse managers and executives.

Finally programs for the preparation of managers and nurse executives, whether for service or academic settings, should include a research agenda for nursing administration. Henry, O'Donnell, Pendergast, Moody, and Hutchinson (1988) have reported a study on the development of such a research agenda. Cost containment is a major theme. McCloskey (1989) notes that to date little research has been conducted on "costing out nursing." However, she points out that some data are emerging that indicate that nursing care is not responsible for the high cost of health care. The emphasis placed on cost efficiency and quality of care by the contributing authors in this text would indicate that substantial research should be conducted regarding issues of productivity, high-quality care, and cost containment. Other research relating to needs of nursing services that should be addressed concern the processes of decision making and change. It might be noted that these same topics are appropriate for research in academic administration. Finally the design of organizational structures, governance systems, and change in academia also are critical areas requiring data-base research, which might be obtained through evaluation and experimental design types of studies.

NURSING ADMINISTRATION—ACADEMIC

The management of nursing education in schools of nursing today offers unprecedented challenge by virtue of complex, simultaneous needs and demands. Significant issues of concern involve (a) the quality, quantity, and type of programs; (b) student recruitment and expected outcomes for practitioners; (c) faculty resources and qualifications; (d) technology and support services; and (e) the organizational structure and governance of academic units. Further challenges include first, obtaining essential revenue, and then subsequently employing sound financial management to operationalize high-quality, cost-effective, productive, and successful programs. Elaboration follows on five major concerns relating to academic administration of nursing education: (a) faculty governance, (b) structure design, (c) faculty resources, (d) academic culture, and (e) change.

Faculty Governance

The organizational structure for governance in academic units and the design for conducting the academic and administrative functions are major issues in higher education today. In this text, various models for governance are explored by Hegyvary (Chapter 58) and Baker (Chapter 60). Starck (Chapter 72) further enlarges on the issues. The point is made that resources, both human and financial, are in scarce supply. Furthermore desire, need, and demand for joint determination of policy in academe are increasingly evident. A joint venture of faculty and administration commonly is advocated for decision-making and policy-making processes. However, administration generally reserves the right to manage and implement policies.

Numerous changes in higher education and nursing as an academic discipline have caused the academic role of faculty to be not well understood at times. The reader is referred for a discussion of the faculty role to a handbook by Pennington (1986). At times it appears that the domains of administration and faculty are clouded. Generally problematic is the lack of clarity and definition of interfaces that exist between faculty and administration roles, rights, responsibilities, and authority. It is not unusual that the difficulty becomes exacerbated in decision-making activities, such as in the recruitment and hiring of new faculty or the selection of a new computer system in the school.

The following general guideline is offered, a general principle advocated essentially by the Vroom and Yetton model for decision making (Gibson, Ivancevich, and Donnelly, 1988). To the extent that a decision may directly affect faculty or that faculty need to be involved or be depended on to implement the decision, faculty then need to be participants in the decision-making process from the initial consideration through the final process of implementation. Methods and criteria for evaluation of faculty and merit salary increases are examples in which where faculty participation is essential. Fairness is a quality that must pervade all management decisions.

Structure Design

A second major aspect of organizations to be discussed here pertains to the structure of an organization. First, a thorough assessment and evaluation of the present structure and design of an organization should be conducted before the planning, design, and implementation of a contemplated change. Contributing authors Hegyvary (Chapter 58) and Baker (Chapter 60) concur that the organization should be evaluated in terms of its mission, purposes, goals, objectives, programs, and the resources needed to fulfill its mandate. Needing to be considered are the advantages and disadvantages of organizing on the basis of departments versus programs versus conceptual curriculum foci, such as health promotion and nursing systems. Students, faculty, and programs also are critical dimensions of the organization to be noted when evaluating its design. The question to which organizational design always should be responsive is how can students best be served; that is, how may the student best be provided substantive high-quality content and facilitated to progress successfully through a program that meets the individual's needs and desires.

To what extent should the organization be decentralized? At least two perspectives may be considered—one, in terms of major functions or services that may be decentralized; another, from the point of view of decision making. Ideally, as is commonly known, decision making should occur at the lowest possible level within an organization. Numerous variables determine what this organizational level will be; these include the type of decision to be made and the experience and qualifications of participants in an organization. In addition to the centralization concern, two other dimensions characteristic of all organizations must be considered in the design and structure of the academic unit, namely, complexity and formalization (Hall, 1987). The three elements of complexity most often considered are (a) horizontal differentiation—the subdivision of tasks to be performed; (b) vertical differentiation—the number of hierarchical authority levels; and (c) spatial dispersion—the extent personnel, activities, and power centers are separated in space. Formalization is concerned with the degree of specificity of behavior required by rules, procedures, and policies. According to Hall (1987), since formalization involves organizational control, it has an ethical and political meaning besides being a structural component of organizations.

Other factors that must be considered in the design of structure are (a) span of control for a manager; (b) diversity and degree of specialization among faculty; (c) size of the academic unit (students and faculty); and (d) technology. In addition to the writings of the contributing authors and the text by Hall (1987), the reader is referred to texts by the following authors for further substantive content concerning the design and structure of organizations, such as academic units: Arnold and Feldman (1986); Cherrington (1989); Gibson, Ivancevich, and Donnelly (1988); Hunsaker and Cook (1986); and Randolph and Blackburn (1989).

Faculty Resources

Faculty resources and qualifications are a continuous, problematic fact for most academic administrators. Felton (Chapter 61), Yeaworth (Chapter 62), and Fagin (Chapter 66) have explored many of the concerns. One guiding principle may be applied—

to capitalize on the positive strengths that faculty have to offer in the present and nurture those strengths in planning for the future. The type and mix of faculty as to kinds of degrees, academic preparation, and clinical background are matters for serious consideration. In this text, although Lenz (Chapter 16), Felton (Chapter 61), and Fagin (Chapter 66) may concur that diversity in faculty preparation is desirable, these writers appear to be in agreement that further discussion is warranted. Perhaps a more critical issue is how to ensure that doctorally prepared faculty maintain and develop their clinical competence. Given that most doctoral programs emphasize research rather than clinical practice, a potential problem exists if doctoral students do not maintain their clinical skills as they progress through their doctoral programs. Later as doctoral faculty, inadequate skills pose a real problem in providing quality, clinical education for undergraduate students.

There are at least two strategies that might be offered to resolve this potential dilemma. One would be to recruit and hire doctoral students as teaching assistants in the clinical areas for undergraduate program content and clinical laboratory experience. Another, a two-track system might be considered for faculty. Such a system could capitalize on the two-track type of system that was proposed for doctoral programs in nursing previously suggested in the part of this summary chapter addressing education. Clinical expertise needs to be fostered, maintained, advanced, and ensured for high quality in nursing programs. Higher education institutions need to investigate seriously other organizational designs to accommodate faculty in clinical disciplines, such as nursing. Alternative requirements (*not* lesser) for promotion and tenure that address the critical expertise needed for both research and clinical teaching also might preclude some instances of burnout. Dick (1986) found that collegial support, positive feedback from the dean, and a participatory management style are more important for protecting faculty members from burnout than attention to their work load. Alternative structures in governance and design should be an excellent means to support faculty.

Academic Culture, Climate, and Environment

The organizational climate in an academic institution has an impact on faculty and students alike. Administrators are increasingly being held accountable for the climate that they establish, support, and essentially must nourish (Haussler, 1988). Providing a work environment and climate that encourages and supports both personal and professional growth should be the goal of every nursing education administrator (Haussler, 1988).

Farrell (Chapter 59) emphasizes the need for viewing and conducting the work in academia as big business. Her points and suggestions are well advised. At the same time, a word of caution might be in order. While promoting the type of "tender power" that is advised by Cohen (1989) for women executives, Ray (1989) supports the need for the executive team to possess knowledge of organizations as businesses. However, Ray also urges that the human side of nursing be fostered and advanced in the structure of health care organizations and academic institutions. Christensen (1988) targets the need for academic administrators to foster an environment that supports ethical reasoning.

Hechenberger (1988) presents a number of ideas that are reinforced in the writings of Conway-Welch (Chapter 65) and Starck (Chapter 72). Hechenberger insists that professional values can best be instilled by the example of leaders in nursing education. It is essential that academic nurse administrators are committed to demonstrate, and persist in reinforcing, appropriate professional values. Then, in the view of these writers the future of nursing academic education administration will be in good hands.

Change

Change is a given in academic administration and higher education. Baker (Chapter 60) offers a model for planning and implementing change. When and if change is to occur, critical involvement of faculty in the planning, timing, *pacing*, communication, and evaluation of change is essential. Sufficient time needs to be allowed to ensure an effective process. Emphasis on process—with such values and criteria of openness, honesty, directness, humanism, and accountability—are all vital in the change process. Effective sustained planning and ongoing evaluation are intrinsic to a productive, successful administration that is changing for the future.

Emphasis in planning for change should be placed on selecting a strategic "site" for the change within the organizational system. For example, it is advisable to initiate change at the point where (a) the site selected for change is not the most critical nor weakest point in the system and (b) one can be assured of a reasonable degree of success in instituting the change. It further is highly advisable to initiate change in steps and stages. Peters's *Thriving on Chaos* (1987) has been subject to some misinterpretation. Although Peters provides numerous prescriptions for successful change, he does not advocate literally turning an organization upside down. Rather, the principles he proposes assume that most organizations are *already* in a state of chaos. If the milieu of the corporate structure between the business world and higher education are indeed comparable, the emphasis should be on *thriving—not* striving for chaos.

The need for successful and effective change frequently brings with it a demand for new leadership. Chaska (Chapter 63) has responded to the uncertainty and inconsistency frequently reflected in the search process, offering specific information and direction applicable to the search for qualified administrators. Given the paucity of accessible creditable information on this topic, an additional guide to recruiting administrators is suggested—a handbook sponsored by the American Association for Higher Education (Marchese, 1987). Furthermore Gilmore (1988) offers significant information regarding making organization leadership transitions successfully. Gilmore also corroborates the challenge and process of leadership that a number of contributing authors have addressed in this volume.

THE FUTURE OF NURSING
Professionalization

A fore-century thinker in relating a conversation between certain symbolic characters concerning life, learning, and persons charged the characters with being prisoners of their own doctrine (Schrum, 1985). Schrum applied this reference to nurses and nursing in asking the question, "How can I speak to you of the future of nursing, if you limit your knowledge [to] its past?" (p. 183). That admonition appears to this author to be well-advised. Nursing needs to be open to new approaches, methods, and ideas. Openness, trust, and respect for the thoughts and ideas of others will help form a vision for the future and a kaleidoscope for nursing.

Another quality that may be advisable to nurture in nursing is the ability to laugh—to laugh at oneself, to laugh at oneself with others, and to laugh with others at ourselves. It seems at times that nurses and nursing may tend to take themselves too seriously. Witness the tension that occasionally is experienced at social functions when a remark intended in jest is taken seriously. On such occasion, one might note that it is time to escape into a "regenerative moment of bracketed time," as described by Barnum (1989), that has a different reality. (Barnum writes on the function of laughter and humor.) It would appear that such brief regenerative moments might greatly assist nurses and nursing to keep their perspective and balance, while yet endeavoring to attain their goals.

Nursing's professional future will depend on its identifying and owning its role in society. "Owning" in this context implies a process whereby the profession and its professionals are in various stages of attaining something that takes a lifetime to complete. Owning one's identity as a professional will require a commitment to the profession of nursing as a person, first and then as a professional. It will require further a commitment on the part of the profession to resolve numerous issues of concern, such as resolving the many definitional issues that nursing has faced throughout its history. Specifically, the nursing profession must come to grips with defining professional nursing practice. Halloran (Chapter 71) clearly urges nursing to renew its commitment to the essence of nursing, as originally defined and taught by Virginia Henderson. Resolution of these issues will determine whether or not we will realize our potential as a profession in the future.

Nursing Education

Recruitment, retention, and the future. Problems related to recruitment, retention in nursing, and the nursing shortage most certainly have taxed nursing's capacity for humor. A number of the contributing authors have addressed aspects of these issues in this volume, for example, Donley and Flaherty (Chapter 64). Previously Aiken and Mullinix (1987) provided an initial comprehensive special report on the nursing shortage, which served as a basis for additional subsequent analysis.

Donley and Flaherty (1989) have further analyzed the demand-caused elements of the shortage. These writers also discussed the final report of the Secretary's Commission on Nursing (Department of Health and Human Services [DHHS], 1988) and examined findings that conditions in the workplace are a factor in the nursing shortage. Donley and Flaherty (1989) stated that "wage compression is perhaps the most serious economic impediment to a career in nursing" (p. 185). The expectation that earning power should increase with education and experience is far from realized in nursing. In more than half of its 16 recommendations, the Commission's report (DHHS, 1988) addressed the reorganization of the work environment for nursing. Donley and Flaherty (1989) summarized its recommendations and the changes that need to be implemented in the work setting, if the nursing shortage is to be ameliorated. In essence, their substantial reinforcement for the strategies that have been proposed by numerous contributors to this text, namely, Haller (Chapter 26), Lyon (Chapter 34), Dracup and Marsden (Chapter 37), Wolf (Chapter 49), Porter-O'Grady (Chapter 51), Weaver (Chapter 53), Andreoli and Tarnow (Chapter 67), Clifford (Chapter 70), and Halloran (Chapter 71). Recruitment into the profession and retention for nursing practice will remain an issue for some time. Thus the suggestions of Graham and Sheppard (Chapter 52) and evaluation of methods (Jolma & Weller, 1989) will prove to be extremely valuable.

Collaborative models for education and practice. Increasing the partnership between education and service is another method that may be utilized to attract persons into nursing and retain them within the profession. Andreoli and Tarnow (Chapter 67)

focus on the establishing of models shared between nursing and education as a priority for nursing. Conceivably, such shared models might also resolve a number of the definitional issues that have plagued nursing. Collaborative models also may assist nursing in redefining its educational roots, as advised by Conway-Welch (Chapter 65). The academic clinician, in a type of joint practice, may assist in the advancement of high-quality care and stimulate faculty to maintain a high level of clinical competence (Cook and Finelli, 1988; Reisch, 1987). Options for faculty practice, as described by Lyon (Chapter 44), are increasing; these may also serve as a basis for developing research programs, as advocated by Stevenson (Chapter 68).

Alternative methods of teaching students are strongly urged by Duffy (Chapter 12). This goal for the clinical area may be achieved through cooperative partnerships between nursing education and service (Donius, 1988). Preceptorship programs, as described by Donius (1988) and Mundinger (1988), may also facilitate faculty practice, research, and curriculum.

Predictions for undergraduate programs. Associate degree programs are likely to evolve into 3-year programs and baccalaureate programs will be redesigned as 5-year programs. (The programs to prepare licensed practical nurses may either go out of existence in the near future or progress into the associate degree program. The knowledge and skill that is increasingly needed to provide direct nursing care seems virtually impossible to provide in 1 year.) Diploma programs are likely to become extinct or evolve into 3-year associate degree programs. The burgeoning knowledge and skill base that is projected to be needed in the roles of associate (technical) and professional future practice will demand lengthened programs.

Educators and practitioners long have stated that the present content and length of preparation is inadequate, given the current technology and the knowledge and skill base that is expected in practice. The cry for extensive preparation in liberal arts, understanding of persons, and the human sciences may be expected to continue (Watson & Bevis, Chapter 14; Stember & Hester, Chapter 22).

Demand for more liberal arts content is already apparent in the chapters in the education part of this text.

New models are being demanded for baccalaureate programs designed for the future. These are being considered seriously and some already have been implemented. In addition to those suggested by a number of the contributing authors and the model proposed in Table 73-1, it is expected that many others will be developed and offered for consideration.

Graduate education: master's, doctoral, post-doctoral, interdisciplinary. One can expect to see the development of graduate programs in nursing as generalist-specialty programs at the master's level with subspecialty areas at the doctoral level. However, there is evidence that postdoctoral education increasingly will be demanded. Margretta Styles (1987) posed seven unanswered developmental questions regarding doctoral programs in nursing for the future. One of these concerned whether doctoral study should serve as a part of a learning continuum and as a prelude to postdoctoral study. In line with the latter projection, the National Center for Nursing Research has developed a trajectory of research training and career development awards. Research training is a career commitment. The trajectory identifies and supports the importance of federal funding for training and nursing research (Hinshaw, 1989).

Evidently there also will be an equivalent demand to prepare clinicians, at the doctoral level, predominantly for practice as clinicians, nurse administrators, or nurse educators. Two-track systems within one doctoral (PhD) program in nursing appears to be gaining in consensus.

Interdisciplinary graduate programs, particularly at the doctoral level, may soon be in demand owing to the increased awareness that health is a complex phenomenon. In academia and nursing, attempts are made to understand health fully and make findings accessible to those who might apply them. The perspectives of any individual discipline, or group of cognate disciplines, may be inadequate to the task. Thus a comprehensive approach and expertise from numerous disciplines, such as philosophy and the social sciences combined with nursing, might encompass the research perspectives necessary to address solutions to significant contemporary health "problems," for example, stress and AIDS. Such is the underlying theme of a prospectus for a proposed interdisciplinary PhD program, developed by a joint committee (Chaska & Jackson, 1988). Interdisciplinary programs will be a definite part of the nursing educational system in the future.

International nursing. The final aspect of nursing education for the future that warrants comment is international nursing. Undergraduate and graduate programs of nursing are direly needed in a number of countries. Jensen and Lindeman (Chapter 18), Rosenblum (Chapter 19), and Brown (Chapter 48) discuss numerous issues in international nursing education and practice. A common ground for nursing education on an international basis needs to be clearly identified. It is to be hoped that a clear definition of the essence of nursing will be the common denominator that is advanced. Then, collaboration on an international basis may occur effectively and successfully in planning and developing nursing education programs. Different countries have different questions that need to be addressed by virtue of native systems of education, research, and practice. There may also be similar questions addressed but different approaches offered for resolving issues.

Leininger (1989) advances the role of the transcultural nurse specialist. Her vision resulted in the establishment of a field called transcultural nursing. Leininger's goal is to develop knowledge specific to diverse cultures and the needs of clients from many cultures.

Meleis (1989) emphasizes the need for cross-national studies and collaboration to develop nursing science that has worldwide application. Although Jensen and Lindeman (Chapter 18) set the stage for international nursing education, Rosenblum (Chapter 19) and Brown (Chapter 48) poignantly describe practice, some of the education needs, and experiences. It is clear that with the increasing numbers of nursing students, patients, and clients from numerous cultures and with the development and expansion of a professional nursing role internationally, opportunities and obligations to facilitate the promotion of health and prevention of illness in other countries are significant.

In meeting needs in international nursing, critical issues must be raised and resolved. For example, the identification of expectations for nursing education of all involved is imperative. Critical resources must be defined in terms of faculty, personnel, sociocultural adaptations that need to be considered, methods of communication, education materials, and library sources. The provision of international nursing education requires monitoring and evaluation.

National center for nursing education. The expansion of nursing education internationally and the previously cited needs for evaluating models for baccalaureate education and graduate programs require that a center (or centers) for nursing education be developed nationally and internationally. Models of various types of nursing education may then be tested, evaluated, and recommended for implementation. A center for nursing education might provide for a unique core of experts and an organizing unit for a planned evaluation approach to nursing education, design, curriculum, and projected outcomes.

Knowledge Development: Research and Theory

Florence Downs is credited with the following statement at the 11th National Forum for Doctoral Programs in Nursing: "Nursing research is replete with sophisticated methodologies applied to sophisticated content" (Downs, 1987). Martha Rogers states that "unless the core of our programs are rooted in an organized body of knowledge specific to nursing, there is no point in a doctoral program for nursing" (Personal communication, June 5, 1989).

Kemp (Chapter 69) provides direction for developing a body of abstract knowledge. Kemp emphasizes the need for synthesized theory that originally is borrowed from other disciplines. There is growing consensus that both the "received" and "perceived" views of theory building are being advocated for the future. Gender-sensitive issues, not limited to feminism, need to be addressed. Tolerance for diversity in the approaches to development of knowledge is advocated. The reader is referred to Schultz and Me-

leis (1988) for a thorough discussion regarding the essence and criticalness of nursing epistemology for the future of nursing as a discipline.

Definitions and conceptualizations of health and caring are essential in the development of nursing science and knowledge. It is critical that in the future arguments for a particular view regarding the approach and development of knowledge be substantiated (C. Deets, EdD, RN, personal communication, June 7, 1989). This justification is essential for the development of nursing as a science.

Stevenson (Chapter 68) presents specific means for meeting the challenges posed by Downs and Rogers (Downs, 1987; M. Rogers, personal communication, June 5, 1989). Stevenson offers concrete suggestions to develop a research career. Steps and stages in the process of developing a research program are made clear. Research development through joint ventures and collaborative models between nursing service and education are encouraged. Stevenson advances a model that incorporates this area as a stage in the progression of nursing research and science. The model for nursing science that she offers should significantly promote research. Finally Stevenson's portrayal of the future of knowledge development in nursing is a timely response to the research challenge.

Nursing Practice

Challenges in future nursing practice are great. Projections of the Secretary's Commission on Nursing (DHHS, 1988) are not encouraging. Evidence suggests that the demand for RNs will continue to increase, and a continued imbalance with supply is anticipated. A probable solution to this problem will be the development of models for practice that emphasize autonomous nursing practice and the restructuring of nursing care delivery systems, as suggested by Lyon (Chapter 34) and Clifford (Chapter 70).

However, it is imperative that the interfaces between the autonomous, the interdependent, and the dependent roles of nursing be clearly addressed. Given the total focus in nursing on health and illness care, focusing only on one nursing role and excluding other roles might well inhibit further development of nursing practice and provision of high-quality nursing care. Clearly the verbalization and practice of the *autonomous nursing role* has had minimal exposure to the public, and professional nurses as well. This limitation is partly due to overemphasis historically on the *dependent role* of nurses, particularly in acute care settings. The *dependent role* has been linked erroneously to a type of "handmaiden" expectation in relation to medical practice. The *interdependent nursing role* more recently has been recognized mutually by physicians and nurses as essential to provision of total care for a patient. The time has come to delineate and operationalize the autonomous role, but at the same time not negate or deny either the interdependent or dependent nursing role. Multifacet roles in nursing are bound to increase, given the well and illness population. The time also has finally come for clear explication of *all* professional nursing roles.

The testing, evaluation, and practice of nursing and the further development of nursing practice should occur in restructured models and settings for care. As Donley and Flaherty (Chapter 64) have pointed out, nursing care in the future is most likely to be provided increasingly in health clinics and for illness prevention. A business orientation to education and care is highly advocated (Farrell, Chapter 59; Donley and Flaherty, Chapter 64), but *not* at the expense of humanistic approaches in care.

Administration: Services and Academic

This summary chapter began with highlighting the importance to nursing of values, a moral commitment, and the professionalization of leadership. The chapter ends with a similar theme as the challenge and plea for the future of the profession. Starck (Chapter 72) clearly points out that values in nursing and the value of nursing in society are inherent to the future of the profession of nursing. Priorities in nursing leadership need to be established.

In a study concerning managers who were both successful and effective, it was found that such managers used a balanced approach to their activities (Luthans, 1988). However, the investigators found that very few managers were both successful and ef-

fective. This author believes that it will be important to incorporate the concepts of both ethics and the art of empowering others in future studies of management, administration, and organizations.

Management literature continually has focused on strategies and tactics that are used to increase power and influence (Conger, 1989). Quality, efficiency, effectiveness, productivity, and cost-effectiveness will always be great concerns of managers and administration. Performance problems may always be an issue. There is one final strategy—empowerment—that, if employed successfully, may either preclude or resolve many problematic situations.

Conger notes (1989) that managers must think of empowerment as the act of strengthening an individual's belief in his or her sense of effectiveness. However, empowerment is more than a set of external actions; it is a process of changing the internal beliefs of persons. Conger cautions that managers should constantly test reality and be alert to signs of "group think." Furthermore his thesis is that it is only those leaders who feel secure about their own power who are able to see the empowerment of subordinates as a gain, rather than a loss, and not be threatened.

Empowerment requires security as well as skill on the part of the leader. Sun Tzu (1963) advises the skillful leader to subdue the enemy's troups without any fighting. The masterpiece of Mushashi (1982) shows Japanese management and strategy techniques as a means to empower. Empowerment practices demand time, confidence, an element of creativity, and a sensitivity to one's environmental context to be effective (Conger, 1989). However, the practice of empowerment is an important strategy for nursing leaders in service and academia to move organizations past difficult transitions to higher goals. Success in empowering others—encouraging, nurturing, and advancing their empowering process—may well be the real criterion for effective management and the professionalization of leadership in nursing for the future.

CONCLUSION

Finally, many questions remain to be asked and many more to be answered. Each major part of this text—each identified kaleidoscope in nursing—has been highlighted in this summary chapter. New kaleidoscopes (patterns) are being developed every day and yet-unborn visions for each area of nursing will emerge. It is not easy to anticipate at what degree of perfection these may arrive nor how they may differ. Who knows what thrilling colors and unexpected patterns are yet to be viewed in visions of the future? It is hoped that this volume will prove to be a new beginning—a turning point and contribution toward the formation of one whole kaleidoscope for nursing.

REFERENCES

Aiken, L.H., & Mullinix, C.F. (1987). Special report: The nurse shortage—myth or reality? *New England Journal of Medicine, 317* (10), 641–646.

Arnold, H.J., & Feldman, H.J. (1986). *Organizational behavior*. New York: McGraw-Hill.

Baker, C. (1987). *Through the kaleidoscope . . . And beyond*. Annapolis, MD: Beechcliff Books.

Barnum, B. (1989). Losses and laughter. *Nursing and Health Care, 10* (2), 59.

Beckstrand, J. (1984). A reply to Collins and Fielder: The concept of theory. *Research in Nursing and Health, 7,* 189–196.

Chaska, N.L. (1983). Theories of nursing and organizations: Generating integrated models for administrative practice. In N.L. Chaska (Ed.), *The nursing profession: A time to speak* (pp. 720–730). New York: McGraw-Hill.

Chaska, N.L., & Jackson, B. (Co-chairs.). (1988). *Prospectus for an interdisciplinary Ph.D. program*. Unpublished paper.

Chaska, N.L., & Markel, R. (1989). Introduction: History and guidelines. In *Proceedings of the 1989 National Forum on Doctoral Education in Nursing*. Indianapolis, IN: The School of Nursing, Indiana University.

Cherrington, D.J. (1989). *Organizational behavior*. Boston: Allyn & Bacon.

Christensen, P.J. (1988). An ethical framework for nursing service administration. *Advances in Nursing Science, 10* (3), 46–55.

Cohen, S.S. (1989). *Tender power*. Reading, MA: Addison-Wesley.

Commission on Organizational Assessment and Renewal. (1989). Summary of COAR report. *The American Nurse, 21* (4), 17–20.

Conger, J.A. (1989). Leadership: The art of improving others. *Academy of Management EXECUTIVE, 3* (1), 17–24.

Cook, S.S., & Finelli, L. (1988). Faculty practice: A new perspective on academic competence. *Journal of Professional Nursing, 4* (1), 23,29.

Department of Health and Human Services. (1988). *Secretary's Commission on Nursing. Final report, Vol. 1*. Washington, DC: U.S. Government Printing Office.

Dick, M.J. (1986). Burnout in nurse faculty: Relationships with management style, collegial support, and workload in collegiate programs. *Journal of Professional Nursing 2* (4), 252–260.

Donius, M.A. (1988). The Columbia: Building a bridge with clinical faculty. *Journal of Professional Nursing, 4* (1), 17–22.

Donley, Sr. R., & Flaherty, Sr. M.J. (1989). Analysis of the market driven nursing shortage. *Nursing and Health Care, 10* (4), 183–187.

Downs, F. (1987). Toward the future. *In Proceedings of the 1987 Forum on Doctoral Education in Nursing, June 24–26, 1987* (pp. 62–66). Pittsburgh: University of Pittsburgh, School of Nursing.

Ellis, L.A. (1989). Capturing nursing's future leaders. *Journal of Professional Nursing, 5* (3), 118, 168.

Ethridge, P., & Lamb, G.S. (1989). Professional nursing case management improves quality, access and costs. *Nursing Management, 20* (3), 30–35.

Fawcett, J. (1989). *Analysis and evaluation of conceptual models of nursing* (2nd ed.). Philadelphia: F.A. Davis.

Feldman, M.J., Ventura, M.R., & Crosby, F. (1987). Studies of nurse practitioner effectiveness. *Nursing Research, 36* (5), 303–308.

Gibson, J.L., Ivancevich, J.M., & Donnelly, J.H. (1988). *Organizations: Behavior, structure, processes* (6th ed.). Plano, TX: Business Publications.

Gilmore, T.N. (1988). *Making a leadership change*. San Francisco: Jossey-Bass.

Hackett, J.T. (1989, January 6). Keeping up with higher tuition bills. *The Indianapolis Star*, p. A19.

Hall, R.H. (1987). *Organizations: Structure, processes, and outcomes* (4th ed.). Englewood Cliffs, NJ: Prentice-Hall.

Hamilton, C.C., & Wilson, C.N. (1989). The new medicare catastrophic coverage act: Will it affect nursing? *Nursing and Health Care, 10* (1), 31–34.

Haussler, S. (1988). Faculty perceptions of the organizational climate in selected top-ranked schools of nursing. *Journal of Professional Nursing, 4,* 274–278.

Hechenberger, N. (1988). The future of nursing education administration. *Journal of Professional Nursing 4*(4), 274–278.

Henry, B., O'Donnell, J.F., Pendergast, J.F., Moody, L.E., & Hutchinson, S.A. (1988). Nursing administration research in hospitals and schools of nursing. *Journal of Nursing Administration, 18* (2), 28–31.

Hinshaw, A.S. (1989). *Trajectory for research training and career development*. Bethesda, MD: National Center for Nursing Research, National Institutes of Health. Abstract presented at the 1989 National Forum on Doctoral Education in Nursing, June 7–9, School of Nursing, Indiana University, Indianapolis.

Hunsaker, P.L., & Cook, C.W. (1986). *Managing organizational behavior*. Reading, MA: Addison-Wesley.

Jennings, B.J., & Meleis, A.I. (1988). Nursing theory and administrative practice: Agenda for the 1990's. *Advances in Nursing Science, 10* (3), 56–69.

Jenny, J. (1989). Classifying nursing diagnosis: A self-care approach. *Nursing and Health Care, 10* (2), 83–89.

Jolma, D.J., & Weller, D.E. (1989). An evaluation of nurse recruitment methods. *Journal of Nursing Administration, 19* (4), 20–24, 38.

Knafl, K.A., Pettengill, M.M., Bevis, M.E., & Kirchhoff, K.T. (1988). Blending qualitative and quantitative approaches to instrument development and data collection. (1988). *Journal of Professional Nursing, 4* (1), 30–37.

Laudan, L. (1977). *Progress and its problems*. Berkeley, CA: University of California Press.

Laudan, L. (1984). *Science and values: The aims of science and their role in scientific debate*. Berkeley, CA: University of California Press.

Leininger, M.M. (1989). The transcultural nurse specialist: Imperative in today's world. *Nursing and Health Care, 10* (5), 251–256.

Lindeman, C. (1989). Curriculum revolution: Reconceptualizing clinical nursing education. *Nursing and Health Care, 10* (1), 23–28.

Luthans, F. (1988). Successful vs. effective real managers. *Academy of Management EXECUTIVE, 2* (2), 127–132.

Marchese, T.J. (1987). *The search committee handbook: A guide to recruiting administrators*. Washington, DC: American Association for Higher Education.

Martin, E. (1989). The prestige of today's nurse. *Nursing Management, 20* (3), 80.

McCloskey, J.C., (1989). Implications of costing out nursing services for reimbursement. *Nursing Management, 20* (1), 44–49.

McCloskey, J.C. & McCain, B. (1988). Variables related to nurse performance. *Image, 20* (4), 203–207.

Mechanic, H.F. (1988). Redefining the expanded role. *Nursing Outlook, 36* (6), 280–284.

Megel, M.E., Langston, N.F., & Creswell, J.W. (1988). Scholarly productivity: A survey of nursing faculty researchers. *Journal of Professional Nursing, 4*, (1), 45–54.

Meleis, A. (1988). Doctoral education in nursing: Its present and its future. *Journal of Professional Nursing, 4* (6), 436–446.

Meleis, A.I. (1989). International research: A need or a luxury. *Nursing Outlook, 37* (3), 138–142.

Mundinger, M.O. (1988). Three dimensional nursing: New partnerships between service and education. *Journal of Professional Nursing, 4* (1), 10–16.

Mushashi, M. (1982). *The book of five rings* (B.J. Brown, Y. Kashiwagi, W.A. Barrett, & E. Sasagawa, Trans.). New York: Bantam Books.

Neilsen, R.P. (1989). Changing unethical organizational behavior. *Academy of Management EXECUTIVE, 3* (2), 123–130.

Northrop, C.E. (1989). The nursing shortage and nursing's legal scope of practice. *Nursing Outlook, 37* (2), 104.

Omachonu, U.K., & Nanda, R. (1989). Measuring productivity: Outcome vs. output. *Nursing Management, 20* (4), 35–40.

Orlando, I.J., & Dugan, A.B. (1989). Independent and dependent paths: The fundamental issue for the profession. *Nursing and Health Care, 10* (2), 77–80.

Pennington, E.A. (Ed.). (1986). Understanding the academic role: A handbook for new faculty (Publication No. 15-2163). New York: National League for Nursing.

Peters, T. (1987). *Thriving on chaos*. New York: Harper & Row.

Pointer, D.D., & Pointer, T.K. (1989). Case-based prospective price reimbursement. *Nursing Management, 20* (4), 30–34.

Porter, R.T., Porter, M.J., & Lower, M.S. (1989). Enhancing the image of nursing. *Journal of Nursing Administration, 19* (2), 36–40.

Randolph, W.A., & Blackburn, R.S. (1989). *Managing organizational behavior*. Homewood, IL: Irwin.

Ray, M.A. (1989). The theory of bureaucratic caring for nursing practice in the organizational culture. *Nursing Administration Quarterly, 3* (2), 31–42.

Reilly, D.E. (1989). Ethics and values in nursing: Are we opening Pandora's box? *Nursing and Health Care, 10* (2), 91–95.

Reisch, S.K. (1987). Academic clinician: A new role for nursing's future. *Nursing and Health Care, 8* (10), 583–586.

Rosenfeld, P. (1987). Nursing education in crisis—A look at recruitment and retention. *Nursing and Health Care, 8* (5), 283–286.

Schrum, M. (1985). Out of the past and into the future. *Journal of Professional Nursing, 1* (4), 183.

Schultz, P.R., & Meleis, A.I. (1988). Nursing epistemology: Traditions insights, questions. *Image, 20* (4), 217–221.

Sigma Theta Tau International (STTI). (1988). *Attitudes, values and beliefs of the public in Indiana toward nursing as a career: A study to enhance recruitment into nursing.* Indianapolis: Sigma Theta Tau International.

Staff. (1989, May 5). Cover story: Nursing shortage cases: AHA data. *Hospitals,* pp. 32–37.

Staff. (1989, June 5). Cover story: Hospitals must budget by DRG's payers. *Hospitals,* pp. 34–39.

Styles, M. (1987). History as a strategy for shaping educational policy. In *Proceedings of the 1987 Forum on Doctoral Education in Nursing, June 24–26, 1987* (p. 11). Pittsburgh: University of Pittsburgh School of Nursing.

Styles, M. (1989). As I see it article on COAR. *American Nurse, 21* (4), 16.11). Pittsburgh: University of Pittsburgh School of Nursing.

Tzu, Sun. (1963). *The art of war* (S.B. Griffith, Trans.). New York: Oxford Press.

Wall, L.L. (1988). Plan development for a nurse recruitment-retention program. *Journal of Nursing Administration, 18* (2), 20–26.

Werley, H., & Leske, J.S. (1988). Pinning down the tracks to doctoral degrees. *Nursing and Health Care, 9* (5), 239–243.

Wohlert, H. (1987). Recruiting for nursing: Whose responsibility? *Journal of Obstetrics, Gynecologic, and Neonatal Nurses, 16* (3), 155–156.

Index

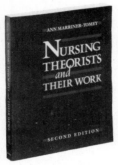
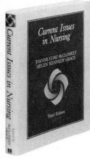